CLINICAL
DERMATOLOGY

CLINICAL DERMATOLOGY

Ramesh Chandra Gharami MD

Professor, Deptt. of Dermatology
Medical College, Kolkata

New Central Book Agency (P) Ltd

LONDON
HYDERABAD ERNAKULAM BHUBANESWAR
NEW DELHI KOLKATA PUNE GUWAHATI

NCBA

REGD OFFICE
8/1 Chintamoni Das Lane, Kolkata 700 009, India
email: ncbapvtltd@eth.net

OVERSEAS
NCBA (UK) Ltd, 149 Park Avenue North, Northampton, NN3 2HY, UK
email: ncbauk@yahoo.com

EXPORT
NCBA Exports Pvt. Ltd, 212 Shahpur Jat, New Delhi 110 049
email: ncbaexports@ncbapvtltd.com

BRANCHES

212 Shahpur Jat
New Delhi 110 049
email: ncbadel@ncbapvtltd.com

Shop Nos. 3 & 4, Vinayak Towers
681/B Budhwar Peth, Appa Balwant Chowk
Pune 411 002
email: ncbapune@ncbapvtltd.com

Shop No. 15, Bharati Towers, Ground Floor
Forest Park, **Bhubaneswar** 751 001
email: ncbabub@ncbapvtltd.com

House No. 3-1-315, 1st Floor
Nimboliadda, Kachiguda, **Hyderabad** 500 027
email: ncbahydb@ncbapvtltd.com

GSS Shopping Complex, 1st Floor
Opposite College Post Office, Convent Road
Ernakulam 682 035
email: ncbaernk@ncbapvtltd.com

Radhamayee Complex (Second Floor)
Opp. SBI, Panbazar, Jaswanta Road
Guwahati 781 001
email: ncbaguwahati@ncbapvtltd.com

CLINICAL DERMATOLOGY • Ramesh Chandra Gharami

First Published: April 2007

Thoroughly Revised and Updated Second Edition: January 2014

Reprinted July 2014

PUBLISHER AND TYPESETTER
New Central Book Agency (P) Ltd
8/1 Chintamoni Das Lane, Kolkata 700 009

PRINTER
New Central Book Agency (P) Ltd
Web-Offset Division, Dhulagarh, Sankrail, Howrah

COVER DESIGNER
Soumen Paul

PROJECT TEAM
Prabir Ghosh, Prabhat Jas`

ISBN 978 81 7381 522 5

Price: ₹ **985.00**

Dedication

Swami Vivekananda

&

Srila A C Bhaktivedanta Swami Probhupada

CONTENTS

Part D: MISCELLANEOUS DERMATOSES

Part E: DERMATOSURGERY

Part F: MULTIPLE CHOICE QUESTIONS (MCQs)

PREFACE TO THE SECOND EDITION

The book CLINICAL DERMATOLOGY, 2nd edition, is my small Savings Account. Whatever I have gleaned from the field of Dermatology for last five years, I have garnered here and now it is open to all.

The present edition is divided into six parts. New chapters like Differential Diagnosis, Classification and Comparative Dermatology will be immensely helpful to all PGTs. The chapter Mental Block is designed solely for an academic exercise. A lot of photographs are added to understand the dermatological cases more clearly.

- Part A is designed for Dermatology Quiz Competition and PG Entrance Examination.
- Part B is designed for all undergraduate and postgraduate students to understand the basics of Dermatology.
- Part C consists of the most common dermatoses for the undergraduate students.
- Part D and Part E are designed mainly for the postgraduate students and advanced undergraduate students.
- Part F consists of Short-Questions and Answers in the form of MCQs.

7th October 2013
Kolkata

R C Gharami

PREFACE TO THE FIRST EDITION

'Education', as Swami Vivekananda would often say, 'is the manifestation of the perfection already present in man.' And I have every reason to believe in such an aphorism. Once, I remember, I happened to have come across the writings of Galileo Galilei where I marked one line which left a lasting influence on me: 'You cannot teach a person anything, you can help them find it within themselves.' While penning this book those lines have repeatedly occurred to me. A small man, in comparison to those giant stalwarts as I am, my little and humble endeavour has always been to awaken the knowledge lying dormant in the students in the subject of Dermatology. I have never hesitated to bow down before the big names whom I have repeatedly consulted while writing this book, and they have pretty generously permitted me to utilise their knowledge and experience in my book. Naturally, I have every intention to express my heartfelt appreciation and gratitude to all of them. I will be failing in my duties if do not show my indebtedness to all my patients, who have permitted me to take their clinical photographs, which have been incorporated in this book. For this act of documentation I am grateful to Dr GC Das without whose help it would have been impossible for me to venture into this book.

I acknowledge my humble gratitude to Prof. Manoj Chowdhury, Dr Goutam Bandyopadhyay, Dr Tapas Chatterjee, Dr JN Sarkar, Dr Anirban Sengupta, Dr Pradipta Mistry, and Dr Sahila Khatoon for their constant encouragement. At the same time I must not forget to convey my regards to Dr Aparesh Ch Patra and Manoj Kr Mandal, for their kind inspiration. I stand indebted to my colleagues in my department in general and to Prof. PK Datta, Dr NK Das and Dr AK Haldar, in particular, for their support and cooperation.

Jaivardhan, Aparajita, Shivashis, Sourav, and Amanatulla—my beloved postgraduate students—have never been reluctant to share their enthusiasm about this book with me. I cannot forget any of their suggestions and the way they have actively participated in the project.

My special thanks to Shri Prabir Ghosh for meticulous typesetting. I am grateful to Shri Amitabha Sen, Director, and all the support staff of New Central Book Agency (P) Ltd for their honest and sincere endeavour in bringing out this book in the shortest possible time.

I do not know how to give vent to my feelings for my wife Maitreyee and daughter Srija for their silent sacrifice to provide me with time to finish this project.

I sincerely hope this book will be of immense help to the students and teachers of Dermatology.

15th May 2007
Kolkata

R C Gharami

ACKNOWLEDGEMENTS

I am grateful to all my patients who are my real teachers to learn dermatology. I have no words to express my gratitude to the authors of various dermatology books, my teachers and senior colleagues from whom I have acquired my knowledge—the sole capital of the book.

I am indebted to all my undergraduate and postgraduate students and colleagues of past and present whose time to time interactions have enriched my knowledge.

Dr Piyush Kumar, one of my best students, provided me with a number of important photographs without which the book would have remained incomplete.

My sincere thanks to Dr Aparesh Patra, Dr Abanti Saha, Dr NK Das and Dr Kaushik Shome who inspired me incessantly.

An evergrowing thanks to my postgraduate students, specially to Anupam, Anupama, Dipti, Dhiraj, Tirthankar, and Vivek who performed sincerely the most assiduous job of proof-reading.

I am beholden to Professor Debabrata Bandyopadhyay for his magnanimity and generosity and only for him I was enable to overcome all the departmental repugnances to complete my work smoothly.

My Pathology Professor, Dr Monoj Chowdhury, has showered his incessant blessings on me.

I am thankful to Mr Shibu Garai, the medical book shop-keeper in Bankura, and to Mr Sisir (Bharat) Kundu for his fulltime service with a smiling face.

I am grateful to my wife, Maitreyee, and daughter, Srija, for their sacrifice.

I am grateful for the sincere devotion and helpful cooperation provided by the publisher—Mr Amitabha Sen, the project supervisor Mr Prabir Ghosh, and others who successfully completed this most vital task of seeing the book through the press.

PART A

GEMS OF DERMATOLOGY FOR PG ENTRANCE

- Chapter–A1 Historical Landmarks in Dermatology
- Chapter–A2 Dermatology at a glance
- Chapter–A3 Signs & Phenomenons in Dermatology
- Chapter–A4 Rapid Fire

CHAPTER A1

HISTORICAL LANDMARKS IN DERMATOLOGY

1400 BC – Phototherapy was first reported from India for treatment of *vitiligo* with some plant extract and sunlight exposure.

460-377 BC – Hippocrates described psoriasis and leprosy as Lopoi as a single entity.

300-200 BC – First evidence of *leprosy* in Egypt was found.

129-99 BC – Galen described psoriasis and eczema as psora.

1313 – Phlip de Fair ordered to burn the psoriasis patients like leprosy victims.

1485 – da Vinci stressed upon the use of lenses to view small objects.

1500 – Earliest mode of treatment of leprosy was chaulmoogra oil, derived from Hydrocarpus tree and was used in Japan and China.

1610 – Galileo invented *Simple microscope.*

1660 – Samuel Hafenreffer first defined pruritus which elicited a *desire to scratch.*

1665 – Robert Hooke invented compound microscope and observed box-like compartments during examining a slice of cork and those he termed as *cells.*

1723 – Leeuwenhoek, first time studied structures of bacteria, protozoa, spermatozoa, RBCs, etc.

1753 – Sir James Lind found citrus fruits were helpful in *scurvy.*

1801 – Hospital Saint-Louis, the first skin hospital was established.

1802 – First lecturer in dermatology was appointed.

1806 – First *Atlas of Dermatology* was edited by Jean-Louis–Alibert.

1808 – Willan coined the term *palpable purpura.*

1809 – Willan accurately described *Psoriasis.*

1810 – First professor in dermatology was appointed.

1817 – Willan and Bateman published their *Atlas of Dermatology* which was most instructive.

1839 – E.Becquerel discovered *ultraviolet light.*

1841 – Hebra separated *Psoriasis* from *Leprosy.*

1846 – Eichsted first described *Pityriasis versicolor.*

1850 – Rudlof Virchow first noticed *Brown bodies* in lepra cells.

1850 – Arsenic was first introduced into US Pharmacopia.

1853 – Robin first isolated fungal elements from the lesion of *Pityriasis versicolor* and named the organism as *Microsporum furfur*.

1854 – Mouat confirmed Chaulmoogra as an effective mode of treatment of leprosy.

1854 – Rudlof Virchow described *Leiomyoma cutis*.

1855 – Nageli & Cramer coined the term cell membrane.

1856 – Hebra published his atlas in which painters were physicians.

1860 – Hebra coined the term *Pemphigus vulgaris*.

1868 – Hebra used the term *Exfoliative dermatitis* for *erythroderma*.

1869 – Wilson first introduced the term lichen planus. Hebra described lichen planus as *Lichen rubber* before Wilson.

1873 – Hansen discovered *Mycobacterium leprae*.

1874 – Malassez isolated *yeast cells* from the scale of the dandruff.

1874 – James Paget, first reported mammary *Paget's disease*.

1876 – Heinrich Koebner first described *Koebner phenomenon* or *isomorphic phenomenon* in *psoriasis*.

1877 – Ehrlich described *mast cells*.

1882 – Robert Koch isolated *Mycobacterium tuberculosis*.

1882 – Mcleod first described *Donovanosis* in India.

1882 – Flemming introduced the term *mitosis*.

1884 – Duhring first described dermatitis herpetiformis.

1885 – Brocq first introduced *pseudopelade*.

1886 – Koebner first used the term *epidermolysis bullosa*.

1888 – Hutchinson first described *chilblains* or *perniotic lupus erythematosus*.

1889 – Radcliffe Crocker first reported *extrammary Paget's disease*.

1889 – Baillon included yeast cells found in dandruff scale under the group of *Malassezia* to bestow honour to Malassez.

1891 – Waldeyer-Hartz coined the term *neuron*.

1893 – Mibelli first coined the term *Porokeratosis*.

1893 – Robinson first described *eccrine hydrocystoma*.

1894 – First Leper Home for leprosy patient was established in Carville, USA.

1894 – Brocq first introduced the term *fixed drug eruption*.

1894 – Radcliffe-Crocker used the term *erythema elevatum diutinum*.

1895 – Colcott Fox first described *granuloma annulare*.

1895 – Kofman first described *nevus comedonicus*.

1896 – Fordyce first described *scrotal angiokeratoma*.

1898 – Benjamin Schenk, a medical student described sporothrix.

1900 – Klippel and Trenaunay first described *KT syndrome*.

1902 – Radcliffe-Crocker introduced the term *granuloma annulare*.

1903 – Niels Finsen got Nobel prize for his therapeutic result with UV radiation in *lupus vulgaris* and he was the only dermatologist ever been awarded by the Nobel committee.

1903 – Robert W.Wood invented *Wood's lamp*.

1904 – Sabouraud considered *Malassezia* yeast was the cause of dandruff and new name was given as *Pityrosporum malassez*.

1905 – Donovan first described *Klebsiella granulomatis* as a causative agent for granuloma venereum from Madras (Chenni), India.

1905 – Einhorn first introduced *procaine* as the modern local anesthetic agent.

1905 – Adamson first described *juvenile xanthogranuloma* and the term was implied by Helwig and Hackney.

1906 – Toyama described *Pityriasis rotunda*.

1907 – Ehrman first originally described *Sneddon's syndrome*.

1909 – Hyde first described prurigo nodularis.

1911 – Darier first described features of *Gottron's syndrome*.

1913 – Snow first described acute hemorrhagic edema of infancy.

1915 – Burns described *KIP syndrome* and acronym was coined by Skinner et al in 1981.

1916 – Hans Reiter first described *Reiter's syndrome* in a young soldier with conjunctivitis, urethritis and arthritis.

1916 – Sutton popularized leukoderma acquisitum centrifugum, which was nothing but halo nevus, originally described by Hebra.

1919 – Mees described *Mees' line* of nail.

1920 – First National Leprosarium was established by conversion of First Leper Home for leprosy patients in Carville, USA.

1922 – UN Brahmachari, first described *post kala-azar dermal leishmaniasis* (PKDL).

1922 – Progressive symmetric erythrokeratoderma was named after Gottron as *Gottron's syndrome*.

1922 – *Stevens Johnson syndrome* was first described by Stevens and Johnson.

1925 – Nicolau first time described *Nicolau syndrome* following use of bismuth salts for the treatment of syphilis.

1925 – Margarot and Deveze first used *Wood's lamp* to detect *fungal infection* of hair.

1927 – Guido Fanconi, first described *Fanconi anemia*.

1927 – Olmsted first described features of *Olmsted syndrome*.

1928 & 1930 – Melkersson and Rosenthal respectively described triad of *Melkersson-Rosenthal syndrome*.

1930 – Brunsting et al, first described *pyoderma gangrenosum*.

1931 – Plowe coined the term *plasmalemma*.

1933 – Cornelia de Lange was credited for description of *Cornelia de Lange syndrome*.

1933 – Haxthausen first described chronic actitic dermatitis.

1936 – Thore Brandt first introduced *acrodermatitis enteropathica*.

1936 – Behcet included eye changes in Behcet's syndrome.

1939 – Ota first described *nevus of Ota*.

1939 – Chatterjee and Lowe from Kolkata, India, first described Tattoo inflicted leprosy.

1939 – Wegener described Wegener's granulomatosis.

1941 – Gottron first repoted acrogeria in two siblings.

1941 – Norman Gregg, first identified *congenital rubella syndrome*.

1943 – Lofgren introduced *lidocaine* as the most popular present day local anesthetic agent.

1945 – Meischer first described *granulomatous cheilitis*.

1946 – Beau described transverse depression at nail plate due to temporary interruption of mitotic activity of proximal nail matrix and known as *Beau's line*.

1946 – Nuremberg trial for devaluation of human life by leading academicians and scientists in the guise of medical research, was held.

1947 – World Medical Association was formed.

1947 – Tzanck first used *cytology* in cutaneous disorders.

1948 – Ackerman first described *verrucous carcinoma*.

1949 – Cochrane et al, first introduced *DDS* (Dapsone) as 1.25g IM twice weekly for treatment of leprosy and orally by Lowe and Smith in same year.

1950 – Bernard Thomus first coined the term *erythema multiforme major*.

1952 – Greither first described Greither disease, a form of hereditary palmoplantar keratoderma.

1952 – Gammel described erythema gyratum repens.

1952 – Lowe first introduced *corticosteroid* in *ENL*.

1952 – Sulberger and Witten first introduced compound F or *hydrocortisone* as topical corticosteroid in Dermatology.

1953 – Japan introduced *leprosy prevention law* which prescribed segregation and isolation of leprosy patient as a part of treatment and *abolished* the law only in 1996.

1953 – Lever differentiated bullous pemphigoid from pemphigus.

1953 – Howard & Pele divided cell cycle into G_1, S, G_2 and M phase.

1954 – Konwaler and Weiss first reported *nodular fasciitis*.

1956 – Lyell first described *toxic epidermal necrolysis*.

1956 – Baron et al, first reported *Hartnup disease*.

1956 – Sneddon and Wilkinson described *subcorneal pustular dermatosis*.

1957 – Sjogren and Larson, described Sjogren syndrome.

1958 – Ross first described *segmental hypohidrosis* with areflexia of lower extremities and tonic pupil.

1959 – G Panja and S Sen first reported *cutaneous histoplasmosis* in India.

1960 – Kitamura described erythromelanosis follicularis faciei.

1960 – Laser was first introduced and Leon Goldman is known as the father of laser medicine.

1962 – Goltz first described *focal dermal hypoplasia* or *Goltz syndrome*.

1962 – Schreiner and Wolff observed *lamellar granules* had the role in *physiological water barrier*.

1962 – Browne and Hogerzeil from Nigeria first introduced clofazimine for leprosy.

1963 – Opromolla first introduced Rifamycin SV as i.m. injection for leprosy.

1963 – Lloyd and Dennis, described *Cowden disease* and named after the name of the first patient.

1964 – Leiker coined the term *granuloma multiforme*.

1964 – Bazex syndrome was described.

1965 – Browne first described anti-inflammatory role of clofazimine.

1965 – Sheskin from Israel first introduced thalidomide in leprosy reaction.

1965 – Sneddon named a neurocutaneous disorder after his name.

1966 – *Bart syndrome* was described.

1968 – Hardy and Anderson termed hyper-eosinophilia syndrome.

1968 – Hitch and Lund described *disseminated* and *recurrent infundibulofolliculitis* (DRIF).

1968 – Cleaver JE, first recognized the defective repair of DNA, damaged by the ultraviolet light in xeroderma pigmentosa.

1968 – Bart et al, coined the term *acquired digital fibrokerotoma*.

1969 – Yarbro first reported the efficacy of hydroxyurea in treatment of refractory *psoriasis*.

1969 – Wells and Whimster originally described *angiolymphoid hyperplasia with eosinophilia*.

1969 – Ive introduced the term *actinic reticuloid*.

1970 – Rees et al, first introduced *oral Rifampicin*.

1971 – Agnello described *urticarial vasculitis*.

1973 – Dupre et al, first time reported *uncombable hair syndrome*.

1974 – Paget described Paget's disease of the breast.

1974 – Lawrence Shulman, first described *eosinophilic fasciitis*.

1974 – Parrish et al, were first used PUVA in *psoriasis*.

1974 – The term pheohyphomycosis was coined.

1977 – Rulon and Helwig first described *papillary eccrine adenoma*.

1977 – Pearson et al, did first trial of *MDT* at Malta.

1978 – Wiskemann first introduced broadband UVB phototherapy for *psoriasis* and *uremic pruritus*.

1979 – Michael Cohen Jr. first identified *Proteus syndrome*.

1979 – *Chronic actinic dermatitis* appeared as global term.

1979 – Sontheimer, Thomas and Gilliam were first to report *SCLE* (*subacute lupus erythematosus*) as a separate entity of cutaneous lupus erythematosus.

1979 – Pye et al, first described *erosive pustular dermatosis of the scalp.*

1981 – Birth year of AIDS.

1982 – Levy and Goldsmith coined the term *peeling skin syndrome.*

1983 – Rudolf Wiedenmann coined the term Proteus syndrome after the *Greek God Proteus* which indicated polymorphous nature of the disease.

1984 – Lucky et al, described *eosinophilic pustular folliculitis in infancy.*

1984 – Yarrow and Ahearn recommended the term *Malassezia* over the term *Pityrosporum* and was accepted as the generic name of the fungus.

1984 – Lokich and Moore first reported *hand-foot syndrome* with 5-*flurouracil.*

1985 – Wolf et al, first introduced the term *Isotopic response.*

1985 – *Microdermabrasion* was first used in Italy.

1985 – Huff described IgA pemphigus.

1986 – Dowd et al first used *nifedipine* in treatment of *chilblains.*

1988 – Weelden et al and Green et al, first introduced narrow band UVB (NB-UVB) phototherapy.

1989 – FDA approved botulinum toxin type A for treatment of *strabismus* and *blepharospasm.*

1989 – *Linear focal elastosis* was first described by Burket.

1990 – Ciaccio and Rebora reported first case of *lichen planus* associated with hepatitis B vaccine.

1991 – Irvine described the term skin failure.

1995 – Shelley first time reported estrogen dermatitis.

1995 – OMIM or online Mendelian Inheritance in Man was set up.

1997 – Westerhof et al, first introduced narrow band UVB (NB-UVB) phototherapy in *vitiligo.*

1997 – *Eruptive lingual papillitis* was first introduced by Lacour and Perrin.

2000 – FDA approved botulinum toxin type A for treatment of *cervical dystonia.*

2002 – FDA approved botulinum toxin type A for treatment of *glabellar wrinkles.*

2006 – Marathi film Nital was released, based on life of a *vitiligo* patient.

- Lucio phenomenon was under the name of Rafael Lucio (1819-86), a Mexican Dermatologist.
- GHA Hansen (1841-1912) noted tiny rods in lepra/Virchow cell in 1871-72, published the discovery in 1874 and declared as lepra bacilli, causative agent for leprosy in 1875.
- Freudenthal termed keratoacanthoma.
- Scleroderma: First described by Hippocrates and later by Carlo Carzio.

Memorable Days in Dermatology

- 31st January: World Leprosy Day
- Last Sunday of January: Indian Leprosy Day.
- 19th May: Vitiligo Day.
- 29th October: World Psoriasis Day.
- 1st December: World AIDS Day.

Origin of Terminology

- In atopic dermatitis, the term atopic, derived from atopy, means no place.
- In Cowden syndrome, the word *Cowden* was the name of the first patient.
- The word craquele of *eczeme craquele* is a French word, means marred with cracks.
- Cytology is derived from Greek word kytos means *hollow vessel.*
- Galli-Galli disease: The word *Galli-Galli* derived from the family name of first two patients who were brother in relation.
- Hartnup disease: The word *Hartnup* derived from the family name of the first patient.
- Heliotrope means a violet color flower, characteristically seen around the eyes in dermatomyositis.
- In Job syndrome, the word Job is derived from the Bible.
- Nummular dermatitis, the word nummular derived from latin word nummularis which means like a coin.
- The German word mauserung in mauserung phenomenon, means moulting.

- Phakomatosis is originated from Greek word *Phakos* which means *mother spot* or *mole*.
- Scleroderma is derived from Greek word scleros which means hard or indurated.
- The term schenki of *Sporothrix schenkii*, derived from the name of the medical student Banjamin Schenk.
- Pityriasis versicolor was previously called as tinea versicolor because in 1853 when Robin first isolated the fungal elements identical to dermatophyte *Microsporum auduoinii* and so the term ***tinea*** came in tinea versicolor.
- In erythema multiforme, the multiforme indicates various forms of skin lesions like macules, papules, vesicles and bullae.
- Pellagra: It is an Italian word, has two parts-pelle means skin and agara means rough.
- Pemphigus is originated from Greek word ***pemphix***, means blister or bubble.
- Larva currens, here currens stand for running or racing.
- Mitosis is derived from Greek word *mitos*, means *thread*.
- In tinea imbricata, the term imbricata is derived from imbrex, means shingle and shingles are like overlapping tiles of the roof.
- Cell, the term derived from Latin word *cella*, means *hollow space*.
- Melasma derived from Greek word which means black spot.
- Chloasma derived from Greek word which means green spot.
- Erythrasma, derived from Greek language, means red.
- The word berloque in berloque dermatitis, derived from French language, means pendant-like.
- In hibernoma, fat cells contain vacuolated spaces which are also found in normal fat cells of animals, habituated to undergo hibernation.
- The term effluvium in telogen or anagen effluvium, is a Latin word, means flowing out.

DERMATOLOGY AT A GLANCE

CHAPTER A2

Tumoral melanosis

- During regression of vertical growth of melanoma, melanophages may be collected within the mass of melanoma instead of melanoma cells, this collection is known as tumoral melanosis.

Relation between TIL (Tumor infiltrating lymphocytes) and prognosis of melanoma

- If TIL is present, prognosis is better and if absent prognosis is worst.
- Non-infiltrating lymphocytic infiltration doesnot have any prognostic value.
- TIL may be brisk and non-brisk.
- Brisk infiltration is defined by presence of continuous band-like infiltration or diffuse infiltration.
- Non-brisk infiltration is defined by discontinuous band like infiltration.
- Brisk infiltration has best prognosis and non-brisk infiltration has intermediate prognosis.

Hot spot in melanoma

- The site where maximum amount of mitotic figures are found is called hot spot.
- If mitotic figures in a hot spot is > $6/mm^2$, prognosis is worst.

Satellites in melanoma

- Discontinuous foci of tumor metastasis within 5 cm distance of the original tumor are called satellites and if they are at a distance > 5 cm, then called as in-transit metastasis.

Microscopic satellites in melanoma

- Nests at reticular dermis, subcutaneous tissue or within blood vessels > 0.05 mm in diameter are known as microscopic satellites.

AEC syndrome

- Ankyloblepharon
- Ectodermal defects
- Cleft lip/-palate

ANOTHER syndrome

- Alopecia
- Nail dystrophy
- Ophthalmic complications
- Thyroid dysfunction
- Hypohidrosis
- Ephelids and enteropathy
- Respiratory tract infection

BAD syndrome

- Black locks
- Albinism
- Deafness

CREST syndrome

- Calcinosis cutis
- Raynaud's phenomenon
- Esophageal dysmotility
- Sclerodactyly
- Telangiectasia

CHIME syndrome

- Colobomas of the eye
- Heart defects
- Ichthyosiform dermatosis
- Mental retardation
- Ear defects

CHILD syndrome

- Chondrodysplasia punctata
- Congenital hemidysplasia
- Unilateral ichthyosiform erythroderma
- Limb defects

EEC syndrome

- Ectodermal dysplasia
- Ectrodactyly (congenital partial or complete absence of a digit)
- Cleft lip-palate

GAPO syndrome

- Growth retardation
- Alopecia
- Pseudoanodontia (unerupted teeth)
- Optic atrophy

Hair-An syndrome

- Hyperandrogenism
- Insulin resistance
- Acanthosis nigricans

HID syndrome

- Hystrix-like ichthyosis
- Bilateral sensory neural deafness

KID syndrome

- Keratitis
- Ichthyosis
- Deafness

PAPA syndrome

- Pyogenic sterile arthritis
- Pyoderma gangrenosum
- Acne

PHACES

- Posterior fossa malformation
- Hemangioma
- Arterial anomaly
- Cardiac defect
- Eye abnormality
- Sternal defect

SAPHO syndrome

- Synovitis, Acne
- Palmo-plantar pustulosis or pustular psoriasis
- Hyperostoses
- Osteitis

Pattern of antinuclear antibodies (ANA)

- Homogenous pattern in systemic lupus erythematosus (SLE)
- Rim pattern in SLE
- Fine speckled pattern in SLE, SLE with nephritis, Sjogren's syndrome, mixed connectve tissue disorder, scleroderma and myositis.

- Coarse speckled pattern in CREST syndrome.
- Nucleolar pattern in scleroderma.

Amyloidosis

- The disease occurs due to deposition of amyloid into various organs including skin.
- Amyloid is the extracellular proteinaceous material, having distinctive physical properties.
- It appears amorphous, eosinophilic and hyaline.
- Ultrastructurally, amyloid consists of polypeptide fibrils, having cross-beta-pleated sheet conformation.
- These fibrils are 8-12 nm in width and intermediate in length.
- There are 16 different types of amyloid and historically AL amyloid is associated with primary cell dyscrasias and AA amyloid is associated with secondary systemic amyloidosis.
- Source of cutaneous amyloid is degenerating keratinocytes.
- Amyloid takes brick-red stain and apple-green birefringence with Congo-red.
- It stains metachromatically with crystal violet and methyl violet stains.

ANCA association in vasculitis

pANCA positive:
- 60% in microscopic polyangiitis and in Churg-Strauss disease.
- 10% in Wegener's granulomatosis.

cANCA positive:
- 80% in Wegener's granulomatosis
- 30% in microscopic polyangiitis and Churg-Strauss disease.

Arsenicism

- **Water and urine contents:** > 50 µg/L
- **Nail content:** > 1.5 mg/Kg
- **Hair content:** > 1 mg/Kg

Anagen effluvium

- Sudden loss of actively growing or anagen hairs.
- Severe disruption of mitotic activity of matriceal cells due to acute insults like chemotherapy, radiation, heavy metal poisoning or other toxins.
- Trichogram shows 100% hairs are in telogen phase.

Acrokeratosis of Bazex

- It is a paraneoplastic condition having psoriasiform plaques.
- It affects all parts of hands and feet except mid palms and arches of the feet.

Acropigmentation of Dohi

- It is a rare pigmentary disorder, primarily occurring in Japan and also in India, Europe and Caribbean with autosomal dominant or sometimes autosomal recessive inheritance.
- Features are progressive pigmented and depigmented macules which often mix in reticular fashion.
- Common sites are dorsal surfaces of the extremities.
- Though the lesions appear in infancy or early childhood but no further spreading after adolescence and last for remaining life.
- Freckle-like macules at face may be associated.

Acropigmentation of Kitamura

- Autosomal dominant pigmentary disorder, characterized by reticulate pigmentation in the form of confluent 1-4 mm pigmented macules.
- It affects both volar and dorsal aspect of hands and feet.

Acute generalized exanthematous pustulosis (AGEP)

- It is characterized by sudden onset of generalized non-follicular pustular eruptions.
- Leukocytosis including neutrophilia and eosinophilia is the usual finding in circulation as well as in skin. This is due to some neutrophil attractant cytokines like IL3, IL8, G-CSF, etc.

- Commonest offending drugs are penicillin, cephalosporin, macrolides, doxycycline, vancomycin, etc.

Agminate folliculitis

- It is a form of tinea capitis, less severe than kerion.
- It is characterized by sharply defined dull red plaques, studded with follicular pustules.

Alopecia areata

- Clinically shows exclamation sign.
- Histologically shows pencil point hair shaft.

Angioid steaks: These are most common ophthalmologic finding in pseudoxanthoma elasticum. It may also be seen in following conditions:

- Sturge-Weber syndrome
- Ehler-Danlos syndrome, neurofibromatosis, tuberous sclerosis
- Diabetes mellitus, hemochromatosis
- Hypercalcemia, hyperphosphatemia
- Sickle cell anemia, thalassemia, hemolytic anemia
- Pituitary disease
- Myopia, traumatic choroidal rupture

Zebra-like pigmentation: Linear and whorled nevoid hypermelanosis along Blaschko's line, appearing in infancy or early childhood and thereafter usually remaining stable.

Acquired melanocytic nevus

- Dermal nevus is dome shaped, elevated, without hyperpigmentation and with or without hair growth.
- Compound nevus is dome shaped, hyperpigmented and usually with hair growth.
- Junctional nevus is nonelevated and non-hairy but pigmented.
- Nevus cells are arranged in a polarized form as round cells in upper dermis, ovoid cells in mid-dermis and spindle cells in the lower dermis.

Acute arsenic toxicity

- Gastrointestinal discomfort, nausea, vomiting, and diarrhea and death potential.
- Edema arsenicalis may be present with swelling of the face and eyelid.
- An asymmetric peripheral neuropathy may develop which resembles Guillain-Barre syndrome.
- White transverse lines are present at all fingernails which are known as Mees' lines detectable after 2 months of exposure. Sometimes a brown pigmentation of nails may occur.
- Permissible arsenic level in ground water is not more than 50 µg/liter.

Atrophie blanche

- Atrophy
- Telangiectasia
- Pigmentation

Acrocyanosis

- Persistent bilateral dusky and mottled discoloration of hands, feet and face.
- It is aggravated by cold exposure.
- Skin may be bright red if temperature is very low.
- No pain or trophic changes.
- Chronic vasospasm of cutaneous small vessels, followed by secondary dilatation of capillaries and subpapillary venous plexuses, stasis in capillary loops, aneurysmal dilatation of digital tips, redistribution of blood flow to the subpapillary venous plexuses, compromised erythrocyte flexibility and increased platelet adhesiveness.
- Tissue is less sclerotic than Raynaud's.
- If it occurs in elderly for the first time, myeloproliferative disorders must be exluded.

Alefacept

- It decreases CD4 count, but it is the safest among the biologicals with minimal risk of immunosuppression.

Adalimumab

- It causes reactivation of latent tuberculosis, congestive heart failure, development of lymphoma and demyelinating disease.

Azathioprine

- Its dose should be adjusted according to the serum level of thiopurine methyltransferase (TPMT).
- It causes bone-marrow suppression, pancytopenia, leukopenia, thrombocytopenia, hepato-toxicty, nausea, etc.

Benzyl benzoate

- It causes irritant contact dermatitis.
- It should be avoided in children and pregnancy.

Baboon syndrome

- The term is used when sharply defined erythematous rashes of systematized allergic contact dermatitis develops at buttocks, anogenital region, flexurals and eye lids.
- It occurs due to exposure to mercury, nickel and ampicillin.

Bart syndrome: Localized absence of skin in epidermolysis bullosa in association with pyloric or duodenal stenosis.

Blood hound facies: Down slanting palpebral fissure, redundant eyelids, broad flat nose, large ears, etc., seen in *cutis laxa*.

Blue berry muffin lesions: These are blue-red infiltrative papules and nodules, 2-8 mm in size, and arc seen in following conditions:

- Cogenital rubella, toxoplasmosis, cytomegalo virus, enterovirus and parvovirus B19 infections.
- Erythroblastosis fetalis, inherited hemolytic disorders, twin twin transfusion.
- Neuroblastoma, leukemia, histiocytosis, alveolar rhabdomyosarcoma.

Barber's pole: It is one of the early diagnostic feature of early congenital syphilis, characterized by alternatc spiral streaks of red, blue and white color at umbilical cord.

Black hairy tongue

- It usually occurs in adults or adolescents without any definite cause, but frequently associated with prolonged antibiotic therapy.
- Hypertrophic and elongated filliform papillae form a dense black to blue-black surface on the mid portion of the dorsal surface of the tongue.

Book syndrome: It is characterized by premature graying of hair, hyperhidrosis of palms and soles, and aplasia of premolar tooth.

Bronze baby syndrome: It is characterized by gray discoloration of skin, following phototherapy for hyperbilirubinemia and it is cleared by 2-3 weeks.

Bowenoid papulosis

- Asymptomatic, skin colored or pigmented or depigmented or lichenoid papules and plaques develop at genitalia.
- Histopathology shows uniform proliferation of squamous cells with occasional mitotic change.

Bromhidrosis/Malodorous sweat

- Nonspecific odor due to garlic, penicillin, bromides, dimethyl sulfoxide, etc.
- Only axillary apocrine glands produce malodorous sweat and no odor from apocrine apparatus of other areas.

Bubonulus: Bubo-like abscess formation from lymphangitis at the shaft of the penis in lymphogranuloma venereum.

Beau's lines: Transverse grooves at nails due to sudden arrest of the growth of the nail plates in association with acute illness.

Mechanism of bulla formation

- Acantholysis, seen in pemphigus.
- Cytolysis, seen in malignancy.
- Spongiosis, seen in dermatitis.

- Ballooning and reticular degeneration, seen in herpes/varicella infection.
- Basement membrane degeneration, seen in epidermolysis bullosa, bullous pemphigoid, dermatitis herpetiformis, epidermolysis bullosa acquisita, bullous SLE/lichen planus, porphyria cutanea tarda.

Basement membrane

- It is the homogeneous band, composed of filamentous structure, lies beneath the basal cells.
- It is 35-45 nm in thickness.

Cutaneous features of breast carcinoma

- Alopecia neoplastica
- Inflammatory carcinoma
- Carcinoma en cruirasse
- Telangiectasia
- Nodular metastasis
- Metastasis at eyelids.

Basement membrane zone

- It lies between the epidermis and dermis.
- It is about 20 times thicker than basement membrane and thickness varies from 500-1000 nm.
- It is not homogeneous and composed of basement membrane, lamina lucida, lamina densa and sublamina densa.
- It is visible under light microscope when stained with PAS.

Connexins

- Pores are the specialized transmembrane channels that connect the cytoplasm of neighbouring cells.
- They are ubiquitous in multicellular organisms and facilitate communication from cell to adjacent cells through arrays of 10-1000 intercellular channels, each of which directly connects the cytoplasm of one cell to another.
- The status of the channels (open/closed) is controlled by several mechanisms including *voltage*, *calcium* concentration, *pH* and *phosphorylation*.
- Each gap junction channel is composed of integral membrane proteins called connexins (Cx).
- Six connexins monomers oligomerize to form an annular hemichannel called a connexon.
- Connexons then cluster at plasma membrane to dock with the connexons of an apposing cell to form functional channel.
- The half life of each connexin is short, i.e., matter of hours, which results in a constant state of assembly and degradation of channels.
- Connexins have a distinct tissue distribution in the body and the pattern of expression in the skin is specific and it changes during development and differentiation as well as in response to stmuli.

Vertically oriented collagen

- Prurigo nodularis
- Acral fibrokeratoma
- Digital fibromatosis of childhood
- Collagenous and elastotic plaques of the hand.

Colloid: Homogeneous eosinophilic material of variable composition.

Chilblains/Perniosis/Pernio

- It is a localized inflammatory disease due to cold above freezing point and characterized by sudden onset of purplish or erythematous swellings or blister and ulceration, affecting the fingers and toes.
- Dampness and wind which increase thermal conductivity and convection, may play a role to develop this entity.
- Cooling effect in nonadaptive tissue is more important than absolute temperature.
- More common in temperate region where winter presents with occasional cold and dampness and less common in very cold areas.
- It may not occur during severe cold.
- It is common in persons with low body mass index and in middle aged women. But may occur in children and elderly.

- Spontaneous remission in spring but may relapse in winter.
- Tight garments, stockings, shoes may aggravate symptom like pruritus and burning sensation.

Café-au-lait spots, seen in:

- 2% Of all new borns.
- In neurofibromatosis, lesions may be bilateral with regular margin, known as coast of California.
- Ataxia telangiectasia
- Bloom's syndrome
- Café-au-lait macules of *Albright syndrome* are unilateral and do not cross the midline and their margins are irregular, known as coast of Maine.

Cellular blue nevi

- Usually 1-3 cm in size, larger than blue nevi.
- Common sites are buttocks and sacrococcygeal region.
- Surface is smooth/irregular and cells are basically melanocytes.
- Histopathology shows a *dumble pattern* when cellular islands penetrate into subcutaneous fat and form a bulbous expansion there.

Cellulite/gynoid lipodystrophy

- There is an alteration in the architecture of epidermal-dermal interface.
- Extracorporeal pulse activation therapy (EPAT) improves skin elasticity and produces intense dermal remodelling by inducing tissue damage through delivery of high pressure acoustic energy.

Cimicosis: It is a bed bugs induced dermatosis and characterized by grouped and linear lesions.

Collodion baby

- A form of ichthyosis where the infant is born with covering cellophane or oiled parchment-like membrane, resembling collodion.
- 60% Cases turn into nonbullous ichthyosiform erythroderma and lamellar ichthyosis, and 5% cases the membranes shed and apparently become normal (self-healing collodion).
- Tautness of the covering causes distorted face, ears, eyelids, lips, vulvae and extremities. It also causes difficulty in sucking and expansion of chest.
- Though the membrane is thick but has poor barrier function and thus causes cutaneous and systemic infection, and fluid-electrolyte imbalance and temperature instability.

Chondrodermatitis hallucis nodularis

- It is having painful, erythematous, globular or nodular lesions and sometimes crusted erosions may develop.
- Size of the lesions vary from 0.5-2 cm.
- It involves the helix, specially upper pole of right ear.

Congenital cartilaginous rest/wattles: Small fleshy appendages on anterior neck or at lower half of the sternocleidomastoid muscle.

Costello syndrome

- Deep creases at palms, is a prominent finding.
- Redundant folds of skin at palms, soles, fingers and neck are also seen.

Coat's disease

- Retinal telangiectasias
- Ipsilateral facial port-wine stain.

Chromhidrosis

- It means excretion of colored sweat from apocrine sweat glands.
- Minimal amount of sweat required for color is 0.001 ml/follicle.
- Face is the commonest site.
- Color of the sweat may be black, violet, blue, brown, yellow or green.

Cutaneous horn

- It is a hard and horny projection on either normal skin or on some other dermatoses.
- Associated dermatoses are viral wart, molluscum contagiosum, epidermal nevus, discoid lupus erythematosus, keratoacanthoma, seborrheic keratosis, trichilemmal or epidermoid cyst.

Colloid bodies

- These are formed by apoptotic keratinocytes with deposition of immunoglobulins like IgG, IgM, IgA, etc.
- Size is about 10-20μm and shape is oval to round.
- These are commonly seen in lichen planus, lupus erythematosus, lichenoid keratosis, fixed drug reaction, poikiloderma, etc.

Cutaneous small vessels vasculitis (CSVV)

- Palpable/nonpalpable purpura, petechiae.
- Urticarial papules, pustules, vesicles.
- Erythema multiforme-like lesions

Cutaneous medium vessel vasculitis (CMVV)

- Livedo reticularis, retiform purpura
- Subcutaneous nodules
- Ulcer and digital necrosis

Cutaneous metastatic sites of prostatic carcinoma

- Inguinal area, lower abdomen, thighs.
- Face and scalp.

Cutaneous metastatic site of pancreatic carcinoma

- Umbilical area.

Cutaneous metastatic sites of thyroid carcinoma

- Abdomen and head.

Cutaneous metastatic sites of ovarian carcinoma

- Umbilical area, vulvae and back.

Cutaneous metastatic sites of renal carcinoma

- When it occurs at head and neck region, the sufferer is almost always a male.

Cutaneous metastatic sites of gastrointestinal carcinoma

- Abdomen, perineal and head-neck region.

Cutaneous metastatic sites of Lung carcinoma

- Chest wall and posterior abdomen.
- Oat cell carcinoma metastasis has a predilection for skin of the back.

Frequency of CK 20 positivity

- 100% – In all colorectal carcinoma and Merkel cell carcinoma.
- 60% – In pancreatic carcinoma
- 50% – In gastric carcinoma
- 40% – In cholangiocarcinoma
- 30% – Transitional cell carcinoma.

Cytokines secreted by karatinocytes

- Proinflammatory: IL_1, IL_6, IL_8, TNFα, etc.
- Anti-inflammatory: IL10 and TGFβ.
- Immune regulatory: IL7, IL12, IL15, IL18-20, IL23, GM-CSF, G-CSF.

Cuticle of nail: Long cuticles of nails are seen in keratosis follicularis spinulosa decalvans and Kindler syndrome.

Cutaneous adverse effects of systemic corticosteroid

- Easy bruisability, ecchymosis, striae
- Hypertrichosis, acne
- Edema, moon facies, buffalo hump
- Candidiasis, dermatophytic infection, boil, carbuncle.
- Conversion of plaque psoriasis into generalized pustular psoriasis.

Cutaneous adverse effect of topical corticosteroid

- Striae, depigmentation
- Acne, perioral dermatitis, hypertrichosis
- Conversion of tinea into tinea incognito, conversion of plaque psoriasis into localized pustular psoriasis.

Systemic corticosteroid induced noncutaneous adverse effects

- Psychosis, vertigo, tetany

- Posterior subcapsular cataract, glaucoma
- Hypertension, hyperglycemia, hyperlipidemia
- Adrenal insufficiency, irregular and profuse menstrual bleeding
- Gastrointestinal ulcer
- Development or reactivation of pulmonary tuberculosis
- Osteoporosis

Cutis laxa

- It is characterized by lax skin due to an unknown etiology.
- It may develop following various dermatoses like urticaria, angioedema, sarcoidosis, syphilis, systemic lupus erythematosus, etc.
- Skin becomes inelastic and hangs as redundant folds.
- When face is involved, patient appears as blood hound.
- Heart and lungs also may be affected.

Cylindroma

- These are multiple firm, smooth, pedunculated and reddish tumors develop usually at scalp.
- Histopathology shows collection of mosaic-like closely set cells that separated from each other by a thin stroma.

Chloroquine

- It binds with DNA and stabilizes lysosomal membrane.
- It inhibits lysosomal enzymes and synthesis of prostaglandins.
- It prevents chemotaxis.

Chlorambucil

- It causes bone-marrow suppression, neutropenia, nausea, vomiting, nephrotic syndrome, etc.

Cyclophosphamide

- It causes alopecia, teratogenicity, infertility.
- It causes hemorrhagic cystitis, anemia, pancytopenia, neutropenia, leukopenia, thrombocytopenia.
- It causes interstitial pneumonitis and syndrome of inappropriate antidiuretic hormone hypersecretion (SIADH).

Cyclosporine

- It causes hypertrichosis, gingival hyperplasia,
- It causes nephrotoxicity, hypertension, hepatotoxicity, nausea, etc.
- Management of cyclosporine induced hypertension is done by 25-50% reduction of the dose and use of calcium channel blockers like irsadipine or amlodipine, beta-blockers and angiotensin converting enzyme inhibitors.
- In cyclosporine induced hypertension, nifedipine should be avoided for the risk of gingival hyperplasia and potassium sparing diuretics should be avoided for the risk of hyperkalemia as cyclosporine also causes it.

Dapsone

- It causes exfoliative dermatitis, toxic epidermal necrolysis, peripheral neuropathy.
- It causes anemia, agranulocytosis, methemoglobinemia, hepatotoxicity, acute tubular necrosis.
- Glucose-6-phosphate dehydrogenese (G6PD) level (4-14U/gm hemoglobin) is to be checked prior to dapsone therapy.

DISH syndrome

- Anterior spinal ligament calcification
- Formation of osteophytes.
- Bony bridges without narrowing of the disc spaces.

Duncan's disease

- It is an X-linked lymphoproliferative disorder.

Congenital erythropoietic porphyria: Due to *uroporphyrinogen III synthase* deficiency.

Erythropoietic protoporphyria: Due to *ferrochelatase* deficiency.

Dermatopathia pigmentosa reticularis

- Autosomal dominant inheritance.
- It is having a triad of generalized reticulate hyperpigmentation, non-cicaticial alopecia and onychodystrophy.

- Other features include hypo/hyperhidrosis, palmoplantar hyperkeratosis, adermatoglyphia, nonscarring blister on dorsa of hands and feet.

Dermatosis papulosis nigra

- A form of early onset seborrheic kerotosis, having pinpoint to pinhead dark brown and mild elevated dome shaped papules, involving face, neck and upper chest.
- Treatment includes electrosurgery or chemical cautery.

Disseminated intravascular coagulation (DIC)

- It occurs in 100% cases of acute promyelocytic leukemia.

Desmosome

- Focal thickening of cell membrane forms specialized attachment plaques between two keratinocytes.
- Actually one half from each of the of two adjacent keratinocytes makes a complete round structure.
- It contains many attachment proteins like *desmoplakin*, *plakoglobin* and *plakophilin.*
- Desmosomes integrate the intermediate filaments of cytoskeleton into the cell membrane and establish the tight adhesive points between apposing cells.
- These are vital to maintain the mechanical integrity and stress resistance of individual cells and multicellular sheet.

Eczema herpeticum

- It occurs, usually after 10 days of a viral infection, specially in atopic dermatitis.
- Commonest of viral infection is herpes virus infection.
- Widely disseminated vesicles which gradually turn into hemorrhagic or crusted lesions. Pustular lesions also develop.
- Face is predominantly affected with development of profuse edema.
- Other areas like trunk and extremities are also involved.
- It is often associated with fever and regional lymphadenopathy.

Eczema marginatum

- It is a form of superficial fungal infection caused by *Epidermophyton floccosum.*
- It is featured by scaly plaques with well demarcated borders and multiple vesicopustules.

Eruptive xanthoma

- Pinhead to larger yellowish papules with an erythematous base, develop in crops at buttocks, arms and extensor surfaces of limbs.
- It mimics lepromatous leprosy and sarcoidosis.

Erythema chronicum migrans

- It is having a solitary annular erythema, very large in size and occurs following a tick bite.

Erythema gyratum repens

- It is having concentric waves of erythema, appearing as wood-grain.
- It is associated with malignancies of breast and lung.
- Lesions only disappear just before death.

Erythema marginatum rheumaticum

- It occurs in rheumatic fever.
- It is characterized by annular erythema appearing at afternoon.
- Lesions may fade within 2-3 hours.
- Recurrence is common and occurs at different sites.

Eruptive lingual papillitis

- It commonly occurs in spring season among the children 3-4 years of age and is associated with fever, difficulty in feeding and intense salivation.
- Affected tongue shows inflammatory hypertrophy of the fungiform papillae at tips and dorsolateral aspect of it.
- Other features are submandibular and cervical adenopathy and angular stomatitis.
- Spontaneous recovery occurs within 1-2 weeks.

Erysipeloid

- The area between distal to wrist and proximal to metacarpophalangeal joints of upper limb is classically affected.

Histopathology of electric burn

- Subepidermal blister.
- Fringe of elongated, degenerated cytoplasmic processes, protruding from the under surface of the detached basal cells into subepidermal space.
- Nuclei of these cells arrange and stretch vertically.
- Upper dermis becomes homogenized due to coagulation necrosis.
- In first degree burn basal layer remains viable and upper epidermis shows coagulation necrosis with cells having pyknotic nuclei and perinuclear halo. In advanced stage nuclei stain faintly eosinophilic or remain unstained. This is known as architectural ghost.

Eccrine squamous syringometaplasia

- Presented with widespread polymorphic lesions from vesicles to large erythematous plaques or localized lesions at intertriginous areas and extremities.

Erythema infectiosum/Fifth disease

- It is caused by parvovirus B19, the only parvovirus infecting human.
- It occurs in school-going children, between 4-10 years of age, during winter and spring.
- Incubation period is 4-14 days.
- Virus binds to erythrocyte P antigen and enhances blood cell destruction or reduction with a transient aplastic crisis.
- Following a mild prodromal features, initial exanthema develops, consisting of bright red macular erythema of the cheeks, sparing nasal bridge and circumoral area. This is known as slapped cheek appearance.
- After 1-4 days of initial exanthema, secondary lesions appear at extremities and then at trunk with reticulate pattern of erythematous maculopapular eruptions.
- Papular purpuric gloves and socks syndrome (PPGSS) may develop.
- Lesions may be aggravated by sunlight or heat and may be associated with arthralgia.

Erythrocyanosis

- It is characterized by nodular lesions with dusky cyanotic discoloration like chilblains.
- It affects thighs and legs, the areas containing thick layer of subcutaneous fat.
- Adolescent and middle aged females are commonly affected.
- It is often associated with keratosis pilaris, angiokeratoma and telangiectasia.
- Lesions spontaneously improve after few years.

Erythromelalgia/Erythermalgia

- It is characterized by feeling of warmth and burning discomfort or pain with erythematous skin at the extremities.
- Pain is intensified when limbs are lowered or heat is applied.
- Pain is reduced when limbs are elevated and cold is applied.
- In primary idiopathic type, blood flow is increased through thermoregulatory arteriovenous shunt.
- It may occur secondary to thrombocythemia, related to myeloproliferative syndrome.
- Treatment includes acetylsalicylic acid, mexiletine, venlafaxine, topical or iv lidocaine, topical amitriptyline and ketamine, and sympathectomy.

Efalizumab and infliximab

- These cause reactivation of latent tuberculosis, lymphoma, demyelinating disease, congestive heart failure, progressive multifocal leukoencephalopathy, etc.

Etanercept

- It causes reactivation of latent tuberculosis, lymphoma, demyelinating disease, congestive heart failure, etc.

Fanconi anemia

- Cutaneous features are generalized dusky or olive brown pigmentation, specially at flexures, neck and lower trunk and scattered rain drop like depigmented and hyperpigmented macules.
- Sometimes *café-au-lait macules* are also seen.

Erythroplasia of Queyrat

- It is characterized by well-defined, glossy and erythematous plaque with irregular margin.
- Gradually erosion and crusting form.
- Treatment includes topical 5% cream of 5-Fluorouracil or radiotherapy.

FACE (Facial Afro-Caribbean childhood erythema)

- Self-limiting monomorphic flesh colored or hypopigmented papules around mouth, eyelids and ears in Negroid children.

Morphology of deep fungus

- Aspergillosis: 2-4 μm septate hyphae with dichotomous branching at 45° angle.
- Histoplasmosis: 2-4 μm spores with narrow necked budding and clear halo, appearing as pseudocapsule. They lie within the cytoplasm of large histiocytes.
- Subcutaneous pheohyphomycosis: 2-25 μm pigmented and loosely arranged hyphae with infrequent branching.
- Alternariosis: 3-10 μm oval spores with double contours and 5-7 μm septate brownish hyphae with variable branching.
- Sporotrichosis: 4-6 μm round to oval spores.
- Cryptococcosis: 4-12 μm and 2-4 μm spores.
- Chromoblastomycosis: 6-12 μm, dark brown spores with thick wall.
- Paracoccidioidomycosis: 6-12 μm narrow necked spores with single or multiple buds. Large size upto 60 μm spores appear as Mariner's wheels.
- Rhinosporidiosis: 7-12 μm spores, but sporangia upto 300 μm.
- Zygomycosis/mucormycosis/phycomycosis: 7-30 μm hyphae with variable branching and angling.
- Blastomycosis: 8-15 μm thick walled spores with single broadbased buds.
- Lobomycosis: 9-10 μm lemon shaped spores with single budding and arranged in chains.
- Coccidiodomycosis: 10-80 μm spores with thick wall and granular cytoplasm. Larger spores contain endospores.

Freckle

- Controlling gene is melanocortin 1 receptor gene (MC1R).
- It is related to fair skin, red hair, melanoma and non-melanoma skin cancer.

Frost bite

- Tissue freezes following exposure to extremely cold air, liquids or metals and leads to death of the tissue as in cryosurgery.
- Rate of freezing determines level of cellular death.
- Slow freezing causes extracellular and fast freezing causes intracellular ice formation.
- Formation of ice-crystal at 0°C within fat globules and cell membranes leading to alteration of osmotic property and flow of water and electrolytes through the cell membranes.
- Thawing may cause more damage due to intracellular flooding of water.
- Slow thawing causes enlargement of ice-crystal and leads to more damage and cells are exposed to high concentration of electrolytes for longer period.
- Peripheral vessels constrict due to cold exposure and leads to increased venous pressure,

reduced capillary perfusion, thrombus formation, hypoxia, damage of the capillaries and surrounding tissues, segmental vascular necrosis and axonal degeneration.

- Mealanocytes are damaged irreversibly at –4 °C to –7 °C.
- Bone, cartilage and nerve sheath are resistant to cold injury.
- Cooling has three stages as first stage shows massive vasoconstriction with rapid fall of temperature, second stage shows hunting reaction with cyclic rise and fall of temperature and third stage shows that temperature falls to ambient temperature.
- Common sites are fingers, toes, ears, nose and cheeks.

Good prognostic signs of frost bite

- Large clear blebs, extending to tip of the digits.
- Rapid return of sensations and normal temperature.
- Short capillary filling time following pressure blanching.
- Pink skin after rewarming.

Poor prognostic signs of frost bite

- Hard, white, cold and insensitive skin.
- Cold and cyanotic skin without any bleb after rewarming.
- Dark hemorrhagic blebs.
- Presence of constitutional sign of tissue necrosis like fever and tachycardia.
- Cyanotic or dark red skin persists after pressure.
- Freeze-thaw-refreeze injury.

Histopathology of friction blister

- Intraepidermal cleft due to cytolysis and necrosis.
- Roof is formed by statum corneum, stratum granulosum and amorphous cellular debris.
- Base is formed by pale colored degenerated keratinocytes and undamaged cells present at deeper part.

Stages of cooling of frost bite

- Rapid fall
- Cyclic fall and rise
- To approach surrounding temperature (ambient temperature).

Frey's syndrome

- Gustatory hyperhidrosis at the area supplied by auriculotemporal nerve following injury or operation of parotid region, causing regrowth of parasympathetic fibers into sympathetic nerves.

Galli-Galli disease

- It is having slightly keratotic papules, red to dark brown in color.
- Lesions coalesce focally to make a reticular pattern.
- Common sites are flexurals including axillae, groins, neck, and trunk, upper limbs and scrotum.

Gamma benzene hexachloride

- It causes aplastic anemia, neurotoxicity and excretes into breast milk. But no report of fetal malformations or abortion has been noted after use of it in pregnancy.

Gottron's papules

- These are flat-topped, polygonal, violaceous lesions on knuckles and are seen in dermatomyositis.

Glomus bodies

- They allow shunting of blood directly from arteriole to venule bypassing the capillary bed.
- They are abundant at acral skin areas like fingers, toes, nailbeds, nose and ears to regulate temperature.
- Each body is having one arterial segment, known as Sacquyet-Hoyer canal and a venous segment.
- Sacquyet-Hoyer canal: This segment is having narrow lumen and thick wall. Wall contains

endothelium, surrounded by 3-6 layers of modified smooth muscle cells, known as glomus cells.

- Each glomus cell has a uniform ovoid nucleus, pale staining cytoplasm and indistinct cell margin. These cells are innervated by unmyelinated adrenergic nerves.
- Venous segment: It is thin-walled and has larger lumen. It drains into subpapillary venules.

Glomus tumor

- It is characterized by a painful purple nodule with a variable size from 1 mm to 10 mm and usually develops at nailbed.
- Direct pressure on the lesion or change of temperature elicits pain.

Gorham-Stout disease

- Massive osteolysis and limb hypertrophy with overlying cutaneous venous and/or lymphatic malformation.

Griselli syndrome: The hallmark is silvery hair.

Good syndrome: It is associated with immunodeficiency and thymoma.

Growth rate

- Scalp hair: 1-3 cm/month.
- Finger nail: 3 mm/month.
- Toe nail: 1 mm/month.
- Hair growth maximum in March and minimum in September.

Granuloma gluteale infantum

- Purple red skin nodules at groin, lower abdomen and inner thighs, develop usually following application of topical corticosteroids.
- Candidal infection and maceration aggravate the lesions.
- Lesions resolve spontaneously within a period of several months.
- Intralesional triamcinolone may be given in resistant cases.

Histamine receptors

- H1 receptors-present in skin
- H2 receptors-present in skin and gastric mucosa
- H3 receptors-present in autonomic nerve terminals
- Hic receptors-present witin the cells for promotion of cell and tissue growth.

Human papilloma virus (HPV)

- Plane wart: HPV3, –10
- Palmoplantar wart: HPV1, –2, –4, –27, –57
- Common wart: HPV1, –2, –4
- Pigmented wart: HPV4, –60, –65
- Condyloma acuminata: HPV6, –11, –16, –18
- Condyloma acuminata with malignant potency: HPV16, –18
- Epidermodysplasia verruciformis: HPV5, –8, –(19-25).

HPV vaccine

- Almost 90-100% benefit is observed in cervical intra-epithelial neoplasia associated with HPV viral types which are included in the HPV vaccine.
- It is more or less confirmed that vaccination confers protection against vaccine type-related cervical neoplasia.

Types of HPV vaccine

- Prophylactic
- Therapeutic.

Half and half nail

- Proximal half is white and distal half is red to brown and the two halves are sharply demarcated.
- This is seen in chronic renal failure.

Hand and foot syndrome

- It is seen in sickle cell anemia and characterized by painful nonpitting edema of hands and feet due to infarction of small bones.

Hair follicle units at scalp (contents of upper dermal transverse section of a 4 mm punch biopsy):

- It contains 10-12 follicular units.
- About 40 hair of which 20-35 are terminal and 5-10 are vellus with a ratio of 3-4:1.
- Each follicular unit contains 2-5 terminal hair, 0-2 vellus hair, sebaceous gland and arrector pili muscle.

HIV infection

- Pruritic papular eruption is the most common cutaneous feature.
- Herpes is one of the most common cutaneous opportunistic infection.
- Oral hairy leukoplakia is seen only in 25% cases. White, verrucous and confluent plaque develops at lateral aspect of the tongue.
- Molluscum contagiosum develops when CD4+ cell count is below 100/cmm.
- Most common bacterial infection is staphylococcal infection.
- Kaposi's sarcoma lesion is painless whereas bacillary angiomatosis lesion is painful.
- Oral candidiasis is one of the early manifestation.
- Scabies is the most common parasitic infection.
- Seborrheic dermatitis is seen in 85% cases in comparision to only 2-4% in normal population. Its severity correlates with CD4+ cell count.
- Xerosis/ichthyosis vulgaris-like ichthyosis is seen in 30% cases.
- Kaposi's sarcoma is the most common malignancy and 95% cases are associated with HHV8 infection.

Acute HIV infection

- Occurs in 50% cases after 2-6 weeks of infection.
- Transient macular or morbilliform eruption is seen in 40-80% cases.
- ELISA or Western blot test is negative but P24 antigen is positive.

Hair growth factors

- Epidermal growth factors
- Transforming growth factors
- Fibroblast growth factors
- Bone morphogenic proteins
- Neurotrophins.

Initiation factors of hair growth

- Signal from hair papillae to epithelial stem cells is carried probably by Noggin.
- Onset of anagen is heralded by STAT-3.
- Key catagen controller is Hairless gene.

Morphogenetic factors of hair follicle

- Regulation of Wnt
- B catenin
- Hedgehog signaling pathways

Hyaline

- It is a PAS-positive and diastase-resistant material, mainly composed of glycoprotein.
- It is seen in:
  - Hyalinosis cutis et mucosae
  - Porphyria
  - Cylindroma

Hematohidrosis

- It is excretion of bloody sweating due to constriction of vascular networks around the sweat glands under extreme level of stress and when the stress is passed away, the vessels dilate so much that they rupture and thus bleed in and around the sweat glands.

Dermatoses with hoarseness of voice

- Secondary syphilis
- Lepromatous leprosy
- Lipoid proteinosis
- Generalized euptive keratoacanthoma
- Relapsing polychondritis

Hemidesmosome

- Half of the desmosome, which attaches a basal keratinocyte with the basement membrane.

Ichthyosis bullosa of Siemens

- A variant of bullous ichthyosiform erythroderma, having more superficial blisters.
- Lesions appear intermittently with tendency of molting known as mauscrung phenomenon.

Causes of acquired ichthyosis

- Old age
- Leprosy, tuberculosis, HIV
- Sarcoidosis, scleroderma
- Hypothyroidism
- Lymphoma
- Drugs like clofazimine, lipid lowering agents, retinoids, hypervitaminosis or hypovitaminosis A.

Ichthyosis hystrix

- This is a form of epidermal nevus.
- Characterized by porcupine-quill-like verrucous hyperkeratosis.

Immunosurveillance in skin, carried out by

- Langerhans' cell
- Tissue resident T cells
- Macrophages
- Dermal dendritic cells

Carcinoma lung

- It is the commonest cause of death among men and women.
- Associated with tripe palm.

Immunoistochemistry

- Desmin and vimentin, positive in leiomyoma sarcoma.
- EMA (epithelial membrane antigen), positive in epitheloid sarcoma.
- S100 and vimentin, positive in desmoplastic melanoma.
- Vimentin, positive in atypical fibroxanthoma.
- Vimentin and CD34, positive in dermatofibro sarcoma protuberans.
- Factor XIIIa, positive in dermatofibroma and positive for veil cells.

Immunofluorescence with linear pattern, seen in

- Epidermolysis bullosa acquisita.
- Bullous lupus erythematosus.
- Dermatitis herpetiformis.

Intraluminal giant cell, seen in

- Melkerson-Rosenthal syndrome
- Recurrent genitocrural infection
- Cutaneous histiocytic lymphangitis
- Rosai-Dorfman disease.

Mechanism of vesicle formation in incontinentia pigmenti

- Deficiency of NF$\kappa\beta$ in some keratinocytes due to mutation of NEMO gene (Nuclear factor essential modulation).
- NF$\kappa\beta$ prevents apoptosis.
- So, NF$\kappa\beta$ deficient keratinocytes undergo rapid apoptosis, leading to cytolysis.
- Marked blood eosinophilia causes influx of eosinophilis in the epidermis.
- Proteases, released by eosinophils cause further cytolysis and resulted in vesicle formation.

Incubation period

- Granuloma inguinale: Average is 3 to 4 weeks and ranges from 19 days to 90 days.
- Primary syphilis: Average is 3 to 4 weeks and ranges from 9 to 90 days.
- Lymphogranuloma venereum: Average is 2 to 3 weeks and ranges from 3-30 days.

Job syndrome

- Freckles, red hair and blue eyes
- Hyperextensible joints
- Hypergammaglobulinemia E

Jordon anomaly

- Leukocytes, plasma cells and macrophages contain fat droplets at their cytoplasm in Chanarin-Dorfman syndrome.

Juvenile xanthogranuloma

- It is having a few or multiple, small, coppery colored, shiny papules.

- Lesions erupt suddenly in early age and resolve spontaneously.
- Common sites: Face, neck, scalp and upper trunk.

Generalized eruptive form of keratoacanthoma

- It commonly affects 40-70 years of age and is often associated with severe pruritus.
- Papules with central crater appear suddenly and persist for several months before regression with atrophic scars.
- Number of lesions may be more than 100.
- Koebner phenomenon may be seen.
- Other features are mask like facies, ectropion and hoarseness of voice.

Familial generalized eruptive form of keratoacanthoma

- It is an autosomal dominant condition and affects children and young adults.
- Papules with central crater appear at sunexposed areas and regress spontaneously.

Keratinocytes

- These are the structural and functional units of the epidermis.
- Physiological keratinocytes
  - Horny keratinocyte or corneocyte
  - Granular keratinocyte
  - Spinous keratinocyte
  - Basal cell
  - Stem cell
- Pathological keratinocytes
  - Acantholytic cell
  - Balloon cell
  - Dyskeratotic cell
  - Koilocyte
  - Multinucleated cell
  - Malignant cell

Keratin

- Soft keratin is found in the stratum corneum of the epidermis. It is due to rapid keratinization with lacking of disulfide bonds.
- Hard keratin is found in hair cortex and nail. It is due to slow keratinization with presence of disulfide bonds.

Keratohyaline granules are basophilic granules, present in the granular layer and contain proteins including involucrin, loricrin (80%) and profilaggrin.

Langerhan's cell: This dendritic cell recognizes the antigen, processes the antigen and presents the antigen to T lymphocyte.

Leg ulcer

- Seen in 3-5% of population over age of 65 years.
- Venous insufficiency is responsible in 45-60% cases of leg ulcers.
- Arterial insufficiency is responsible in 10-20% cases.
- Diabetes mellitus is responsible in 15-25% cases.
- Combined causes are seen in 10-15% cases.
- Smoking and obesity increase the risk.

Keratinocyte derived antimicrobial agents

- Antileukoprotease (ALP)
- Dermicidin (DCD1)
- Human B defensins (HBD1-4)
- Human cationic antimicrobial peptide (hCAP18)
- Lysozyme
- Psoriasin
- RNase

Langerhans cell

- Becomes ATPase positive after 50 days of gestation.
- Becomes CD1a positive after 60 days of gestation.
- After 90 days of gestation both ATPase and CD1a become positive.
- Extremities are having more concentration of Langerhans cell than trunk.
- Average concentration of Langerhans cell is 4% of epidermal cell population and 400-600/ mm^2.

Lactic acid in skin: It attracts mosquito to bite.

Leiomyoma sacroma: Immunohistochemistry shows positivity for desmin and vimentin.

Stages of nerve involvement in leprosy

- Stage of parasitization
- Stage of host response
- Stage of clinical involvement
- Stage of nerve damage
- Stage of nerve destruction

Onset and progress of nerve damage in leprosy

- Insidious onset and gradual progress
- Episodic onset and saltatory progress
- Catastrophic onset and catastrophic progress
- Late onset and silent progress

Residual signs of leprosy for which no treatment is required

- Post inflammatory wrinkling, hypo/hyperpigmentation, scar, etc.
- Persisting or even increment of anesthesia due to silent fibrosis of nerve trunk.
- Thickened nerve without tenderness.
- Presence of deformities.

Mechanism of down regulation of cell mediated immunity (CMI) in leprosy

- Macrophages directly inhibit T cell proliferation.
- Macrophages produce prostaglandin E2 (PGE2), which indirectly inhibits T cells.
- Defective macrophages cannot produce IL1 to sensitize T cells and also cannot present the antigen to sensitized T cells.
- Macrophages produce reactive nitrogen intermediators (RNI) which inhibit T cell.

Mechanism of *M.leprae* to become virulent to the host

- Lipoarabinomannan (LAM), a cell wall protein, inhibits interferon gamma (IFN γ) mediated signal transduction.
- Phenolic glycolipid1 (PGL1), modifies formation of superoxides.
- Bacilli produce superoxide dismutase which again modifies superoxides.
- LAM and PGL1 act as scavenger to remove the superoxides.

Leukoplakia: Hydrated keratin layer is responsible for white color.

Drugs responsible for lichenoid drug eruption

- Antimalarials
- ACE inhibitors, B-blockers and thiazide diuretics
- Proton pump inhibitors
- NSAIDS and sulfasalazine
- Penicillamine, gold and viagra

Clinical features of lichenoid drug eruption

- Larger sized lesions
- Less monomorphic with presence of scale, crust, oozing and ulceration.
- No Wickham's striae in the lesions.
- Sparing of classical sites like flexors, mucous membrane and genitalia.

Histopathology of lichenoid drug eruption

- Confluent parakeratosis with neutrophils.
- Extravasated RBCs in the epidermis and paler superficial layers of the epidermis.
- Necrosis of the keratinocytes.
- Perivascular and periappendageal infiltration with eosinophils and plama cells.

Lipoid proteinosis: Facial skin appears as *pig-skin leather*.

Livedo reticularis

- Bilateral symmetrical
- Regular
- Reversible

Livedo racemosa

- Unilateral
- Broken/irregular
- Irreversible

Lipoatrophy: It appears as round or band like depression following loss of subcutaneous fat, commonly involving thighs, legs, buttocks and face.

Lipoid proteinosis: Bilateral sickle-shaped opacity at sella turcica is seen due to calcification.

Lobomycosis: Can occur in animal other than human is Dolphin.

Lozenge cells: These are lozenge shaped keratinocytes, seen in plasma cell balanitis.

Lenalidomide is *nonteratogenic* and 50,000 times more potent than thalidomide for inhibition of TNFα.

Lyme disease

- Caused by *Borrelia burgdorferi*, a spirochete and borne by tick.

Mazzotti test: Diethylcarbamazine 50 mg is administered orally and positive result is shown by developing mild and transient pruritic rash within 15 minutes, in a case of onchocerciasis.

Mees' lines

- Whitish transverse line at nail plate resulting from abnormal keratinization due to transient injury to the nail matrix.
- Related to acute *arsenic poisoning*, severe *stress*, *systemic illness* and drugs like *sulfonamide*.

Melioidosis

- Acute unilateral suppuration of parotid gland, seen in childhood form.

Melorheostosis

- Roughening of one surface of long bones underlying linear morphoea and radiographically characterized by a picture suggestive of wax flowing down the side of the candle.

Melkersson-Rosenthal syndrome

- Recurrent facial paralysis
- Soft non-pitting edema of the lips
- Scrotal tongue

Muehrcke's line: Narrow and white transverse bands in pairs, seen on nails in chronic hypoalbuminemia.

Positive markers of Merkel cell carcinoma

- CK 20
- Chromogranin A
- CD 56
- Synaptophysin

Negative markers of Merkel cell carcinoma

- Lymphocyte common antigen (LCA).

Metastatic calcification: It is associated with *chronic renal failure*, *sarcoidosis* and *malignancy*.

Morbihan's disease: It is characterized by solid facial edema as an unusual and disfiguring complication of acne.

Morbilliform eruption

- Associated with *rubella*, *Epstein-Barr virus* and *human herpes virus*-6 *infections*.

Metastatic adenocarcinoma

- Small groups of tumor cells.
- Cells lie in large pool of mucin.

Metastatic gastric carcinoma

- Tumor cell are anaplastic, infiltrating, variable cellularity.
- Cells lie in loose stroma.
- Varying amount of signet ring cells are present.

Metastatic mucinous carcinoma

- Gastrointestinal carcinoma
- Lung/breast carcinoma

Molluscoid pseudotumor: Bluish gray spongy nodules due to herniation of subcutaneous fat in classical *Ehlers Danlos syndrome*.

Mondor's disease: Thrombophlebitis occurs in subcutaneous veins of anterolateral and thoraco-abdominal areas.

Mucin

- Alcian blue positive at pH 2.5 and negative at pH 0.4.

- Stains metachromatically with toluidine blue at pH 3.0 and negative at pH 2.0.
- PAS positive, diastase resistant.
- Mucicarmine positive.

Merkel cell

- An epidermal touch receptor, originates at 8-12 weeks of gestation and is present in skin and oral mucosa.
- It is connected with neighbouring keratinocytes by the help of tonofilaments like intermediate fibers and occasionally by desmosomes.
- It contains *neuron-specific enolase* in the cytoplasm, but does not have any neurotransmitter as such.

Metastasis to the skin from internal malignancies

- Incidence is 5-10% of all metastasis.
- Relative frequencies are 69% from breasts, 9% from large intestine and 4% from lungs and ovaries.
- Relative frequencies in men are 24% from lungs, 19% from large intestine, 12% from oral cavity, 6% from kidneys, 6% from stomach and 13% from melanoma.
- Relation with age is that older persons are commonly affected than youngs and in youngs common causes are neuroblastoma and rhabdomyosarcoma.
- Relation with site is that it occurs near the primary source except scalp and scalp involvement is 5% of all cutaneous metastasis.
- Umbilicus is involved commonly in adenocarcinoma of stomach, breasts, ovaries and endometrium.
- Umbilicus is the commonest site of cutaneous metastasis from gastric carcinoma.
- Relation with sex is that cutaneous metastasis from rectum/colon, in men abdomen, periumbilical region, head and neck are commonly affected.
- Relation with pattern is that zosteriform pattern at abdomen/chest is associated with carcinoma of breasts, lungs, stomach, bladder, prostate and ovaries.

Rare causes of cutaneous metastasis

- Thyroid, neuroendocrine system
- Liver, pancreas, gall bladder
- Urinary bladder, endometrium
- Prostate, and testes.

Metastasis appearing as first sign

- Lung carcinoma
- Renal carcinoma
- Ovarian carcinoma

Cutaneous metastasis through lymphatic channels

- Breast
- Oral cavity

Methotrexate

- It causes mucosal ulceration, tender, eroded psoriatic lesions with hepatic, hematologic and pulmonary toxicity.

Mycophenolate mofetil

- It causes teratogenicity, progressive multifocal leukoencephalopathy, nausea, vomiting, dyspepsia, diarrhea, constipation, neutropenia, infection, renal toxicity, etc.

Mosaicism patterns

- Lines of Blaschko
- Checker board pattern
- Phylloid pattern

Morbilliform drug erution: Commonest cause is antibiotic therapy.

Types of morphea

- Guttate
- Plaque
- Linear
- Segmental
- Subcutaneous/morphea profundus
- Generalized morphea

Cutaneous features of medium vessel vasculitis

- Livedo reticularis

- Retiform purpura
- Ulceration
- Subcutaneous nodules
- Digital gangrene

Muir-Torre syndrome

- Presence of keratoacanthoma and sebaceous neoplasia.
- Associated with colonic carcinoma

Neutrophilic eccrine hidradenitis

- Occurs after 7-14 days of chemotherapy with cytarabine, methotrexate and zidovudine, GM-CSF, etc.
- Painful edematous polymorphic papules and plaques at trunk and face.
- Lesions may be linear, annular, erythema multiforme like, purpuric and even pustular.
- Histopathology shows hydropic changes in the secretory part of the sweat glands with neutrophilic infiltration.

Necrolytic erythema, associated with

- Acrodermatitis enteropathica
- Glucagonoma syndrome
- Necrolytic acral erythema
- Hartnup disease

Necrolytic acral erythema

- Associated with Hepatitis C.
- Presence of eroded erythematous to violaceous patches.
- Tender flaccid blisters, and eroded hyperkeratotic plaques.
- Commonest site: Lower limb.

Necrobiosis lipoidica

- It is seen only in 0.3% of diabetic patients but 75% of patients of this condition suffer from diabetes.
- Lesion starts as well circumscribed, round, dull red, firm papule or plaque.
- Gradually size and number of the lesions increase and they may coalesce to become irregular or serpiginous. Later center of the lesion becomes atrophic and shiny but periphery becomes brownish.
- Ulceration, telangiectasia, sclerosis and comedo-like lesions may develop within the lesion.

Nicolau syndrome (embolia cutis medicamentosa)

- Livedoid pattern of cutaneous necrosis following injection of phenylbutazones, corticosteroids, local anesthetics and antibiotics.

Neimann Pick disease

- It is an autosomal recessive entity with deposition of sphingomyelin due to sphingomyelinase deficiency.
- Sphingomyelin derived ceramides are reduced in the stratum corneum, leading to defective barrier function.
- Skin lesions are facial papules, brown hyperpigmentation and indurated brown plaques.
- Xanthoma and juvenile xanthogranuloma are also seen.

Onychauxis

- Thickening of the nail plate.
- Characterized by hyperkeratosis, discoloration, loss of translucency and subungual hyperkeratosis.
- Complications are distal onycholysis, increased susceptibility of onychomycosis, pain, subungual hemorrhage and ulceration.

Onychocryptosis

- Characterised by overcurvature, subcutaneous ingrowing and hypertrophy of the lateral nail folds.
- Other associated features are inflammation of the nail folds, pain on ambulation and with or without granulation tissue.
- Causes are improper cutting of the nails, external pressure due to poorly fitted footwear or high heeled shoes, abnormal long toes and pointed toes, imbalance between the nail plate and the

nail bed, poor hygiene and hyperhidrosis, congenital excessive curvature of the nail plate, congenital malalignment of great toe nail, etc.

Nondermatophytic causes of onychomycosis

- *Fusarium/Aspergillus/Acremonium spp.*, producing superficial white pattern.
- *Scopulariopsis brevicaulis*, having lemon-shaped conidia and atypical hyphae and producing lateral yellow brown discoloration.

Onychoclavus/Subungual heloma/Subungual corn

- Subungual hyperkeratotic dark spot with elevated or splitted nail plate due to anatomical defect or mechanical changes in foot function.
- Pressure with a probe produces intense pain but does not yield.
- X-ray confirms the diagnosis.

Odland bodies or lamellar granules

- These are derivatives of Golgi apparatus of the upper spinous cells.
- Odland bodies contain baskets of lipids, polysaccharides and hydrolytic enzymes.
- Odland bodies contribute to form outer lipid layer of the cornified envelop of corneocytes.
- This lipid layer contains ceramides (50%), cholesterol (35%) and free fatty acids (15%).

Psoriasis

- Oil drop or oil spot phenomenon reflects an exocytosis of leukocytes beneath the nail plate.
- **Koebner phenomenon** in psoriasis is seen in 25% cases and time required for developing koebner phenomenon following trauma is 2-6 weeks.

Pseudoxanthoma elasticum

- Yellowish papules which may remain discrete or may coalesce.
- Common sites are neck, axillae and groins.
- Intermittent claudication is seen in an early age.
- Gastrointestinal bleeding may occur.
- Reduced visual acquity is due to angioid streaks.

Plasma cells

- These are tissue (dermis) bound cells, derived from B lymphocytes and not found in circulation.
- Coarse and condensed chromatin of the nucleus of plasma cell appears as cartwheel or clock face.

Perivascular plasma cell infiltration

- Syphilitic chancre
- Condyloma lata
- Scleroderma/morphea
- Kaposi's sarcoma
- Rosacea
- Perioral dermatitis
- Erythema chronicum migrans.

Painful tumors and tumor-like conditions of the skin:

- Angiolipoma
- Neurofibroma and neurilemmoma
- Glomus tumor
- Eccrine tumor (Spiradenoma)
- Leiomyoma
- Adiposis dolorosa
- Chondrodermatitis nodularis helicis
- Erythema nodosum

Painless ulcers

- Neuropathic ulcers
  # Diabetes
  # Leprosy
  # Syringomyelia
  # Alcohol and drugs
- Neoplastic ulcer
- Chancre of syphilis
- Buruli ulcer
- Venous ulcer.

Cold induced panniculitis

- Children are more affected than adults.
- Children are having higher amount of saturated fatty acids, resulting in solidification at less cold temperature.
- Tender erythematous subcutaneous nodules develop 1-3 days after cold exposure and commonly affected sites are cheeks and legs.
- Challenge by putting ice cube for 10 minutes, leads to develop erythematous plaque after 12-18 hours.
- Histopathology shows perivascular mixed cell infiltration with neutrophils, lymphocytes and histiocytes at dermal-subcutaneous junction, followed by necrosis and abscess formation.
- Lesions usually subside by 2 weeks.
- It should be differentiated from nodular erythrocyanosis, sclerema neonatorum, subcutaneous fat necrosis of the newborn.

Histopathology of porphyria cutanea tarda

- Reduplication of epidermal or vascular basement membrane.
- Festooning of the basement membrane.
- Lightly eosinophilic hyaline materials deposit in and around small vessels in upper dermis.
- Fibrillar and amorphous materials deposit around superficial venules and at dermoepidermal junction, known as caterpillar bodies.

Porphyria without skin manifestation

- ALA dehydratase deficiency
- Acute intermittent porphyria.

Porphyria, autosomal dominant type

- Acute intermittent porphyria
- Hereditary coproporphyria
- Variegate porphyria

Peripheral thickened nerve, seen in

- Leprosy
- Neurofibromatosis
- Amyloidosis
- Pachydermoperiosteosis
- Familial hypertrophic interstitial neurosis
- Physiologically in wrestler or porter.

Periorificial dermatitis, associated with

- Acrodermatitis enteropathica
- Methylmalonic acidemia
- Propionic acidemia
- Selenium deficiency
- Biotin deficiency

Pityriasis rotunda

- It is a rare, asymptomatic, chronic and persistent form of acquired ichthyosis, usually occurs in Japanese, Africans and West Indians. It is characterized by circular or oval, brown, scaly patches at trunk and extremities.
- It commonly affects age group 20-45 years.
- Lesions are well defined nummular scaly plaques with hyper- or hypopigmented background and lesions persist for months to years.
- Number of the lesions varies from 1 to 100.
- Size may be more than 2 cm.

Pigmentary demarcation lines

- Type A (Futcher's/Voigt's lines)–Most common types, seen at dorsoventral aspect of the arms.
- Type B–Appear during pregnancy at lower limbs and disappear after delivery.
- Type C–Present at sternum extending from clavicle to the lower border of the sternum.
- Type D–Postero-median lines along the spine.
- Type E–Periareolar hypopigmented macules.
- Type F–Periorbital hyperpigmentation.

Perleche/angular cheilitis

- It is a common disorder, characterized by fissuring, maceration, exudation and crusting at the angle of the mouth.
- It is basically due to collection and maintenance of a moist environment and not due to nutritional deficiency.

- Predisposing factors are lip-licking, ill fitting dentures or dental malocclusion.
- Infection with bacteria or candida is a secondary phenomenon.

Phakomatosis

- A group of disorders which must affect central nervous system and retina of the eye.
- Phakoma or tumor develops at retina.
- There are four prime disorders under it:
  - Neurofibromatosis
  - Tuberous sclerosis
  - Sturge-Weber syndrome
  - Von Hippel-Lindau syndrome.

Pityriasis amiantacea (asbestos-like)

- Having large plates of scale firmly adherent to the hair and scalp, associated with focal hair loss and secondary infection.
- It commonly affects teenagers.
- About 2-15% cases turn into classical psoriasis.

Features of prolidase deficiency

- Childhood onset
- Recalcitrant leg ulcer
- Premature graying of hair
- Telangiectasia
- Photosensitivity
- Lymphedema
- Rare development of squamous cell carcinoma.

Proliferating trichilemmal cyst/proliferating pilar tumor

- Usually single subcutaneous nodule and commonest site is scalp.
- Gradually enlarges, becomes lobulated and undergoes ulceration when mimics squamous cell carcinoma.

Pseudoalbinism: It is related to selenium deficiency.

Pseudo-ochronosis: It is seen among *Jewelry workers.*

Pseudo melanoma: It is a recurrent tumor following incomplete surgery of a melanocytic nevus.

Pseudo-Kaposi's sarcoma: It is related to *stasis dermatitis.*

Pseudo-Darier's sign: It is associated with leiomyoma cutis. When the lesion comes in contact with cold substance, it becomes more prominent and painful.

Pseudolymphoma: It is often induced by drugs like thiazides, penicillin and sulfonamides.

Pseudochromhidrosis: It refers to the condition in which initial colorless sweat, later becomes colorful due to action of chromogenic bacteria, specially *Corynebacteria.*

Pseudocellulitis: Lesions of the Sweet syndrome or contact dermatitis mimicking cellulitis.

Pseudoichthyosis: Pityriais rotunda is named as such.

Pseudolepromatous face: It is seen in diffuse acute cutaneous leishmaniasis.

Pruritus is relieved by scratching only for 15-25 mins.

Variants of pruritus

- Creeping eruption/Sandworm eruption/Plumber's itch/Duck-hunter's itch: It is caused by movement of the hookworm larvae through the skin.
- Copra itch/Grocer's itch: It is caused by *Glycyphagus domesticus* and characterized by intensely pruritic papules and papulovesicles at exposed part of the body and commonly occuring to dockers, storekeepers and shopkeepers.
- Dew itch/Ground itch/uncinarial itch: It is caused by penetration of skin by the larvae of the hookworms and characterized by transient eruption with variable amount of itching.
- Dhobie itch/Eczema marginatum: It is nothing but tinea cruris, caused by dermatophytes.
- Dogger bank itch/Seabathers eruption: It is caused by contact with seaweeds, jelly fish, sea anemones, corals, etc. and characterized by irritant or toxic contact dermatitis.

- Grain itch/Barley itch/Straw itch/Cotton-seed dermatitis/Acrodermatitis urticarioides/Shoveller's itch: It is caused by *Pyemotes tritichi* mite and characterized by contact dermatitis like lesions when a person comes in contact with grain or straw, infested with the mites.
- Scrub itch/Trombidiosis: It is caused by larvae of *Trombiculids* and characterized by dermatitis.
- Swimmer's itch/Sedge-pool itch/Cercarial dermatitis: It is caused by free living cercarial stage of non-human schistosomes.
- Scabitic itching: Itching in scabies aggravated at night due to hypersensitivity reaction to mites and mites' products.

Penicillium marneffei

- A dimorphic fungus, causes fatal infection in HIV infected person.
- Tropical climate with high humidity and rainfall is favourable for fungal growth.
- Microscopic examination shows septate hyphae with lateral and terminal conidiospores and chains of oval conidia.

Pigmentation of skin

- Acanthosis nigricans: *Hyperkeratosis* is the cause of pigmentation.
- Melanin is the cause of reticular pigmentation in Partington syndrome/Familial amyloidosis.
- Melanin is the cause of facial pigmentation in *hereditary hemochromatosis*.
- In acanthosis nigricans, pigmentation is due to hyperkeratosis.
- In Peutz Jegher's syndrome hyperpigmentation is due to increased number of melanocytes.
- In Piebaldism and Waardenburg's syndrome, hypopigmentation is due to decreased number of melanocytes.
- Azelaic acid causes hypopigmentation by inhibiting melanocyte *tyrosinase enzyme*.
- In hemachromatosis, pigmentation is due to deposition of melanin and not due to iron.

Pterygium colli

- Congenital folds of skin extending from mastoid region to acromion on the lateral aspect of the neck.
- These are associated with LEOPARD syndrome, Down syndrome, combined immune deficiency syndrome and Turner syndrome.

Raynaud's phenomenon

- It occurs secondary to some other dermatoses like scleroderma, lupus erythematosus, etc. and characterized by palor, cyanosis and erythema.

Raynaud's disease

- It is not associated with other dermaoses and presents as a primary phenomenon.

Retapamulin

- A novel pleuromutilin derivative for topical therapy, effective against skin and soft tissue infection, caused by *Staphylococcus aureus* and *Streptococcus pyogenes* which are resistant to commonly used topical antibiotics.
- Pleuromutilin is derived from Pleurotus mutilin, an edible mushroom.
- A C21 keto group is essential for antimicrobial activity. It inhibits bacterial protein synthesis at 50s ribosome.
- It is bacteriostatic drug and may be -cidal with high concentration.
- Adverse effects:
  - Pruritus, burning, redness, swelling, blister, dermatitis.
  - Headache, diarrhea
- It is under pregnancy category B.

Recessive dystrophic epidermolysis bullosa

- It is one of the most severe form of genodermatosis, affecting children and young adults.
- Patient suffers from lifelong severe blistering of skin and mucosa, followed by scarring.
- Hands and feet are more commonly affected organs and digits may be fused.
- Aggressive squamous cell carcinoma may develop and cause death.

Rickettsial pox

- It is caused by *Rickettsia akari*, borne by house mouse mite and characterized by varicella-like eruptions with lympadenopathy and splenomegaly.

Rowell's syndrome, requires 3 major and one minor criteria for diagnosis:

* Major criteria:

- Lupus erythematosus-like lesions
- Erythema multiforme-like lesions
- Speckled pattern antinuclear antibody

* Minor criteria:

- Chilblains
- Anti Ro/anti La antibody
- Positive rheumatoid factor

Frequency of cutaneous lesions in rheumatic fever

- Nodules-90-100%
- Ulcers-30-60%
- Livedo reticularis-0-20%
- Digital infarction-0-5%

Rocky mountain spotted fever

- Caused by *Rickettsia rickettsii*, borne by tick.
- Rash spreads centripetally.
- Treatment of choice is doxycycline.

Biologicals and pregnancy

- Pregnancy cat C: Efalizumab
- Pregnancy cat B: Alefacept, etenercept, infliximab, adalimumab.

Pathogenesis of Raynaud's phenomenon

- Reduced blood flow through the digital blood vessels due to local abnormal vascular reaction and subsequently compromised perfusion.
- Vasoconstriction due to hyperreactivity to sympathetic nervous system.
- Enhanced localized production of vasoconstrictors and reduced production of local vasodilators.

Pathogenesis of Raynaud's phenomenon in scleroderma

- Activation and damage of the endothelial cells.
- Induction of fibrinolysis and activation of platelet.
- Failure to reopen arteriovenous anastomosis.

Raynaud's phenomenon

- Episodic attacks last for minutes to hours.
- Well demarcated white-blue digits induced by cold exposure or emotional stimuli.
- Only portion of a digit is affected and often thumbs are spared.
- Classical color changes are pallor, cyanosis and hyperemia.
- Proximal parts of the digits are pink and warmer but distal parts are cold.
- In some cases only blanching, followed by feeling of numbness.
- In some cases, one or more fingers or toes may be numb and described as dead.
- Digits become bright red on reworming with or without throbbing pain.
- Prominent pain and persistent ischemic attack, indicates presence of secondary cause.
- Fingers and toes are commonly affected but nose, earlobes and nipples may be affected.
- Digital ulccr or gangrene in extreme cases, are very painful, specially at night.
- Other secondary changes are small pitted scars, atrophic, thin and tight skin, loss of hair over dorsal surfaces of the digits, and brittle and deformed nails.

Scrub typhus/tsutsugamushi fever

- Caused by *Orientia tsutsugamushi*, borne by *Trombiculid mite* (chiggers)
- Treatment of choice is *doxycycline*.

Systemic drug related intertriginous and flexural exanthema (SDRIFE)

- Occurs after exposure to systemic drugs.
- Sharply demarcated erythema of buttocks and v-shaped erythema of the thighs.

- Erythematous areas are studded with papules, vesicles, bullae and pustules.
- Symmetrical involvement of at least one flexural region.
- No systemic symptoms.
- Drugs are penicillins, cephalosporins, erythromycin, allopurinol, etc.

Sarcoidosis

- Activated CD4 cells produce cytokines mainly IL2 and IFNγ.
- Lymphopenia at peripheral blood is due to compartmentalization of monocytes and T cells within tissue.

Smoker's patch/stomatitis nicotina

- It occurs in middle aged persons, having a history of heavy smoking.
- Clinical features are distinct umbilicated papules at palate, ostia of mucosal ducts appearing as red, pinpoints and surrounded by a milky white, slightly elevated asymptomatic papules.
- Intervening mucosa becomes white and thickened with a tendency to desquamate at places as raw beefy areas or even ulceration.

Sclerema neonatorum

- Newborns normally have more saturated fat and desaturation is failed due to prematurity and immaturity of the enzyme system.
- Also sepsis, dehydration, chilling, infection and other stresses further inhibit the enzyme system.
- Exposure to cold is not very important.
- Prematurity is seen in 50% cases.
- It is characterized by rapidly spreading diffuse hardening of the skin and subcutaneous tissue. Lesions start at buttocks and trunk, usually within first week of life.
- Palms, soles and scrotum are spared.
- Histopathology shows greatly enlarged adipocytes and wide fibrous band, no fat cell necrosis, but fat cell may contain needle like cleft.

Subacute lupus erythematosus

- Annular and psoriasiform lesions without scarring are the commonest features.
- Rare features are erythroderma, pityriasis rubra pilaris–like lesions, toxic epidermal necrolysis like and erythema gyratum repens-like lesions.

Subcutaneous fat necrosis of newborn

- There is no clear relation with cold, but there may be a defect in fat composition.
- Other precipitating factors are hypothermia, poor nutrition and various physical stresses.
- It occurs in premature or fullterm baby and is precipitated by forceps or cesarian section.
- Within few days to weeks of age, indurated, erythematous to violaceous mobile plaques and nodules appear and some may discharge caseous material.
- Common sites are back, thigh and cheeks.
- Histopathology shows fat necrosis, crystallization with ganulomatous infiltration and foci of calcification.
- Though it is benign and self-limiting, sometimes hypercalcemia and death may occur.

SCORTEN in toxic epidermal necrolysis (TEN):

Each parameter is having a score, valued 1

- Clinical parameters
  - Age more than 40 years.
  - Pulse more than 120/minute.
  - Associated with malignancy.
  - Involvement more than 10% of body surface area.
- Blood parameters
  - Sugar more than 14 mmol/L
  - Urea more than 10 mmol/L
  - Bicarbonate less than 20 mmol/L
- Score vs mortality rate
  - Score 1 indicates about 3% mortality
  - Score 2 indicates about 10% mortality
  - Score 3 indicates about 35% mortality
  - Score 4 indicates about 60% mortality
  - Score 5 indicates about 90% mortality.

Systemic lupus erythematosus (SLE)

- ANA test is positive in 95% cases
- DDS (dapsone) is the drug of choice in bullous form.

Sporotrichoid lesions, seen in

- Atypical mycobacterial infection
- Nocardiosis
- Sporotrichosis

Syphilis, false positive serological test:

- Serological test may be falsely positive when titer is </=1:8 and seen in following conditions:
  - Old age
  - Autoimmune diseases including systemic lupus erythematosus and rheumatoid arthritis.
  - Viral infections including herpes, HIV and immunization.
  - Following use of parenteral drugs.

Systemic mastocytosis

- It occurs in adult with features of abdominal pain, nausea, vomiting, diarrhea, gastrointestinal hemorrhage, etc.
- Internal organs involved: Gastrointestinal tract, skeletal system, lungs, kidneys, lymph nodes, heart, liver and spleen.
- Skeletal lesions may be radio-opaque or radiolucent or both.

Tache noire

- It is nothing but the hemorrhagic eschar developed at the site of tick bite in rickettsia.

Transit time

- 13 days from basal layer to spinous layer
- 14 days from spinous layer to granular layer
- 14 days from granular layer to corneal layer
- 14 days to shed off from the corneal layer as invisible scales.
- From basal layer to shedding of corneal layer is variable from 50-70 days.

Non-antibiotic activities of Tetracyclines

- Inhibition of lipase production.
- Inhibition of chemotactic factor production.
- Inhibition of protein kinase C.
- Inhibition of proteases.
- Inhibition of leukocyte movement.
- Inhibition of angiogenesis and metastatic activity.
- Inhibition of granuloma formation.

Transport media for biopsy sample

- For immunofluorescence mapping
  - If storage is required for <24 hours
    - # normal saline (0.9%)
    - # liquid nitrogen
  - If storage is required for 24 hours to 6 weeks.
    - # Michel medium
- For electron microscopy
  - 2.5% gluteraldehyde solution.

Telangiectasia

- Permanent dilatation of capillaries, venules or arterioles which may disappear on gentle pressure with a microscopic slide (diascopy).
- Mat telangiectasia is seen in scleroderma.
- Papular telangiectasia is seen in hereditary hemorrhagic telangiectasia.
- Linear telangiectasia at face is seen in solar damage, rosacea and carcinoid syndrome.
- Photodistributed telangiectasia is a rare complication of *nifedipine*.

Tonofilament

- Fine fibres running from desmosome to cytoplasm within a keratinocyte and maintain the structure of the cell, like the pillars of the house. But tonofilaments are not present in melanocytes.
- During keratinization tonofilaments turn into bundles at spinous layer as tonofibrils.

Telogen effluvium

- Falling of telogen hairs.
- Precipitating factors:
  - Child birth

- High fever, HIV infection
- Major surgery, life-threatening trauma
- Restricted diet, nutritional deficiency, iron deficiency anemia
- Hypothyroidism, hormonal drugs
- Onset of androgenetic alopecia
- Allergic contact dermatitis
- Psychological stress

Telangiectasia macularis eruptiva perstans (TMEP)

- It is an adult onset mastocytosis, presenting with small, redbrown, telangiectatic macules at trunk and extremities.
- It shows little or no tendency toward urtication.

Stages of trophic ulcer

- Concealed ulcer
- Threatened ulcer
- Overt ulcer

Types of trophic ulcer

- Acute
- Chronic
- Complicated
- Recurrent

Topological frequency of plantar ulcer

- Forefoot: 70-90%
- Big toe: 30-50%
- Heel and mid lateral border: 5-10%
- Tips of toes: 5%.

Thyroid transforming factors (TTF1)

- Positive in small cell carcinoma of lung.
- Negative in Merkel cell carcinoma.

Trichilemmoma

- Lobulated proliferation with palisaded periphery.
- Abundant clear cells at outer root sheath (ORS) due to glycogen content.

Terry nail

- Distal 1-2 mm is having normal pink color but proximal part is white.
- This is seen in cirrhosis, congestive cardiac failure and adult onset diabetes mellitus.

Tinea capitis

- Infection of skin as well as hair of the scalp.
- Most common world-wide causative species is *Trichophyton tonsurans*.

Tinea imbricata

- It is caused by *Trichophyton concentricum*, a dermatophyte.
- It is characterized by scaly, polycyclic patch with concentric rings.
- Parallel lines of scales overlap each other and appear as tiles of the roof or shingles.

Tinea incognito: Steroid modified tinea, characterized by indurated erythematous papules within the previous patch.

Toll-like receptors (TLRs)

- These receptors recognize various antigenic molecules and sensitize defence mechanism like a gate-keeper.
- There are 12 members of TLR family, designated as TLR1, TLR2, ... upto TLR12.
- Particular TLR binds with a ligand, resulting in activation of a common signaling pathway, involving the transcription factors like NF-$k\beta$ (nuclear factor kappa-β) and mitogen-activated protein kinases (MAPKS). This activation leads to release of proinflammatory cytokines.
- This activation is crucial for both innate and adaptive immunity.
- TLR3 specially recognizes viral particles.
- TLR12 plays a vital role in contact hypersensitivity.
- TLRs and their ligands:
  - TLR1 binds with triacylated and diacylated lipoproteins.
  - TLR2 binds with triacylated lipoproteins and peptidoglycans.

- TLR3 binds with dsDNA.
- TLR4 binds with lipopolysaccharides.
- TLR5 binds with flagellin.
- TLR6 binds with diacylated lipoproteins.
- TLR7 binds with imidazoquinolones.
- TLR8 binds with ssRNA.
- TLR9 binds with cpGDNA.
- TLR10 binds with ?
- TLR11 binds with ?
- TLR12 binds with ?

Telogen club

- It is having a brightly eosinophilic trichilemmal keratinization.

Telogen germinal unit

- This is seen at mid to upper dermis and just below the telogen club hair when vertical section is examined.
- It is having follicular epithelium with radial projections and also having the shape of a daisy.

Tinea nigra

- It is caused by the black yeast-like mould, *Phaeoannellomyces werneckii* and characterized by asymptomatic, light to dark brown or black macule or patch with sharply defined margin.
- Lesion rarely contains visible scales.
- It commonly affects palms and soles and sometimes dorsal surfaces of the hands.
- It may be mistaken as malignant melanoma.

TNF-α in toxic epidermal necrolysis

- It has a dual role in toxic epidermal necrolysis as initially induces inflammation, apoptosis and cell damage.
- But in later it causes promotion of cell growth, resists apoptosis and suppresses inflammation.
- Thus, thalidomide a potent TNF-α inhibitor is not effective in toxic epidermal necrolysis.

Trichoschisis: The term is used for green-stick fracture of hair and it is associated with trichothiodystrophy blastysis.

Trichoptilosis: The term is used for longitudinal splitting of hair shaft.

Frequency of lesions in Tuberous sclerosis

- Ash leaf macules–90-100%
- Shagreen patch–40-50%
- Periungual fibroma–30-60%
- Pitted enamel–>90%
- Seizure–70-95%.

Causes of acute urticaria

- 50%–Idiopathic
- 40%–Upper respiratory tract infection
- 9%–Drugs
- 1%–Food.

Causes of chronic urticaria

- 35%–Physical urticaria
- 25%–Autoimmune urticaria
- 25%–Idiopathic
- 5%–Urticarial vasculitis
- 5%–Pseudoallergy
- 5%–Infection.

Cold induced urticaria

- It comprises 2% of all forms of urticaria.
- Most of the cases are idiopathic and some are associated with serologic abnormalities like elevated IgE and IgM.
- Some of the idiopathic cases are familial
- Histamine is the main mediator, but leukotriene and platelet activating factor are also may be.
- It occurs at the sites of localized cooling, specially during rewarming.
- It is clinically characterized by persisting edematous papules and plaques with or without dermatographism and cholinergic urticaria.
- It may be associated with headache, fever, arthralgia, etc. with leukocytosis.
- Swelling of the oral mucosa or esophagus may occur due to ingestion of cold drinks.
- Rarely histamine shock develops as an alarming sign and leads to loss of consciousness.

- Sometimes death may occur during cold water swimming.
- Ice cube test is done for diagnosis by wrapping a ice bag on skin for 30 seconds to 10 minutes and wheal develops on rewarming. But water at 7°C is more fruitful in some cases as it causes less severe vasoconstriction.

Variegate porphyria

- Autosomal recessive disorder with protoporphyrinogen oxidase deficiency.
- South Africans, ages between 30-50 years are commonly affected.
- Clinical features are photosensitive blisters, hyperpigmentation and scarring.

Vorner palmoplantar keratoderma

- It is a form of epidermolytic hyperkeratosis.

Whipple's disease

- It is caused by *Tropheryma whippelii*, a type of actinomycetes.
- Skin lesions include hyperpigmented sunexposed areas, scars, erythema nodosum and subcutaneous nodules.

SIGNS & PHENOMENONS IN DERMATOLOGY

CHAPTER A3

Albright sign: Shortening of digits with dimple, seen in Gorlin syndrome/Basal cell nevus syndrome.

Antenna sign: Slightly long strands of keratin are often coming out from the affected follicles in *keratosis pilaris* and these glint when examined with side light. This is known as Antenna sign.

Auspitz sign: When a psoriatic papule or plaque is scraped with the edge of a glass slide, after removal of basal plasma membrane (Buckley's membrane), a few bleeding points may appear and this is known as Auspitz sign. The test is known as Grattage test.

Angry back phenomenon: If patch test is done before complete remission of the allergic contact dermatitis with same allergen, the dermatitis may relapse.

Beevor phenomenon: When metacarpophalangeal joints remain stable in flexion, the interphalangeal joints become extended by long extensors.

Bare under belly sign: In some cases of mycosis fungoides, lymphocytes are present on upper or epidermal side of vessels.

Black dot sign: It is a features of poison ivy reaction.

Beighton sign: Passive apposition of the thumb to the flexor aspect of the forearm in *Ehlers Danlos syndrome*.

Big boss sign: Lymphocytes of epidermis are larger than that of dermis in mycosis fungoides.

Branham sign: Application of tourniquet often results in reduction of volume of the pulse of the arterio-venous fistula and this helps to differentiate Klippel-Trenaunay syndrome from Parkes-Weber syndrome.

Buerger's sign: It is seen in the arterial disease of the lower limb. When leg is elevated, pallor develops at the sole due to marked ischemia and while on dependency it results in delayed but exaggerated hyperemia at dorsum of foot.

Butterfly sign: Sparing of a butterfly shaped interscapular area in biliary pruritus and the area is difficult to reach by hand.

Corn flake sign: If epidermoid cyst ruptures, keratin of the cyst induces a foreign body reaction and produces giant cell. This giant cell contains silver like keratin and known as Corn flake sign.

Crowe's sign: Axillary freckles in neurofibromatosis.

Cullen sign: Hemorrhagic discoloration around the umbilicus in ectopic pregnancy and pancreatitis or due to any retroperitoneal hemorrhage.

Dirty fingernail sign: It is seen in histopathology of dermatofibroma.

Deck chair sign: Papuloerythroderma of Ofuji is characterized by flat-topped papules with widespread distribution, and striking-sparing of body folds.

Dimple sign/Fitzpatrick sign: A dimpling is produced when the lesion of dermatofibroma is pressed downward or laterally.

Dubois sign: Shortening of little finger in congenital syphilis.

Drip sign: In dermatitis artefacta lesions develop along the site of dropping produced by corrosive liquids.

Darier's sign: Following stroking of a flat lesion of urticaria pigmentosa the lesion becomes erythematous, edematous and even vesiculates. It is due to degranulation of mast cells.

Exclammation sign: Short hair with thin proximal part and broad distal part, seen in alopecia areata. Presence of it indicates that the disease is active.

Fettucini sign: Lymphocytes are interspersed between thick and wiry collagen fibers in mycosis fungoides.

Flag sign (1): Alternate light and dark color band in hair due to protein energy malnutrition.

Flag sign (2): It is seen in histopathology of actinic keratosis.

Fournier's sign: Bowing of the tibia in syphilis, yaws and osteitis deformans.

Fox's sign: Pancreatitis associated purpura or hemorrhage below the level of inguinal ligament.

Forschheimer's sign: A maculopapular eruption during prodromal period or early stage of rubella on soft palate.

Friar tuck sign: When major part of the crown is affected in trichotillomania, the appearance is known as Friar tuck sign.

Frank sign: Acquired diagonal crease in ear lobules of adults, indicates a risk of atherosclerotic coronary artery disease.

Gorlin's sign: Ability to touch the tip of the nose by extension of the tongue in *Ehlers Danlos syndrome*.

Garland sign: Reticulate erythema of the extensor surfaces of the arms in erythema infectiosum (Fifth disease).

Gottron's sign: Erythematous and violaceous papules at metacarpal and proximal interphalangeal joints, seen in dermatomyositis.

Groove sign: It is formed due to inflammation of lymph glands of either side of inguinal ligament in lymphogranuloma venereum.

Grey Turner's sign: Bruise-like discoloration of skin of left flank in acute pancreatitis.

Gaunlet and boot sign: Dermatitis of hands and feet with a demarcation line in pellagra.

Hanging curtain sign: If a lesion of pityriasis rosea is stretched along its long axis, scales show a tendency to become folded across the lines of stretch.

Hamburger sign: Collection of protein and erythrocytes within the splitted follicles in trichotillomania.

Hoigne sign/pseudoanaphylactic reaction: Intramuscular penicillin injection in cardiovascular tertiary syphilis causes hypertension, tachycardia, fear of eminent death, unusual taste sensation, auditory or visual disturbances, neuromuscular twitching, occasional seizure and even loss of consciousness. It occurs in less than 0.1% cases and lasts rarely more than 30 minutes.

Heuck-Gottron sign: Loss of nail cuticle and presence of telangiectasia in scleroderma.

Head light sign: Prominent facial pallor over both cheeks, perinasal and periorbital areas in atopic dermatitis.

Heliotrope sign: Violaceous erythema around the eyes, seen in dermatomyositis.

Hanging groin: Degenerative changes in long standing onchocerciasis, leads to loss of dermal elastic fibers and along with inguinal huge lymphadenopathy, groin appears like hanging.

Hertoghe's sign: Lateral thinning or absence of eyebrow, seen in atopic dermatitis.

Holster sign: Pruritic, symmetric, confluent, macular violaceous erythema at lateral aspects of thighs and hips in dermatomyositis.

Hutchinson's sign (1): In herpes zoster, vesicles at the tip of the nose indicates involvement of nasocilliary nerve of thc ophthalmic branch of the trigeminal nerve. This suggests the risk of eye involvement.

Hutchinson's sign (2): A longitudinal melanotic streak on nail-plate accompanied by periungual pigmentation indicates presence of subungual malignant melanoma.

Isomorphic phenomenon/Koebnerphenomenon: This is characterized by development of lesions along the line or site of trauma. In 1990, Boyd and Neldner classified this into 4 groups.

- Type 1/true isomorphic phenomenon: This is reproduced with a variety of insults and seen in psoriasis, lichen planus and vitiligo.
- Type 2/pseudoisomorphic phenomenon: This is seen in infective conditions like viral wart and molluscum contagiosum.
- Type 3: Diseases may be localized at the site of trauma such as lichen nitidus, erythema multiforme, Darier's disease, Hailey Hailey disease, perforating folliculitis, reactive perforating collagenosis and Kaposi's sarcoma.
- Type 4: Rarely seen where single or few reports were published, such as anaphylactoid purpura, bullous pemphigoid erythrokeratodermia variabilis, lichen amyloidosis, urticaria pigmentosa, dermatitis herpetiformis, multicentric reticulo histiocytosis and eruptive xanthoma.

Jellinek sign: Eyelid pigmentation in thyrotoxicosis.

Kaposi-Stemmer sign: Failure to pinch or pick up a fold of skin at the base of the second toe, indicates lymphedema.

Knee-cut sign: Deep linear fissure along skin creases at anogenital region, seen in Crohn's disease.

Lambda sign: In sarcoidosis, Gallium 67 scan uptake is seen by bilateral hilar lymphadenopathy and right paratracheal nodes.

Last week sign: Return of normal basket weave orthokeratosis under the huge parakeratosis.

Lowenbach's sign: Reduced or absent granular layer in histopathology of pityriasis rosea.

Lutz sign/bulla spreading sign: Peripheral extension of a bulla beyond the marked margin following smooth pressure given over it by a finger.

Lucio phenomenon

- It is associated with diffuse form of non-nodular lepromatous leprosy or Lucio leprosy and mostly encountered among Mexicans.
- It is due to massive invasion of endothelial cells of the arterioles by profuse number of lepra bacilli.
- Initially, it was named as lepra manchada.

Leser-Trelat sign: Sudden onset of numerous seborrheic keratosis, in association with gastrointestinal adenocarcinoma or transitional carcinoma of the bladder.

Marquee sign: Organisms of cutaneous leishmaniasis tend to localize at the periphery of the macrophages.

Asboe-Hansen sign: When the blister is small, intact and tense and shows positive bulla spreading sign.

Mechanic's hand sign: Hyperkeratosis of the ulnar side of the thumb and radial side of the index finger, seen in dermatomyositis.

Mauserung phenomenon: It is a form of Nikolsky sign and present in *ichthyosis bullosa of Siemens*.

Meyerson phenomenon: Eczematous changes around a halo nevus.

Meirowsky's phenomenon: Immediate but transient pigmentation of the skin, following exposure to ultraviolet radiation. It lasts for 10-20 minutes.

Munson sign: The lower eyelid is distorted when the patient direct the gaze downwards, seen in atopic dermatitis with advanced stage of keratoconus.

Nikolsky sign: It is a pathognomonic sign in pemphigus and it indicates presence of acantholysis.

- Marginal Nikolsky sign: When the test is positive at perilesional skin.
- Direct Nikolsky sign: When it is positive over normal looking skin at a distant site.
- Nikolsky phenomenon: When superficial layer of epidermis is felt to be moved over deeper layer without immediate formation of erosion but later a blister develops.
- Modified Nikolsky sign: When peripheral extension of a blister occurs following giving a pressure over it.
- Pseudo-Nikolsky sign/epidermal peeling sign: When the test is positive in involved or erythematous skin. It is seen in Stevens-Johnson syndrome, toxic epidermal necrolysis, bullous ichthyosiform erythroderma and some cases of burn.

Oil drop sign: When psoriatic lesion develops entirely within the nail bed it appears as oil drop.

Ollendorf's probe sign: When papular lesions of secondary syphilis are pressed with a blunt probe, it elicits pain.

Olfleck's phenomenon: Subungual hyperkeratois due to collection of parakeratotic stratum corneum, results in brownish discoloration of nail plates.

Osler's sign: Pigmented sclera in alkaptonuria.

Panda's sign: Following laser treatment of nevus of Ota, persistence of pigmentation in periorbital location.

Panda sign: In sarcoidosis, Gallium 67 uptake by bilateral parotids and lacrimal glands.

Pelkan sign: Metaphyseal spurs and marginal fracture in scurvy.

Pathergy phenomenon: Development of neutrophilic infiltration at the site of a needle prick. It is seen classically in 20% cases of pyoderma gangrenosum.

Pemberton sign: Facial plethora during lifting of the arm above the head due to large retrosternal goiter.

Wrist sign: Overlapping of the thumb and the fifth finger when these encircle the opposite wrist in *Marfan syndrome*.

Promontory sign: Protrusion of normal blood vessels from the wall of the newly formed vessels in Kaposi's sarcoma.

Pseudo-Koebner's phenomenon: Infective disorder may occur along the line of scratch.

Example: Viral wart and molluscum contagiosum.

Pseudo-Darier sign: Firm stroking on the lesion of congenital smooth muscle hamartoma or leiomyoma cutis, may provoke fasciculation or temporary induration giving a cobblestone or goose flesh appearance.

Pseudo-Hutchinson sign:

- Black streaks of pigmentation may be normally seen at proximal nail folds in dark individuals.
- Histopathology shows small clusters of melanocytes at suprabasal zone of distal nail matrix and visible macroscopically through transparent cuticle.
- It demands exclusion of subungual malignant melanoma.

Prayer sign: Some patients of diabetes mellitus can't bring their palms completely together and they can't bend their fingers backward. This occurs due to thick, indurated and waxy skin of fingers and this is known as diabetic cheiroarthropathy.

Radiation recall phenomenon: It is associated with administration of methotrexate within 3 weeks of radiation therapy and development of erythematous, edematous and necrotic lesions in skin.

Rope sign: Linear, erythematous or skin colored nodules arranged like a cord, extending from upperback to axilla in rheumatoid arthritis.

Ramana's sign: Unilateral eyelid edema and lacrimal gland inflammation, seen in Chaga's disease or American trypanosomiasis, caused by *Trypanosoma cruzi*.

Raccoon sign: Periorbital purpura, seen in primary systemic amyloidosis.

Round finger pad sign: When viewed from the side, normal peaked contour of the pulp appears as a rounded hemisphere due to loss of pad of fat in scleroderma.

Rumpel Leede sign: Due to capillary leakage, showers of purpura develop distal to sphygmomanometer cuff, when the pressure is released. It is seen in drug induced erythema multiforme.

Russel's sign: Abrasions and scars at knuckle pads due to repeated trauma for induced vomiting in anorexia nervosa or bulimia.

Sabouraud's sign: Presence of erythrocytes at papillary dermis as well as in epidermis in histopathology of pityriasis rosea.

Sarcophagus sign: Hypertrophic periosteal cloaking of the bone encasing the entire shaft with layers of marrow trapped in between due to perisoteal reaction in congenital syphilis.

Sheklakov sign/False Nikosky's sign: When peripheral remnant of roof of a ruptured blister is pulled, resulting in extension of the erosion on the surrounding normal appearing skin. It is seen in:

- Bullous pemphigoid
- Herpes gestationis
- Dermatitis herpetiformis
- Linear IgA bullous dermatosis
- Epidermolysis bullosa acquisita
- Junctional and dystrophic epidermolysis bullosa
- Porphyria
- Bullous systemic lupus erythematosus

Shawl sign: Symmetric, confluent, macular, violaceous erythema overlying posterior shoulder and neck, deltoids, extensor arms and forearms in dermatomyositis.

Slapped cheek sign: Erythematous cheeks along with pharyngitis, fever and lymphadenopathy in erythema infectiosum, caused by *Parvo virus* B19.

Snowflake sign: Ultrasonographic findings of amniotic fluid when the fetus is suffering from epidermolysis bullosa.

Starburst phenomenon: Appearance of livedo reticularis in cutaneous polyarteritis nodosa.

Shotgun appearance: Seen in bowenoid papulosis.

Staphne's sign: Periodontal thickening detected by X-ray, seen in scleroderma.

Steinberg sign/thumb sign: Extension of the thumb past the ulnar border of the hand when apposed to the palm in *Marfan syndrome*.

Tent sign: Stretching of pilomatricoma lesion, the surface shows multiple facets and angles like a tent.

Teeter tottor sign: When one side of the pilomatricoma nodule is depressed, the other side lifts up.

Thinker's sign

- Asymptomatic, diffuse, dry, hyperpigmented and hyperkeratotic plaques on the lower third of the front of the thigh in chronic obstructive pulmonary disease.
- This is due to chronic intermittent irritation secondary to characteristic dyspnoeic posture habituated by the patient.

Thumb sign: Completely apposed thumb in the clenched hand crosses the ulnar border.

Thumb print sign: Unique pattern of periumbilical purpura, resembling multiple thumb prints in disseminated strongyloidiasis.

Tongue sign: In uremia tongue may be large and pale with prominent impression of teeth along the margin.

Toy soldier sign: Lymphocytes are aligned as single units having >4 in number in each, along the basal layer of the epidermis in mycosis fungoides.

Trousseau sign: Recurrent and migratory nature of thrombophlebitis is due to hypercoagulable state. About 50% cases are associated with carcinoma of pancreas, stomach and lungs. Trousseau himself faced his own sign and died of that.

Turner sign: Bluish patch of discoloration at the flank due to bleeding at subcutaneous level in pancreatitis.

Tree frog sign: It is a posture of tree frog, associated with mandibuloacral dysplasia.

Unna's sign: Eczematoid histopathological form of pityriasis rosea.

Ugly duckling principle/sign: A helpful guideline in children having multiple nevi where the lesions that stand as odd from the rest i.e., the lesion may have darker pigmentation, irregular texure or irregular border, warrant to consider for exision.

V sign: Confluent, macular, violaceous and erythematous lesions over V area of upper chest and neck in dermatomyositis.

Walzel's sign: Development of livedo reticularis like lesions at abdomen and trunk in association with acute and chronic pancreatitis.

Walking dandruff sign: Excessive dandruff develops on the back of dogs and cats when infested with *Cheyletiella mites*.

Wimberger sign/cat bite sign: Sawtooth appearance of metaphysis of tibia in X-ray of the baby, having early congenital syphilis.

Winter bottom sign: Pronounced enlargement of posterior group of lymph nodes in Gambian form of African trypanosomiasis.

Wrist sign: Thumb and little finger overlap each other when they wrap the opposite wrist in Marfan syndrome.

RAPID FIRE

CHAPTER A4

Abbreviations

- **SCOT:** Scleroderma cyclophosphamide or transplantation.
- **STEPS:** System for Thalidomide Education and Prescribing Safety programme.
- **FOX:** Fork head box.
- **FABP:** Fatty acid binding protein.
- **JAK:** Janus kinases.
- **PEODDN:** Porokeratotic eccrine osteal and dermal ductal nevus.
- **STAT:** Signal transducer and activator transcription.
- **SOX:** Sry related HMG box.
- **ATPC1 gene:** ATP binding cassette 1 gene.
- **SAMPUS:** Superficial atypical melanocytic proliferation of uncertain significance.
- **NEMO:** Nuclear factor κβ essential modulation.
- **DISH:** Diffuse skeletal hyperostosis.

Genetic mutations

- **Charcot–Marie-Tooth disease,** the first human connexin disorder: Gene encodes *connexin* 32 (Cx32).
- **Clouston syndrome:** JB6 gene, encodes *connexin* 30.
- **Epidermolytic palmoplantar keratoderma:** Gene encodes *keratin* 9, expressed at palms and soles.
- **Erythrokeratodermia variabilis:** Gene encodes *connexin* 31 (Cx31) and *connexin* 30.3 (Cx30.3).
- **Epidermolytic hyperkeratosis:** Gene encodes K1 and K10.
- **Hidrotic ectodermal dysplasia:** Gene encodes *connexin* 30 (Cx30).
- **Hartnup disease:** Gene encodes SLC6A19.
- **Hailey Hailey disease:** ATP2C1 gene encodes Ca^{2+} Mn^{2+} ATPase protein 1.
- **Ichthyosis bullosa of Siemens:** Gene encodes K2e.
- **KIP syndrome:** Gene encodes *connexin* 26 or *connexin* 30.
- **Lymphedema praecox:** Gene encodes FOXC2.
- **Mal de Meleda:** ARSB gene encodes SLURP1.
- **Naxos disease:** JUP gene encodes desmosomal component of *plakoglobin.*
- **Netherton syndrome:** SPINK5 gene encodes *lymphoepithelial kajal type serine protease inhibitor* (LEKTI).

- Nonepidermolytic palmoplantar keratoderma: Gene encodes *keratin*1, *keratin*6a and *keratin*16.
- Neurofibromatosis 1 (NF1): Gene encodes neurofibromin.
- Neurofibromatosis 2 (NF2): Gene encodes MERLIN.
- Palmoplantar keratoderma with deafness: MTTS1 gene encodes *mitochondrial tRNA*.
- Papillon-Lefevre syndrome: CTSC gene encodes *cathepsin C*.
- Primary lymphedema: Gene encodes FABP4 and SOX17.
- Pseudoxanthoma elasticum: Gene encodes ATP binding cassette transporter protein C6 (ABCC6) or multidrug resistant protein 6 (MRP6).
- Recessive dystrophic epidermolysis bullosa: Gene COL7A1, encodes type VII collagen.
- Recessive X-linked ichthyosis: ARSC1 gene encodes *steroid sulfatase*.
- Striate palmoplantar keratoderma: Gene encodes *desmoplakin* or *desmoglein* 1.
- Vohwinkel syndrome: GJB6 gene encodes *connexin* 26(Cx26), associated with hearing impairment.
- Lamellar ichthyosis: Gene encodes *transglutaminase* 1 (TGase 1).

Autosomal dominant (AD) inheritance

- Neurofibromatosis
- Epidermolysis bullosa simplex (Koebner type, herpetiform type and mottled pigmented type).
- Dystrophic epidermolysis bullosa
- Hailey-Hailey disease
- Ichthyosis vulgaris
- Epidermolytic hyperkeratosis
- Progressive symmetric erythrokeratodermia
- Erythrokeratodermia variabilis
- Darier's disease
- Acrokeratosis verruciformis
- Hidrotic ectodermal dysplasia
- Piebaldism
- Waardenburg syndrome
- Tuberous sclerosis
- Dyschromatoses (Reticulate acropigmentation of Dohi and dyschromatosis universalis hereditaria).
- Peutz-Jeghers syndrome
- Porphyria cutanea tarda
- Acute intermittent porphyria
- Hereditary coproporphyria
- Variegate porphyria

Autosomal recessive (AR) inheritance

- Ataxia-telangiectasia
- Epidermolysis bullosa simplex with muscular dystrophy
- Junctional epidermolysis bullosa
- Dystrophic epidermolysis bullosa
- Lamellar ichthyosis
- Nonbullous congenital ichthyosiform erythroderma
- Ichthyosis linearis circumflexa
- Refsum syndrome
- Xeroderma pigmentosa
- Cockayne syndrome
- Trichothiodystrophy
- Bloom syndrome
- Rothmund Thomson syndrome
- Hartnup disease
- Erythropoietic porphyria
- δ-Aminolevulanic acid delydratase porphyria
- Hepatoerythropoietic porphyria
- Lipoid proteinosis
- Harlequin ichthyosis

X-linked recessive (XLR) inheritance

- X-linked ichthyosis
- Anhidrotic ectodermal dysplasia
- Angiokeratoma corporis diffusum

X-linked dominant (XLD) inheritance

- Incontinentia pigmenti
- Goltz syndrome
- CHILD syndrome

Mixed inheritance

- Epidermolysis bullosa simplex (AD/AR)
- Dystrophic epidermolysis bullosa (AD/AR)
- Harlequin fetus (AD/AR)
- Erythropoietic protoporphyria (AD/AR)
- Hypohidrotic ectodermal dysplasia (XR/AR/AD).

Special appearances and structures

- Checkerboard parakeratosis of *pityriasis rubra pilaris* is due to presence of focal parakeratosis with a regular arrangement both vertically and horizontally.
- Coral beads are seen in *multisystem reticulohistiocytosis.*
- Coral red in *erythrasma* on Wood's lamp examination is due to presence of porphyrin.
- Coat sleeve appearance: Tight aggregation of lymphocytes around the vessels in erythema annulare centrifugum.
- Dirty finger appearance: It is associated with hyperpigmented basal layer in dermatofibroma.
- Erisipela de la costa: Erythema of face and upper trunk in onchocerciasis of young adults.
- Frog spawn: Appearance of lesions of lymphangioma circumscriptum.
- Great wall of China: This is nothing but the double edged railway track like elevated margin of the lesion of porokeratosis.
- Gyrate or cerebriform lesion is seen in *cutis verticis gyrata.*
- Jigsaw puzzle like appearance is present in histopathology of cylindroma.
- Hanging groin or elephantiasis of genitalia: It is seen in onchocerciasis.
- Lizard skin/elephant skin/leopard skin: It is seen in chronic stage of onchocerciasis.
- Mal morado: Violaceous papules and plaques of onchocerciasis leading to leonine facies in older patient.
- Moroccan leather/plucked chick appearance is seen in pseudoxanthoma elasticum.
- Pig skin leather at face: It is seen in lipoid proteinosis.
- Sawtooth rete ridges are seen in histopathology of lichen planus.
- Valley reef/Relief map: Arrangement of the lesions of Reiter's disease appear like such.
- Rocky island pattern succulent plaque: It is seen in Sweet syndrome.
- Star burst livedo reticularis is seen in cutaneous polyarteritis nodosa.
- Cytoplasmic zebra bodies are seen in Neimann-Pick disease.
- String of beads: These are seen in lipoid proteinosis.
- String of pearls: These are seen in CBDC, linear IgA dermatosis and vesicular bullous pemphigoid.
- Tapioca pudding-like clear lesions are seen in dyshidrosiform dermatitis of palms and soles.
- Music box keratoderma is seen in punctate keratoderma of palms and soles.
- Target like lesion: It is seen in erythema multiforme.
- Windblown appearance: Epidermal change in histopathology of Bowen's disease.
- Goose bumps appearance: Confluent papules, pierced by hairs in disseminated and recurrent infundibulofolliculitis.
- Snow flake opacity: It is seen in cornea due to dead microfilaria induced tissue reaction.
- Honeycomb pattern palmoplantar keratoderma is seen in Vohwinkel syndrome. Pseudoainhum leads to amputation of distal digits in Vohwinkel syndrome.
- Starfish like keratoderma at knuckles is seen in Vohwinkel syndrome.

- Whistling face: It is a feature of Freeman-Sheldon (craniocarpo tarsal) syndrome.
- Starburst pattern on dermoscopy is seen in spitz nevus.
- Bean bag cell: This is cytophagic histiocyte, seen in lymphomatous cytophagic panniculitis, Rosai-Dorfmann syndrome and sometimes in Sweet syndrome.
- Civatte bodies are homogeneous eosinophilic structures formed by apoptotic keratinocytes.
- Clear cells: These are seen in carcinoma of renal, bladder, prostate, breast, sebaceous gland and in melanoma.
- Chunks of coal: Some large atypical lymphoid cells within a heavy mixed infiltrate in lymphomatoid papulosis.
- Flower cell is seen in adult T-cell lymphoma.
- Floret giant cell is seen in pleomorphic lipoma.
- Kamino bodies are seen in spitz nevi.
- Marine pilot's wheel spores are seen in of paracoccidiodomycosis.
- Lemon shaped spore is seen in lobomycosis.
- Michaelis-Gutmann bodies are seen in malakoplakia.
- Touton giant cell is seen in juvenile xanthogranuloma.
- Small multinucleated cells, known as Montgomery giant cells are seen in chronic actinic dermatitis (CAD).
- Shadow cell is seen in pilomatricoma and epidermoid cyst of Gardner syndrome.
- Shadow in shadow cell is due to unstained area of absent nucleus.
- Stacks of plate appearance is multilayered necrobiosis, seen in necrobiosis lipoidica diabeticorum.
- Safety pin like structures of *Calymmatobacterium granulomatis* are seen within large macrophages in granuloma inguinale.
- Caterpillar bodies are seen in 50% of porphyria cutanea tarda and these are PAS and collgen IV positive basement membrane and colloid bodies at basal layer.
- Swarm of bees appearance is due to collection of lymphocytes around the follicle, seen in alopecia areata.
- Strap cell is seen in rhabdomyosarcoma.
- Epidermal vacuum cleaner: Acanthotic epidermal downgrowth serves as cleaner to eliminate elastotic material in *Pesudoxanthoma elasticum.*
- Lafora bodies: These are inclusion bodies, seen at excretory ducts of sweat glands of clinically normal areas of the skin in Lafora's disease.
- Weibel-Palade bodies: Presence of electron-dense rod-shaped cytoplasmic structures, size 0.1 × 0.3 µm, consisting of longitudinally oriented tubules, embedded in a dense matrix.
- Comma shaped bodies: Seen in juvenile xanthogranuloma within the nucleus of histiocytes.
- Russel body: Plasma cells are laden with immunoglobulins and classically are seen in rhinoscleroma. Size is twice the plasma cell and may be upto 20 µm. They are gram positive, PAS positive and diastase resistant.
- Cigar shaped nuclei, seen in smooth muscle fibers and myofilaments are cytoplasmic contents of smooth muscle. Myofilaments are only 5 nm in diameter.
- Ghost cell/Shadow cell: Seen in pilomatricoma and matriceous basal cell carcinoma.
- Iccosome bodies within follicular dendritic cell membrane contain *antigen-antibody complex.*
- Henderson-Paterson bodies: These are cytoplasmic inclusion bodies, seen in molluscum contagiosum.
- Oncocytic morophages: These cells are having abundant eosinophilic and granular cytoplasm, often a ground glass appearance, seen in multicentric reticulohistiocytosis.
- Worm like bodies are seen in *benign cephalic histocytosis.*
- Michaelis-Gutmann bodies are cytoplasmic PAS and Alcian blue positive granules and develop within phagolysosomes. Bacteria, calcium and iron depositions are responsible for these granules.

Miscellaneous information

- Sodium hyaluronate biopolymer is essential for maintaining the hydration and elasticity of the skin.
- Hyaline fat necrosis is a distinctive feature of lupus panniculitis.
- Ectodermal dysplasia is related with nuclear factor (NF-κβ) activation.
- EEC syndrome is associated with mutation of p63 gene and scarring folliculitis is seen during puberty.
- AEC syndrome is associated with mutation of p63 gene and often erosive scalp dermatitis develops at an early age.
- Hair cycle:
  - Catagen: 10-14 days
  - Telogen: 3-4 months
  - Exogen
  - Kenogen
  - Anagen: 2-6 years.
- Keratinocyte size: 11-20 μm.
- Lower lip pits are seen in:
  - Van Der Wounde syndrome
  - Popliteal pterygium syndrome
  - Orofacial digital syndrome type I
- Imiquimod upregulates Th1 cytokines like IL1, IL6, IL8, IL12, IFNα and TNFα. But IL2 remains unchanged as well as TH2 cytokines like IL4 and IL5 are downregulated.
- TLR2 plays a role in atopic dermatitis.
- Pulicosis is caused by human flea, *Pulex irritans*.
- Treatment of biotin deficiency: 10 mg biotin per day.
- Melanoma originates from melanocytes and nevus cells.
- Melanoma lesion at the hairy part of the limbs has better prognosis than lesion at the palms, soles, trunk, head and neck.
- Prevalence of psoriasis in HIV seropositive population is 1.3 to 2.5%.
- Loose anagen hair shows rumpled sock cuticle.
- Whisker or kinky hair may be the first sign of male pattern baldness.
- Receded frontal hairline at both sides is known as professor angle.
- Baldness does not occur in congenital 5α reductase type 2 deficiency.
- In androgenetic alopecia, hair growth suppression is mediated by androgen sensitive TGF-β1, derived from dermal papilla cells.
- Caseation necrosis clearly differentiates erythema induratum from erythema nodosum.
- Migratory poliosis of scalp is characterized by migrating circular patches of white hair without any alopecia and it histologically resembles alopecia areata.
- Hypertrichosis is defined by excess hair growth including androgen independent areas.
- Hirsutism is defined by excess hairgrowth in females at androgen dependent areas.
- Plaqule: Poorly defined dermal thickening, which is classically seen in morphea.
- Raccoon sign: Periorbital ecchymosis in primary systemic amyloidosis.
- Content of epidermal/sebaceous cyst has foul smell but pilar/trichilemmal cyst does not have.
- Ceruloderma is characterized by excess melanin in dermis and pigmentation is not accentuated under Wood's lamp.
- Riehl's melanosis is considered as a form of pigmented contact dermatitis.
- Azelaic acid is antiproliferative and cytotoxic to melanocyte and is a weak competitive inhibitor of tyrosinase.
- Hori's nevus is characterized by late onset, bilateral symmetrical distribution and sparing of mucosal surfaces.
- Periorbital pigmentation is now considered as extension of pigmentary demarcation lines of the face.
- Erbium:YAG laser is most effective laser for melasma.
- Exogenous ochronosis is a complication of long term hydroquinone therapy.

- Addisonian pigmentation is characterized by involvement of light exposed areas, flexures, creases and mucous membranes.
- Kligman formula contains hydroquinone 5%, tretinoin 0.1% and dexamethasone 0.1%.
- Liver biopsy is indicated in methotrexate therapy if aminoterminal of procollagen III (PIIINP) assay shows:
  - Pretreatment level >8.0 μg/L
  - Three abnormal levels >4.2 μg/L over 12 months period.
  - In two consecutive levels >8.0 μg/L
- Synonym:
  - Pigmented spindle cell nevus as Reed nevus.
  - Measles as first disease and rubeola.
  - Rubella as third disease and German measles.
  - Erythema infectiosum as fifth disease.
  - Roseola infantum as sixth disease and exanthem subitum.
  - Milker's nodule as pseudocowpox.
  - Focal epithelial hyperplasia of oral mucosa as Heck's disease and fourth disease.
  - Carney complex as NAME or LAMB.
- Ecthyma contagiosum is caused by virus.
- Epstein-Bar virus is a member of Herpes virus.
- Enanthem in exanthema subitum is known as Nagayamai's spot.
- Vitiligo macule developing at the site of post inflammatory hyperpigmentation is known as blue vitiligo.
- Acquired lentigene is caused by PUVA.
- Melanocyte-keratinocyte ratio in epidermal melanin functional unit is 1:32 and in structural unit is 1:10.
- Skin chromophores are melanin for brown color, hemoglobin for red and blue colors, and porphyrin for yellow color.
- IL1α and β therapy can cause mucositis and phlebitis.
- IL2 therapy can cause diffuse erythema, aggravation of psoriasis and autoimmune diseases.
- IL3 therapy can cause flushing.
- IL4 therapy can cause edema.
- IL6 therapy can cause erythematous eruption.
- GM-CSF therapy can cause diffuse eruption.
- G-CSF therapy can cause neutrophilic dermatosis and vasculitis.
- TNFα therapy can cause erythroderma.
- IFNα therapy can cause alopecia.
- IFNβ therapy can cause vasculitis.
- IFNγ therapy can cause aggravation of graft vs host disease.
- Molluscum contagiosum in HIV occurs when CD4 cell count <100/cmm.
- Bacillary angiomatosis is painful in contrast to Kaposi's sarcoma which is painless.
- In normal population the incidence of seborrheic dermatitis is 2-4%, whether in HIV it is >85%.
- Elongated vascular channels in myopericytoma are having prominent branching, appearing as stag-horn.
- Hemangiopericytoma shows concentric layer of tumor cells around vascular channel, appearing as onion peel.
- Some cells in glomangiopericytoma show central punched out nuclei and pale eosinophilic cytoplasm.
- In Chediak-Higashi syndrome, giant lysosomal granules are seen in neutrophils, melanocytes and Langerhans cells.
- Giant melanosomes within the keratinocytes are seen in Chediak-Higashi syndrome and these melanosomes are poorly dispersible.
- Neutrophils in Chediak-Higashi syndrome are lacking of Cathepsin G, a potent antimicrobial agent and so lysosomal killing defect occurs.
- Erythema gyratum repens is associated with carcinoma of esophagus and breast and it can spread upto 1 cm/day.
- In Chediak-Higashi syndrome, intracellular killing defect is due to unavailability of primary lysosomes.
- *Parvovirus* is known as erythrovirus because it has tropism for erythroid progenitor cells.

* Cellular receptor for *Parvovirus* B19 is a globoside, also known as blood group P antigen.
* Single stranded viruses are rubella, measles, hepatitis C, hepatitis A and Hand-foot-mouth disease virus.
* Slapped cheek appearance is associated with erythema infectiosum or fifth disease.
* Papular purpuric gloves and socks syndrome (PPGSS) is associated with parvovirus infection.
* Frequency of café-au-lait spot:
  - 1% in newborns
  - 25% among 1-5 years age-group
  - 25-35% among 5-15 years age-group.
* Silvery hair syndromes:
  - Chediak-Higashi syndrome
  - Griscelli syndrome
  - Elejalde syndrome
* Treatment of choice in silvery hair syndromes is bone marrow or stem cell transplantation.
* Presence of iris translucency and foveal hypoplasia is the pathognomonic sign of albinism.
* Edema of the face is the hallmark of DRESS syndrome.
* Non-freezing injury of the skin occurs at temperature 15°C.
* Trench foot in wet condition with temperature above freezing point is associated with limb immobility and constrictive foot wears.
* Pulling boat hand is characterized by erythematous macules and plaques followed by vesicles formation, and pain and buring sensation due to prolonged cold exposure with high humidity and wind.
* Immersion foot occurs like trench foot but usually at shipwreck.
* In erythema multiforme, a history of herpes simplex infection may be present in 50% cases.
* Erythema multiforme (EM) minor means skin lesions involving less than 30% of body surface area without mucosal involvement.
* EM major or Stevens-Johnson syndrome means involvement of less than 30% body surface area with mucosal affection.
* Toxic epidermal necrolysis means skin invovement more than 30% of body surface area.
* EM minor is usually caused by herpes simplex or other viral infection.
* EM major or SJS is caused by drugs in 90% cases.
* Individual keratinocyte necrosis at basal layer is the hallmark of erythema multiforme.
* Satellite cell necrosis is characterized by intraepidermal keratinocyte necrosis, closely surrounded by lymphocytes.
* Drug induced erythema multiforme shows widespread keratinocyte necrosis, microscopic cleft formation and pronounced pigment incontinence.
* Herpes simplex induced erythema multiforme shows more exocytosis, liquefaction degeneration of basal layer, papillary dermal edema and in some cases presence of eosinophils or concentration of apoptotic keratinocytes at acrosyringium.
* Commonest cause of malignancy associated ITP is lymphoma (Hodgkin and chronic lymphoid leukemia).
* In erythema multiforme, epidermis is infiltrated with CD8 + T cells and dermis is infiltrated with CD4 + T cells.
* TNFα is responsible skin necrosis in drug induced SJS or TEN.
* CD4 + T cells produce INFγ and initiate inflammatory cascade in herpes simplex induced erythema multiforme.

Measurement

1 mm = 1000 µm

1 µm = 1000 nm

1 nm = 10 Angstrom (10Å).

Peak age of onset

- Erythema toxicum neonatorum: 2 Days
- Acropustulosis of infancy: 3-6 Months.

- Kawasaki disease: 2 Years.
- Granulosa rubra nasi: 7-12 Years.
- Erythromelanosis faciei: 10-20 Years.
- Pseudoxanthoma elasticum: 10-30 Years.
- Lichen aureus: 10-30 Years.
- Body dysmorphic phenomenon: 20-40 Years.
- Lichen planus: 40-60 Years.

Commonest site

- Annular lichen planus: Axillae > penis
- Eosinophilic pustular folliculitis: Scalp > neck > face > trunk.
- Erythomelanosis faciei: Lateral aspect of cheeks.
- SCLE like annular lesions of neonatal LE: Face.

* Investigation of choice is rectal biopsy in primary systemic amyloidosis.
* Lymphedema distichiasis syndrome is associated with double rows of eyelashes.
* Shell nail is a feature of bronchiectasis.
* KL6, a mucin like glycoprotein, increases in serum of scleroderma in childhood, complicated with pulmonary fibrosis.
* Tunga penetrans is *a jigger flea*.
* PAS-positive granules are seen in outer layer of sweat ducts in Lafora's disease.
* Size of sweat glands is reduced in uremia.
* Viral particles are seen in lumen of sweat gland tubules in Ebola hemorrhagic fever and in severe acute respiratory distress syndrome (SARS).
* Vacuolar degeneration of secretory cells or ductal cells of sweat apparatus is seen in lymphoma, multiple myeloma and heat stroke.
* In hypothyroidism, PAS positive and diastase resistant granules are seen in secretory cells of sweat glands.
* Membrane bound vacuoles are seen in secretory cells of sweat glands in mucopolysaccharides, mucolipidoses, acid maltase deficiency and adrenoleukodystrophy.
* Lipid inclusions are seen in secretory sweat gland cells in sphingolipidoses.
* Only apocrine glands of axillae produce bromhidrosis and it is associated with ingestion of garlic, asparagus, curry, penicillin, bromide, dimethyl sulphoxide, etc.
* Skin changes in POEMS syndrome:
    - Diffuse hyperpigmentation
    - Hypertrichosis
    - Thick and tight sclerodermoid skin
    - Glomeruloid hemangioma
* Papillary dermis is primarily composed of type III collagen.
* Elastic fibers appear in dermis by 22nd week of gestation.
* Total number of sweat glands: 3 million.
* Weight of each sweat gland: 35 μg.
* Sweat production: 1.8 liter/100 g sweat gland/hour.
* Dimethyl glyoxime test is done to detect the presence of nickel in a product.
* Consort dermatitis indicates allergic contact dermatitis develops to spouse from the partner.
* Mottled hyperpigmentation is a feature of progeria.
* Floppy ears is a late stage feature of polychondritis.
* Rock hard skin is seen in sclerodermoid chronic graft vs host disease.
* Cutaneous features of Sipple syndrome/MEN 2A are notalgia paresthetica and macular or lichen amyloidosis.
* Regularly spaced clumps of melanin in hair are seen in Chediak-Higashi syndrome.
* Eczema, thrombocytopenia and immuno deficiency are seen in Wiskott Aldrich syndrome.
* In tuberous sclerosis, TSC1 gene encodes Hamertin and TSC2 gene encodes Tuberin.
* Molluscum pendulum is seen in tuberous sclerosis.
* Onset of Cowden syndrome is adulthood and commonest associated malignancy is breast carcinoma.
* In Lhermite Duclos disease, hamartoma affects cerebellum.

* Sebaceous tumors in Muir Torre syndrome appear in the 6th decade and commonest associated malignancy is colorectal carcinoma.
* DNA viruses, from largest to smallest size: Pox virus > Herpes virus > Adenovirus > Papovavirus > Parvovirus.
* RNA viruses, from largest to smallest size: Paramyxo virus > Orthomyxo virus > Rhabdo virus > Reovirus > Toga virus.
* Terra firma is characterized by reticular pigmentation due to retention of keratin.
* Subcutaneous nodules in Gardner syndrome
  * Follicular cysts
  * Lipoma
  * Fibroma
* In Gardner syndrome, intestinal polyps turn into adenocarcinoma at around 39 years of age.
* Ecthyma contagiosum is a parapox viral infection.
* Endemic typhus is caused by *Rickettsia typhi*, borne by rat flea.
* Parrot's paralysis is painful movement due to osteochondritis in early congenital syphilis.
* Orthonyx is the field of mechanical nail correction.
* Epidemic typhus, caused by *Rickettsia prowazeki*, borne by *pediculosis humanus var corporis*, is characterized by truncal macular eruptions which spread distally, sparing face, palms and soles.
* Erosio interdigitalis blastomycetica is characterized by erythematous, itchy or slightly painful erosion, developing between digits by a budding fungus.
* White line of Frankel is the widening of provisional zone of calcification in scurvy.
* Laboratory test of scurvy is the detection of leukocytic ascorbate level.
* Earliest cutaneous feature of scurvy is follicular keratosis.
* TNFα therapy can cause erythroderma.
* IFNα therapy can cause alopecia.
* IFNβ therapy can cause vasculitis.
* GM-CSF therapy can cause neutrophilic dermatosis and diffuse eruption.
* IL6 therapy can cause erythematous eruption.
* IL4 therapy can cause edema.
* IL3 therapy can cause flushing.
* IL2 therapy can cause diffuse erythema and aggravate psoriasis.
* IL1 therapy can cause mucositis and phlebitis.
* Desmosomal plakoglobin, plakophilin and desmoplakin between two adjacent keratinocytes are connected by desmoglein and desmocollin.
* Cytoplasmic α catenin and β catenin of two adjacent keratinocytes are connected by cadherins (E, P and N).
* Extradigital sites of Raynaud's phenomenon are earlobes, nose and nipples.
* Thumb is usually spared in Raynaud's phenomenon.
* Two main features of secondary Raynaud's phenomenon are pain during ischemic phase and persistent ischemia.
* Bosentan is the endothelial receptor antagonist.
* Halofunginase inhibits collagen I.
* Desmoplakin is dumble shaped.
* Troker cell are normal clear cell of the breast.
* HPV60 produces plantar nodules, containing cheesy material and visible rete ridges.
* Hydroxyurea induced dermopathy commonly affects the hand and feet with scaly, lichenoid and erythematous papules, after several years of therapy.
* In 50% cases of Paget's disease do not have any underlying mass.
* Effects of UVR exposure on melanocytes:
  * Single exposure increases tyrosinase activity and increases size of the melanocyte.
  * Repeated exposures increase transfer of stage iv melanosomes to keratinocytes and increase number of active melanocytes.
  * Chronic exposure increases density of melanocytes twice than unexposed areas.

- Genes responsible for normal color variation in human skin:
  - MC1-R
  - SCL24A5
  - OCA2(P)
- Agouti signaling protein (ASP), is responsible for alternating production of eumelanin and pheomelanin in some animals.
- Spiral hyphae are seen in *Trichophyton mentagrophyte*.
- Pectinate hyphae are seen in *Microsporum audounii*.
- Antler hyphae are seen in *T. schoenleinii*.
- Acetone acts as *nail-polish* remover.
- Smell in bromhidrosis is due to 3-methyl-2-hexenoic acid.
- Pulicosis is a flea induced dermatosis.
- Redman syndrome is typically caused by vancomycin.
- Palpable purpura is the hallmark of cutaneous-vasculitis.
- Waxy, wrinkled and thickened knuckles in children is pathognomonic in erythropoietic protoporhyria.
- Bleeding following paring of plantar wart, is diagnostic of plantar wart.
- Red color urine and erythrodontia are characteristic features of *congenital erythropoietic porphyria*.
- Tufts of wooly hair at the pore is diagnostic in Trichofolliculoma.
- Hair within the follicle becomes soft, deformed and swollen in trichotillomania is known as trichomalacia and it is the pathognomonic feature of trichotillomania.
- Glomeruloid hemangioma is a characteristic cutaneous feature of POEMS syndrome.
- Plantar wart with hyperpigmentation is caused by HPV65.
- Whitish plantar wart is caused by HPV63.
- Commonest cause of deep-seated plantar wart is HPV1.
- Large irregular homogeneous eosinophilic cytoplasmic inclusions bodies as well as intranuclear small round eosinophilic inclusion bodies are seen in mosaic wart.
- Butcher wart is caused by HPV6.
- Laryngeal carcinoma is associated with HPV30.
- Buschke Lowenstein wart is caused by HPV6.
- Esophageal squamous cell carcinoma is caused by HPV16.
- Edema of the face is the hallmark of DRESS (Drug reaction, eosinophilia and systemic symptoms).
- Nevus of Ota occurs bilaterally in 10% cases.
- Mongolian spot is uniform but nevus of Ota is speckled.
- Nevus of Ota is distributed at supraclavicular, scapular and deltoid regions.
- Nevus of Ota may affect periorbital, temple, forehead, malar regions as well as sclera, conjunctiva, cornea, retina, oral mucosa and nasal mucosa.
- Cytokines related with localized alopecia areata are IL1α and IL4 (Th2 pathway).
- Cytokines related to universal alopecia areata are IFNγ and IL2 (Th1 pathway).
- Tryptase level is increased by 4 folds in normal skin of atopic dermatitis.
- From red purple to gray color changes of the skin lesion is pathognomonic in necrotizing fasciitis.
- Cornoid lamella is the hallmark of porokeratosis.
- Adamson's fringe is the zone of the stem of the follicle above which keratinization starts and so superficial fungal infection remains above this zone.
- Auber's line is the line drawn through the maximum bulge area of the hair bulb and most of the germinative epithelial cells lie below this line.
- Fibrous streamer is the concentrically arranged collagen, containing numerous vessels and increased number of mast cells and is formed during miniaturization or catagen hair follicle formation.

* KL6, a mucin like glycoprotein in serum, increases in childhood type of scleroderma complicated with pulmonary fibrosis.
* Cryoglobulins are immunoglobulins which precipitate when serum is cooled and redissolve upon rewarming.
* Type I cryoglobulin is monoclonal, either IgA or IgM type, seen in lymphoma, leukemia, Waldenstrom macroglobulinemia and multiple myeloma.
* Type II cryoglobulin is a combination of polyclonal and monolclonal antibody complex where one acts as antigen and another one as antibody.
* The most common paraneoplastic vasculitic association lies between polyateritis nodosa and hairy cell leukemia.
* Histopathology of catagen hair follicles shows eosinophilic glassy membrane and lack of hair shaft.
* IgA deposition is seen at capillaries in Henoch-Schoenlein purpura.
* Botulinum toxin is under pregnancy category C and contraindicated in myasthenia gravis and in concomitant use with medications like aminoglycosides, penicillamine, quinine and calcium channel blockers.
* Waterglass is sodium silicate.
* Plica polonica is matted hair due to pus and exudates in severe cases of pediculosis capitis.
* Pityriasis rosea like eruptions are associated with metronidazole, clonidine, captopril and ketotifen.
* In active stage bulla of urticaria pigmentosa is subepidermal and at healing stage it is intraepidermal.
* Band like mast cell infiltration is seen in erythrodermic diffuse mastocytosis.
* Vesicle of incontinentia pigmenti is intraepidermal and single cell keratinization is seen within a whorl of epidermal cells at intervesicular area.
* Pattern of dermal necrosis is wedge shaped in Degos' disease.
* Cryopyrin induces inflammation in Muckle Well syndrome.
* Benzoic acid may cause nonimmunologic urticaria.
* Bite like dermal inflammatory infiltrate is seen in caterpillar bite.
* *Curvularia lunata*, one of the causative agents of mycetoma, has four celled curved macroconidia.
* Linezolid inhibits 23s subunit of 50s ribosome.
* Accumulation of trimethylamine is responsible for odor of decaying fish in fish odor syndrome or trimethylaminuria.
* Glycogen in cell is best stained with PAS when Carnoy's solution is used as fixative.
* Autofluorescent yellow-brown pigment is seen at affected cells in Neuroid-ceroid-lipofuscinoses.
* Diameter of shaft and inner root sheath (IRS) are equal in vellus hair.
* Incontinentia pigmenti is a X-linked dominant disorder.
* Cytokines IL6, IL18, TNF-α, IFNγ and Fas are responsible for toxic epidermal necrolysis.
* Psammoma bodies are seen in ovarian carcinoma and thyroid papillary carcinoma.
* In all porphyria, histopathology shows hyalinization around the vessels.
* Thalidomide is a potent inhibitor of TNFα and IL6.
* Lenalidomide, a derivative of thalidomide is 50,000 times more potent to inhibit TNFα.
* Treatment of choice in pediculosis corporis is cleaning and ironing of clothes and bed linens.
* Oid-oid disease (Sulzberger-Gabre syndrome) is a variant of nummular dermatitis having larger lesions and intense pruritus.
* Pediculosis humanas corporis transmits typhus, trench fever and relapsing fever.
* Bull's eye phenomenon is associated with eye-complications in chloroquine therapy.
* Oil acne presents as folliculitis like lesions at arms and thighs due to contact with industrial oil, cutting oil, oil-soaked clothings and air borne oil mists.

* Coal tar or pitch acne appears as comedonal acne at malar regions due to contact with coal tar oil, creosote oil, pitch, etc. among construction workers.
* Chloracne is characterized by closed comedone and straw colored cysts at malar cresents, retroauricular folds, posterior neck, trunk, extremities, buttocks, scrotum and penis due to percutaneous absorption or ingestion of halogenated hydrocarbons.
* Giant molluscum contagiosum develops in HIV infection when CD4 cell count comes below 50/cmm and disseminated lesions develop when the count is below 250/cmm.
* Pigmentation in urticaria pigmentosa is due to melanin, derived from melanocytes, stimulated by mast cells, except in nodular urticaria pigmentosa where pigmentation is derived from melanosomes present within the mast cells.

Blue light (410 nm) therapy in acne

* It acts through photosensitivity of porphyrin, generated by *Propionibacterium acne* and thus provides a bactericidal action and reduces inflammation.

Newer drugs for scleroderma

- Bosentan: Endothelial dual receptor antagonist, given 12 mg twice daily in patient with pulmonary hypertension. It prevents digital ulcer.
- Halofunginone: Inhibits collagen I synthesis.
- Ximedan: Uscful in localized scleroderma and used with electrophoresis.
- Urokinase: Increases skin elasticity and softness and reduces Raynaud's phenomenon.
- Quinapril: Dose is 80 mg/day for at least 3 years.
- Sildenafil: Helps to endothelial mediated vasodilatation.
- Imatinib mesylate: Inhibits platelet derived growth factor.

Minimal inhibitory concentration (MIC) in leprosy

- DDS 0.03 μg/ml
- Rifampicin 0.3 μg/ml
- Ofloxacin 0.2 μg/ml
- Minocycline 0.2 μg/ml
- Clarithromycin 0.0125 μg/ml.

* IVIg in TEN: 0.4-0.75 g/kg/day for 3 days
* Leukovorin in methotrexate toxicity: 20 mg iv 6 hourly till plasma level of methotrexate comes down to 5×10^{-8} mmol/L.
* Propranolol is a beneficial treatment in adrenergic urticaria.
* Aluminium chlorohydrate is the least irritant *antiperspirant*.
* Concentration of 8-MOP (0.75% solution) in bath PUVA is 1 ml/2 L of water.
* Minimal inhibitory concentration (MIC) of nevirapine in HIV is 0.1 μg/ml.
* Cold urticaria is a sign of Muckle-Well syndrome.
* Acral erythema is most commonly induced by doxorubicin, cytosine arabinoside and 5-fluorouracil.
* Minoxidil is the only FDA approved topical therapy for androgenetic alopecia.
* Imiquimod increases expression of IFNα, IL6 & IL8 in keratinocytes.
* Red color sweat is due to lipofuscin.
* Glomumab is self injectable TNF inhibitor, useful in psoriatic arthritis.

Cimetidine is useful in following conditions:

- Chronic mucocutaneous candidiasis
- Mucocutaneous herpes simplex infection
- Molluscum contagiosum

* Dasatinib is a tyrosine kinase inhibitor which may cause lobular panniculitis.
* DCD is the abbreviation of dynamic cooling system, used in granuloma inguinale of tibia.
* Jack/Stat inhibitor: A future drug in psoriasis, as STAT is highly expressed in psoriasis by the keratinocytes and mediates cell proliferation.
* Thalidomide is the drug of choice in type 2 lepra reaction.
* Myofibroblasts in infantile digital fibroma have

pathognomic cytoplasmic eosinophilic hyaline globules.

* Adverse effects of systemic retinoids are cheilitis, teratogenicity, hypertriglyceridemia, periungual granuloma pyogenicum and hyperostosis.
* Drug induced SLE has no cutaneous manifestations when it is caused by drugs like hydralazine, INH, procainamide and minocycline.
* Podophyllin is contraindicated in pregnancy.
* Sorafenib, a multikinase inhibitor (VEGFR2, PDGFR-B, Flt-3, cKit), causes painless subungual splinter hemorrhage.
* Sunitinib, a multikinase inhibitor (VEGFR2, PDGFR-3, Flt-3), causes reversible hair depigmentation after 5-6 weeks of therapy.
* Vibrating tools (30-300 Hz) may cause numbness, tingling, blanching and stiffness of the fingers with weakness of the intrinsic muscles of the working hand.
* Pathognomonic feature of Tangier disease is enlarged yellow tonsils and low plasma cholesterol level.
* Echinocandins (caspofungin and micafungin) are inhibitors of glucan synthesis of fungal cell wall and effective against candida and aspergillus.
* Fatty food helps absorption of griseofulvin and itraconazole.
* Terbinafine is less effective against candida, microsporum and malassezia.
* Voriconazole is effective against yeast form of fungus.
* Posaconazole is effective against candida.
* Frost nip is characterized by reversible numbness and pain with erythema at cheeks, ears and nose.
* Halocarboxylase synthetase deficiency causes ichthyosis and erythematous eruptions at scalp and eyebrows.
* Hypomastia, the term is used when the volume of adult female breast is 200 ml or less.
* Palmoplantar hyperhidrosis may be associated with chloracne.
* Bottom heavy filtration is seen in cutaneous lymphoma, herpes folliculitis and hidradenitis suppurativa.
* Cold erythema differs from cold urticaria by presence of pain and absence of urticaria.
* Familial polymorphous cold eruption, an autosomal dominant rare condition is characterized by childhood onset of nonpruritic urticaria and influenza like symptoms.
* In pityriasis rubra pilaris, at least 14 days is required to develop alternate parakeratosis.
* Ustekinumab is IL-12 and IL-23 inhibitor, useful in psoriasis.
* Needle-shaped clefts are seen within the adepocytes in sclerema neonatorum.
* Neonatal acne is caused by *Malassezia sympodalis*.
* Nevus spilus/speckled lentiginous nevus, a variant of congenital melanocytic nevus initially presents as café au lait macule and later lentigines appear.
* The pox viruses like variola vaccinia and cowpox are brick-shaped and size of the virus is (300 × 240) nm.
* Imiquimod 5% cream may be effective in erosive recalcitrant lichen planus of the lip.
* Methotrexate induced ulceration, localized to the lesion is due to higher uptake of the drug.
* Niacin is ineffective in Hartnup disease.
* Argentaffin, the term is used when some substances like phenolic group of melanin reduces silver salt into metallic silver and produces a black stain.
* Guargum, an oral preparation, used for pruritus in intrahepatic cholestasis.
* Natural source of glycolic acid is sugarcane and of salicylic acid is wilow bark.
* SSKI works in sporotrichosis as immunomodulator.
* In cystinosis, skin and hair pigmentation is reduced due to impaired pigment production within melanosomes.

- Omeprazole can cause urticaria, erythema nodosum, lichen planus and pityriasis rosea like lesions.
- Kligman formula:
  - Hydroquinone-5%
  - Tretinoin-0.1%
  - Dexamethasone-0.1%.
- One fingertip unit (FTU) = 0.5 g.
- Foam sclerotherapy is done by sodium tetradecyl sulfate.
- Rubella and measles viruses are single stranded RNA viruses.
- Parvo virus is a single stranded DNA virus.
- Hyperpigmented skin at birth is present normally at scrotum and distal phalanges.
- Heck's disease, caused by HPV13 & 32, is commonly seen in Eskimos.
- Phagolysosomes are formed in leishmaniasis but cannot kill the protozoa.
- Phagolysosomes are not at all formed in tuberculosis.
- Phagolysosomes are formed in leprosy but lepra bacilli can bypass them.
- Wooly scalp hair is a feature of Noxos diasease.
- Exanthem is the maculopapular eruptions of the skin, induced by viral infection.
- Duke's disease is also known as "fourth disease".
- Erythema multiforme is a group of disorders often induced by herpetic infection and drugs with a classical target or targetoid lesions.
- Tuberculin test is to be done prior therapy with infliximab, adalimumab and efalizumab.
- Enanthem is the maculopapular eruption of the oral mucosa, induced by viral infection.
- Funisititis is the inflammation of the umbilical cord.
- Ichthyosis hystrix is associated with epidermolytic hyperkeratosis and epidermal nevus.
- Alkali test is used to detect iiritant substance in case of irritant contact dermatitis.
- Buehler test is used to detect allergen in allergic contact dermatitis.
- Dick test is done to produce delayed hypersensitivity reaction to streptococcal antigen.
- Draize test is done to assess eye-safety of any shampoo.
- Floppy sock is the microscopic appearance of plucked hair as ruffling of hair cuticle in loose anagen hair.
- Guthrie's test is the screening test to detect phenylketonuria.
- Hess test is used to detect capillary fragility in purpura.
- Hair pull test plucks a bunch of 20-25 hairs.
- Fernandez test, a type of lepromin test, detects delayed hypersensitivity reaction to the soluble component of leprous extract and reading is taken after 48 hours.
- Mitsuda test, a type of lepromin test, detects delayed hypersensitivity reaction to the particulate form of leprous extract and reading is taken after 3-4 weeks.
- Leishmanin test is negative in Indian form of post kala-azar; but positive in African form.
- Lutidine test is used to diagnose formaldehyde induced allergic contact dermatitis.
- Machhado-Guenerio test is done in Chagas' disease.
- Mazzotti's test is done in onchocerciasis with diethylcarbamazine challenge.
- Montenegro test is an indradermal test to detect leishmaniasis.
- Monilethrix is characterized by nodes with intervals of 0.7-1 mm and narrow internodal spaces.
- Magnussen and Kligman test (MK) is done in guineapig to detect human allergen.
- PMA-NBT test (Phorbol-myristate acetate stimulated nitroblue tetrazolium dye test) can detect chronic granulomatous disease.
- Roat (Repeat open application test) is used to identify offending cosmetics.
- Pressure test is done to differentiate between plantar wart and corn.
- Ross Miles test is used to detect foaming power of a shampoo.

* Soret band is spectrum of ultraviolet light (400-410 nm) and excites porphyrins to emit red fluorescence.
* Simple sweat test readily differentiates leprosy lesion from nonleprosy lesion, on comparing the temperature felt by dorsum of the finger.
* Sabin-Feldman dye test detect IgG antibody in toxoplasmosis.
* Schirmer's test is a screening test for keratoconjunctivitis sicca in Sjogren's syndrome.
* Schultz-Charlton reaction shows blanching of rash in scarlet fever, around the point of injection of antitoxin.
* Sandwich test shows presence of fungi between orthokeratotic upper layer and parakeratotic lower layer of the epidermis.
* Whiff test is done with 10% KOH in bacterial vaginosis.
* Pastia's line are accentuated petechial exanthema at flexural areas in scarlet fever.
* Black galactorrhea is associated with drugs like phenothiazines and minocycline.
* Adenoma sebaceum is a form of angiofibroma and there is no relation with sebaceous gland.
* Apple jelly nodules are seen in granulomatous diseases like lupus vulgaris and sarcoidosis.
* Ashleaf macules are seen in tuberous sclerosis.
* Botryomycosis is most commonly caused by *Staphylococcus aureus* and rarely by Pseudomonas; but there is no relation with fungus.
* Barber's pole is an appearance of umbilical cord in congenital syphilis, having alternating red, pale blue and chalky white bands.
* Baghdad boil/Delhi boil/Aaleppo boil/Oriental sore is a form of cutaneous leishmaniasis.
* Café-au-lait macules in neurofibromatosis have regular margin and known as coast of California.
* Café-au-lait macules in Albright syndrome have irregular margin and known as coast of Maine.
* Chizzole macule is feature of industrial fluoride toxicity.
* Corkscrew hair is characterized by circular and spiral shape, seen in scurvy.
* Chancre redux is development of new syphilitic ulcer on the healed scar of previous attack.
* Pseudochancre redux is development of a lesion of some other dermatosis on the healed scar of syphilitic ulcer.
* Canites is graying of hair and premature canites occurs below age of 20 years in black and 30 years in white.
* Distribution of pityriasis rosea lesions appears as Christmas tree.
* In erythroplakia red color is due to absence of keratin layer.
* Echthyma gangrenosum is having an extremely painful ulcer and caused by *Pseudomonas aeruginosa*.
* Elkonyxis is an isolated large pit in nailplate, seen in Reiter's disease.
* Familial dysbetalipoproteinemia shows yellow lines or infiltrations along the palmar creases and it is the pathognomonic feature.
* Famial hypercholesterolemia shows a unique yellowish xanthoma in the interdigital spaces.
* Flagellate pigmentation occurs after a cumulative dose of *bleomycin* ranging between 90 to 285 mg.
* Corneal verticillate is a feature of Fabry's disease.
* Fox-Fordoyce disease, is an apocrine gland disease having extremely pruritic papules at axillae and areolae.
* Fordyce's spots are nothing but ectopic sebaceous glands at vermilion border of lips, buccal mucosa, glans penis and labia minora.
* Hoarseness of voice is associated with lepromatous leprosy, lipoid proteinosis, secondary syphilis and sarcoidosis.
* Herald patch or mother patch is seen in pityriasis rosea.
* Herpes iris of Bateman is classically seen in herpes simplex induced erythema multiforme.
* Iris pearls are seen in lepromatous leprosy.

* Impetigo herpetiformis is a form of pustular psoriasis in pregnancy and there is no relation with pyogenic infection.
* Jarisch-Herxheimer reaction (JH reaction) is seen in early syphilis, treated with penicillin within 6-8 hours of therapy. It is also seen in onchocerciasis for diethylcarbamazine therapy or in strongyloidosis for thiabendazole therapy.
* Janeway lesions are faint macular lesions at thenar and hypothenar eminences in bacterial endocarditis.
* Koenen's tumors are periungual fibroma, seen in tuberous sclerosis.
* Lupus means lesion having an eroded or gnawed quality, resembling the bite of a wolf.
* Beau's lines are transverse grooves due to temporary halting of nail growth, associated with severe form of systemic illness.
* Mees' lines are transverse whitish bands due to acute arsenic toxicity.
* Myiasis is caused by larvae of house-fly.
* Majocchi's granuloma is caused by fungi.
* Majocchi's disease in a form of pigmented purpura with an annular pattern.
* Martorell's ulcer is a form of hypertensive ulcer.
* Myrmecia is a form of plantar wart, caused by HPV1.
* Maculae caerulae are blue-gray macules near the base of lashes or pubic hair, following bites of crub lice (pthiriasis).
* Main succulente is swollen and edematous hand in syringomyelia.
* Neopolitan nail shows white, brown and red bands in aged person.
* Onycholysis is the separation of nail plate from distal nail bed.
* Onychomadesis is the separation of nail plate from proximal nail bed.
* Onychoschizia is transverse lamellar splitting of free edge of nail plate, seen in polycythemia.
* Osler's nodes are erythematous tender lesions at pads of fingers and toes in subacute bacterial endocarditis.
* Ophiasis is alopecia areata along the hair margin.
* Pearly penile papules are flesh colored or whitish lesions of angiofibroma.
* Poliosis is focal graying of hair, seen in vitiligo, Piebaldism and Waardenburg syndrome.
* Plica polonica is a bunch of crusted and matted hair, is associated with pediculosis capitis.
* Poikiloderma is characterized by atrophy, dyspigmentation and telangiectasia.
* Pingpong patch is formed due to repeated trauma from a table tennis ball.
* Pili incarnate are ingrowing hair causing pseudofolliculitis.
* Pityriasis means branny scaling.
* Pityriasis alba is characterized by illdefined mild scaly hypopigmented oval to round patches, commonly occurring at face of the child.
* Pityriasis versicolor, a superficial fungal infection, is caused by *malassezia furfur*, characterized by hypo-to hyperpigmented fine scaly macules and patches at bath areas.
* Pityriasis rosea is characterized by oval shaped small annular patches with peripheral collorette of scales and an inverted far tree like distribution at the trunk.
* Pityriasis simplex/furfuracea, a form of early seborrheic dermatitis, has fine loosely adherent scales.
* Cradle cap is a form of infantile seborrheic capitis with thick adherent crust.
* Pityriasis steatoides is a form of pubertal or post pubertal seborrheic capitis with greasy adherent mounds.
* Pityriasis amiantacea is characterized by masses of adherent silvery scales along with bunch of hair shafts, laying like tiles of a roof.
* Pityriasis circinata et marginata of Vidal is a variant of pityriasis rosea with single or few large lesions, usually occurring at axillae or groins of adults.

* Pityriasis lichenoides is a form of inflammatory dermatosis of unknown etiology and sometimes considered as parapsoriasis.
* Pityriasis lichenoides et varioliformis acuta (PLEVA), an acute form of pityriasis lichenoides, is characterized by sudden onset of edematous and erythematous papulopustular eruptions with subsequent central necrosis.
* Pityriasis lichenoides chronica is characterized by insidious onset of numerous papules with central mica like scales and subsequent development of hypopigmented macules.
* Pityriasis nigra/tinea nigra, caused by *Phaeoannelomyces werneckii*, is characterized by asymptomatic nonscaly well defined, brown, to black macules or patches at palms.
* Pityriasis rotunda, a form of acquired ichthyosis, is characterized by sharply defined ichthyotic patches at trunk, thighs and buttocks.
* Pityriasis rubra pilaris, a chronic papulosquamous disorder of unknown etiology, presents with scaly follicular papules as discrete and coalesced lesions.
* Pityriasis folliculorum, caused by *Demodex folliculorum*, is characterized by diffuse facial erythema, and follicular scales appearing as nutmeg grater.
* Pinch purpura is a characteristic feature of primary systemic amyloidosis.
* Pterygium unguis is fusion of proximal nail fold with nail plate which extends distally along the growth of the nail, seen in lichen planus.
* Reverse pterygium is fusion of hyponychium with distal end of nail plate, seen in scleroderma.
* Cartilage erosion in multicentricreticulo histiocytosis is caused by urokinase.
* Pangeria is a generalized form of premature aging.
* Melanocytes are irreversibly damaged at temperature <–4 °C.
* Progeria is characterized by premature senility with hypertrichosis, bird facies, dry and wrinkled skin.
* Multiple halo nevi after the age of 40 years may be associated with ocular or cutaneous malignant melanoma.
* Acrogeria shows premaurity or features of senility at acral areas.
* Pomade is a scented cosmetic in which apple extract is an ingredient.
* Parrot's paralysis is seen in congenital syphilis.
* Poikiloderma of Civatte is characterized by reddish-brown reticulate pigmentation, telangiectasia and atrophy, occurring at cheeks and neck of middle aged women, following use of phototoxic cosmetics.
* Ring of Woronoff is hypopigmented ring around a subsiding psoriatic lesion.
* Racket nail is seen in hyperparathyroidism.
* Shin spots/diabetic dermopathy is characterized by dull red papules at the shins.
* Turkey ear is a massive earlobe, seen in lupus pernio, a form of sarcoidosis.
* Therapeutic paradox is associated with cardiovascular tertiary syphilis, characterized by deterioration of the disease following penicillin therapy.
* Vagabond's disease/morbus errorium is hyperpigmented skin associated with chronic infestation of pediculosis corporis.
* Veldt's sore/desert sore is characterized by shallow and crusted ulcers, probably caused by Corynebacterium, seen in desert.
* Vulgaris, the word denotes widespread.
* Wheal less urticaria is a form of localized or generalized itching without apparent physical sign of urticaria.
* Wickham's striae are whitish linear streaks on the surface of lichen planus.
* Zoster sine herpete is characterized by pain without skin rash in herpes zoster.

- Gloves-stocking anesthesia is seen in lepromatous leprosy.
- Cornoid lamella is a parakeratotic column, seen in histopathology of porokeratosis and it corresponds with the thread like margin of a lesion.
- Cerebriform/scrotal tongue is seen in Melkerson-Rosenthal syndrome, midline lymphedema and pemphigus vegetans.
- Intravenous immunoglobulin (IVIG) can cause aseptic meningtis, headache and nausea.
- Integrin extracellular matrix receptors anchor the basal cells with the basement membrane.
- Subcutaneous nodules in Churg-Strauss disease are commonly seen at scalp and extremites.
- Histopathological hallmark of Churg-Strauss disease is presence of eosinophils.
- Acral peeling skin syndrome is associated with reduced transglutaminase 5 (TG5).
- Orchitis is a common feature of polyarteritis nodosa (PAN), associated with hepatitis B viral infection (HBV).
- Starburst livedo reticularis is a feature of polyarteritis nodosa (PAN).
- Average duration of non-complementeric urticarial vascultis is 3 years.
- Deflazacort is the bone-sparing corticosteroid.
- Oral hairy leukoplakia is associated with HIV, EBV, HPV and candidal infections.
- Systemic tacrolimus causes herpetic infection, paresthesia, headache, tremor, delirium, coma, nephrotoxicity, hypertension, hyperglycemia, hyperkalemia, diarrhea, respiratory or urinary infection, lymphoma and drug-drug interaction.
- Thalidomide causes cutaneous eruptions, peripheral neuropathy, teratogenicity, phocomelia, bradycardia, anemia and thrombosis.
- Keratinocytes do not secrete IL2, IL4 and IFNγ.
- Size of LD body is only 1-5 μm.
- Acne scar best treated with Diode laser (1450 nm).
- Carbon dioxide laser (10600 nm) can be used in presence of pacemaker.
- Argon laser (488 nm and 514 nm) is useful for vascular and pigmentary disorders.
- The operator can change the wavelength, spot size and exposure time with tunable pulsed dye laser.
- Flash lamp pulsed dye laser causes no effect at surrounding due to very short pulses (300-400 μs) and it is useful in children.
- Neodynium-YAG laser (1060 nm) has highest penetrating power (>5 mm) and is useful for deep vascular lesion, subcutaneous lesion and recalcitrant keloid.
- Excimer laser (248 nm and 308 nm) makes an ultra thin incision and targets the melanocytes.
- Ruby laser (694 nm) is useful for tattoo and nevus of Ota.
- Helium-Neon laser (633 nm) is known as soft laser.
- KTP laser (532 nm) is useful for epidermal pigmentation and superficial vascular lesion.
- Q-switched Alexandrite laser (720-850 nm) is useful for dermal and epidermal pigmentation.
- Re-epithelialization following ablative laser resurfacing takes 3-10 days.
- Usually 5 treatment settings are required for non-ablative laser resurfacing.
- IPL laser is best for photoaging.
- Skin laxity is best treated with radiofrequency.
- Cryogen spray is required for protection of epidermis in non-ablative laser resurfacing.
- Target temperature of the dermis attained during nonablative laser resurfacing with 1320 nm Nd:YAG laser is 408 °C.
- Pulse duration of laser, used in ablative laser resurfacing should not exceed 1 ms.
- The penetration depth of CO_2 laser depends on presence of water.
- Nd:YAG laser (1064 nm) is used for lipolysis.

* Pulsed dye laser (585 nm) does not produce any scar when port-wine stain (PWD) is treated with it.
* Hair removal lasers (RAD-N)
  - Ruby (694 nm)
  - Alexandrite (755 nm)
  - Diode (800 nm)
  - Nd:YAG (1064 nm)
* Laser for pigmented epidermal lesion (KNC)
  - Krypton, green (512 nm, 531 nm)
  - Frequency doubled Nd:YAG (532 nm)
  - Copper vapour, green (511 nm)
* Trummer field lines or scurvy lines are radiolucent transverse lines at metaphysis of long bones of extremities.

PART B

BASIC DERMATOLOGY

ANATOMY, PHYSIOLOGY, BIOCHEMISTRY, PATHOLOGY AND PHARMACOLOGY

CHAPTER B1

Skin as an organ: It is the outermost and largest organ of the human body.

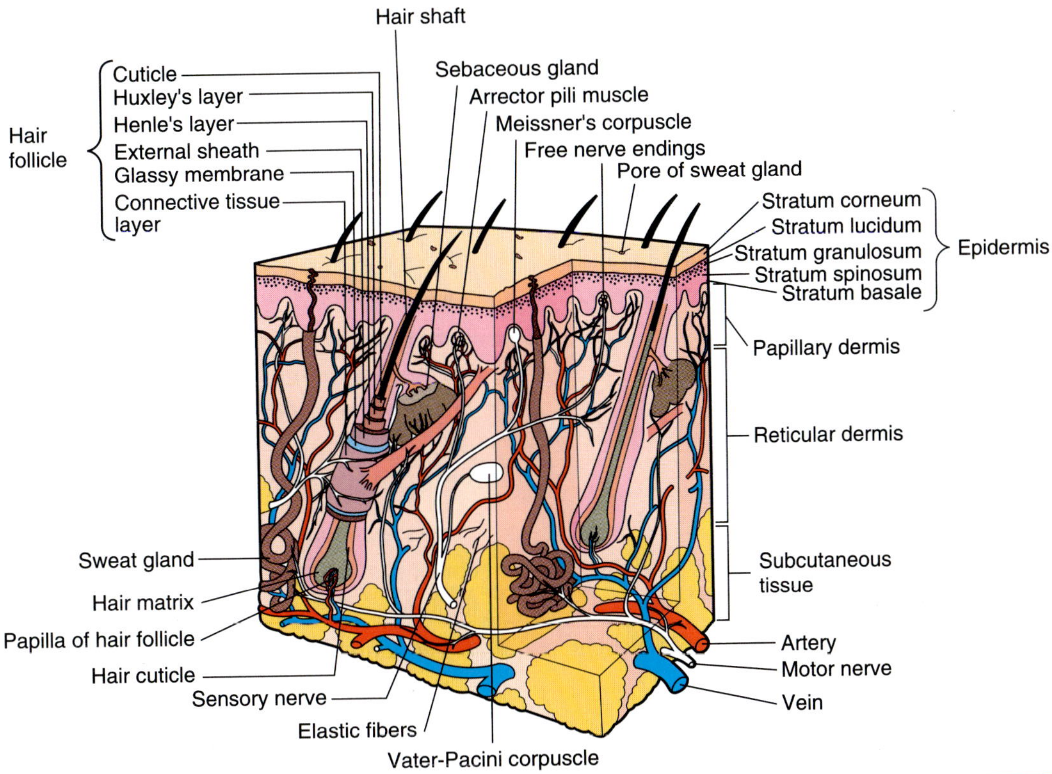

Fig. 1: Structures of the skin

Parts of the skin

- Epidermis
- Dermis
- Hypodermis/subcutaneous tissue

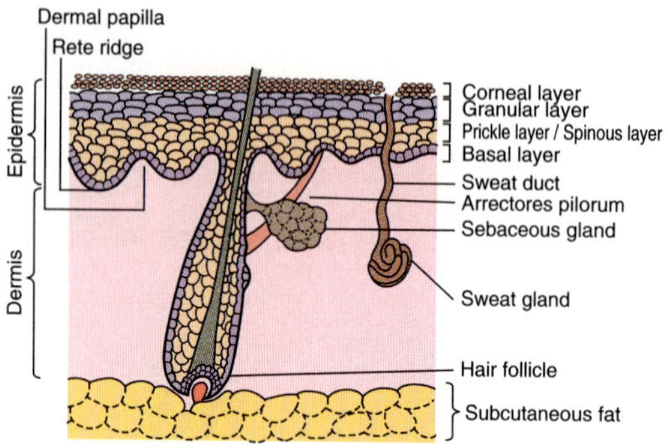

Fig. 2: Structures of the skin

Layers of the epidermis

- Stratum corneum/corneal layer/horny layer
- Stratum lucidum
- Stratum granulosum/granular layer
- Stratum basalis/basal layer
- Malpighian layer: It is the viable part of the epidermis and contains nucleated keratinocytes. It consists of all layers of epidermis except corneal layer. Vitamin D is synthesized in this layer. Thickness of the viable part is 100 μm.

Unique features of the skin

- Total area: 1.5-2 m^2
- Weight: 4-7 kg
- pH: 5.7
- Fluid content: 1/3rd of total body fluid
- Blood circulation: 1/4th of total circulation
- Length of arterial plexuses: 240 km
- Subcutaneous fat: 10% of total body weight
- Perceptible minimum weight: 50 μg
- Tolerable temperature: Varying from –18 °C to + 45 °C
- Nerve conduction velocity: 2m/s
- Only 20% loss of the skin is enough to cause death due to fluid and electrolytes imbalance. But a person can survive for about 40 days, solely depending on subcutaneous fat.
- Normal exfoliation: 1 gm per day and 4 kg per year. But in erythroderma, this is raised to 30-50 gm per day.
- Thickness of epidermis: (50-150) μm.
- Structural and functional unit of epidermis is keratinocyte.
- Surface density of nucleated keratinocytes: 50,000/mm^2.
- Basal layer keratinocytes proliferate and differentiate into other layers. This gradual process of conversion ultimately forms the flattened anucleated keratinocyte containing keratin fibers and the process is known as keratinization.
- These anucleated keratinocytes, formed by the process of keratinization are known as corneocytes.
- Each corneocyte covers an area of 25 basal keratinocytes.
- Keratinization shows both qualitative and quatitative changes within the cells.
- Average time for keratinization is 4 weeks.
- Time for exfoliation of cornified layer is about 2 weeks.
- Time taken by a basal cell to pass through keratinization and ultimate exfoliation is 56-72 days. This time comes down to 7-10 days in psoriasis.

Development of the skin

* Weeks, mentioned below against different parts/contents of the skin, indicate gestational age of the fetus.
  - Periderm, the single layered epidermis: 3rd to 4th week.
  - Two layered epidermis consisting of periderm and basal layer: 6th to 8th week.
  - Three layered epidermis: 9th to 11th week.

- Four layered epidermis: 18th to 22nd week.
- Periderm covers the embryo at 6th week and sheds off between 19th to 21st week of gestation.
- Keratinization: 15th to 21st week.
- Langerhans cell: 6th week.
- Melanocyte: 7th week.
- Merkel cell: 11th week.
- Dermoepidermal junction: 8th week.
- Hair follicle: 9th to 16th week.
- Sebaceous gland: 13th to 16th week.
- Apocrine sweat gland: 30th week.
- Eccrine sweat gland: 16th to 22nd week.
- Hair: 19th to 21st week.
- Nail: 19th to 21st week.
- Elastic fibers: 22nd to 24th week.
- Dermis and hypodermis: 3rd week.

Functions of the skin

- Protection from external injuries of physical, chemical, thermal, electrical, radiologic and microbial origin.
- Barrier function for selective entry and exit.
- Immune response to both external and internal stimuli.
- Antimicrobial action.
- Thermoregulation.
- Neurological response.
- Synthesis of vitamin D.
- Maintenance of body image.

Stratum corneum/corneal layer/horny layer

- It is the outermost layer and formed by a specialized process, known as keratinization.
- It is thinnest at eyelid (10-15 μm) and thickest at soles (100 μm).
- It is made up of piled-up layers of flattened anucleated keratinocytes, known as corneocytes.
- It appears as a brick wall where the corneocytes are the bricks, and a mixture of lipids and proteins is like that of cement and sands.
- Single corneocyte covers the area of 25 basal keratnocytes.
- An average human body sheds about 50-60 billion corneocytes per day.

Stratum lucidum

- It is an electrolucent layer lies between corneal and granular layers.
- It is most appreciable at palms and soles.

Stratum granulosum/granular layer

- It consists of 1-3 layers of keratinocytes.
- These cells are having cytoplasmic granules and so the name is implied.
- Keratinocytes of this layer contain basophilic granules, known as keratohyaline granules.
- Keratohyaline granules contain various proteins including involucrin, loricrin and profilaggrin.
- During keratinization, phosphatase enzyme converts profilaggrin into filaggrin and forms a thick and tough peripheral envelope of the corneocytes.
- Transglutaminase (TG) enzymes make a mixture of structural proteins like loricrin and involucrin, and lipids like ceramides.
- This mixture of proteins and lipids acts as glue like cementing substance which is capable to bind corneocyte one to another.

Stratum spinosum/spinous layer

- It consists of polygonal keratinocytes and they are interlocked with each other through cytoplasmic processes, appearing as spines and so the name is implied.
- Cells of upper of spinous layer contain Odland bodies or lamellar granules, synthesized by their Golgi apparatus.
- Odland bodies contain baskets of lipids, polysaccharides and hydrolytic enzymes. These lipid contents contribute to form outer layer of the cornified envelope of corneocytes.

- Lipid layer contains ceramides (50%), cholesterol (35%) and free fatty acids (15%).

Stratum basalis/basal layer

- It consists of single layer of cuboidal or columnar cells which continuously proliferate to replenish the pool of epidermal cells.
- Basal layer is not straight like corneal layer. It is undulating, having upward and downward projections.

Basal cell regeneration time

- Each basal cell divides in every 4 days and thus renews itself.

Growth fraction

- Basal cells which are prepared for division at a time are known as stem cells.
- Stem cells are also present at the bulge of the hair follicle, above which the arrector pili muscle is attached.

Cell cycle time

- Average cell cycle time is 311 hours. It comes down to only 11 hours in psoriasis. So, in psoriasis basal cells proliferate 28 times more than normal. But some believe only 7-10 times.

Rete ridges

- These are the downward projections of the epidermis into the dermis.

Dermal papillae

- These are the upward projections of the dermis into the epidermis.

Epidermal keratinization

- It is a complicated process through which the basal cells follow a series of proliferation to differentiate into spinous cells, granular cells, horny cells (corneocytes) respectively and at the end, corneocytes shed off.
- It involves following major changes:
  - Synthesis of distinctive proteins like keratin, filaggrin and involucrin and lipids containing lamellar granules.
  - Alterations of nuclei, cytoplasmic organelles, plasma membranes and desmosomes.
  - Keratins are lacking disulfide cross-links and embedded in sulfur-rich amorphous matrix. Thus a degree of flexibility and elasticity is maintained in the cornified layer.
  - Phosphatase enzyme converts profilaggrin into filaggrin in corneal layer. These protein contents form the thick and tough peripheral envelope of the corneocytes. Loricrin and involucrin are structural proteins which blend with ceramide by the help of transglutaminase enzyme.
  - Corneocytes are packed up with keratin filaments and lacked of all other organelles including nucleus.
  - The organelles are destroyed by hydrolytic and degrading enzymes stored in the odland bodies and by lysosomes.

Regional variation of skin

- Slightly verrucous surface is seen at eyelid, axilla, elbow and knee.
- Relatively thickened skin is seen at elbow and knee.
- Thickened stratum corneum is seen at palm and sole.
- Apocrine glands are predominantly present at axilla.
- Closely packed sebaceous glands are seen at nose.
- Anagen follicles descend deeply into subcutaneous tissue.
- Numerous vellus hair follicles are seen at eyelid.

Contents of the epidermis

- Keratinocyte
- Melanocyte
- Langerhans cell
- Merkel cell
- Epidermal parts of eccrine and apocrine ducts
- Epidermal parts of pilosebaceous unit.

Contents of the dermis

- Amorphous ground substance: It consists of mucopolysaccharides.
- Fibrous structures: These are collagen tissue, elastic tissue and arrector pili muscle.
- Cellular structures: These are fibroblasts, mast cells, dermal dendrocytes and macrophages.
- Special structures: These are hair follicles, sebaceous glands and apocrine/eccrine sweat glands.
- Blood vessels and lymphatics
- Sensory apparatus: Free nerve endings, Meissner's corpuscles, Merkel disc, Pacinian corpuscles and Ruffini corpuscles.

Keratinocytes

- These cells are the structural and functional units of the epidermis and constitute 80-90% of the epidermal cells.
- These originate from ectoderm by 3rd week of gestation as a single layer. These turn into two layers by 5th week, three layers by 10th week and four layers by 19th week of gestation.
- Other ultrastructures like desmosome, hemidesmosome, basement membrane develop between 6th to 12th week of gestation, and tonofilaments develop by 16th week.
- Size, shape, composition, orientation and functions of keratinocytes are variable from one layer to another layer of epidermis.
- The concentration of keratinocytes in the epidermis is 50,000 cell/mm^2 of the surface area.
- Like other mammalian cells, each cell contains actin, tubulin and intermediate filaments of 7-10 nm in size.
- Actin is composed of microtubules of 20-25 nm in diameter.
- Intermediate filaments of keratinocyte is known as keratin.
- Keratin, derived from the Greek word Keras means horn. It is a family having more than 30 members. They are the production of two different Gene families, one is responsible for basic keratin and one is for acidic keratin.
- Each keratin is having three parts:
  - Nonhelical N-terminal head and C-terminal tail
  - Helical body
- Keratin filaments exist in pairs, like 1 & 10 or 5 & 14. Each pair consists of one acidic and one basic filament. Interwining adjacent filaments make thicker fibrils. During keratinization, different stages of differentiation shows expression of different types of keratin.
- There are 54 genes to control the production of different types of keratins with specificity.
- Keratins of hair and nails are modified and composed of large amounts of amino acid cysteine with several cross-links.
- Retinoid levels, growth factors and hormones may regulate keratin gene expression.

Distribution of keratins

- K5/K14 keratins are expressed in stratified epithelium.
- K1/K18 keratins are expressed by nonkeratinized epithelium.
- K1/K10 keratins are expressed at suprabasal cells, indicating epithelial differentiation.
- K15 keratin is expressed at basal cells of hair follicle bulge regions where pluripotent stem cell are present.

- K9 keratin is expressed at palmoplantar epidermis.
- K2e keratin is expressed at superficial interfollicular epidermis.
- K6/K16/K17 keratins are expressed at suprabasal cells during epidermal hyperproliferation as in psoriasis or during wound healing.

Functions of keratins

- To maintain cytoskeleton.
- To play roles in cell signaling, stress response and apoptosis.

Changes of keratinocytes during keratinization

- Basal cells are columnar or cuboidal in shape and contain larger oval nuclei and more basic cytoplasm.
- Suprabasal keratinocytes contain desmosomal processes to form spinous cells.
- Cytoplasm of each basal cell and lower spinous cell contain abundant rough endoplasmic reticulum, ribosomes, Golgi apparatus and mitochondria. These cells also synthesize tonofilament/keratin intermediate filaments of 7.0 nm in diameter and later these tonofilaments are converted into keratinous proteins, known as keratin which fill up the corneocytes in the outer most layer.
- Tonofilaments are oriented along the long axis of the cells. They modulate the shape of the cells and maintain the central position of the nucleus as well as cell to cell contact via desmosomes.
- As the cells pass toward outermost layer, these filaments are aggregated into bundles.
- Molecular weight of the tonofilament fiber is also changed 50-58 kilodalton at basal layer to 56.6-67 kilodalton at suprabasal layer keratinocyte.
- Upper spinous keratinocytes contain keratohyaline granules. They become more prominent at granular layer. These granules are electron-dense bodies and devoid of internal structure.
- Keratohyaline granules are rich in profilaggrin proteins which are converted into filaggrin (filament aggregating proteins) in the corneal layer.
- Filaggrin is a histidine rich protein which act as glue to aggregate and to align keratin filaments within the cornified cells.
- Keratohyaline granules also contain cysteine rich-proteins having disulfide bonds. These bonds contribute chemical inertia and strength of the cornified layer.
- All these proteins make an amorphous protein matrix which embeds keratin fibers in the cornified layer.
- Upper spinous layer also contain lamellar granules or Odland bodies.
- These bodies originate near the Golgi apparatus, migrate to the cytoplasm and fuse with plasma membrane. From there they discharge their contents into intercellular spaces.
- Size of individual body is 300 nm in diameter.
- They possess highly ordered lamellar structures containing free sterols, phospholipids and sphingophospholipids, and several hydrolytic enzymes like lipases, glycosidases and acid phosphatases.
- Lipases and glycosidases convert the polar lipids (phospholipids and sphingophospholipids) into more hydrophobic, nonpolar, neutral lipids like ceramides and free fatty acids. Thus intercellular spaces are made into an effective water-proof crystalline sheets.
- Acid phosphatases dissolve adhesive intercellular coatings and thus desquamation occurs.
- Keratinocytes in the corneal layer lose their nuclei and most of the cytoplasmic organelles.

- Lysosomal enzymes degrade all these organelles except tonofilaments and keratohyaline granules.
- Following enzymatic degradation nucleus is replaced by histones and other proteins.
- Plasma membranes of these anucleated keratinocytes become thickened to form marginal band or cornified cellular envelope which are oriented parallel to the skin surface. This band is about 15 nm thick. This is the most resistant part to any injurious agent and having many disulfide bonds. Epidermal transglutaminases play a vital role to form this marginal band.
- Calcium dependent enzymes cross link various precursor proteins within the membrane by forming isopeptide bonds.
- Marginal band is surrounded by a lipid envelop which determines the cohesiveness of the stratum corneum.
- These two envelopes are interlinked with ester linkages.
- Throughout the process of cornification, the intercellular junctional areas or desmosomes continuously breakdown and reform when the keratinocytes move upward from their basal position.
- Contractile intracellular actin filaments help each keratinocyte to pull the nearby keratinocytes by extending adhesion.
- In the upper most cells of the granular layer and cells of the cornified layer, marginal bands and desmosomes form a continuous layer.
- Cholesteryl sulfate acts as an intercellular cement substance. Hydrolysis of this enzyme results in cleavage between the desmosomes and ultimately corneocytes desquamate.
- Thickness of statum corneum is variable from 15-30 cell layers.

Contents of the cornified envelope

- Outermost layer contains lipids:
  - Ceramide (50%)
  - Cholesterol (35%)
  - Free fatty acids (15%)
  - Molar ratio = 1:1:1.
- Inner layer contains following proteins:
  - Involucrin, loricrin (80%), filaggrin
  - Periplakin, invoplakin
  - Elafin, cystatin, repetin
  - Transglutaminase 1,3 & 5 (TGs)
  - Small proline-rich protein, late envelope protein/XP-5
  - Keratin 1,2 & 10.

Cell-cell junction

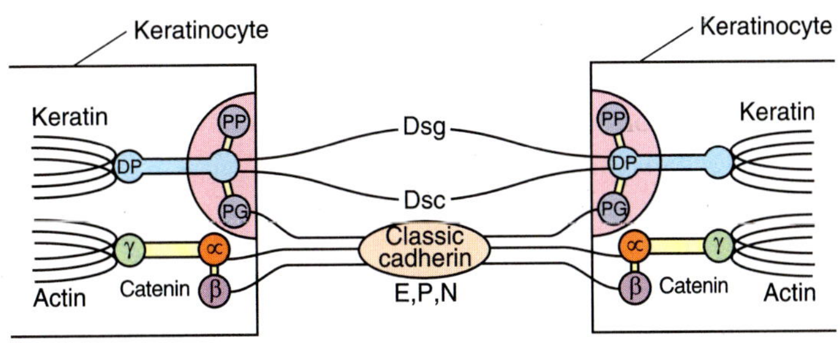

Fig. 3: Ultrastructures of cell-cell junction

Types of cell-cell junction

- Desmosomal junction
- Adherens junction
- Gap junction
- Tight junction

Desmosomal junction: Keratin fibers bind with following desmosomal intracellular proteins:

- Plakoglobin (PG)
- Plakophilin (PP)
- Desmoplakin (DP)

* All these desmosomal intracellular proteins of two opposing cells bind with following transmembrane proteins:
  - Desmoglein (Dsg)
  - Desmocollin (Dsc)
* Adherens junction: Actin filaments bind with following intracellular proteins:
  - α Catenin
  - β Catenin
  - γ Catenin
* All these adherens junctional proteins bind with transmembrane proteins:
  - Classic cadherin (E, P, N).
* Desmoglein, desmocollin and classic cadherin are the members of a single family, known as Cadherin family.

Gap junction

- It contains **connexins** to make pores at cell membrane for communication between two cells.
- Specialized transmembrane channels are formed that connect the cytoplasm of neighbouring cells.
- Each gap junction channel is composed of integral membrane proteins called connexins (Cx).
- Six connexins monomers oligomerize to form an annular hemichannel called a connexon.

Tight junction

- Cementing material sealed such a way that free passage is inhibited.

Dermoepidermal junction

* It is the interface between epidermis and dermis which connects the both.

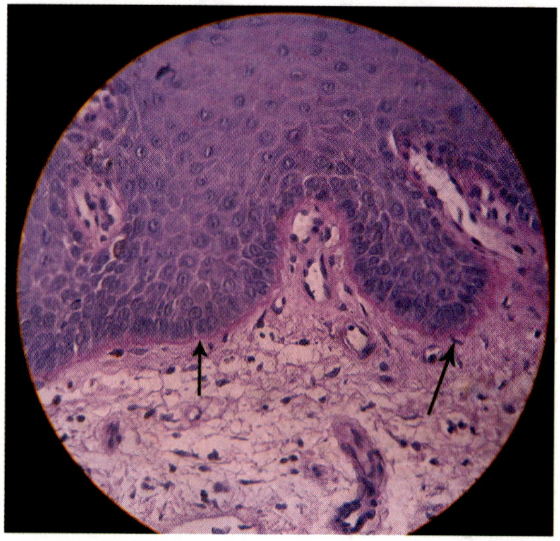

Fig. 4: Thickened basement membrane

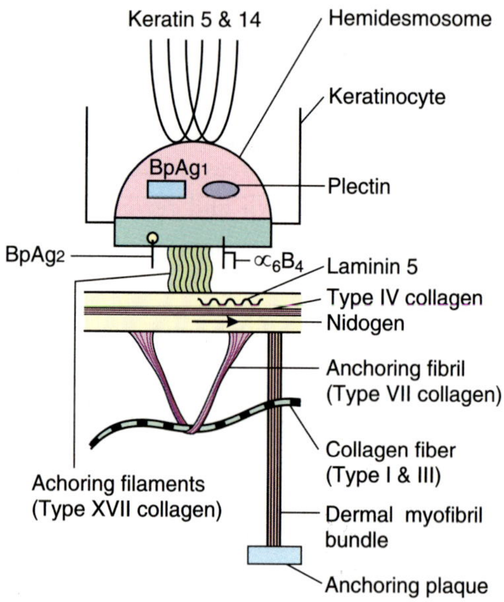

Fig. 5: Ultrastructures of dermoepidermal junction

* It consists of followings:
  - Basal lamina of basal cells.
  - Hemidesmosome which is nothing but thickened basal lamina, having inner plaque and outer plaque.

- Keratin 5 & 14, remain attached with hemidesmosome.
- Inner plaque contains BP230 (BPAg1) and plectin proteins.
- Outer plaque contains BP180 (BPAg2) and ∝6β4-integrin.
- Lamina lucida contains anchoring filaments (collagen XVII), and parts of BP180 and ∝6β4-integrin.
- Lamina densa contains laminin 5(Epiligrin), nidogen and collagen IV.
- Sublamina densa contains anchoring fibrils (collagen VII), anchoring plaque, elastin, fibulins, linkin, latent TGF binding protein (LTBP) and heparan sulfate proteoglycans (HSPG).
- Thickness of the basement membrane is 35-45 nm.
- Thickness of the basement membrane zone is 0.5 µm-1µm.

Function of dermoepidermal junction

- To maintain the attachment between the epidermis and the dermis.
- To support the epidermis.
- To regulate the permeability across it.
- To regulate embryonal differentiation.

Relation of keratins with diseases

- Keratin 5 & 14:
  - Epidermolysis bullosa (EB) simplex
- BPAG1 (BP 230 Kd):
  - Bullous pemphigoid (BP)
- BPAG2 (BP 180, type XVII collagen):
  - BP
  - Pemphigoid gestationis (PG)
  - Cicatricial pemphigoid (CP)
  - Linear IgA bullous dermatosis (LABD)
  - Generalized atrophic benign epidermolysis bullosa.
- Integrin (α6β4), subunit β4:
  - Ocular CP
  - Junctional EB with pyloric atresia
- Laminin 5:
  - Antiepiligrin CP
  - Junctional EB-Herlitz
- Type VII collagen:
  - EB acquisita
  - Bullous systemic lupus erythematosus
  - Dystrophic EB

Melanocytes

- Melanocytes are dendritic cells of the epidermis and capable to produce pigmentation.
- Melanoblasts are the precursor cells of melanocytes.
- These melanoblast cells are originated from neural crest and migrate at skin in a cephalo-caudal direction at 3rd to 4th month of gestation.
- Melanosomes are seen in melanocyte at 8th to 10th week of gestation.

Physical properties

- These cells are present at skin, inner ear, and choroid and iris of the eye.
- Exceptionally melanocytes at choroid/uveal tissue are nondendritic.
- Melanocytes constitute 10% of basal cells with a varying melanocyte:keratinocyte ration of 1:10 in the epidermis and 1:5 in the hair follicle.
- One melanocyte can transfer melanin to about 36 keratinocyte and this functional unit is known as epidermal melanin unit.
- Melanocytes lie between the basal cells with the help of E-cadherin.
- Follicular melanocytes are of two types, differentiated melanocytes and melanocyte stem cells.

Microscopic properties

- Each cell has a small, dark staining nucleus and clear cytoplasm. Cytoplasm appears clear due to shrinkage but all clear cells at basal layer are not melanocytes.
- It does not have any tonofilaments.

Physiological properties

- Growth factors of melanocyte are Wnt, endothelin and steel factor.
- Growth inhibiting factor of melanocyte is bone morphogenic protein (BMP).
- Histochemical markers are S100 and HMB 45.
- Melanocytes possess melanocyte specific receptors, like melanocortin 1 and melatonin receptors.
- Melanocytes also possess other receptors like Frizzled 5, c-Kit (receptor tyrosine kinases), HGF (hepatocyte growth factor receptor). These are important for cell signaling pathways like RAS/RAF/MEK/ERK and P13K/AKT and these are essential for melanoma cell survival.
- Melanin pigment is produced by melanocytes. It requires oxidation of tyrosine by tyrosinase enzyme.
- Pigment is of two types, such as brown or black color eumelanin and yellow or red color, pheomelanin.
- Pheomelanin is converted into eumelanin by activation of melanocortin 1 receptor.
- Melanin is stored in melanosomes and subsequently transferred to keratinocytes of the epidermis and shaft of the growing hair.
- Melanosomes are assembled by NCKX5 protein, encoded by SLC24A5 genes.
- Melanin turns into black when stained with silver.
- Melanophages are the dermal macrophages containing melanin pigmentation.
- Melanophores are melanosome which are unable to transfer melanin to keratinocytes.
- Melanin protects the skin from harmful ultra-violet light.
- It acts as a signal man at optic chiasma of the optic nerve and maintains K^+ pump within endolymph of cochlea in ears.

* Reduced number of melanocytes in:
  - Piebaldism
  - Waardenburg's syndrome
* Defective pigment production in:
  - Albinism, Griscelli syndrome
  - Vitiligo, Elejalde syndrome
* Defective pigment processing in:
  - Hermanskey-Pudlak syndrome
  - Chediak-Higashi syndrome
* Defective Notch signaling in:
  - Graying of hair.
  - Development or progression of melanoma.

Merkel cells

* These epidermal cells serve as mechanoceptors and respond to touch sensation.
* Origin of Merkel cells, is not yet clear but most accepted view is from the neural crest cells at 6th-7th week of gestation.
* These constitute 0.5-2% of epidermal cells and density is 50/mm^2.
* Cells are clustered around the unmyelinated sensory nerve endings to make touch spots at the bottom of the rete ridges and at the outer root sheath of the follicles around the attachment site of the arrector pili muscles.
* Sites of distribution:
  - Amongst basal keratinocytes and mostly found in hairy skin.
  - Tactile areas of glabrous skin, lip, anal canal and tongue.
  - Eccrine sweat glands.

* Number of Merkel cells are twice at sun exposed skin than covered area.
* They make a close connection with nearby sensory nerve endings and known as Merkel cell-neurite complex. This complex acts as mechanoceptor for touch sensation.
* They have an immunoreactivity for various neuropeptides like Met-encephalin, vasoactive intestinal polypeptide, enolase, synaptophysin and pancreastatin.
* They contain chromogranin.
* Electron microscopy
  * Merkel cells are oval in shape, about 15 µm in length along the long axis and oriented parallel to the basement membrane.
  * Each cell has a large bilobed nucleus and clear cytoplasm due to scarcity of intracellular organelles.
  * It contains lot of neurosecretory granules and each granule is 50-160 nm in size.
* Merkel cell in various dermatoses
  * Number is reduced or absent in vitiligo.
  * Hyperplasia is seen in association with:
    (a) nevus sebaceous, trichoblastoma, trichoepithelioma and nodular hidradenoma.
    (b) neurofibroma, neurilemmoma, nodular prurigo and neurodermatitis.
  * Autoantibodies against these cells are found in pemphigus vulgaris and graft-versus-host disease.

Langerhans cells

* These are antigen presenting dendritic epidermal cells, derived from monocyte precursors of bone marrow.
* These cells are present at spinous layer of the epidermis, outer root sheath of hair follicle, secretory duct of the sebaceous gland and epithelium of the tonsillar crypts.
* Electron microscopy:
  * Lobulated nucleus and relatively clear cytoplasm.
  * Containing cytoplasmic rod or racquet shaped granules, known as Birbeck granules.
  * These granules store Langerin protein.
* Function:
  * Phagocytosis and processing of antigens.
  * Antigen presentation and interaction with lymphocytes.
  * To release cytokines, like interleukin 1(IL1), to promote chemotaxis and to activate lymphocytes.
  * To balance immunological response and peripheral tolerance.
  * To initiate Th2 response than Th1.
  * To regulate the proinflammatory activity of the keratinocytes.
  * To carry skin-specific components to draining lymph nodes during non-inflammatory state of the skin to maintain peripheral tolerance against epidermal self-determinants.

Mast cells

* Ovoid or spindle shaped cells present in skin, bronchus, nasal mucosa and gut.
* These cells play a dominant role in adaptive and innate immunity.
* They are having a unique capability to stain metachromatically with basic aniline dyes.
* In skin, cells are mostly distributed in the subpapillary dermis with a concentration of $7000/mm^3$. They are also present close to blood vessels, nerves and appendages.
* Growth, maturation and differentiation are influenced by stem cell factor (SCF), nerve growth factor (NGF), and cytokines like IL3, IL4, IL6, IL9 and IL10.
* Mast cell proliferate by influence of IgE-dependent activation and IL4.
* Expression of Kit (CD117), a tyrosine kinase transmembrane receptor, encoded by KIT gene, dictates survival, differentiation, chemotaxis and signaling of mast cell activation.

* Two types of mast cells, connective tissue type and mucosal type, are present.
* Connective tissue type mast cells produce tryptase and chymase both but mucosal type mast cells produce only tryptase.
* Microscopic features
  - Mast cells, larger than eosinophils and basophils.
  - Usually mononuclear nucleus, occasionally binuclear and rarely having mitosis.
  - Cytoplasm containing numerous round granules.
* Mast cell activation, following crosslinking with:
  - High affinity IgE receptors.
  - Non IgE mediated activation through complement receptors.
  - Toll-like receptors.
  - IFN-γ through IgG mediated aggregation of high affinity IgE receptors.
  - SCF, complement (C3a and C5a), neuropeptides (substance P), adenosine and scavenger receptors.
* Released preformed chemicals
  - Histamine, serotonin and proteases.
* Released newly formed chemicals
  - Leukotrienes, prostaglandins, cytokines and chemokines.
* Results of mast cell activation
  - Increased vascular permeability.
  - Smooth muscle contraction.
  - Increased fibroblast activation, leading to collagen deposition.
  - Activation of B cells to synthesize IgE.
  - Recruitment of neutrophils and eosinophils.
  - Activation of basophils to produce histamine.
  - Differentiation of T cells into TH2 phenotype.
* Skin disorders related with mast cells
  - Urticaria pigmentosa
  - Allergic contact dermatitis and atopic dermatitis.
  - Immunobullous disorders and chronic graft-versus-host disease.
  - Scleroderma.
* Role of mast cell in atopic dermatitis
  - Increased number of mast cell.
  - Pruritus in atopic dermatitis is contributed by activation of PAR2 receptor (proteinase activated receptor 2) and tryptase.
  - Chymase may elicit and maintain inflammation by increasing spongiosis and compromising skin barrier.
  - Interaction of mast cell and nerves resulting in inflammation mediated by neuropeptides like substance P, NGF, calcitonin, gene related peptide and vasoactive intestinal polypeptide (VIP).

Hair follicles and hair

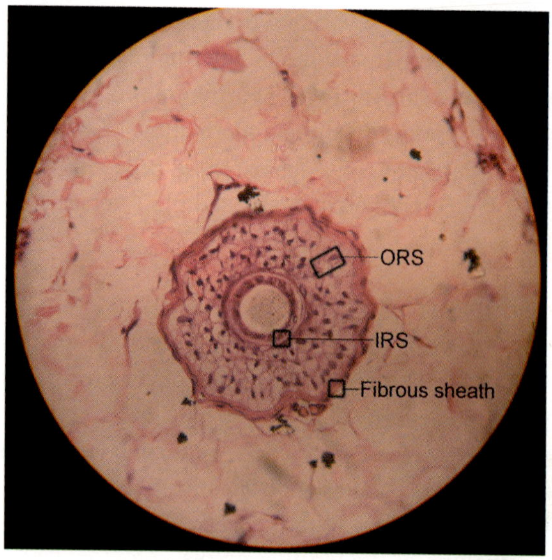

Fig. 6: Catagen follicle with apoptotic ORS, surrounded by crinkled fibrous sheath and hair shaft at the center and thin IRS between the ORS and the shaft

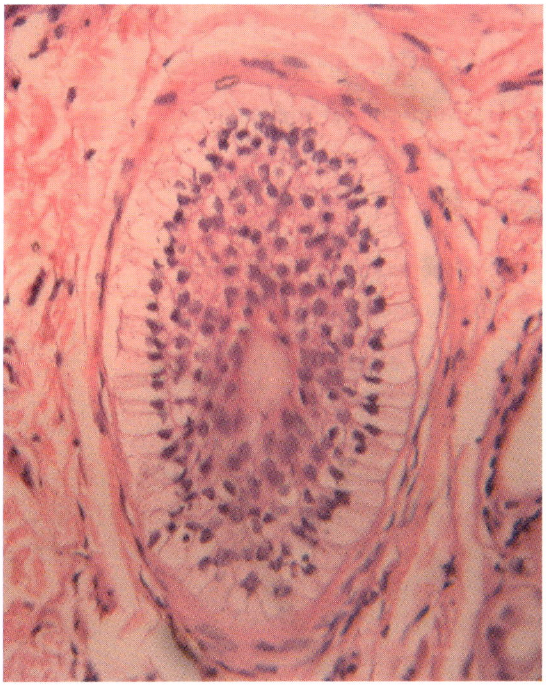

Fig. 7: Anagen follicle with broad ORS and prominent glycogen riched outer most basal layer of the ORS

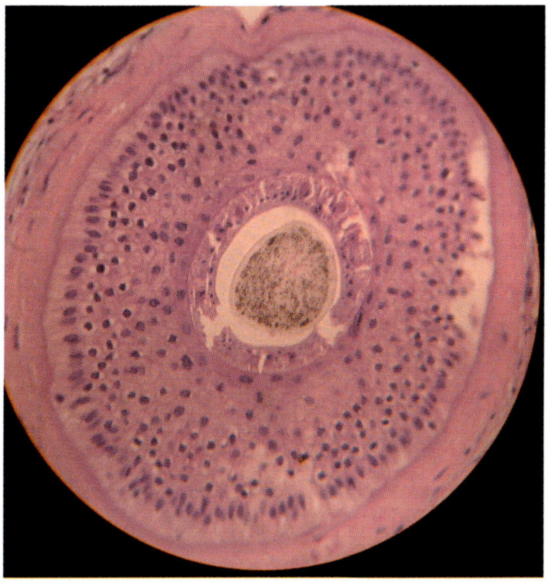

Fig. 8: Cross section of follicle at lower isthmus level showing hair shaft at the center, disintegrated IRS and broad ORS, surrounded by fibrous sheath

- Hair follicles start to develop at 9th week of gestation and hair is exposed on the surface at 20th week.
- Adamson's fringe is the distinct border between the keratinized and nonkeratinized parts of a follicle.
- Auber's line passes through the maximum diameter of the dermal papilla. Germinative basal cells lie below this line.
- Arrector pilorum muscle is attached obliquely at the mid region of the follicle, so that hair becomes erected when the muscle contracts.

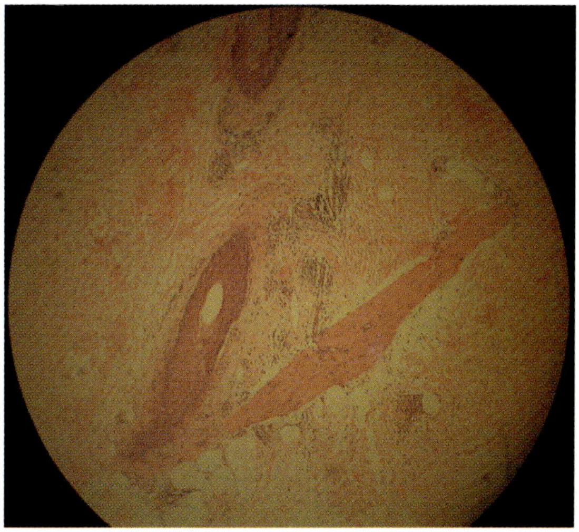

Fig. 9: Attachment of arrector pilorum muscle with the follicle

- Number of hair follicles
  - Whole body: 5 million
  - Scalp: 1 lac.
- Hair grows in a cyclic way, i.e., each hair grows to a maximum length, then regresses and falls.
- Phases of cyclical hair growth
  - Anagen phase: Hair grows in an average for 3 years and 80-90% scalp hairs remain in this phase.
  - Catagen phase: Hair follicle regresses and in an average it lasts for 3 weeks. Only 1% scalp hairs remain in this phase.

- Telogen phase: Hair rests and prepares for anagen. In an average, it lasts for 3-4 months and 10-15% scalp hairs remain in this phase.
- Exogen phase: Hair falls.
- Kenogen phase: Lag period before starting anagen.

* Growth rate of hair
  - Scalp hairs: 1.5 cm/month.
  - Hair growth maximum in March and minimum in September.

* Types of hair
  - Lanugo hair/prenatal hair: They are fine, soft, unmedullated, usually unpigmented and shed in utero at 32nd to 36th week of gestation.
  - Vellus hair/postnatal hair: They are soft, unmedullated, usually pigmented and seldom more than 2 cm in length.
  - Terminal hair: They are longer, coarser, medullated and pigmented.

* Development of hair follicle
  - Formation of follicular placode/anlarge: Aggregation of basal cells by dermal influence is the presumptive hair follicle. These are first seen at scalp and face at 10-12 weeks of geststional age.
  - Formation of dermal papilla: Follicular placode stimulates dermal aggregation at the base of the follicular placode and subsequent proliferation and downward elongation.
  - Formation of hair peg: Base of the placode invaginates dermal papilla at 12-14 weeks of gestational age.
  - Two bulges appear at 13-16 weeks of gestation. Superficial one is for development of sebaceous gland and distal one is for attachment of arrector pili muscle.
  - Complete hair canals are formed and hairs are visible on the surface at 19-21 weeks of gestation.

* Morphogenesis of hair follicle depends on
  - Regulation of Wnt
  - B catenin
  - Hedgehog signaling pathways.

* Growth of hair is maintained by
  - Epidermal growth factors
  - Transforming growth factors
  - Fibroblast growth factors
  - Bone morphogenic proteins
  - Neurotrophins.

* Function of hair follicle
  - To produce hair.
  - To protect the newly formed hair.
  - To guide the hair to come out of the skin.

* Parts of the follicle: Follicle extends from surface of the epidermis to deep dermis or dermo-subcutaneous junction.
  - Infundibulum, extending from surface to opening of sebaceous gland.
  - Isthmus, extending from opening of sebaceous gland to insertion site of arrector pili muscle.
  - Stem, extending from isthmus to Adamson's fringe.
  - Bulb, extending from Adamson's fringe to lower end of the follicle.

* Segments of hair follicle
  - Transitory segment/lower segment: Segment of the follicle beneath the isthmus, includes stem and bulb of the follicle. It is transitory because it disappears during catagen phase and reappears during anagen phase.
  - Fixed segment/upper segment: This includes isthmus and infundibulum, and it is not actively involved in hair cycle.

* Changes of hair follicle at catagen phase
  - Loss of metachromasia from the follicular papillae, indicating loss of mucin.
  - Matricial cells stop proliferation.
  - Melanocytes in the bulb regress, and stop to produce and transfer melanin to keratinocytes.

- Melanin instead of taken by keratinocytes, is engulfed by macrophages present at the papillae and nearby dermis.
- Many of the individual keratinocytes of the outer root sheath (ORS) undergo necrosis, as a part of the programmed cell death or apoptosis. This cell necrosis is indicated by karyorrhexis or fragmented nucleus.
- Due to this apoptosis, ORS is turned into a keratinizing sac, identical to ORS of the isthmus and the follicle becomes club shaped.
- A thin column of epithelial cells connects the hair papilla with the club follicle. This is surrounded by a thickened and corrugated glassy basement membrane zone.
- Perifollicular fibrous tissue sheath also becomes thickened, wrinkled and folded.
- At the end of the catagen whole of these altered basement membrane zone and fibrous sheath are reabsorbed and reappear during anagen.

* Changes during telogen
  - Epithelial cells of the club follicle further regress and the club steadily moves upwards along with the papilla.
  - As the papilla goes up and the column of epithelium shortens, a streamer of fibrous tissue is formed along the perifollicular fibrous sheath.
  - Ultimately the club is reached at the site of insertion of arrector pilorum muscle where the germ cells are present for future production of hair follicle.
  - Cross section of the club follicle appears as a rectangle and closely set basaloid cells are arranged in a palisaded fashion at the periphery of the rectangle. These cells act as germ cells which proliferate and differentiate into new follicle at the beginning of the anagen.

* Changes during anagen
  - Re-establishment of the intimate relation between the papilla and germ cells of the club hair reconstitutes the matrix.
  - This newly formed matrix enlarges, elongates and moves downward along the previous fibrous streamer.

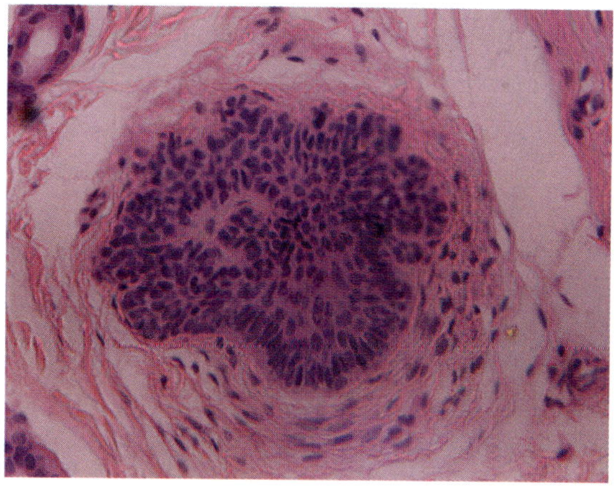

Fig. 10: Cross section of a club follicle.

  - As it goes down the lower end becomes bulbous to invaginate the papilla. Thus a new follicular bulb is formed.
  - Melanocytes get back their dendritic form and start melanization.
  - Matricial cells gradually proliferate and differentiate into various layers like outer root sheath, inner root sheath and hair shaft.
  - Newly formed hair goes upward and dislodges the older one which lies within the infundibulum.
  - Root of anagen hair is deeply pigmented and is surrounded by translucent inner sheath.

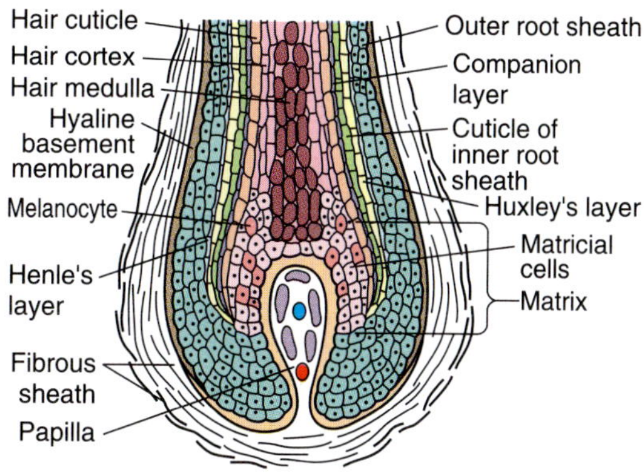

Fig. 11: Ultrastructures of hair bulb

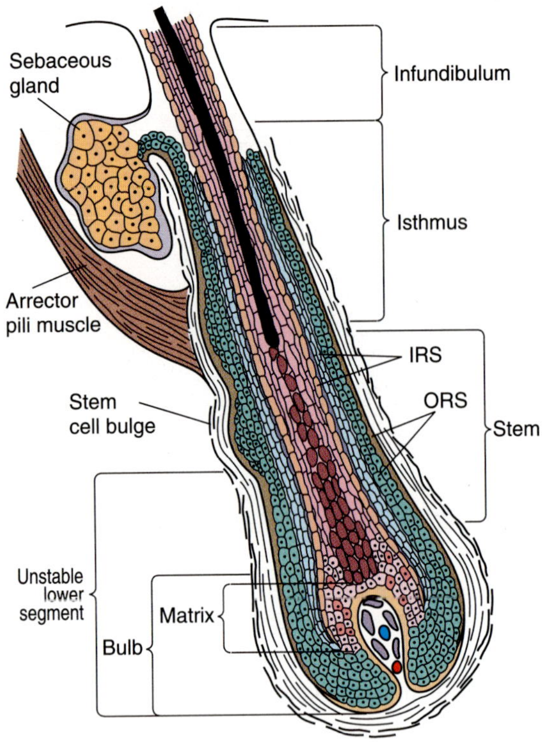

Fig. 12: Structures of the hair follicle

* Layers of the hair follicle
  - Hair shaft
  - Inner root sheath (IRS), extending from bulb to middle of the isthmus to take care of the newly formed tender hair shaft.
  - Outer root sheath (ORS), basically downward extension of the epidermis, covers the entire follicle. It is composed of pale and clear cells. Outermost cells are arranged perpendicular to the basement membrane and it is surrounded by a fibrous sheath.
* Layers of the hair shaft
  - Medulla
  - Cortex
  - Cuticle
* Layers of the inner root sheath
  - Cuticle: It is one cell thick and fully keratinized. It interdigitates with the cuticle of hair shaft.
  - Huxley's layer: It is two cells thick and con tains lot of trichohyaline granules.
  - Henle's layer: It is one cell thick and keratinized first among all other layers.
* **Layers of the follicle at the level of the isthmus:** There are eight concentric rings from inside to outside.
  - Medulla
  - Cortex
  - Cuticle of the hair shaft
  - A companion layer is present between two cuticles.
  - Cuticle of the inner root sheath (IRS)
  - Huxley layer of IRS
  - Henle layer of IRS
  - Epidermal layer of outer root sheath
  - Fibrous sheath
* Hair canal is formed by premature death of central core cells of hair follicle before being keratinized.
* Hair keratinization
  - Henle's layer is keratinized first, followed by two cuticles, Huxley's layer and hair cortex.
  - Medulla is last to be keratinized.
  - Hair cortex is keratinized by losing the nuclei and not from the trichohyaline granules. So, the keratin of cortex is hard.
  - Inner root sheath (IRS) is keratinized from trichohyalin granules which produce soft keratin and known as trichilemmal keratinization. This keratin is bright pink in comparision to epidermal keratin, formed by keratohyaline keratinization.
  - Part of the outer root (ORS) sheath below the isthmus is accompanied by inner root sheath and does not go under keratinization. ORS cells have clear, vacuolated cytoplasm due to presence of considerable amount of glycogen.

- At the middle of the isthmus, where IRS becomes disintegrated, keratinization of ORS starts.
- Infundibular part is keratinized from keratohyaline granules.

Sebaceous glands

- These glands develop from epidermis at 13th-16th week of gestation.

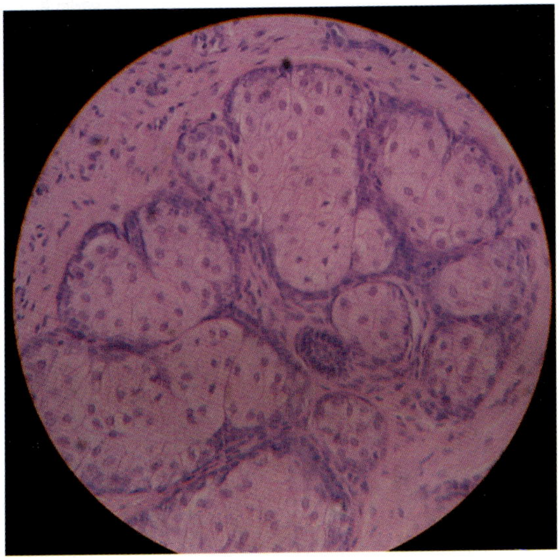

Fig. 13: A pilosebaceous unit contains multilobed sebaceous gland centering a follicle

- So, they are present at birth and produce relatively high amount of sebum but then reduce till puberty.
- At puberty due to influence of androgens, specially 5α-dihydrotestosterone (DHT), again sebum production as well as size of the glands increase.
- At the end of puberty, sebum production remains constant throughout adulthood, and then declines after menopause in females and sixth to seventh decade in males.
- In last stage, androgen receptors are translocated at nucleus and androgens lose its influence.
- These glands are always associated with hair follicles, except those are found at lips and other mucosal surfaces.
- Glands are distributed mostly at scalp, face, upper back, chest, midline of the back, axillae and groin.
- Fordyce spots are nothing but ectopic sebaceous glands present at lips and glans penis.
- Each gland consists of cauliflower like convoluted glandular and ductal parts.
- The ductal part connects the gland with the infundibulum of the hair follicle.
- Sebaceous gland and its duct along with infundibulum and hair make a pilosebaceous unit.
- There are three types of pilosebaceous units:
  - Vellus follicle, having a small sebaceous gland around a short thin hair.
  - Sebaceous follicle, having a large multilobular sebaceous gland around a mid sized hair.
  - Terminal hair follicle, having a fairly large sebaceous gland around a long thick hair.
- Sebaceous follicles are most commonly found at face, upper chest and upper back and these sites correspond development of acne vulgaris.
- Upper part of the infundibulum is keratinized by keratohyaline granules as it is lined by granular layer but lower part is keratinized from trichilemmal granules as it is not lined by granular layer.
- Each gland produces sebum and releases it by holocrine process into infundibular portion of the hair follicle.
- Sebocytes are the structural and functional units of sebaceous gland and their turnover time is about 14 days.
- In a healthy adult, rate of sebum production is 1 mg/10 cm^2 in 3 hours.
- Sebum production less than 0.5 mg/10 cm^2 in every 3 hours, is considered as dry skin and 1.5-4 mg/10 cm^2 in 3 hours is considered as high and clinically induces seborrhea.
- Pilosebaceous unit is having a rich bacterial and fungal flora as a part of normal flora.
  - Desquamated scales of upper infundibulum contains *Malassezia spp*. fungi.

- ♦ Mid portion of the infundibulum contains *Staphylococcus epidermidis* and other micrococci.
- ♦ Deeper portion of the infundibulum contains *Propionibacterium spp.*
- ♦ Hair follicles of elderly person also contains a mite, *Demodex folliculorum*.

* **Composition of sebum:** Sebum is a light yellow viscous fluid, produced by the sebaceous glands and consists of:
    - ♦ Triglycerides, free fatty acids, squalenes,
    - ♦ Wax and sterol esters, and free sterols.
* **Function of sebum**
    - It repels rain from skin and hair.
    - It plays a thermoregulatory function. Emulsification of eccrine sweat, leads to formation of a sweat sheet and thus it prevents loss of individual sweat drops from the skin.
    - It keeps the skin soft and moist.

Eccrine sweat glands

* These glands first appear at palms and soles around 12th week of gestation.
* They are distributed in whole skin sparing mucosae.
* Though the glands are present at birth but they fully function only after age of 2 years.
* The secretory parts of the glands are situated deep to the dermis and subcutaneous tissue and their ducts open directly at the skin surface.
* Ductal part within the epidermis is known as acrosyringium.
* Myoepithelial cells are arranged longitudinally and provide support and help to secrete sweat on cholinergic stimuli.
* **Salient features**
    - ♦ Number of sweat glands: 2.5 million.
    - ♦ Concentration of sweat glands at palms and soles: 620/cm^2.
    - ♦ Total weight of sweat glands: 100 gm.
    - ♦ Sweat is hypotonic and contains sodium, potassium, urea and lactate.
    - ♦ pH of sweat is variable from 4.0-6.8.
    - ♦ Size of each eccrine gland: 20 μm but apocrine gland is 200 μm.
    - ♦ Maximum amount of sweat formation: 1.8 litre per hour and 5 litre per day.

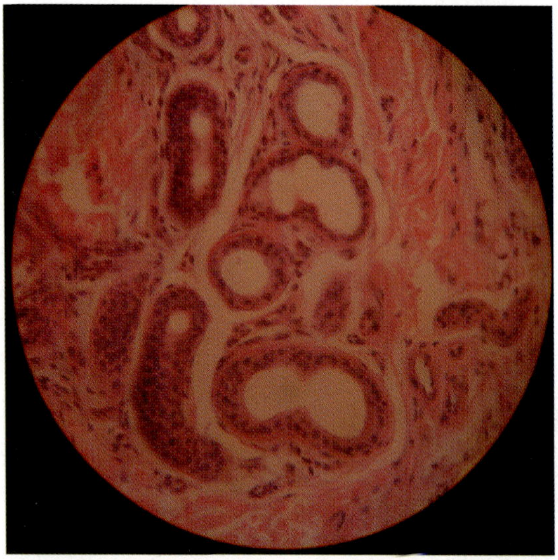

Fig. 14: Eccrine glands

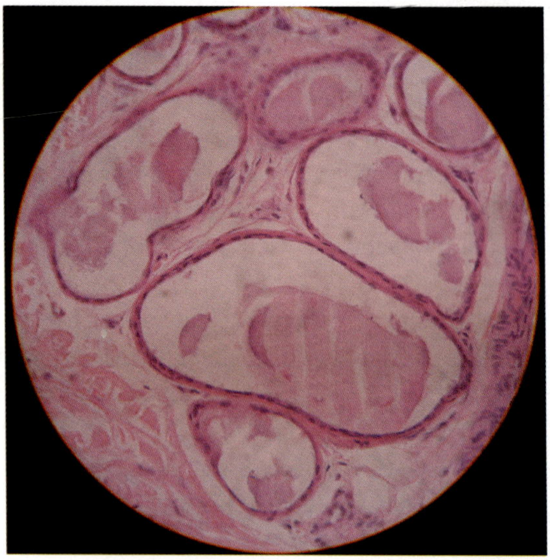

Fig. 15: Apocrine glands

- **Functions of sweat**
  - It helps to cool the skin through evaporation and by convection of heat.
  - It moistens the palms and soles for better grip.

Apocrine sweat glands

- These glands develop between 12th to 15th week of gestation as a part of pilosebaceous unit.

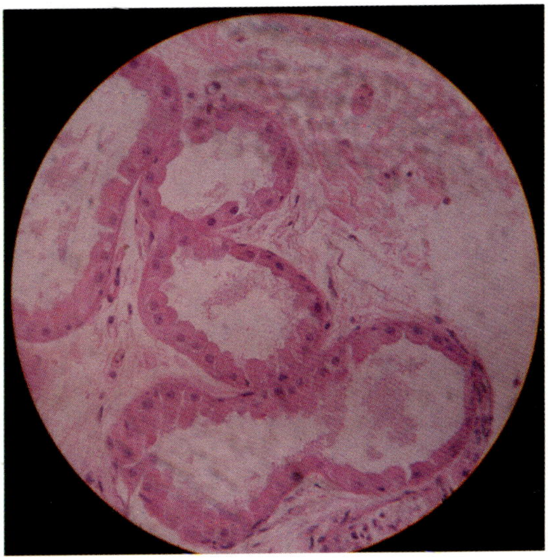

Fig. 16: Large size glands, lined by decapitated secretory epithelium

- Glands are distributed at axillae, areola and perianal regions.
- Secretory part of each gland is situated at subcutaneous tissue and duct opens at infundibulum of the follicle just above the opening of the sebaceous duct.
- The glands secrete odorless oily fluid. But due to bacterial decomposition this may be colored and foul smelling.
- Only axillary glands can produce such odor. The main substance responsible for this odor is 3-methyl-2 hexenoic acid.

Collagen tissue

- This fibrous tissue family is the principal constituent of the dermis.
- There are at least 15 genetically distinct types of collagen.
- It shares 70% of the dry weight of the skin.
- It is synthesized by the fibroblast within the rough endoplasmic reticulum.
- It consists of myofibrils and myofibrils are made of polypeptide chains with a helical arrangement.
- Main aminoacids are hydroxyproline, hydroxylysine and glycine.
- Fine collagen fibers are seen in papillary dermis but coarse fibers are seen in reticular dermis.
- Main function of collagen tissue is to resist the stress.
- Defective collagen synthesis is seen in Ehlers-Danlos syndrome, cutis laxa and osteogenesis imperfecta.
- **Major types of collagen, related to skin**
  - Type I is present in reticular dermis and each fiber has cross-striation at regular interval of 68 nm. It is increased in scleroderma.
  - Type III is present in papillary dermis.
  - Type IV is present in lamina densa of basement membrane zone.
  - Type VII is present in sublamina densa of basement membrane zone as anchoring fibrils. Defective function of this type is seen in epidermolysis bullosa dystrophica, epidermolysis bullosa acquisita and bullous lupus erythematosus.
  - Type XVII is present at lamina lucida of basement membrane zone as anchoring filaments.

Elastic tissue

- It is also synthesized by fibroblasts but differs from collagen tissues both in structurally and chemically.
- It is composed of filamentous protein and amorphous protein, elastin.
- Unique proteins of elastic tissue are desmosine and isodesmosine.

* Elastic fibers are fine in papillary dermis but coarse in reticular dermis.
* Main function is to maintain elasticity of the skin.
* Defective elastic tissue synthesis is seen in Marfan syndrome and pseudoxanthoma elasticum.

Extracellular matrix or ground substance of the dermis

* It is composed of glycosaminoglycans, synthesized by the fibroblasts.
* These glycosaminoglycans are made up of acid mucopolysaccharides, neutral mucopolysaccharides and electrolytes.
* Acid mucopolysaccharides are chondroitin sulfate and dermatan sulfate.
* Hyaluronic acid is a minor mucopolysaccharide but increases in pathological states.
* Hyaluronic acid stains with colloidal iron or stains metachromically with alcian blue and toludine blue at higher pH.
* Acid mucopolysaccharides stain at pH 3.0 and 0.5 with alcian blue and stain metachromically with toluidine blue at both pH 3.0 and 1.5.
* Hyaluronic acid synthesis is increased in lupus erythematosus and dermatomyositis.

Nails

* Nails are rectangular, strong and relatively non-flexible keratinous plates.
* These lie at the distal part of digits and remain firmly attached with the respective nail bed.
* All margins of the nail are partially covered by nail folds except distal one.
* Proximal nail fold covers 1/4th of the nail plate.
* Overhanging minute nail fold is known as cuticle.
* Lunula is the whitish half moon shaped part of the nail at the proximal portion.
* Nail plate is pink due to its relative translucency and rich vascularity of the nail bed.
* Proximal part of the nail bed is known as nail matrix which actually produces the nail plate.
* Nail grows distally and becomes separated from the nail bed at the distal end. This open part between the nail bed and nail plate is known as hyponychium.
* Nail plate is rich in calcium, phospholipid and hard keratin.
* Retained nuclei in the cells of nail plate is known as pertinax bodies.
* Nail matrix also contains melanocytes.
* Dermal collagen fibers are vertically oriented at nail bed and become attached with phalangeal periosteum.
* Nail bed contains vessels, lymphatics, elastic fibers and eccrine sweat glands.
* Arterio-venous anastomosis at the nail bed is known as glomus bodies.
* Glomus bodies serve to maintain circulation during cold weather.
* **Nail growth rate**
    - Finger nail: 3 mm per month.
    - Toe nail: 1 mm per month.
* **Nail keratinization**
    - Dorsal surface of proximal nail fold (PNF) undergoes epidermal type of keratinization and keratin is soft.
    - Ventral surface of PNF undergoes onycholemmal keratinization and keratin is semi-hard.
    - Nail bed undergoes onycholemmal type of keratinization.
    - Nail plate undergoes trichilemmal type of keratinization and keratin is hard due to rich sulfur bonds.
* **Function of nail**
    - Protection of the distal parts of the digits.
    - Pinching and holding fine objects.
    - Self protection.
    - To maintain cosmetic role.

Subcutaneous tissue/hypodermis

- It lies between dermis and fascia of the muscle and contains compact fat cells or adipocytes.
- Adipocytes are arranged in small groups, centering an arteriole, known as microlobules.
- A group of microlobules, separated by fibrous structures or septa is known as macrolobule. Septa houses the dermal structures like blood vessels, lymphatics and nerves.
- Size of each adipocyte is 100 μm, each microlobule is 1 mm and macrolobule is 1 cm.

Nerve supply of the skin

* Nerve supply of skin is derived from:
    - Somatic sensory nervous system
    - Autonomic motor nervous system
* Both the nervous system are developed from neural crest.

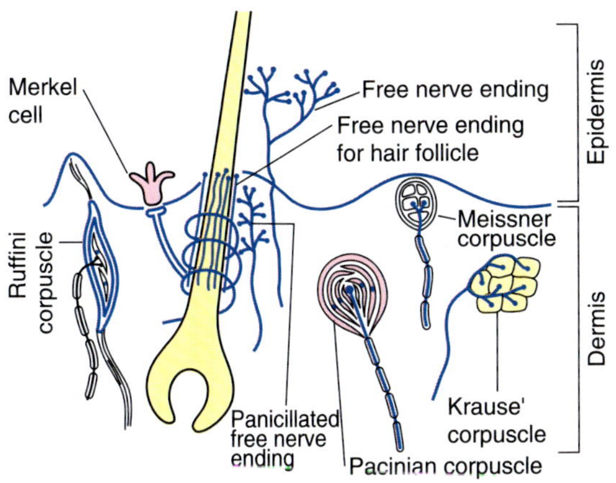

Fig. 17: Neural network of the skin

* This peripheral nervous system is comprised of dorsal root ganglia, sympathetic ganglia, Schwann cells, endonureal sheath cells and the laminar cells of specialized sensory end organs and Merkel cell.
* Skin contains an extensive neural network. This network is composed of following:
    - Cholinergic and adrenergic nerves.
    - Myelinated and unmyelinated sensory fibers.
* Skin also contains several transducers for perception of touch, pressure and vibration.

* **Somatic sensory system**

- It mediates the sensation of pain, itch, temperature, light touch, pressure, vibration, propioception, and epicritical or discriminative sensation of touch.
- Cell bodies of all these nerves remain within the dorsal root ganglion.
- **Autonomic motor nervous system:** It controls
    - Cutaneous vascular tone
    - Pilomotor response
    - Sudomotor activity.

* **Specialized sensory receptors**
    - These possess terminal nerve endings, formed by lamellar condensation of connective tissue and Schwann cells.
    - Merkel cells are present amongst the basal cells.
    - Nerve endings are present along the basement membrane.
    - Meissner's corpuscles and Pacinian corpuscles are present in the deeper dermis.
    - Ruffini corpuscles are present surrounding hair follicles.

* **Pacinian corpuscles**
    - These are present mostly in the deep dermis and subcutaneous tissue at pressure bearing areas like lips, penis, clitoris and nipples.
    - They serve as mechanoceptors and detect the sensation of pressure.
    - Size of each corpuscle is 0.8 × 1.5 mm and supplied by a myelinated axon that makes several turns before entering the capsule to connect the bulbar sensory terminal.
    - This bulbar sensory terminal is devoid of myelin sheath. This is surrounded by laminar cells which are modified Schwann cells. So, the nerve terminal connect the laminar cells directly.
    - The action potential generated during a distortion, is amplified due to the concentric arrangement of the laminar cells.

- **Meissner corpuscles**
  - These are present at tips of dermal papillae and mostly at finger tips.
  - They act as rapidly adapting mechanoceptors that detect light touch.
  - Size of each corpuscle is 50 × 150 μm.
  - It is composed of layers of flattened laminar cells. The axon weaves back and forth between stacks of laminar cells.
  - Some of the laminar cells or axons have direct contact with basal keratinocytes.
- **Mucocutaneous end organs**
  - They are predominantly located in the subpapillary connective tissue of glans penis, prepuce, clitoris, labia minora, perianal area, eyelids and lips.
  - They act as touch receptor.
  - Though Pacinian and Meissner corpuscles may be visualized under light microscope with hematoxylin and eosin stain, these nerve endings are not visible with same method.
  - Size of each nerve ending is about 50 μm in diameter.
  - It consists of loosely arranged branched axon which forms an irregular oval mass. There is no true capsule around the mass. Several myelinated nerve fibers may connect each nerve ending or they connect one end organ with another.
  - It contains a lobular unit formed by concentric lamellar processes.
- **Unspecialized sensory receptors**
  - They are millions in number.
  - Some are associated with follicles and others are not.
  - They may be visualized by light microscopy with special stain like silver salt, methylene blue or cholinesterase.
  - Hair follicles are supplied by highly branched myelinated sensory nerves.
  - Each axon supplies several follicles and similarly one follicle is supplied by several different axons.
  - Isthmus of each follicle exclusively has these neural network.
  - Papillary dermis is supplied by horizontally oriented network of unmyelinated axons, terminated at dermoepidermal junction to make contact between basal lamina of Schwann cell and basal lamina of basal cell.
  - Free nerve endings are profusely seen at glans penis.
- **Transmission of sensations**
  - Heavily myelinated βA fibers of cranial and spinal nerves, having 10-14 μm in diameter, rapidly conduct discriminative sensations of touch, vibration and propioception.
  - Moderately myelinated γA fibers of narrower diameter, conduct light touch and pressure.
  - Thinly myelinated δA fibers conduct pain, temperature and physiological itching. Physiological itching is casual and well localized.
  - Unmyelinated C fibers, having diameter less than 5 μm slowly conduct sensations of pain, temperature and pathological itching. Pathological itching is very unpleasant and poorly localized.
- **Autonomic nervous system**
  - It supplies neuroeffector fibers to the skin.
  - Unmyelinated sympathetic postganglionic nerves, arborize into terminal autonomic plexuses which ultimate innervate smooth muscles of hair follicle, apocrine and eccrine glands, and cutaneous blood vessels.
- **Hair erection**
  - Muscle of hair erection is arrector pilorum muscle, innervated by unmyelinated adrenergic nerves and when impulses originate within the nerves, the muscle contracts and hair becomes erected.
- **Apocrine and eccrine gland secretion**
  - They are supplied by unmyelinated adrenergic and cholinergic nerves.

- Apocrine secretion is mainly controlled by adrenergic activity.
- Widespread eccrine activity is controlled by cholinergic activity to regulate high temperature.

* **Vasoconstriction and vasodilation**
  - Stimulation of adrenergic fibers causes vasoconstriction as it works on α receptors of vascular smooth muscles.
  - Vasodilation occurs in an indirect way, by sympathetic blockade.
  - Arteriovenous shunts or Glomus bodies, present at hands, feet, nose and ears, i.e., acral parts, are supplied by parasympathetic cholinergic nerves and these are controlled by degree of tonic sympathetic vasoconstriction.

Blood supply

* Vascular supply of the skin is embryologically an intricate network of mesenchymal cells which surround arborizing spaces.

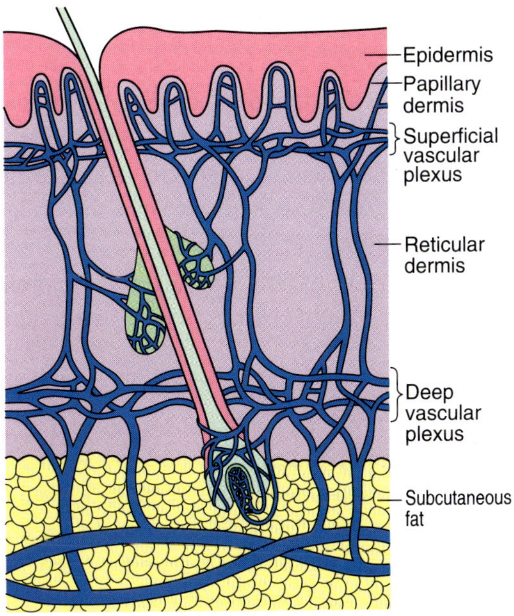

Fig. 18: Vascular network of the skin

* Dermal blood vessels are arranged in
  - Superficial plexus of arterioles and venules
  - Communicating vessels, containing arteries and veins
  - Deep plexus of arterioles and venules.
* Superficial plexus is positioned at the upper part of the papillary dermis, just below the papillary dermis and so, it is known as subpapillary plexus.
* Deep plexus is positioned in the lower part of the reticular dermis.
* These two plexuses lie parallel to the skin surface.
* Communicating vessels are straight, perpendicular to the skin surface, and they communicate the two plexuses and among themselves.
* From the superficial plexus, an arcade of capillary loop goes upward within each dermal papilla.
* Each capillary loop is formed by an arteriole ascending up, followed by a hairpin bend downward to be converted into a venule. This venule drains into postcapillary venule before merging with superficial plexus from there dermal communicating veins draining into deep plexus and after that into subcutaneous small veins.
* Similarly subcutaneous small arteries supply the deep plexus, from where communicating arteries connect the superficial plexus to supply the ascending arteriole of the capillary loop.
* Superficial and deep plexuses anastomose each other profusely, specially around the pilosebaceous unit and sweat apparatus. This arrangement helps an alternative circulation when one of the channel is blocked.
* Cross section of larger arteries of deeper dermis and subcutaneous tissue contains:
  - Intima, composed of endothelial cells and internal elastic membrane;
  - Media, composed of collagen, nonlayered elastic fibers and concentric layers of smooth muscle and external elastic membrane.
  - Adventitia, composed of fibrocytes, type III collagen and elastic fibers.

* **Smaller arteries of superficial dermis**
    - Not have any internal or elastic membranes and their walls contain a discontinuous layer of elastic fibers and smooth muscle cells.
* **Ascending arteriole of the papillary loop**
    - Contains only single layer of endothelial cells, lining a narrow lumen, and surrounded by a discontinuous layer of pericytes.
    - The endothelial cells and pericytes are surrounded by a continuous basal lamina.
* **Descending venous segment of the capillary loop**
    - Lumen is wider and surrounded by numerous pericytes and multilayered basal lamina.
* Gradually walls of the venules become thicker from post capillary venules to subcutaneous veins. Walls of the larger venule contains variable amount of smooth muscle and elastic fibers but no elastic membrane. Large veins have valves and only few are having internal elastic membrane.
* **Post capillary venule**
    - It consists of endothelial cells, pericytes, basal lamina and thin layer of type III collagen.
* Veil cells are flat adventitial cells and present entirely outside the walls of the arterioles, capillaries and venules. They separate the vessels from the surrounding dermis.
* **Electron microscopy of an endothelial cell**
    - Presence of bundles of cytoplasmic filaments, of 7.5-10 μm in diameter.
    - Presence of electron-dense rod-shaped cytoplasmic structures, size 0.1 × 0.3 μm, consisting of longitudinally oriented tubules, embedded in a dense matrix. These are known as Weibel-Palade bodies. They are infrequently seen in endothelial cells of dermal vessels.
* Capillaries of the skin are mostly lined by continuous layer of endothelial cells and they are attached with specialized intercellular junction. Serum fluid and small water soluble particles exchange from lumina to pericapillary tissue via transport through micropinocytic vesicles. Post-capillary venules are the most permeable parts, through which water, oxygen, carbondioxide, nutrients, hormones and toxins are exchanged. So, they are the frequent target of the pathological challenge.
* Fenestrated capillaries are present adjacent to the eccrine glands and follicular bulbs and allow passage of larger molecules, such as plasma proteins, through the gaps between the endothelial cells. These intercellular gaps may be widened by contraction of actin filaments.
* Each pericyte makes tight junction with 2-4 endothelial cells by breaking the basal lamina. These interdigitating contact points between pericytes and endothelial cell, are rich in fibronectin. Pericyte actually control the inter-endothelial cell gaps during any inflammatory process and thus the amount of leakage.
* This function of pericyte depends on many vasoactive substances like prostaglandins and histamines released by leukocytes, mast cells and platelets during inflammation.

Glomus bodies

* They allow shunting of blood directly from arteriole to venule bypassing the capillary bed.
* They are abundant at acral skin areas like fingers, toes, nail beds, nose and ears to regulate temperature.
* Each body is having one arterial segment, known as Sacquyet-Hoyer canal and venous segment.
    - Sacquyet-Hoyer canal: This segment is having narrow lumen and thick wall. Wall contains endothelium, surrounded by 3-6 layers of modified smooth muscle cells, known as glomus cells. Each glomus cell has a uniform ovoid nucleus, pale staining cytoplasm and indistinct cell margin. These cells are innervated by unmyelinated adrenergic nerves.
    - Venous segment: It is thin-walled and has larger lumen. It drains into subpapillary venules.

- Normal skin receives 5-10% of cardiac output. But in extreme temperature to lose heat, it may rise up to 7 folds and come down to zero in extreme cold to conserve heat.
- **Factors causing vasoconstriction**
  - Angiotensin II, vasopressin, epinephrine and local cooling.
- **Factors causing vasodilatation**
  - Ethanol, histamine, prostaglandin E and local heat.

Lymphatic supply

- These are arranged parallel to the vascular plexuses.
- Their function is to clear fluids, macromolecules, cells, foreign materials from the interstitial spaces.
- They provide the passage for immunoglobulins, antigens and Langerhans cells to perform immunological function. So, any aberration of lymphatics, tissues become vulnerable to infection.
- Superficial plexus of lymphatic capillaries are positioned at upper part of the reticular dermis, just beneath the superficial venous plexus and 200 μm below the epidermis.
- Lymphatic vessels are surrounded by elastic fibers.
- Elastic fibers are oriented in such a suitable manner, so that the waste products can pass through the lymphatics easily.
- Lymphatic channels are supported by fine collagen fibrils. They are attached in a right angle to the wall, so that can act as anchoring filaments and thus prevent collapsing. Lymphatic capillaries are lined by attenuated endothelial cell without any fenestrae. They lack pericyte and basal lamina is discontinuous. They are having very few pinocytic vesicles.
- There are wide gaps between overlapping endothelial cells which permit filtration and removal of fluids, macromolecules, inflammatory cells, etc. from the extracellular compartment of the dermis.

Permeability of the skin

- Skin is an essentially impermeable membrane which protects the body from noxious external insults as well as limits water and heat loss to maintain a balance. But truly it is not completely impermeable.
- The permeability of the skin has regional variation and it also varies according to the age.
- For therapeutic purposes, this permeability may be enhanced without disturbing the normal function of the skin.
- Chemical impermeability almost exclusively is served by the stratum corneum and lesser extent by other layers of the epidermis.
- Skin acts as a barrier to absorption of most of the substances and permits entry of some selective substances.
- But this permeability often becomes compromised in various diseases which dictates the prognosis of the diseases as well as options for therapy.

Barriers to absorption

- Principal barrier of percutaneous absorption is the stratum corneum.
- Barrier function depends on thickness of the stratum corneum, concentration of corneocytes and geometrical organization of the corneocytes.
- Stratum corneum follows a bricks and mortar model where protein rich dead cells are bricks and lipid within the intercellular spaces is mortar. Selective permeability depends on the intactness of this model.

Routes of percutaneous absorption

- There are three possible routes:
  - Through stratum corneum
  - Through the pilosebaceous apparatus
  - Through the sweat ducts.
- Absorption through the stratum corneum occurs by diffusion which follows the Fick's law.

This law says that rate of absorption of a chemical is proportional to the concentration difference across a membrane. So, a concentration gradient between the high concentration of a solute on the skin surface and its absence or very low concentration below the stratum corneum produces a driving force and this force allows the substance to enter across the skin.

* Intracellular protein fibers allow the entry of polar or water soluble (hydrophilic) substances and intercellular lipid layer allows the entry of lipophilic substances.
* Hair follicles and sweat ducts act as easy pathways for certain substances like ions, polar compounds, large molecules which cannot pass through the stratum corneum easily.

Factors influencing percutaneous absorption and clinical correlations

* Hyperemic skin, due to increased blood flow as in erythroderma, enhances absorptive power.
* Occlusion and hydration of stratum corneum increases absorption. Hydration increases size of the corneocytes and increases intercellular spaces and thus enhances absorption of both lipophilic and hydrophilic compounds. For irritant substance like tretinoin and aluminum compounds should be applied on dry skin to limit their absorption and on the other hand cytotoxic drugs or antiviral drugs should be applied on moist or hydrated skin for better absorption.
* Denudation of the skin due to disease or chemical influences absorption. In diseases like toxic epidermal necrolysis, Stevens-Johnson syndrome, pemphigus and burns, due to complete or partial loss of epidermis, there is a dramatic change in absorption capacity.
* In disease like psoriasis in which skin barrier is imperfectly formed, enhances absorption.
* Mucous membrane has 10-15 times more absorptive power than skin due to lack of stratum corneum.
* **Regional variations in absorption capacity**
    * Changes of pH influence the absorption as it causes ionization and ionization reduces absorption.
    * Eyelids and scrotal skin have highest absorptive power due to thinnest stratum corneum and the palms and soles have the lowest due to thickest stratum corneum.
    * Absorption also depends on the total area on which a compound is applied.
    * Thickened stratum corneum of neurodermatitis or ichthyosis may act as a reservoir but psoriatic skin does not have this.
* Lipid and lipid soluble substances pass easily than water and water soluble substances. So, chemical quality of a substance influences absorption.
* Smaller molecules are absorbed easily than larger molecules.
* Gaseous state of a compound except carbon monoxide is absorbed faster.
* Metabolic capability and enzymatic activity of skin influence absorption. A highly lipophilic substance following absorption enhances the rate of absorption.
* Nature of the vehicle influences the absorption of the incorporated compound. An ointment maintains hydration of the skin and thus increase the absorption of the incorporated substance. Also the degree of partition coefficient also influences the absorption. Some vehicles injure the stratum corneum and thus increase absorption.

Absorption accelerants

* Passage of some compounds through the skin can be enhanced by some chemical and physical enhancers or accelerants. These are:
    * Stripping of horny layer
    * Heat
    * Ultrasound
    * Iontophoresis
    * Urea, acts by enhancing hydration and by proteolytic effect.

- Salicylic acid acts as keratolytic agent and thus enhances absorption.
- Chemicals like ethanol, propylene glycol, pyrrolidones, dimethylacetamide, dimethylformamide and dimethyl sulfoxide are known enhancer of absorption.
- Other chemical enhancer under experiment are alkyl sulfoxide, phosphine oxide, surfactants, caprolactam and azepines.

Dermatopathology

Orthokeratosis

- Normal basket-weave stratum corneum is termed as orthokeratosis.
- But this normal thickness is variable from site to site of the body skin as thickest at soles and thinnest at eyelids.

Hyperkeratosis

- The term is used when stratum corneum becomes thicker than usual thickness.
- It may or may not be associated with parakeratosis.
- It is commonly seen in psoriasis, lichen planus, keratoderma, wart, etc.

Parakeratosis

- The term is used when nuclei are retained within the corneocytes.

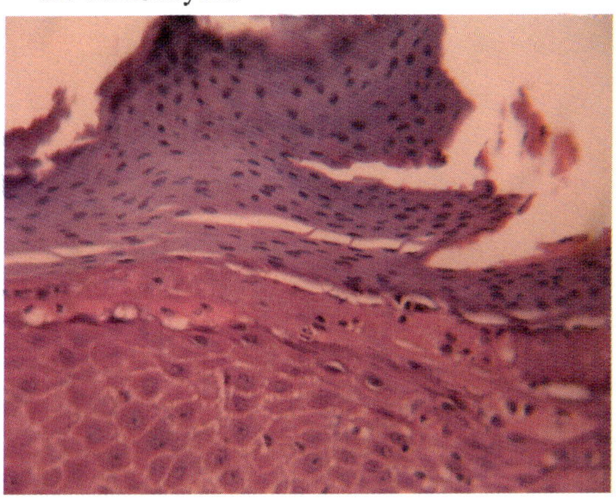

Fig. 19: Confluent parakeratosis

Patterns of parakeratosis

- Focal parakeratosis: Patchy parakeratosis, seen in pityriasis rosea.
- Mound parakeratosis: Focal heaped up parakeratosis seen in Reiter's disease.
- Checker-board parakeratosis: Vertically as well as horizontally and regularly arranged focal parakeratosis, seen in pityriasis rubra pilaris and plantar psoriasis.
- Shoulder parakeratosis: Focal parakeratosis present at shoulder of the follicle, seen in pityriasis rubra pilaris and seborrheic dermatitis.
- Column parakeratosis: A column of parakeratosis is arranged vertically, seen in porokeratosis as cornoid lamella and in verruca vulgaris.
- Alternate parakeratosis: Horizontally or vertically arranged linear parakeratosis alternating with ortho-keratosis, seen in psoriasis and linear verrucous epidermal nevus (ILVEN).
- Sandwich parakeratosis: A band of parakeratosis between orthokeratosis at above and below, seen in tinea corporis. Parakeratotic part embeds fungal hyphae in tinea corporis.
- Confluent/diffuse parakeratosis: Extensive parakeratosis involving full thickness of stratum corneum, seen in psoriasis.
- Granular parakeratosis: In true sense, there is no parakeratosis. Actually external powder or dusts get deposited within stratum corneum, mimicking those as nuclei of keratinocytes.

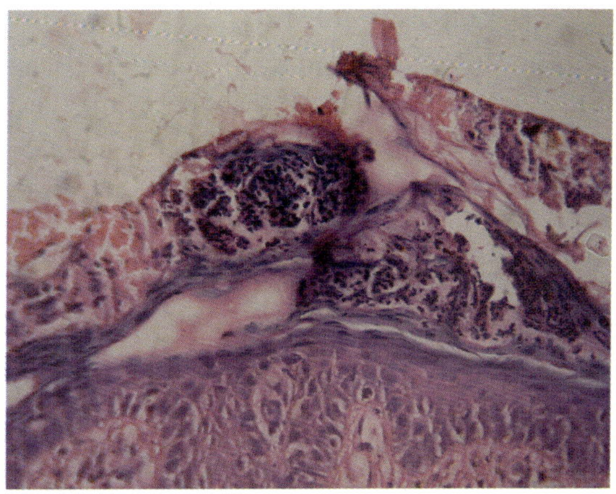

Fig. 20: Mound parakeratosis

- Hypergranulosis: Increased thickness of granular layer, classically seen in lichen planus.

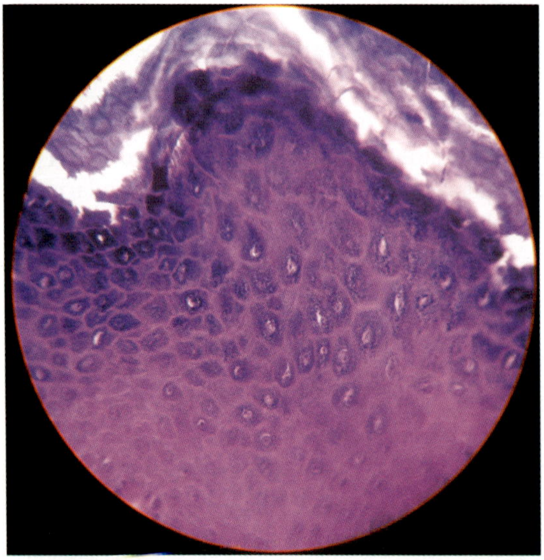

Fig. 21: Profuse thickening of granular layer

- Hypogranulosis: Decreased thickness of granular layer, classically seen in psoriasis and ichthyosis vulgaris.

Papillomatosis

- The term is used when subepidermal papillae go upward leading an undulating skin surface.
- It is classically seen in seborrheic keratosis, verruca vulgaris, tuberculosis verrucosa cutis, verrucous epidermal nevus and chromoblastomycosis.
- In psoriasis, upward prolongation of dermal papillae is present but that does not produce any undulation on the surface.

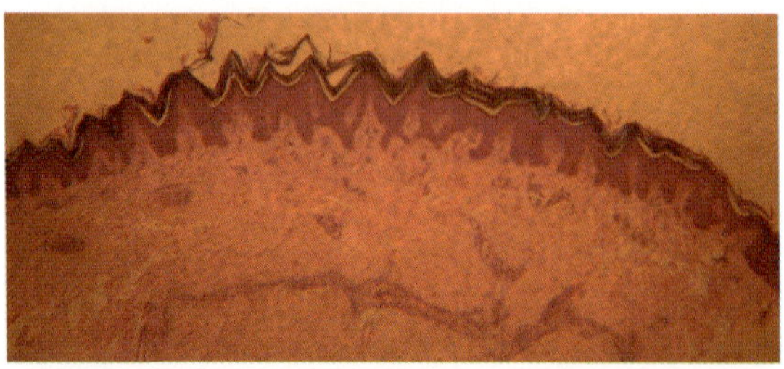

Fig. 22: Papillomatosis in a case of verrucous epidermal nevus

- **Follicular plugging:** Invagination of the stratum corneum, through the pilosebaceous orifice, classically seen in discoid lupus erythematosus.

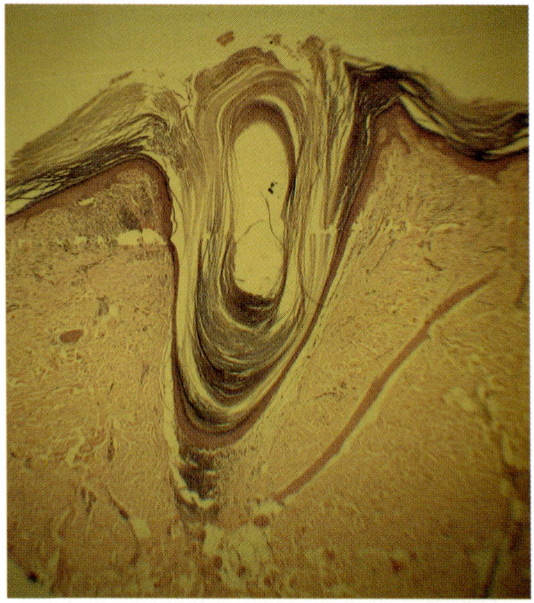

Fig. 23: Follicular keratin plug with an isolated arrector pili muscle

- **Dell:** Small invagination of stratum corneum at non-follicular opening, classically seen in lichen sclerosus et atrophicus (LSA).
- **Keratin cyst:** The cyst develops within the epidermis following complete and abrupt keratinization.

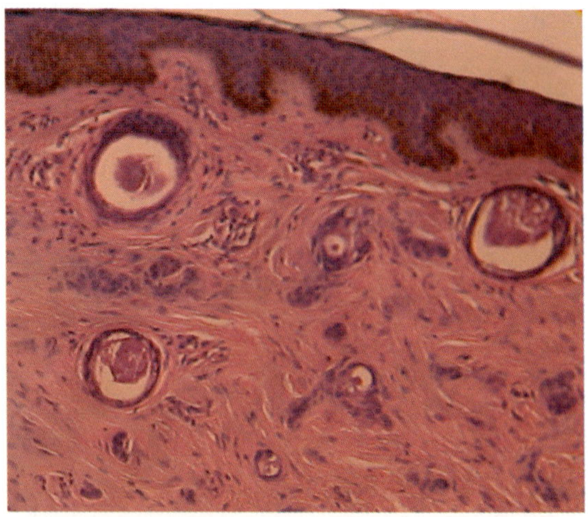

Fig. 24: Multiple cysts in syringoma

* **Pseudohorn cyst:** Following cross section of a follicular plug, a horn cyst is formed. Though it is within the epidermis but it is not formed in situ but formed by invagination and so it is called pseudohorn cyst. It is lined by normal epidermis including granular layer. Quality of horny part is similar to other part of the horny layer.

  Keratin pearl: Here keratin is formed within the epidermis but with a gradual and incomplete fashion.

  Acanthosis: The term is used for thickening of the stratum malpighii or viable part of the epidermis.

Acantholysis

* The term is used to denote the loss of cohecence between the keratinocytes.

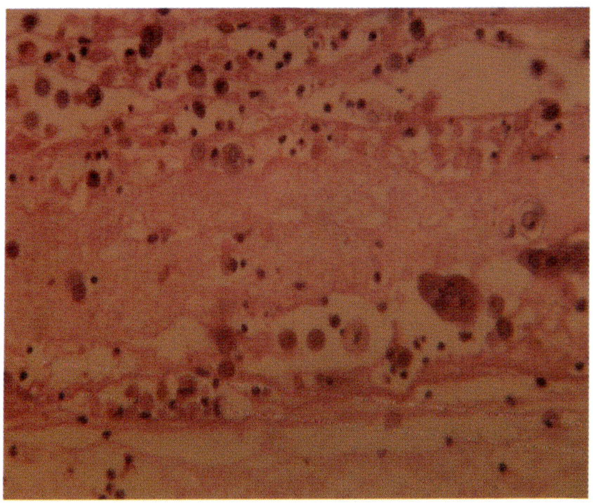

Fig. 25: Isolated and mass of acantholytic cells in pemphigus

* It may be primary or secondary.
* Primary acantholysis is seen in:
  - Pemphigus and its variants
  - Darier's disease
  - Transient acantholytic dermatosis
  - Warty dyskeratoma
  - Incidental focal acantholytic dermatosis.
  - Epidermolytic hyperkeratosis.

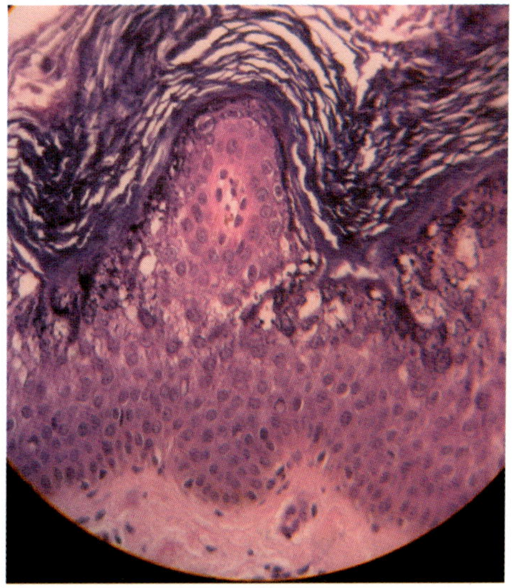

Fig. 26: Focal acantholysis in a case of epidermolytic hyperkeratosis

* Secondary acantholysis is seen in:
  - Herpes
  - Chicken pox
  - Herpes zoster
  - Impetigo and subcorneal pustular dermatosis
  - Adenoid dyskeratotic squamous cell carcinoma.

Acantholytic cell

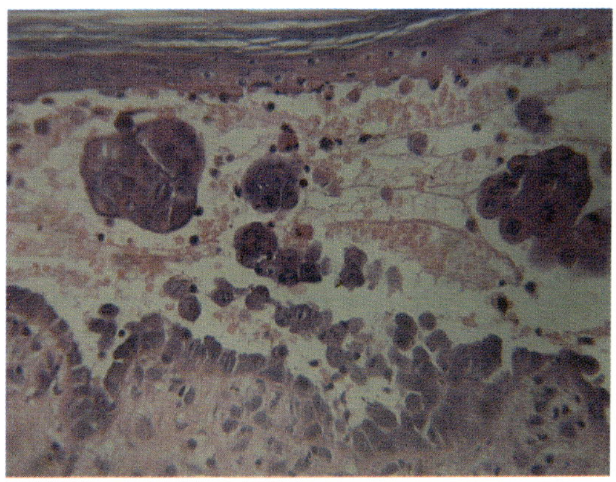

Fig. 27: Multiple acantholytic cells in the cavity of pemphigus vesicle and basal layer is showing classical tomb-stone appearance

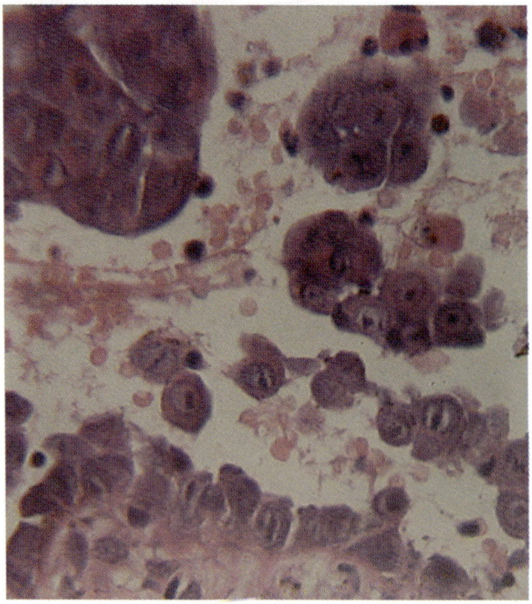

Fig. 28: Multiple acantholytic cells lying singly as well as in clump

- It is nothing but keratinocytes altered by the process of acantholysis.
- Either it exists as an isolated cell or as an isolated small group of cells.
- The cell takes a round shape instead of polygonal shape and has a slightly larger round nucleus with perinuclear halo.

Dyskeratosis

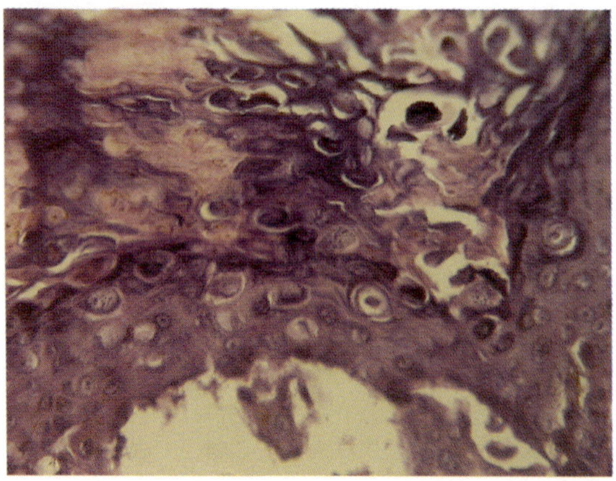

Fig. 29: Grains present in the stratum corneum and corp ronds present at upper spinous and in granular layer

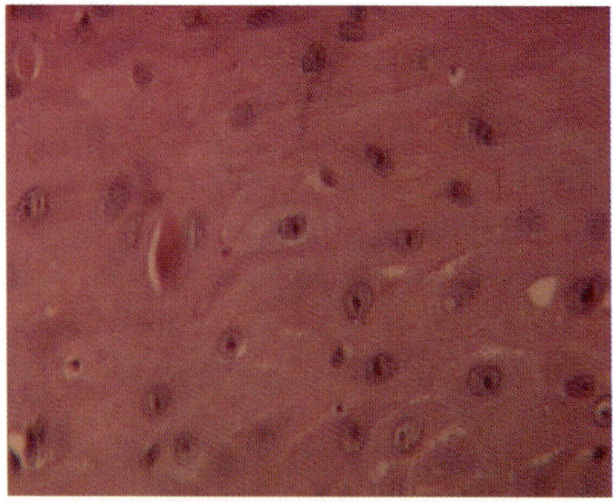

Fig. 30: Individual cell keratinization with a diffuse field of keratinization

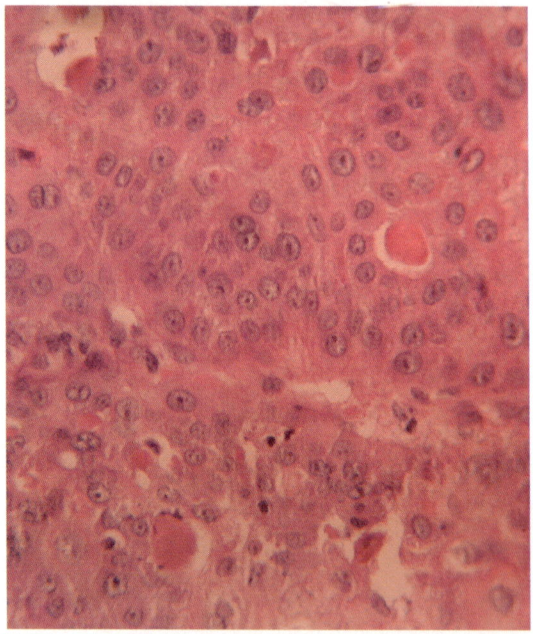

Fig. 31: Multiple large dyskeratotic cells with pink keratin, replacing their nuclei in a moderately differentiated squamous cell carcinoma

- The term is used when individual keratinocyte undergoes faulty and premature keratinization.
- Cytoplasm is replaced by keratin and nucleus is shrunken before replaced completely.
- Two different patterns of dyskeratosis, one is related with acantholytic dermatosis and another one is related with cutaneous malignancy.

- **Corps ronds**
  - These cells are having a basophilic shell of keratin at the periphery and basophilic, homogeneous pyknotic nuclei at the center with a perinuclear halo.
  - They are seen in Darier's disease, warty dyskeratoma, focal acantholytic dyskeratoma, and rarely in transient acantholytic dermatosis and Hailey Hailey disease.
- **Grains:** They have elongated basophilic nuclei:
- Corps ronds and grains both are seen in Darier's disease.
- Grains are present at stratum corneum and corps ronds are present at granular and upper spinous layers.
- In malignant dyskeratosis, cells are having remnants of their nuclei and eosinophilic keratinized cytoplasm.

Spongiosis

- Collection of fluid at intercellular spaces of the keratinocytes, resulting in widening of intercellular spaces.
- Severe edema often produces intracellular edema also and leads to reticular or ballooning degeneration of the keratinocytes.
- It is assocated with many inflammatory dermatoses like acute and subacute dermatitis.

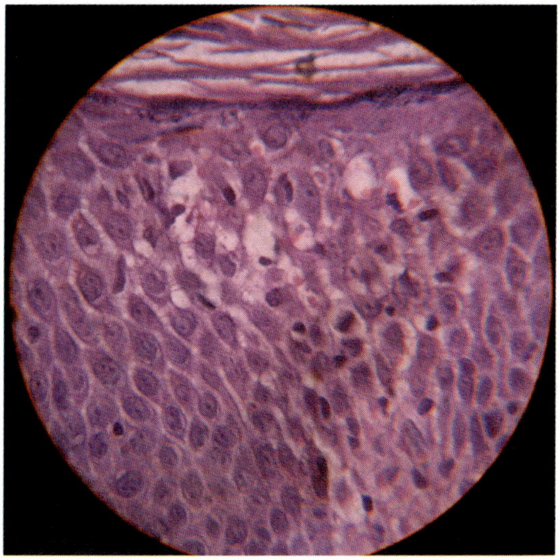

Fig. 32: Spongiosis with exocytosis

Villi: When elongated and tortuous papillae, lined by a single layer of epidermal cells, extend into a bulla, vesicle or lacunae, they are termed as villi.

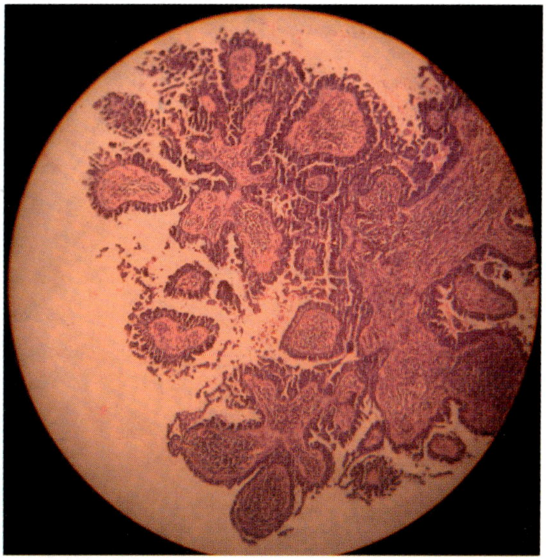

Fig. 33: Multiple villi

Ballooning degeration of epidermis

- Marked swelling of the keratinocytes due to intracellular edema.
- Loss of intercellular bridges, results in acantholysis and formation of vesicle or bulla.
- Commonly seen in viral infection like herpes and chicken pox.

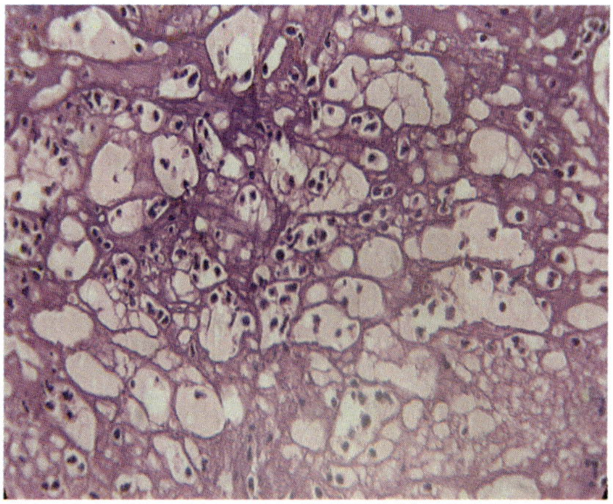

Fig. 34: Ballooning and reticular degeneration

Reticular degeneration of epidermis

- Severe intracellular edema, leads to incomplete rupture of the keratinocyte cell membranes and formation of multilocular bulla.
- Resistant cell walls remain as septae inside the bulla.
- Commonly associated with spongiotic acute dermatitis and blistering viral dermatoses.

Granular degeneration of epidermis

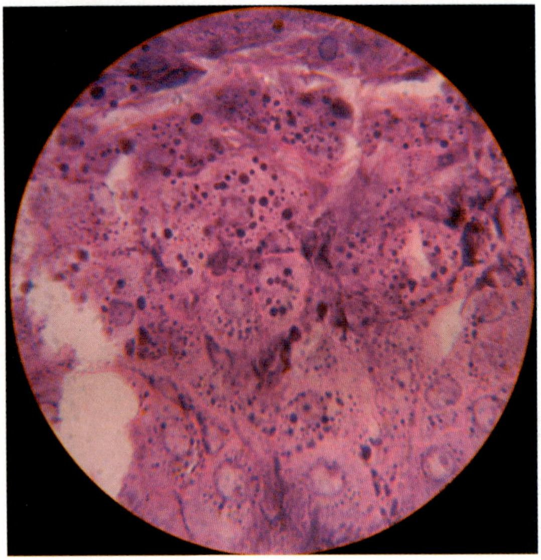

Fig. 35: Granular degeneration in a case of epidermodysplasia verruciformis

- Hyperkeratosis.
- Markedly thickened granular layer and increased number of keratohyaline granules.
- Perinuclear clear spaces.
- Indistinct cell membranes, peripheral to the clear spaces.
- Cell membranes contain lightly staining material or keratohyaline granules.

Liquefaction degeneration of basal layer/ Hydropic degeneration of basal layer

- Vacuolization of the basal keratinocytes leads to pigment incontinence.
- Commonly seen in lupus erythematosus, dermatomyositis, lichen sclerosus et atrophicus, early lichen planus, poikiloderma atrophicans vasculare, erythema dyschromicum perstans.

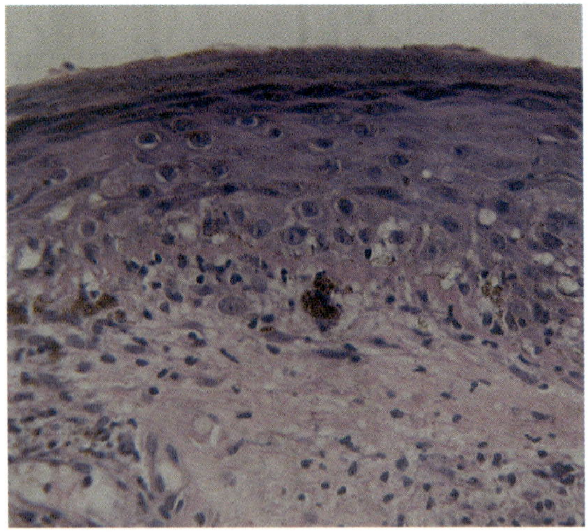

Fig. 36: Interface dermatitis with vacuolar degeneration of basal layer and pigment incontinence

Incontinence of pigment: Dropping of melanin from the degenerated basal cells. The melanin pigment accumulates within melanophages at upper dermis.

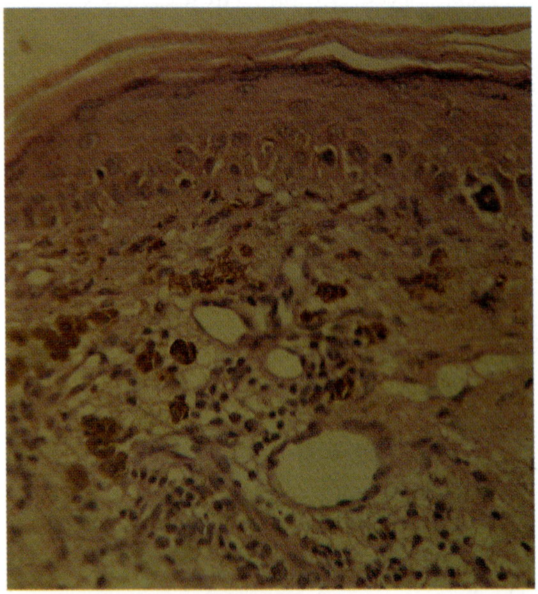

Fig. 37: Basal layer degeneration with pigment incontinence

* It is seen in:
  - Incontinentia pigmenti
  - Lichen planus

- Lupus erythematosus
- Fixed drug reaction
- Poikiloderma atrophicans vasculare
- Erythema dyschromicum perstans

Apoptosis

- It is basically a programmed epidermal cell death.
- The literal meaning of apoptosis is falling of leaves from the tree. In pathology, it is used to denote falling of colloid bodies from the epidermis to the dermis due to degeneration of keratinocytes.
- It is seen in following dermatoses:
  - Lichen planus
  - Benign lichenoid dermatosis
  - Lupus erythematosus
  - Macular and lichenoid amyloidosis
  - Juvenile colloid milium

Colloid/Civatte bodies

- These are round to oval shaped homogeneous eosinophilic material.
- They are formed from degenerated of keratinocytes dropping into the dermis by the process of apoptosis.
- Average size is 10 μm in diameter.
- They are seen at lower epidermis and upper dermis.
- They are present in following disorders but nowhere it is specific.
  - Lichen planus
  - Lupus erythematosus.

Grenz zone

- It is a narrow interface between the epidermis and dermal infiltrate.
- It is see in:
  - Leprosy (LL, BL, BB, BT)
  - Pseudolymphoma
  - B-cell lymphoma
  - Granuloma faciale
  - Lobomycosis.

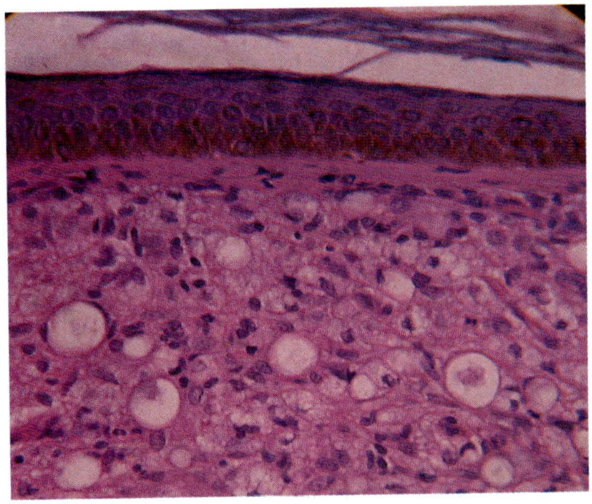

Fig. 38: Grenz zone with foamy macrophages in the dermis in a case of lepromatous leprosy

Macrophage

- Activated or stimulated monocyte is termed as macrophage.
- Monocytes are derived from bone marrow and circulate in blood. To perform a phagocytic function, they enter the skin and other tissues. These tissue bound macrophages are also termed as histiocytes.
- Morphologically monocytes are indistinguishable from the lymphocytes in routine histological process except their size and content of lysosomal enzymes.
- Size of a lymphocyte is 10-12 μm and of a monocyte is 12-15 μm.
- Lysosomal enzymes are lysozyme acid phosphatase, β-glucuronidase and aryl sulphatase. So, histochemically monocytes can be differentiated from lymphocytes, by using special stain for these enzymes. Also monocytes express CD68 but the lymphocytes do not.
- Macrophages are larger than monocytes. Size of a macrophage is variable from 20 μm to 80 μm.
- They are having lightly staining, elongated and vesicular nuclei with clearly visible nuclear membrane.

- In routine staining, very often macrophages are indistinguishable from fibroblasts and endothelial cells except their particular location and phagocytic function.
- Macrophages when ingest melanin are termed as melanophages. They are normally found at papillary dermis in dark skinned persons.
- When they ingest hemosiderin, are termed as siderophages.
- They aggregate for a purpose of phagocytosis and form a granuloma.
- When their nuclei become round in shape and appear as epithelial cells are known as epithelioid cell.
- After completion of phagocytic function macrophages may fuse to form multinucleated giant cell.

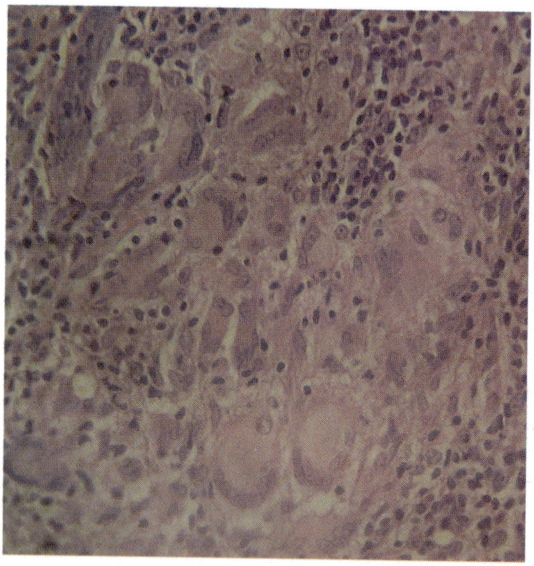

Fig. 39: Multiple larger epitheloid cells with vesicular nuclei at the center of the granuloma and smaller lymphoid cells with dark colored nuclei at the periphery of the granuloma

Histoid cell

- Sometimes endothelial cell or fibroblastic cell resembles a histiocyte and termed as histoid cell.

Lymphoid cell

- The term is used in place of lymphocytes, because histologically lymphocytes and monocytes are indistinguishable.
- During histopathological examination both types of cells show small, round, deeply basophilic nuclei and hardly any cytoplasm.

Plasma cell

* This is an immunologically modified B-lymphocyte.
* The cells are tissue bound and so, not seen in the circulation.
* They are having sharply defined, deeply basophilic, homogeneous and abundant cytoplasm.
* Nucleus is round and eccentrically placed. Nuclear membrane is coarse and contains deeply basophilic chromatin particles which are arranged in a regular fashion. For this arrangement, nucleus takes a cartwheel/clock face appearance.

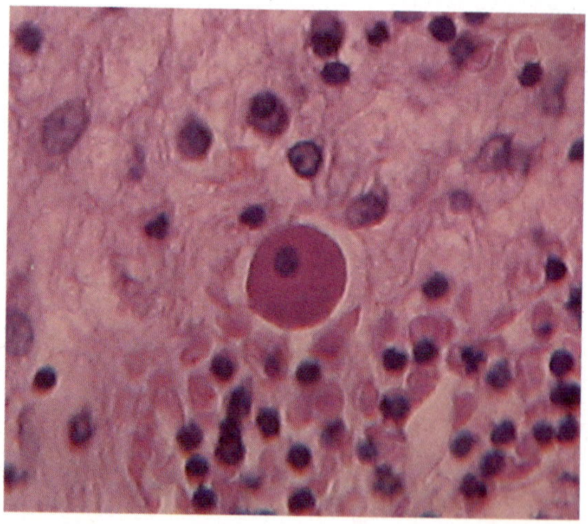

Fig. 40: Plasma cells with Russel body at the center

* Cytoplasm of plasma cell contains extensive networks of flat and irregularly dilated cisternae in their endoplasmic reticulum. Also abundant ribosomes are present at the rough endoplasmic reticulum and cytoplasm. All these ultrastructures synthesize immunoglobulins. When the cisternae are filled up with immunoglobulins, the content is released into extracellular space.

- When a plasma cell produces profuse amount of immunoglobulin, the nucleus may be replaced by eosinophilic and homogeneous material of immunoglobulin, known as Russel body. At last the cell lyses and only the Russel body persists.
- The size of Russel body may be twice that of the plasma cell, as much as 20 μm in diameter. It contains varying amount of glycoproteins and immunoglobulins. It is stained by Gram and PAS stains.
- Plasma cells are predominantly found in
  - Early syphilis
  - Rhinoscleroma
  - Granuloma inguinale
  - Plasmacytoma

Metaplasia: The term is used to denote conversion of one type of tissue in another type. As an example, ossification may be seen in epidermal tumor like pilomatricoma or in dermal nevi.

Dysplasia: The term is used to denote disordered appearance of a cell. It often precedes atypia of the cell.

Anaplasia: Atypical appearance of nuclei in malignant cells.

Pyknosis: The term is used to denote shrinkage of nucleus.

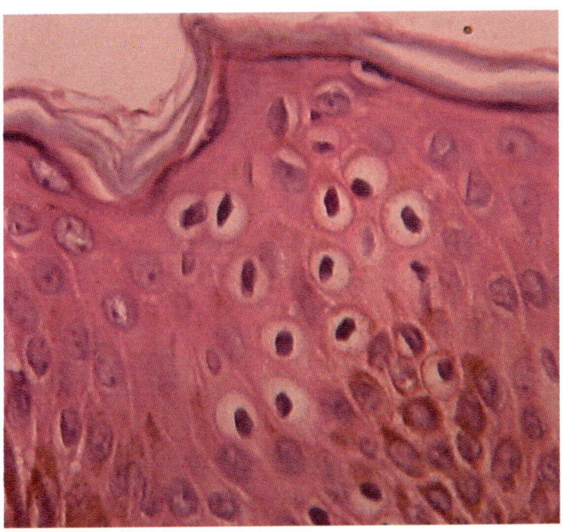

Fig. 41: Keratinocytes with shrunken nucleus

Karyorrhexis: The term denotes fragmentation of nucleus, resulting in nuclear dusts.

Leukocytoclasis: The term is used for disintegration of neutrophils.

Metachromasia

- This is a phenomenon in which color of the original dye is changed when a particular tissue is stained with it.
- It occurs in presence of acid mucopolysaccharides or amyloid.
- Granules of mast cell contains dermatan sulfate, which is a rich component of sulfated acid mucoploysaccharide. When mast cell is stained with methylene blue, toluidine blue or Giemsa, the granules are turned into purple, instead of becoming blue, at pH 3.0 and pH 1.5.
- Dermal mucin in mucinosis contains hyaluronic acid, a major component of nonsulfated acid mucopolysaccharide. It stains metachromically only at pH 3.0, but not at pH 1.5.
- Amyloid becomes red with crystal violet due to metachromasia. It also occurs in colloid milium.

Pleomorphism: The term is used to denote variation in the appearance of nuclei of same type of cells. Nuclei often become large, irregular and hyperchromatic.

Lichenoid tissue reaction: A band like mononuclear inflammatory cells invades the dermoepidermal junction and causes cytolysis of the basal keratinocytes and melanocytes.

Interface dermatosis: The term is used when dermoepidermal junction is obscured by dermal inflammatory cells.

Epidermotropism

- The term is used when mononuclear cells enter the epidermis actively without any spongiosis or with negligible spongiosis.
- Mononuclear cells remain singly or in cluster. These aggregated mononuclear cells are known

as Pautrier microabscess, seen in mycosis fungoides.

Exocytosis

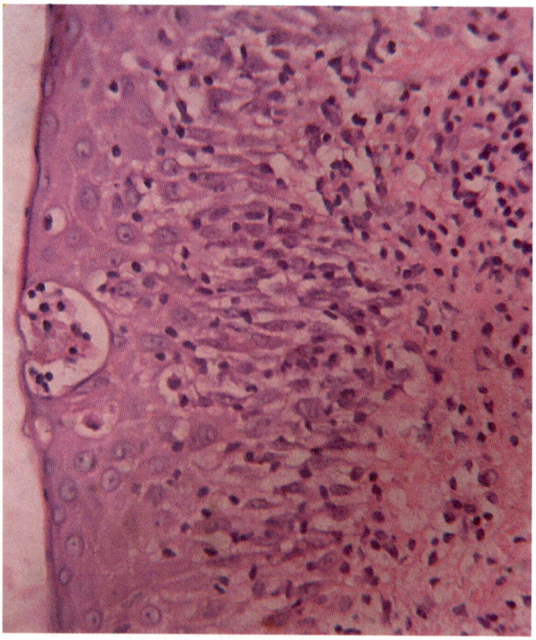

Fig. 42: Mononuclear cell infiltration in the epidermis with spongiosis

- The term is used when mononuclear cells enter the epidermis in presence of spongiosis and this is a passive process.
- It is classically seen in acute and subacute dermatitis.

Giant cell

- Langhans' giant cell: The large multinucleated macrophage in which nuclei are arranged at the periphery in a regular fashion.
- Foreign body giant cell: The large multinucleated macrophage in which nuclei are arranged haphazardly.
- Touton giant cell: The large multinucleated macrophage contains a wreath of nuclei, surrounding a central eosinophilic nonfoamy cytoplasm and a peripheral area of foamy cytoplasm. It is seen in juvenile xanthogranuloma and various other types of xanthoma.

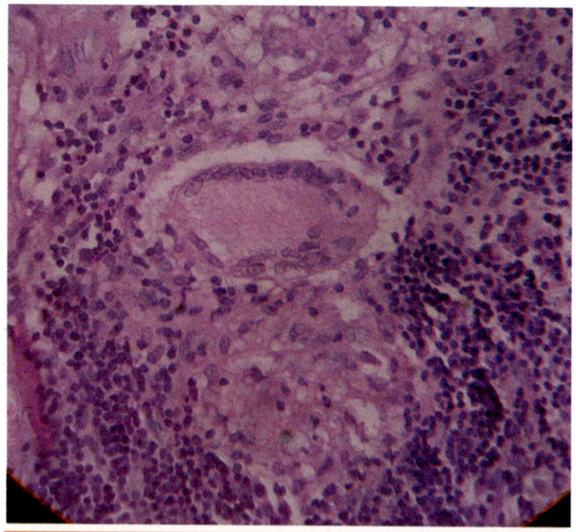

Fig. 43: Granuloma contains a huge giant cell

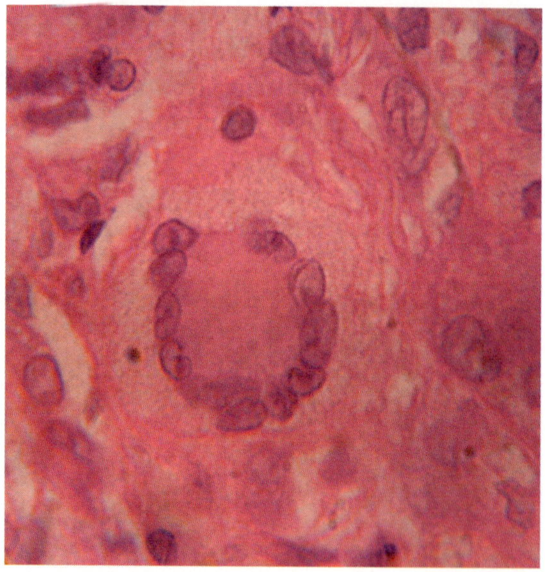

Fig. 44: A classic touton giant cell

- Floret giant cell: Nuclei are arranged like a wreath of flower, seen in pleomorphic lipoma.

Granuloma

- The term is used to denote an aggregation of macrophages for the purpose of phagocytosis.
- It may be due to presence of foreign body which forms a foreign body type of granuloma or it may be due to delayed hypersensitivity reaction which forms allergic type of granuloma.

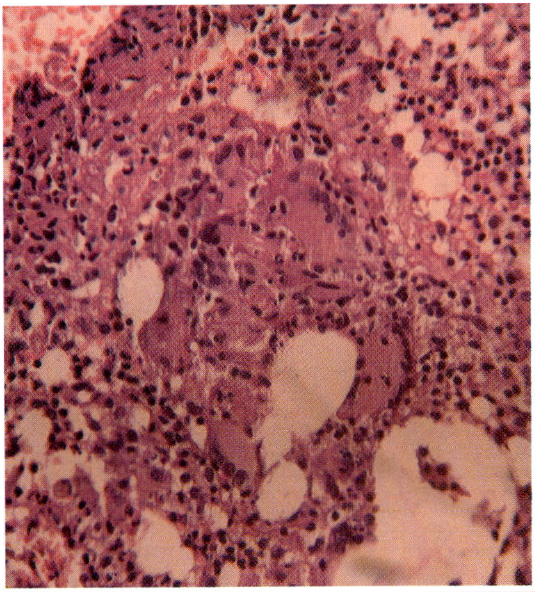

Fig. 45: Caseating granuloma in a case of atypical mycobacterial infection

- Foreign body granuloma
  - Substances like oils, starch and powder enter the dermis from outside or substances like urates and keratins formed endogenously.
  - Granuloma is mostly composed of macrophages, giant cells and scanty epithelioid cells.
  - Giant cells are usually larger in size and contain haphazardly arranged nuclei.
- Allergic granuloma
  - Delayed hypersensitivity reaction to foreign materials or microorganisms which are waiting for phagocytosis.
  - Foreign materials are zirconium, beryllium and tattoo reagents.
  - Common microorganisms are *Mycobacterium leprae*, *Mycobacterium tuberculosis* and deep fungi.
  - Sometimes it may be due to an idiopathic cause as in sarcoidosis or due to a hypersensitivity reaction.
  - Granuloma contains epithelioid cells predominantly.
  - Nuclei in the multinucleated giant cell are arranged at the periphery like a horseshoe pattern and known as Langhans' giant cell.
  - These giant cells are usually smaller than foreign body type of giant cell.
  - Sometimes nuclei of giant cell may be an overlap of both types.

Fibrinoid degeneration of connective tissue

- Collagen is replaced by fibrin which appears homogeneous and brightly eosinophilic.
- It is seen in:
  - Hypersensitivity vasculitis
  - Rheumatoid nodule
  - Lupus erythematosus

  Colliquative necrosis: The term is used when necrosis is associated with formation of pus.

Granulation tissue

- This is newly formed swollen collagen tissue, seen during healing of a wound or ulcer and in chronic inflammatory process.
- It also contains fibroblasts, newly formed capillaries and a dense chronic inflammatory infiltrates including lymphoid cells, macrophages and plasma cells.

  Storiform pattern: Elongated fibroblastic cells intersect at various angles or intertwine and appear as weaving of a doormat. It is seen in dermatofibroma and dermatofibrosarcoma.

  Cartwheel pattern: Elongated fibroblastic cells radiate from a central hub of fibrous tissue in a whorl like fashion and appear as cartwheel pattern. It is seen in various fibrous tissue tumors.

Pseudoepitheliomatous hyperplasia, seen in

- Tuberculosis verrucosa cutis
- Atypical mycobacterial infection

- Deep fungal infection
- Pemphigus vegetans
- Pyoderma gangrenosum
- Pyoderma vegetante
- Halogenoderma
- Keratoacanthoma

Eosinophilic spongiosis, seen in

- Allergic contact dermatitis
- Insect bite reaction
- Allergic drug reaction
- Bullous pemphigoid
- Pemphigus vulgaris
- Transient acantholytic dermatosis

Vasculitis

- Mural inflammation, mostly by the neutrophils
- Deposition of fibrin.
- Endothelial swelling with increased intercellular fenestrations.
- Extravasation of erythrocytes, leukocytoclasia and formation of nuclear dusts.

Vasculopathy

- Perivascular predominant lymphocytic and sparse neutrophilic infiltration.
- No leukocytoclasia and no mural fibrin deposition.
- No endothelial swelling.

Vascular reaction

- Mild mural inflammation, but no fibrin deposition.
- Mild endothelial swelling.
- Mild leukocytoclasia.

Foam cells, seen in

- Atypical mycobacterial infection
- Leprosy
- Other bacterial infections

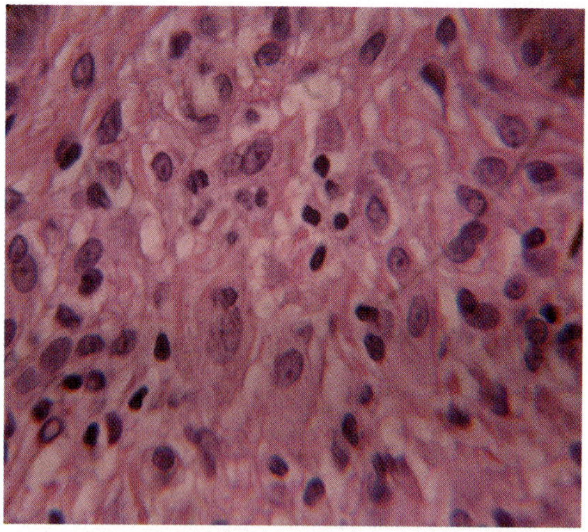

Fig. 46: Foam cells in xanthoma

- Pneumocystosis
- Panniculitis
- Xanthoma
- Juvenile xanthogranuloma
- Necrobiotic xanthogranuloma
- Atypical fibroxanthoma
- Dermatofibroma
- Balloon cell nevus
- Balloon cell hemangioma
- Granular cell tumor
- Hibernoma
- Langerhans cell histiocytosis
- Liposarcoma
- Sebaceous gland tumor
- Schwannoma

Extravasation of RBCs, seen in

- Vasculitis, purpuric dermatoses, vascular tumors
- Pityriasis lichenoides
- Pityriasis rosea (sometimes)
- Stasis dermatitis
- Cellulitis
- Meningococcemia
- Gonococcemia
- Herpes

- Langerhans cell histiocytosis
- Primary systemic amyloidosis.

Indian filing of cells

* The term is used when single row of cells extend between and around collagen bundles.
* It is seen in:
  - Non-Hodgkin's lymphoma
  - Metastatic scirrhous carcinoma
  - Lymphocytoma
  - Granuloma annulare

Fat necrosis

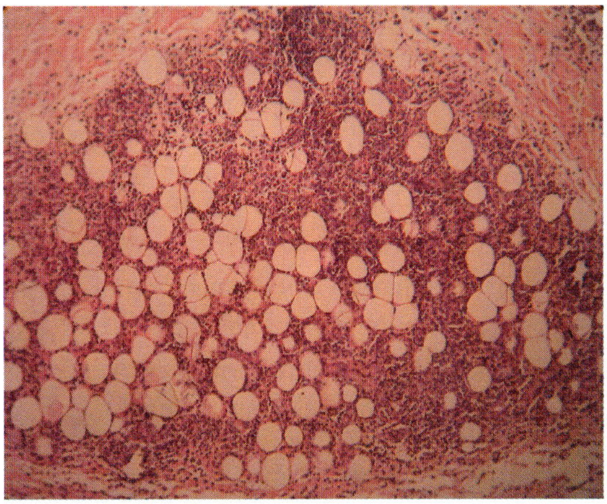

Fig. 47: Lobular panniculitis

* Lipophagic necrosis
  - Necrotic adipocytes are replaced by foamy macrophages.
  - Marophages are filled up with lipid contents of adipocytes.
  - These lipophages are having large, microvacuolated or organic cytoplasm.
  - This is seen in late stage of many panniculitis and classically seen in traumatic panniculitis, lipodermatosclerosis, erythema nodosum and nodular vasculitis.
* Liquefactive necrosis
  - Saponification of lipids of adipocytes by pancreatic lipases and deposition of calcium.
  - This leads to loss of nuclei and granular basophilic cytoplasm.
  - Adipocytes appear as ghost cells.
* Hyalinizing fat necrosis
  - Adipocytes become anucleated and mummified.
  - They are surrounded by glassy homogeneous proteinaceous material and effaced architecture.
  - It is seen in lupus panniculitis, dermatomyositis and lipodermatosclerosis.
* Membranous fat necrosis
  - It is seen in majority of the panniculitis at their late stages.
  - Necrotic adipocytes appear as leathery eosinophilic with hyaline crenulated rim and collapsed cellular organelles.
  - It is seen in lipodermatosclerosis
* Ischemic fat necrosis
  - Adipocytes become necrotic and pallor due to poor blood supply.
  - Necosis starts at center of the lobule and cells appear as ghost cells. These cells are smaller in size with preserved outlines.
  - Interstitium enlarges.
  - It is seen in erythema induratum of Bazin, calciphylaxis, infective panniculitis and cutaneous polyarteritis nodosa.
* Basophilic fat necrosis
  - Necrotic adipocytes intermingle with disintegrated neutrophils and basophilic granular materials.
  - Basophilic granular materials represent aggregated bacteria.
  - It is seen in infective panniculitis.

Necrotizing follicular reaction, seen in

- Mixed cryoglobulinemia
- Behcet's disease
- Rheumatoid vasculitis
- Herpetic folliculitis

- Acute pustular bacterid
- Pustular drug reaction

Sweet-like vascular reaction, seen in

- Bowel associated arthritic dermatoses
- Behcet's syndrome
- Idiopathic pustular vasculitis
- Rheumatoid arthritis
- Acute pustular bacterid
- Sweet's syndrome

Pharmacoloy: Topical preparations

Vehicle: It is the substance through which a drug is dispersed for topical therapy.

Solution

- It is a transparent vehicle, usually made up of water, ethanol or propylene glycol.
- It is useful for hairy and intertriginous areas.
- It many causes stringent or burning sensation when used at intertriginous areas.

Paint

- It is a staining liquid which when applied, the liquid part evaporates and persists as a thin firmly adherent protective layer at the site of application.
- It is useful for mucosal surfaces and intertriginous areas.

Tincture

- It is an alcoholic solution which when applied persists as sticky substance.
- Commonly used drug is podophyllin for genital wart.

Colloidion

- It is made of organic solvent like pyroxilin (cellulose nitrate).
- When it evaporates a flexible film is left and works as a water repellant.

Lotion

- It is a *homogeneous* mixture of water and powder.
- It is useful for widespread areas.
- Commonly used lotion is calamine lotion, which acts as a soothing agent.

Emulsion

- It is a mixture of water and powder which remains as a precipitation and becomes homogeneous on shaking well.
- It is useful for widespread areas.
- Commonly used emulsion is gammabenzene hexachloride for scabies.

Gel

- It is a transparent vehicle, prepared from seaweeds.
- It is costlier, than cream or ointment.
- It is useful for intertriginous and hairy areas.
- It usually does not cause buring sensation when used for intertriginous areas in comparison to solution.

Cream

- It is a biphasic vehicle, made up of oil and water with the help of an emulsifier.
- It is useful in conditions with prominent crusting but minimum oozing.

Ointment

- It is a monophasic vehicle, made of oily or greasy substance.
- It prevents evaporation of water.
- It useful for chronic, dry, scaly and lichenified lesions.

Orabase

- It is a sticky vehicle, useful for oral mucosa.
- It consists of carboxy methylcellulose, pectin and gelatin.
- Commonly used drug is triamcinolone acetonide.

Powder

- It is dust like preparation and a poor vehicle to disperse drug.
- It is useful to absorb oozing but often pro-

duces a cake on the surface which may prevent healing.

Condy's compress

- It is a solution of potassium permanganate (1:8000 dilution) for compression at oozy areas.
- It acts as an astringent and dries up oozing quickly.
- It acts as a scavenger and cleans the crusts.
- It produces nascent oxygen which acts as an antimicrobial agent.
- When water evaporates, it produces a soothing effect.
- It is cheaper, very easily available and easy to prepare.

Burrow's solution

- It is a solution of 6-12% aluminium subacetate.
- It has very effective astringent effect and can dry up the oozy lesions within hours.
- It is not easily available and costlier than potassium permanganate.

EMLA

- It is the eutectic mixture of 50% lidocaine and 50% prilocaine and used as local anesthesia.

Shampoo

- It is designed to clean hair and scalp by removing sebum, scale, microorganisms and environmental dusts.
- The main component is surfactant.
- Shampoo also contains thickeners, foam-boosters, coloring agents and preservatives.
- Baby shampoo contains amphoteric surfactant that does not sting the eyes.

Conditioner

- It enhances compability of wet and dry hair.
- It also increases the volume of fine and straight hair without causing any extra build-up.
- It promotes appearance, fullness, luster and general manageability.
- The main contents are hydrolysed proteins, cationic surfactants, polymers, lipids, glycols and silicons.

Hair dye

- It is used to conceal gray or white hair.
- Usually temporary colors are harmless but permanent colors are notorious to produce severe to mild hypersensitivity reaction.
- Temporary dyes are deposited on the surface of the hair and may be removed by shampoo. These are indolamine, indophenols, derivatives of azo-, azine or thiazine.
- Semipermanent dyes can penetrate hair cuticle. They are derived from nitroanilines, nitrophenelinediamines and nitroaminophenols.
- Permanent dyes are colorless precursors. They react with hydrogen peroxide inside the hair shaft to produce permanent colors. These are p-phenylenediamines or paraaminophenols.

Nail polish

- This is used to beautify nails.
- It is an adhesive film, consists of nitrocellulose resin, plasticizer, solvent and diluents, color and suspending agent.
- Nitrocellulose resin helps to improve the adhesion and glossiness.
- Plasticizer increases flexibility.
- Solvent and diluents modify viscosity.
- Suspending agent prevent settling.
- Usually it is harmless to nail but may produce contact sensitization to other sites, specially eyelids during scratching.

Sunprotective agents

- The solar radiations are absorbed by the cellular DNA, RNA, protein enzyme, membrane lipid of keratinocytes and by the dermis. Then they exert a tissue damaging effect.

- UVA can penetrate deeper than UVB.
- Absorption and filtration of UV radiation occurs at the stratum corneum and prevents further penetration.
- UVA absorbing agents are anthralin, benzophenons and camphor.
- UVB absorbing agents are para-aminobezoic acid (PABA), cinnamate and salicylate.
- UV radiations may be scattered from the epidermis and effective agents are titanium oxide (TiO_2), zinc oxide (ZnO) and melanin.
- TiO_2 and ZnO also can reflect the radiation.
- UV radiation induced reactive free radicals like singlet oxygen, superoxide ions, hydroxyl radicals in the epidermis and dermis can be tackled by anti-oxidants, vitamin C and beta carotenes.
- Physical blocking agents are umbrella, hat and clothing.
- UV radiation induced inflammation may be controlled by antihistaminics, prostaglandin inhibitors and indomethacin.

General principle of topical therapy

- Factors influencing percutaneous absorption:
  - Age of the patient
  - Site of application
  - Intact barrier function
  - Disruption of barrier function
  - Thickness of the stratum corneum
  - Skin hydration
  - Artificial occlusion
  - Active drug concentration
  - Lipophilicity of the drug
  - Composition of vehicle
- Influence of site in percutaneous application:
  - Scrotum and eyelid > Jaw > Forehead > Axilla > Scalp > Back > Palm > Ankle > Sole > Dorsal forearm > Ventral forearm

Drugs which should be taken before food

- Azithromycin, roxythromycin, erythromycin
- Ciprofloxacin, Norfloxacin
- Cephalexin, cephadroxil
- Ampicillin, dicloxacillin
- Sulfonamides
- Rifampicin
- Acetaminophen
- Paracetamol
- H1 antihistaminics
- Psoralen, ideally before food but it is often taken after food due to chance of nausea and vomiting when taken in empty stomach
- D-penicillamine
- Azidothymidine, DDI, indinavir, lamivudine
- General tonics like liver extract, enzymes, etc.

Drugs should be taken with food

- Itraconazole, griseofulvin, potassium iodide
- Cefuroxime, metronidazole
- Clofazimine
- NSAIDS
- Ketotifen
- Retinoids
- Steroids
- Cyclosporine with apple or orange juice but not with grape juice
- Ritonavir, nelfinavir
- Fluoxetine
- Iron preparations

Drugs should be taken after food

- Squinavir
- Aspirin
- H2 blockers
- Ethionamide
- Vitamin B complex
- Antioxidants

Drugs safety in pregnancy

- Level of safety of a particular drug during pregnancy was introduced by FDA (USA).

* All drugs are classified into following categories:

Category A: Adequate well controlled studies in pregnant women have failed to demonstrate any risk to the fetus.

- Vitamin B6
- Folic acid
- Vitamin A (except high dose)
- Vitamin D

Category B: No evidence of risk in humans. Either animal findings show risk and human findings donot or no adequate human studies have been done, but animal findings are negative.

- Chlorpheniramine, diphenylhydramine
- Cyproheptadine, azatadine, cetirizine, loratadine.
- Ciclopirox, nystatin, terbinafine.
- Imiquimod.
- Permethrin
- Penicillin, cephalosporins, erythromycin, azithromycin, clindamycin, sulphonamide (except near term), metronidazole, ethambutol.
- Acyclovir, famciclovir, valaciclovir.
- Lansoprazole, famotidine, cimetidine, ranitidine.
- Ibuprofen (1st trimester)

Category C: Risk cannot be ruled out. Human studies are lacking, animal studies are either positive for fetal risk or lacking as well. However, potential benefits may justify the risk.

- Promethazine, hydroxyzine, astemizole, azelastine, fexophenadine, terfenadine.
- Bacitracin, mupirocin, quinolones, vancomycin.
- Imidazoles, miconazole, selenium sulphide, griseofulvin, ketoconazole, fluconazole, itraconazole.
- Podophyllin
- Clarithromycin, DDS, isoniazid, rifampicin, pyrazinamide, ethionamide, PAS, cycloserine
- Nucleoside reverse trancriptase inhibitors, non-nucleoside reverse transcriptase inhibitors, protease inhibitors.
- Cyclosporine
- Psoralen
- Vitamin C, vitamin B12, vitamin B2, vitamin B1, iron.
- Cisapride, nizatidine, omeprazole.
- Metoclopramide
- Heparin
- Nifedipine
- Promethazine
- Midazolam, doxepin, amphetamine, lorazepam, clomipramine, sertaline, fluoxetine
- Hydroxychloroquine
- Gold salts
- Topical mometasone/fluticasone, systemic cortisone/hydrocortisone/prednisolone/dexamethasone/beclomethasone/betamethasone.
- Aspirin (low dose)
- Benzoyl peroxide, topical metronidazole/tretinoins/adapalene.

Category D: Positive evidence for risk where investigational or postmarketing data show risk to the fetus. Nevertheless, potential benefits may outweigh the potential risk.

- Streptomycin, sulphonamide (near term), kanamycin, tetracycline.
- Vitamin D
- Ketanserin, ibuprofen (2nd & 3rd trimester), aspirin (full dose).
- Potassium iodide
- Diazepam, alprazolam, buspirone, imipramine, amitriptyline.
- Phenobarbital
- Methotrexate, cyclophosphamide, 5-fluorouracil
- Topical calcipotriene
- Topical glucocorticoids
- Topical rofecoxib/ketorolac/other NSAIDs.

Category X: Contraindicated in pregnancy where studies in animal or humans, or investigational or postmarketing data show risk to the fetus. Risk overweighs any benefit to the patient.

- Vitamin A (high dose), systemic retinoids.
- Methotrexate, tazarotene
- Danazol, estrogens, misoprostol, oral contraceptive pills.
- Spironolactone
- Ethanol (large dose).

DCP therapy

* In this therapy suprapharmacological dose of corticosteroid is used along with cyclophosphamide.
* The main aim of this therapy is to avoid steroid induced hypothalamo-pituitary axis (HPA) suppression.
* It is composed of 4 phases.

Phase I:

- On 1st day 100 mg of dexamethasone dissolved in 500 ml of 5% glucose is given as a slow intravenous drip over 2 hours and this to be repeated for another 2 days.
- On 2nd day 500 mg of cyclophosphamide is added in the same drip.
- On 3rd day 50 mg of cyclophosphamide is given orally till next pulse which is introduced exactly after 28 days. This regimen will continue till complete clinical remission and is ready to enter phase II.

Phase II:

- Patient will receive extra 9 pulses and become ready to enter phase III.

Phase III:

- Patient will get only 50 mg cyclophosphamide orally for another 9 months and become ready to enter phase IV.

Phase IV:

- Patient will remain under observation for another 10 years.

Common indications:

- Pemphigus
- Dermatomyositis
- SLE
- Pyoderma gangrenosum

Common adverse effects:

- Fluid and electrolytes imbalance
- Cardiac failure and shock

Photodynamic therapy

* Photosensitiser accumulates in abnormal tissue, absorbs light, produces singlet oxygen by a photochemical reaction and exerts a cytotoxic effect within the tissue.
* Singlet oxygen exerts its cytotoxic effect with a radius of > 0.02μm and its lifetime in biological system is < 0.04 microseconds.
* Photosensitizing chemicals
  - Porfimer: It is used intravenously and there is a risk of cutaneous photosensitivity and so sunexposure should be avoided for at least following therapy.
  - 5-Aminolevulinic acid–It is applied on the skin to be concentrated within the underlying tissue and to be converted into protoporphyrin IX.
* Photosensitisers are believed to be localized within blood vessels, lysosomes, mitochondria, plasma membrane and nuclei of the tumor cells.
* Mechanism of action:
  - Direct destruction by singlet oxygen
  - Damage of the vessels
  - Activation of immune system.
* For more penetration light should have longer wavelength, such as 630 nm can penetrate </=5 mm and 700-800 nm can penetrate </=20 mm. But longer wavelength lacks sufficient energy to activate a useful photochemical reaction.
* Ideal features of a photosensitiser
  - It should be minimally toxic.
  - It should be taken up by the pathological tissue more quickly than surrounding normal tissue. It should be cleared quickly from the normal tissue.

- It should be cleared from the pathological tissue more slowly. Vascularity of the pathological tissue helps to accumulate more within it and poor lymphatic drainage prevents to clear from it.
- Activating wavelength of light should match with required penetration.
- Capable to produce large amount of cytotoxic effect.

Transdermal therapy

- Advantages of transdermal therapy over conventional systemic therapy:
  - Avoidance of peak plasma concentration profiles.
  - Avoidance of first-pass metabolism in the gastrointestinal tract and liver. No patient variation as a result of differences in absorption of drug from gastrointestinal tract.
  - Rapid termination of drug administered.
  - Prolonged duration of action, resulting in less frequent administration and lower total daily dose of the drug.
  - Better patient compliance.
- Limitations of transdermal therapy:
  - Drugs having low molecular weight (<1000 daltons) and having a balanced water and oil solubility, can penetrate the skin adequately. But daily dose should not exceed 5 mg.
  - It requires a delivery device which will control both rate and duration of drug input.
- Drugs already approved for transdermal administration:
  - Glyceryl trinitrate for coronary insufficiency.
  - Hyoscine for motion sickness.
  - Estradiol for estrogen replacement therapy.
  - Clonidine for hypertension.
- Drugs under trial for transdermal therapy:
  - Azatadine, an antihistaminic.
  - Timolol and bupranolol, β-blockers.
  - Fentanyl, an analgesic.
  - Nicotine
  - Testosterone.

Iontophoresis

- It is a non-invasive process to increase drug delivery through the skin by using an electric current.
- As skin is a semi-permeable membrane, allows little amount of drug to pass through it when the drug is applied on the surface.
- Iontophoresis increases the penetration of electrically charged drugs through the skin where the electrical energy facilitates the movement of ions across the stratum corneum by repulsion of like charges and attraction of opposite charges.
- Iontophoresis device has DC voltage delivery system and electrodes.
- It enhances trans-dermal drug delivery through following mechanisms:
  - Ion-electric field interaction provides extra energy that drives ions through the skin.
  - Flow of electric current increases permeability of skin
  - Electro-osmosis produces bulk motion of the solvent that carries ions.
- It is devoid of gastrointestinal incompatibility, uncertain absorption, and first pass metabolism.
- There is no complication due to intramuscular or intravascular injection. But there is possibility of electric burn if electrodes are not properly used or formation of undesirable blisters.
- It has been used for various dermatological disorders:
  - Iontophoresis was most successfully used for treatment of hyperhidrosis. Simple tap water is used for this purpose. The mechanism of action is not yet clear, probably a mechanical blockage is developed at the sweat ducts within the stratum corneum. When stripping of stratum corneum is done, the blockage is also removed and sweating is restored.

- Histamine or zinc oxide iontophoresis was used for treatment of leg ulcers.
- Copper sulfate and potassium iodide iontophoresis were used for treatment of dermatophytosis and sporotrichosis respectively.
- Sodium salicylate iontophoresis was used for treatment of plantar warts and hyperkeratosis with fissuring of palms and soles.
- Idoxuridine iontophoresis was used for treatment of aborting episodes of herpes simplex infection or to reduce the discomfort and healing time of herpes simplex lesions.
- Triamcinolone acetonide iontophoresis was tried for treatment of aphthous stomatitis.
- Methyl prednisolone was used for treatment of lichen planus.
- Iontophoresis of local anesthetic agents was used for oral mucosa. Skin anesthesia was best achieved by using a solution containing 1% and 4% lidocaine with 1:10,000 to 1:50,000 epinephrine.
- Meladine solution 1% iontophoresis was used for vitiligo.
- Hyaluronidase iontophoresis was used for scleroderma and lymphedema.
- Pilocarpine iontophoresis was used for sweat test to diagnose cystic fibrosis.
- Iontophoresis with iron oxide and titanium oxide were used for introduction of artificial skin color.
- Iodine iontophoresis was used to reduce scar tissue.
- Antibiotic iontophoresis was used for treatment of burn patient.

CLASSIFICATION AND DIFFERENTIAL DIAGNOSIS

CHAPTER B2

Immune mechanism

* Innate immunity, exerted by
  * Complements
  * Toll-like receptors
  * Antimicrobial peptides
  * Cytokines
  * Macrophages
  * Neutrophils, eosinophils, basophils
  * Natural killer cells
* Adaptive immunity, exerted by
  * Langerhans cells and other dendritic cells
  * T helper cells
  * Cytotoxic T cells
  * Regulatory T cells
  * B cells

Immunobullous disorders

* Pemphigus
* Pemphigoid
* Dermatitis herpetiformis
* Linear IgA dermatosis
* Epidermolysis bullosa acquisita
* Bullous systemic lupus erythematosus
* Bullous lichen planus.

Mechanobullous disorders

* Epidermolysis bullosa (EB) simplex
  * Generalized EB (*Kobner*)
  * EB Ogna (*Gedde-Dehl*)
  * EB of hands and feet (Weber-Cockyne)
  * Herpetiform EB
  * EB with mottled pigmentation
  * Superficial EB
* Junctional epidermolysis bullosa
  * Lethal (Herlitz)
  * Nonlethal generalized
  * Nonlethal localized
  * Nonlethal inverse
  * Progressive
  * Cicatricial
* Epidermolysis bullosa dystrophica

a. Autosomal recessive type

* Generalized
* Generalized non-mutilating
* Inverse type

b. Autosomal dominant type
- ♦ Hyperplastic (*Cockyne-Touraine*)
- ♦ Albopapuloid (*Pasini*)

Miscellaneous bullous disorders

- ♦ Porphyria cutanea tarda
- ♦ Diabetic bulla
- ♦ Heat induced blister
- ♦ Friction blister
- ♦ Suction blister

Dermal and subcutaneous deep fungal infection

- ♦ Sporotrichosis
- ♦ Mycetoma
- ♦ Chromoblastomycosis
- ♦ Pheohyphomycosis
- ♦ Zygomycosis
- ♦ Lobomycosis

Variants of ACD (allergic contact dermatitis)

- ♦ Purpuric
- ♦ Leukodermic
- ♦ Ichthyosiform
- ♦ Follicular
- ♦ Pustular
- ♦ Dermal
- ♦ Granulomatous
- ♦ Lymphomatoid

Metastatic deep fungal infection

- ♦ Aspergillosis
- ♦ Blastomycosis
- ♦ Cryptococcosis
- ♦ Paracoccidioidomycosis
- ♦ Histoplasmosis
- ♦ Mucormycosis
- ♦ Coccidioidomycosis

Cutaneous adverse drug reactions

- ✶ Immunologic drug reaction
  - ♦ IgE mediated type I reaction, such as anaphylaxis from beta-lactum antibiotic.
  - ♦ Cytotoxic type II reaction.
  - ♦ Immune complex mediated type III reaction, such as serum sickness from antithymocyte globulin.
  - ♦ Delayed cell mediated type IV reaction, such as contact dermatitis from topical antihistamines.
  - ♦ Specific T cell mediated reaction, such as morbilliform rash from sulphonamides.
  - ♦ Fas/fas-ligand mediated reaction, such as toxic epidermal necrolysis and Stevens-Johnson syndrome.
  - ♦ Other reactions, such as lupus-like syndrome.
- ✶ Predictable non-immunological drug reaction
  - ♦ Primary pharmacologic side effects, such as dry mouth from antihistamines.
  - ♦ Secondary pharmacologic side effects such as oral thrush following broadspectrum antibiotic.
  - ♦ Drug toxicity such as oral ulcer following methotrexate.
  - ♦ Drug-drug interaction
  - ♦ Drug overdose.
- ✶ Unpredictable nonimmunologic reaction
  - ♦ Pseudoallergic, such as anaphylactic reaction after radiocontrast media.
  - ♦ Idiosyncratic
  - ♦ Intolerance

Neonatal vesicles

- ✶ Hereditary
  - ♦ Epidermolysis bullosa
  - ♦ Epidermolytic hyperkeratosis
  - ♦ Ectodermal dysplasia
  - ♦ Erythropoietic porphyria
  - ♦ Protein C/S deficiency
  - ♦ Incontinentia pigmenti
  - ♦ Hyperimmunoglobinemia E syndrome
  - ♦ Acrodermatitis enteropathica
- ✶ Acquired
  - ♦ Suction blister
  - ♦ Bullous impetigo

- Staphylococcal scalded skin syndrome
- β-hemolytic streptococcal infection
- Hemophilus influenzae infection
- Congenital syphilis
- Congenital candidiasis
- Herpes
- Varicella/chickenpox
- Miliaria crystalina
- Infantile acropustulosis
- Diffuse mastocytosis
- Self-healing reticulohistiocytosis
- Chronic bullous dermatosis of childhood (CBDC)
- Neonatal systemic lupus erythematosus

Keratoderma of palms and soles (PPK)

* Diffuse involvement
  - Epidermolytic PPK
  - Nonepidermolytic PPK
  - Mal de Meleda
  - PPK with deafness
  - Naxos disease
  - Sclerotylosis
  - Vohwinkel syndrome
  - Clouston syndrome
  - Omsted syndrome
* Focal involvement
  - Keratoderma areata
  - Striate PPK
  - Pachyonychia congenita
  - Keratosis punctata palmaris et plantaris
  - Papillon-Lefevre syndrome
  - Richner Hanhart syndrome
  - Howel Evans syndrome

Leg ulcer

- Malignant ulcer
- Hematologic ulcer
- Vascular ulcer
- Vasculitic ulcer
- Neuropathic ulcer
- Traumatic ulcer
- Infective ulcer
- Inflammatory ulcer
- Miscellaneous ulcer

Dermatofibroma/Benign fibrous histiocytoma (BFH)

- Cellular BFH
- Aneurysmal BFH
- Atypical BFH
- Epithelioid BFH
- Deep BFH

Hyperhidrosis

i. Physiological cause
  - Menopause

ii. Central causes
  - Emotional
  - Spinal injury
  - Stroke

iii. Systemic diseases
  - Tuberculosis
  - Malaria
  - Hyperthyroidism
  - Hyperparathyroidism

iv. Tumors
  - Pheochromocytoma
  - Carcinoid syndrome
  - Lymphoma
  - Leukemia

v. Drugs
  - Insulin
  - Meperidine
  - Emetics
  - Antipyretics

Occupational dermatoses

* Due to mechanical trauma
  - Hyperpigmentation
  - Hyperkeratosis

- Lichenification
- Callus/corn
- Black heel/telon noir, jogger's toe
- Friction blister, erosion and ulcer
- Koebner phenomenon in psoriasis and lichen planus
- Post-traumatic dermatitis

* Due to musical instrument
  - Fiddler's neck
  - Cellist's chest
  - Guiter nipple
  - Flautist's chin
* Due to computer
  - Mousing callus
  - Computer palm
* Due to vibration
  - Paresthesia and acro-osteolysis
* Due to household works
  - Hand dermatitis
  - Pulpitis
* Due to thermal injury
  - Blister
  - Necrosis
  - Ulceration
  - Erythema ab igne
  - Heat urticaria
  - Fern-like electric burn
* Due to chemical
  - Allergic contact dermatitis
  - Irritant contact dermatitis
  - Granulomatous reaction
  - Sclerodermoid changes due to vinyl chloride and silicon
* Due to cold exposure
  - Raynaud's phenomenon
  - Vasoconstriction
  - Hunting reaction
  - Immersion foot
  - Pulling boat hands
  - Acrocyanosis
  - Chilblains
  - Cold urticaria
  - Cold panniculitis
  - Erythromelalgia
  - Raynaud's phenomenon
  - Sclerema neonatorum
  - Subcutaneous fat necrosis of newborn
  - Livedo reticularis
  - Cryoglobulinemia
  - Cold agglutinemia
  - Cryofibrinogenimia
  - Frost bite.

Lupus erythematosus of the skin

* Acute cutaneous lupus erythematosus (ACLE)
  - Malar rash
  - Bullous LE
  - Erythema multiforme like LE (Rowell's syndrome)
  - Erythema multiforme major/TEN-like
* Subacute lupus erythematosus (SCLE)
  - Annular lesions
  - Papulosquamous lesions
  - Pityriasis rubra pilaris like lesions
  - Erythroderma
  - TEN-like lesions
  - Erythema gyratum repens-like lesions
* Chronic cutaneous lupus erythematosus
  - Discoid lupus erythematosus
    #Localized (head and neck)
    #Generalized
    #Hypertrophic
  - Tumid LE
  - Lupus profundus
  - Chilblains lupus

Mastocytosis of the skin

- Mastocytoma
- Urticaria pigmentosa

- Diffuse cutaneous mastocytosis
- Telangiectasia macularis eruptiva perstans

Onycholysis

- Trauma
- Foreign body insertion
- Formaldehyde for nail hardening
- Gasoline for paint removal
- Onychomycosis
- Chronic paronychia
- Secondary syphilis
- Wart
- Psoriasis
- Lichen planus
- Allergic contact dermatitis
- Porphyria cutanea tarda
- Epidermolysis bullosa acquisita
- Bullous pemphigoid
- Pemphigus vulgaris
- Glomus tumor
- Myxoid cyst
- Fibroma
- Melanoma
- Tetracycline
- Chloramphenicol
- Fluoroquinolones
- Quinine
- Phenothiazine
- Thiazide
- Nonsteroidal anti-inflammatory drugs (NSAIDs)
- Psoralen
- Retinoids
- Pregnancy
- Peripheral vascular disease
- Hyperhidrosis
- Yellow nail syndrome
- Hyper-/hypothyroidism
- Iron deficiency

Psychodermatologic disorders

i. Psychophysiologic disorders
- Acne
- Atopic dermatitis
- Psoriasis
- Dyshidrosis

ii. Primary psychiatric disorders
- Trichotillomania
- Delusional parasitosis
- Neurotic excoriations
- Factitial dermatitis

iii. Secondary psychiatric disorders
- Depression due to disfigurement in vitiligo, alopecia areata, etc.

iv. Cutaneous sensory disorders without any organic etiology and with or without any psychiatric disease.
- Unpleasant sensation like itching, burning, stinging, crawling, biting, etc.

v. Purely dermatologic and nonpsychiatric disorders in which psychotropic drugs are more effective than traditional dermatological drugs.
- Icthing in some cases is better controlled by anti-depressive drug doxepin than traditional antihistamine diphenhydramine.

Porphyria

A. Upstairs and downstairs model of hemesynthesis:

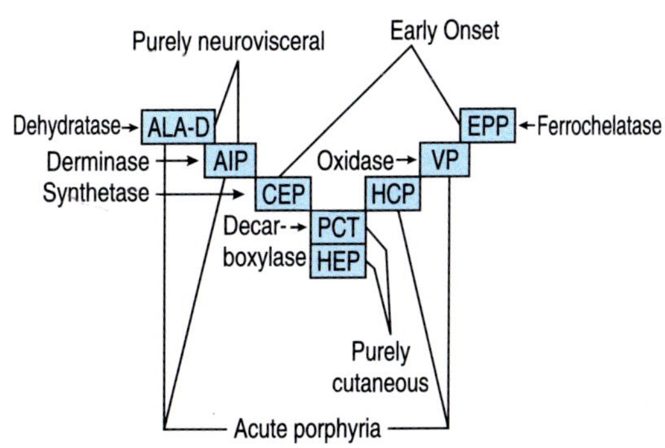

Fig. 1: Upstairs & downstairs model of heme synthesis

B. According to the onset and course

i. Acute porphyria
- ALA dehydratase deficiency porphyria (ALA-D)
- Acute intermittent porphyria (AIP)
- Hereditary coproporphyria (HCP)
- Variegate porphyria (VP)

ii. Chronic porphyria
- Congenital erythropoietic porphyria (CEP)
- Porphyria cutanea tarda (PCT)
- Hepatoerythropoietic porphyria (HEP)
- Erythropoietic protoporphyria (EPP)

C. According to the clinical manifestations:

i. Only cutaneous manifestation
- Porphyria cutanea tarda
- Hepatoerythropoietic porphyria

ii. No cutaneous manifestation but having neuro-visceral features
- ALA dehydratase deficiency porphyria
- Acute intermittent porphyria

iii. Both cutaneous and neurovisceral manifestations
- Congenital erythropoietic porphyria
- Hereditary coproporphyria
- Variegate porphyria
- Erythropoietic protoporphyria

Poikiloderma associated disorders

- Poikiloderma of Civatte
- Rothmund-Thomson syndrome
- Dyskeratosis congenita
- Xeroderma pigmentosa
- Bloom syndrome
- Cockyne syndrome
- Goltz syndrome
- Kindler syndrome
- Porphyria
- Dermatomyositis
- Systemic lupus erythematosus
- Graft versus host disease
- Large plaque parapsoriasis
- Mycosis fungoides
- Hodgkin lymphoma
- Post radiation
- Post steroid
- Arsenic and polycyclic hydrocarbon toxicity.

Primary scarring alopecia

* Neutrophilic
  - Folliculitis decalvans
  - Dissecting folliculitis
* Lymphocytic
  - Pseudopelade of Broq
  - Lichen planopilaris
  - Lupus erythematosus
  - Alopecia mucinosa
  - Keratosis follicularis spinulosa decalvans
* Mixed
  - Acne keloidalis/folliculitis keloidalis
  - Folliculitis necroticans
  - Erosive pustular dermatosis
* Nonspecific
  - End-stage of any of the above
  - Morphea

Pregnancy dermatoses

A. Specific dermatoses with fetal risk
- Pemphigoid gestationis
- Impetigo herpetiformis
- Cholestasis of pregnancy

B. Specific dermatoses without fetal risk
- Polymorphous eruption of pregnancy
- Prurigo of pregnancy
- Pruritic folliculitis of pregnancy
- Atopic eruption of pregnancy

C. Dermatoses modified by pregnancy

* Deterioration:
  - Leprosy
  - Condyloma acuminata
  - Herpes simplex
  - Varicella

- Candida
- Pityrosporum folliculitis
- Trichomoniasis
- Systemic scleroderma
- Systemic lupus erythematosus
- Erythema multiforme
- Dermatomyositis
- Pemphigus vulgaris
- Porphyria cutanea tarda
- Acrodermatitis enteropathica
- Ehler Danlos syndrome, type i & iv
- Pseudoxanthoma elasticum
- Erythrokeratoderma variabilis
- Bowenoid papulosis
- Langerhans cell histiocytosis
- Mycosis fungoides
- Malignant melanoma
- Neurofibroma

* Improvement
  - Hidradenitis suppurativa
  - Fox-Fordyce disease
* Unpredictable
  - Atopic dermatitis
  - Acne vulgaris
  - Psoriasis

D. Physiological cutaneous changes

- Striae distensae
- Chloasma
- Linea nigra

Hair shaft abnormalities

- Trichorrhexis nodosa
- Trichorrhexis invaginata
- Trichonodosis
- Trichothiodystrophy
- Monilethrix
- Pseudomonilethrix
- Pilitorti & associated syndromes
  1. Menke's kinky hair syndrome
  2. Bjornstad's syndrome
  3. Bazex syndrome
  4. Conradi-Hunermann syndrome
  5. Crandall's syndrome
  6. Citrullinemia
  7. Salti-Salem syndrome
  8. Some ectodermal dysplasia
- Pili annulati
- Pili multigemini
- Pohl-Pinkus lines
- Bubble hair
- Stright hair nevus
- Birds nest hair & dread locks
- Woolly hair & woolly hair nevus
- Uncombable hair syndrome
- Loose anagen hair syndrome

Porokeratosis

* Common variants
  - Classical porokeratosis of Mebelli
  - Disseminated superficial actinic porokeratosis
  - Disseminated superficial porokeratosis
  - Porokeratosis Palmaris et plantaris disseminata
  - Linear porokeratosis
* Uncommon variants
  - Facial porokeratosis
  - Giant porokeratosis
  - Punched out porokeratosis
  - Hyperkeratotic verrucous porokeratosis
  - Reticulate porokeratosis

Benign apocrine tumors

- Apocrine nevus
- Apocrine tubular papilloma
- Apocrine cylindroma
- Erosive adenomatosis of nipple
- Apocrine hidrocystoma
- Apocrine hidradenoma papilliferum
- Syringocystadenoma papilliferum

Connective tissue tumors

- Fibrous hamartoma of infancy
- Solitary fibroma
- Pleomorphic fibroma
- Dermatofibroma
- Desmoplastic fibroblastoma
- Atypical fibrohistiocytoma
- Collagenoma
- Sclerotic/plywood collaginoma
- Giant cell collaginoma

Eccrine benign tumors

- Eccrine nevus
- Poroma
- Cylindroma
- Hidrocystoma
- Hidradenoma
- Hidracanthoma simplex
- Syringoma
- Syringo fibroadenoma
- Spiradenoma

Hair follicle tumors

- Trichoadenoma
- Trichoblastoma
- Trichodiscoma
- Tricoepithelioma
- Trichofolliculoma
- Fibrofolliculoma
- Infundibular tumor
- Pilomatricoma
- Trichilemmal horn

Solitary neurofibroma

- Epithelioid cell type
- Dendritic cell type
- Granular cell type
- Pigmented cell type
- Collagenous type
- Myxoid type
- Lipomatous type

T-cell lymphoma

* Mycosis fungoides (MF)
  - Granulomatous slack skin
  - Pagetoid reticulosis
  - Adnexotrophic MF
  - Poikiloderma vasculare atrophicans
  - Psoriasiform MF
  - Subcutaneous panniculitis like MF
  - Sezary syndrome
* Adult T cell lymphoma
* NK T cell lymphoma

Primary B-cell lymphoma

- Follicle centric lymphoma
- Marginal follicular lymphoma
- Diffuse large B cell lymphoma
  - # Leg type
  - # Other type
  - # Intravascular type
- Plasmacytoid lymphoma

Secondary B-cell lymphoma

- CLL (Chronic lymphocytic leukemia)
- NHL (Non-Hodgkin lymphoma)

Lobular panniculitides

* Vasculitic
  - Erythema nodosum leprosum
  - Lucio phenomenon
  - Erythema induratum of Bazin
* Granulomatous
  - Traumatic panniculitis
  - Post-irradiation panniculitis
  - Post-steroid panniculitis
  - Sarcoidal panniculitis
  - Lymphomatous panniculitis
  - Subcutaneous fat necrosis of childhood
  - Lipomembranous fat necrosis
  - Lipodystrophy
  - Lipoatrophy

* Neutrophilic
  - Pancreatic panniculitis
  - Alfa$_1$ (α_1) antitrypsin deficiency
  - Infective panniculitis (bacterial, fungal, protozoal)
  - Foreign body/factitial panniculitis
* Lymphocytic
  - Cold panniculitis
  - Lupus panniculitis
* Sparse/no infiltration
  - Sclerosing panniculitis
  - Calciphylaxis
  - Sclerema neonatorum

Septal panniculitides

* Vasculitic
  - Thromophlebitis
  - Cutaneous polyarteritis nodosa
* Granulomatous with collagen degeneration
  - Necrobiosis lipoidica
  - Necrobiotic xanthogranuloma
* Granulomatous with fibrin degeneration
  - Rheumatoid nodule
* Granulomatous with mucin degeneration
  - Subcutaneous granuloma annulare
* Granulomatous without any degeneration
  - Erythema nodosum
* Lymphocytic/sparse infiltration
  - Deep morphea/morphoea profunda

Leukocytoclastic Vasculitis

* Involvement of cutaneous small vessels
  - Henoch-Schonlein purpura
  - Hypersensitivity vasculitis
  - Urticarial vasculitis
  - Erythema elevatum diutinum
  - Acute hemorrhagic edema of childhood
* Involvement of small to medium vessels

(i) Secondary vasculitis, due to
  - Infection
  - Autoimmune or connective tissue disorders
  - Drug or food additives
  - Malignancy
  - Genetic disorders

(ii) ANCA associated disorders
  - Microscopic polyangiitis
  - Wegener's granulomatosis
  - Churg-Strauss disease

(iii) Cryoglobulinemia associated
  - Type II
  - Type III

* Involvement of medium vessels
  - Polyarteritis nodosa
* Involvement of large vessel
  - Temporal arteritis
  - Takayasu's arteritis

Annular lesions

- Tinea corporis/cruris/imbricata
- Impetigo circinata
- BT, BB, BL leprosy
- Lupus vulgaris
- Tuberculosis verrucosa cutis
- Secondary syphilis
- Creeping eruption
- Granuloma annulare
- Sarcoidosis
- Subacute lupus erythematosus
- Necrolytic migratory erythema
- Elastotis perforans serpiginosa
- Psoriasis
- Lichen planus
- Pityriais rosea
- Porokeratosis
- Keratoacanthoma centrifugam marginatum
- Ichthyosis linearis circumflexa
- Urticaria
- Erythema annulare centrifugum
- Erythema migrans
- Erythema gyratum repens

- Purpura annularis telangiectoides
- Basal cell carcinoma
- Hemangioma
- Tufted hemangioendothelioma

Chancriform ulcers

- Syphilis
- Chancroid
- Yaws
- Tuberculosis
- Leishmaniasis
- Sporotricosis
- Blastomycosis

Cheilitis

- Actinic cheilitis
- Angular cheilitis
- Allergic/irritant contact cheilitis
- Cheilitis exfoliativa
- Granulomatous cheilitis
- Cheilitis glandularis

Cobble stone tongue

- Crohn's disease
- Cowden's disease
- Darier's disease
- Lipoid proteinosis

Earlobe infiltration

- Leprosy
- PKDL
- Multicentric reticulohistiocytosis
- Angiolymphoid hyperplasia
- Chondrodermatitis hallucis nodularis
- Calcinosis cutis
- Steatocystoma

Follicular hyperkeratosis

- Keratosis pilaris
- Keratosis pilaris decalvans
- Keratosis pilaris atrophicans
- Atrophoderma vermiculatum
- Kyrles disease
- Lichen planopilaris
- Lichen spinulosa
- Lichen scrofulosorum
- Atopic dermatitis
- Seborrhoeic dermatitis
- Fiber glass dermatitis
- Id eruption
- Drug reaction
- Scurvy
- Phrynoderma
- Psoriasis
- Pityriasis rubra pilaris
- Reiter's disease
- Sarcoidosis
- Cutaneous T-cell lymphoma
- Pityriasis versicolor
- Pityriasis rosea
- Fox-Fordyce disease

Annular vegetating ulcers

- Lupus vulgaris
- Blastomycosis
- Blastomycosis-like pyoderma
- Pyodermite vegetante
- Pyoderma gangrenosum (superficial spreading type)
- Necrolytic migratory erythema

Leonine facies

- Lepromatous leprosy
- Leishmaniasis
- Lipoid proteinosis
- Papular mucinosis
- Pachydermoperiostosis
- Amyloidosis
- Mastocytosis
- Multicentric reticulohistiocytosis
- Chronic actinic dermatitis

- Actinic reticuloid
- Progressive nodular histiocytosis
- Sezary syndrome
- B-cell lymphoma
- Polyostotic fibrous dysplasia
- Trichoepithelioma
- Neurofibromatosis
- Albright syndrome

Pearly papules

- Molluscum contagiosum
- Cryptococcosis
- Milia
- Sebaceous hyperplasia
- Sarcoidosis
- Granuloma annulare
- Trichoepithelioma
- Trichilemmoma
- Hidrocystoma
- Neuroma (palisading and encapsulated form)
- Malignant fibrous histiocytoma/atypical fibroxanthoma
- Basal cell carcinoma

Lichenoid papules

1. Lichen planus
2. Lichen nitidus
3. Lichen striatus
4. Lichenoid keratosis
5. Lichenoid drug reaction
6. Lichenoid polymorphic light eruption
7. Pityriasis lichenoides chronica
8. Guttate psoriasis
9. Papular sarcoidosis
10. Papular granuloma annulare
11. Lichenoid secondary syphilis
12. Papular mucinosis
13. Graft vs host disease
14. Id eruption
15. Bowenoid papulosis
16. Oid-Oid disease

Periorbital swelling

- Allergic contact dermatitis
- Irritant contact dermatitis
- Allergic gastroenteropathy
- Angioedema
- Urticaria
- Cellulitis
- Erysipelas
- Dental abscess
- Sinusitis
- Herpes
- Infectious mononucleosis
- Mucormycosis
- Trichinosis
- Chagas disease
- Post-infection
- Post irradiation
- Superior venacaval syndrome
- Cavernous sinus thrombosis
- Lymphoma
- Leukemia
- Osteoma
- Dermatomyositis
- Systemic lupus erythematosus
- Sarcoidosis
- Myxoedema
- Melkersson-Rosenthal syndrome

Piebald like lesion

- Piebaldism
- Waardenburg syndrome
- Tietz syndrome
- Albinism-deafness syndrome

Subungual hyperkeratosis

- Psoriasis
- Pityriasis rubra pilaris

- Reiter's disease
- Darier's disease
- Lichen planus
- Hyperkeratotic dermatitis
- Wart
- Onychomycosis
- Norwegian scabies

Subcutaneous cord like lesions

- Mondor's disease
- Panniculitis
- Nephrogenic fibrosing dermopathy
- Eosinophilic fasciitis
- Thrombophlebitis
- Rope sign in rheumatoid arthritis

Splinter hemorrhage

- Trauma
- Trichinosis
- Endocarditis
- Dermatomyositis
- Systemic lupus erythematosus/Scleroderma
- Microscopic polyangiitis

Sporotrichoid lesions

- Nocardiosis
- Sporotrichosis
- Cat scratch disease
- Leishmaniasis
- Tularemia
- Atypical tuberculosis
- Bacillary angiomatosis

Umbilicated papules

- Molluscum contagiosum
- Cryptococcosis
- Keratoacanthoma
- Lichen planus
- Sebaceous cyst

Nonleprotic peripheral nerve thickening

- Neurofibromatosis
- Primary amyloidosis
- Pachydermoperiostosis
- Familial hypertrophic interstitial neuritis
- Charcot-Marie Tooth disease
- Chronic inflammatory demyelinating polyneuropathy
- Cytomegalo virus associated polyneuropathy
- HIV infection-associated polyneuropathy
- Physiological in wrester and coolie

Vegetative lesion of the groin

- Pemphigus vegetans
- Benign familial pemphigus/Hailey Hailey disease
- Darier disease

Warty lesion

- Wart
- Tuberculosis verrucosa cutis
- Verrucous epidermal nevus
- Elephantiasis verrucosa nostras cutis
- Seborrheic keratosis
- Warty dyskeratoma
- Verrucous carcinoma

Diffuse pigmentation

- Addison's disease
- Cushing syndrome
- Hyper-and hypothyroidism
- Chronic hepatitis
- Chronic renal disease
- Hemochromatosis
- Ochronosis
- Metastatic melanoma
- Drugs and heavy metals
- Carbon baby syndrome

Anesthesia without peripheral nerve thickening

- Traumatic or entrapment neuropathy
- Meralgia paresthetica
- Congenital indifference to pain
- Chronic arsenicosis
- Isoniazide or thalidomide therapy
- Diabetes mellitus
- Syringomyelia
- Guillain-Barre syndrome

Reticulated pigmentation

- Erythema ab igne
- Retiform purpura
- Livedo reticularis
- Livedoid vasculitis
- Livedo racemosa
- Dermatopathia pigmentosa reticularis
- Reticuted acropigmentation of kitamura
- Dowling-Degos disease
- Dyskeratosis congenita
- Naegeli-Franceschetii-Jadassohn syndrome
- Clouston syndrome (Hidrotic ectodermal dysplasia)
- Tinea versicolor
- Retained keratin (terra firma)

Idiopathic photodermatoses

- Polymorphous light eruption
- Solar urticaria
- Actinic prurigo
- Hydroa vacciniforme
- Juvenile spring eruption

Photosensitive genodermatoses

- Xeroderma pigmentosa
- Bloom syndrome
- Rothmund-Thomson syndrome
- Cockayne syndrome
- Trichothiodystrophy
- Hartnup disease

Dermatoses aggravated by sunlight

- Photoallergic contact dermatitis
- Photoirritant contact dermatitis
- Phytophotodermatitis
- Lupus erythematosus
- Dermatomyositis
- Porphyrias (congenital erythropoietic porphyria, erythropoietic protoporphyria, porphyria cutanea tarda and pseudo porphyria cutanea tarda)
- Pellagra
- Tinea faciei
- Seborrheic dermatitis of face

Dyschromatoses

- Dyschromatosis symmetrica hereditaria (DSH)
- Dyschromatosis universalis hereditaria
- Acropigmentation of Dohi

Human herpes virus (HHV)

- α-herpes virus
  - HHV_1 (HSV_1)
  - HHV_2 (HSV_2)
  - HHV_3 (Varicella-Zoster virus)
- β-herpes virus
  - HHV_5 (Cytomegalovirus)
  - HHV_6 (HSV_6)
  - HHV_7 (Human T cell lymphotrophic virus)
- γ-herpes virus
  - HHV_4 (Epstein-Barr virus)
  - HHV_8 (Kaposi sarcoma associated virus).

COMPARATIVE DERMATOLOGY

CHAPTER B3

Morphology	Acute dermatitis	Subacute dermatitis	Chronic dermatitis
Vesicles, papulovesicles	+++	+/–	–
Papules	++/+	+/–	+/++
Erosions	+	+/–	–
Oozing	+++	+	–
Crusting	+	+++	–
Scaling	+/–	+/–	++/+
Lichenification	–	–	+++

Features	Nevus cell	Melanocyte	Melanoma cell
Arrangement	Cluster	Solitary	Cluster and sheet
Cytoplasm	Round or spindle	Dendritic	Round or spindle
Nucleus	Small and regular	Small and regular	Large, irregular and hyperchromatic
Mitosis	Rare	Rare	Frequent

Exogenous dermatitis	Endogeneous dermatitis
* Cause is from outside the body	* Cause is from inside the body
* Lesions are usually focal and unilateral * Generalized lesions are distributed asymmetrically	* Lesions are usually multiple and bilateral * Generalized lesions are usually distributed symmetrically
* Course is usually short	* Course is usually long with frequent relapse and remission

Allergic contact dermatitis (ACD)	Irritant contact dermatitis (ICD)
❖ Requires sensitization ❖ A form of delayed hypersensitivity reaction	❖ No need of prior sensitization ❖ A form of direct burn
❖ Slow onset ❖ Symptom: Itching ❖ Lesions: Erythematous papules, papulovesicles, vesicles, erosions, oozing and crusting in acute stage. ❖ Lesions are lichenified papules and plaques in chronic stage ❖ Lesions may extend beyond the area of contact	❖ Rapid onset ❖ Symptoms: Burning sensation and pain ❖ Lesions: Erythematous macules, patches, vesicles. Erosions, ulcerations, necrosis, crusting in acute stage followed by dyspigmentation and scarring. Papules are absent. ❖ Lesions are mild erythematous macules and patches with xerosis, chapping and fissuring in chronic stage ❖ Lesions remain localized within the area of contact

Melanocytes	Nevus cells
Dendritic	Nondendritic
Arrange singly	Lie in cluster or nest
Can transfer melanin to keratinocyte	Can not

Features	Ichthyosis vulgaris	X-linked ichthyosis
Inheritance	Autosomal dominant	X-linked recessive
Deficiency	Profillagrin	Steroid sulfatase
Onset	After 3 months of age	Within 3 months of age
Scale	Fine and lighter	Large and darker
Site	Mostly extensors of the limbs	Extensors along with flexor surfaces of the limbs, face and trunk
Association	Atopic dermatitis	Maternal cataract
Histopathology	Hypo- or absent granular layer	Normal or slightly thickened granular layer
Electron microscopy	Abnormal profillagrin	Nonspecific

Features	Glomus tumor	Glomangioma
Onset	Adolescence to adulthood	Infancy and childhood
Symptom	Painful	Asymptomatic
Number	Solitary	Multiple
Site	Extremities with a subungual predilection	Extremities without any subungual predilection
Histopathology	Solid mass due to proliferation of glomus cells	Dilated vessels, lined by few glomus cells

Features	Granulomatous cheilitis	Cheilitis glandularis
Onset	Sudden onset in adulthood	Insidious onset in infancy and childhood
Site	Starts at upper lip but lower lip is severely affected.	Lower lip is affected first and more severely than upper lip.
Clinical features	❖ Asymptomatic progressive and permanent swelling. ❖ Secondary infection does not occur.	❖ Swelling and eversion of lower lip. ❖ Patulous openings of the mucous ducts. ❖ Mucoid discharge acts as glue which dries to adhere the lips by night. ❖ Mucous glands are palpable with a pebbly feeling. ❖ Secondary infection may occur.
Causes	Unknown	❖ Chronic irritation ❖ Actinic damage ❖ Factitious trauma ❖ Atopy
Histopathology	Tuberculoid granuloma with infiltration of lymphocytes, plasma cells, histiocytes and Langhans' giant cell.	Infiltration of lymphocytes, histiocytes and plasma cells in and around the glands.

Features	Psoriatic erythroderma	Dermatitis induced erythroderma	Drug induced erythroderma	Essential erythroderma
Prior to onset	Psoriatic lesion ++/–	Focal dermatitis ++	Drug intake ++	No history of any other dermatoses
Scaling	+++	++ to +	++ to +	++ to +
Erythema	+++	++ to +	++ to +	+++ to +
Edema	+ to ++	+++	+ to ++	+ to ++
Onset	Usually insidious	Insidious	Dramatic	Insidious to dramatic

Features	Pruritic papular eruption	Eosinophilic folliculitis
Clinical features	❖ Excoriated skin colored papules and prurigo nodularis like lesions. ❖ Pustules are rare. ❖ Post inflammatory hyperpigmentation and scar formation	❖ Edematous papules with few pustules.
Distribution	❖ Symmetrically distributed at extremities, face, trunk, and rarely at palms, soles and digital spaces.	❖ Forehead, eyelids, cheeks, neck, posterior auricular, upper arms and trunk.
Histopathology	❖ Epidermal hyperplasia. ❖ Dermal perivascular and interstitial lymphocytic and eosinophilic infiltration	❖ Follicular spongiosis. ❖ Folliculocentric eosinophilic infiltration. ❖ Presence of flame figures and eosinophilic abscesses.
Investigation in association with HIV infection	❖ CD4 < 100/μL ❖ Increased CD8 cells.	CD4 < 300/μL

Features	Demodex folliculitis (Demodicidosis)	Pityrosporum folliculitis
Clinical features	❖ Rosacea-like erythematous papules with reddish background	❖ Follicular and perifollicular papules and pustules.
Distribution	❖ Head and neck.	❖ Back, chest and shoulder.
Histopathology	❖ Spongiotic infundibular infiltration. Demonstration of Demodex folliculorum	❖ Yeasts may be found.

Features	Plasma cell balanitis	Erythroplasia of Queyrat
Etiology	Unknown	HPV type 16, 18, 31, 35
Lesions	Sharply defined erythematous patch with moist and shiny surface. Never turns into malignancy.	Single or multiple erythematous fixed well defined multiple papules or single plaque with moist smooth or velvety surface. Invasive SCC may develop.
Histopathology	Epidermal atrophy with basal layer degeneration and erosion, lozenge-shaped keratinocytes, lichenoid infiltration with predominant plasma cells.	Epidermal hyperplasia with abnormal keratinocytes.
Treatment	❖ Circumcision ❖ Topical corticosteroid ❖ Laser ablation	❖ 5%-5-FU cream, once daily for 3-12 weeks. ❖ 5% imiquimod, thrice in a week for 3-12 weeks. ❖ Surgery

Features	Inflammatory verrucous epidermal nevus (ILVEN)	Linear psoriasis
Expression of K10	Normal	Reduced
Age	1st Month of life	Later life
Symptom	Very pruritic	Occasionally pruritic
Progress	Slow	Rapid
Response to medical therapy	Poor	good

Features	Urticaria	Urticarial vasculitis
Symptom	Itching	Burning or pain
Morphology	❖ Erythematous and edematous papules and plaques, persisting for < 24 hours. ❖ No residual lesion following subsidence.	❖ Erythematous and edematous papules and plaques, persisting for > 24 hours, along with purpura, vesicle and necrosis. ❖ Hypo- or hyperpigmentation may persist as residual sign.
Distribution	❖ Asymmetrical and at any site.	❖ Symmetrical and mostly at trunk and proximal limbs.
Association	❖ Usually no systemic features present ❖ Angioedema often associated	❖ Usually systemic features present ❖ Angioedema, usually not present.

Features	Acropigmentation of Kitamura	Acropigmentation of Dohi
Morphology	❖ Atrophic reticulate pigmentation at dorsa of the hands and feet. ❖ Breakage of epidermal ridges. ❖ Palmar pits present.	❖ Mixture of mottled hypo- and hyperpigmented, nonatrophic macules at dorsa of the hands and feet, arms, legs, trunk and shoulder. ❖ No breakage of the epidermal ridge-pattern. ❖ No palmar pits.

Features	Raynaud's phenomenon	Raynaud's disease
Etiology	Secondary	Primary
Age of onset	> 25 years	Adolescent/young adult, mean age 14 years
Female : male ratio	4:1	20:1
Number of attacks/day	5-10	< 5
Precipitating factors	Only cold	Cold and emotion
Ischemic changes	Present	Absent
Abnormal capillaroscopy	Present	Absent
Anticentromere antibody	Positive in 50-60% cases	Negative
Antinuclear antibody	Positive in 90-95% cases	Negative
Scl 70	Positive in 20-30% cases	Negative
Platelet activity	Increased in 75% cases	Normal

Features	Lichen nitidus	Lichen planus
Size and color	Pin head size and skin colored or hypopigmented or flesh colored.	Pinhead to larger size and purple to violaceous color, later hyperpigmented.
Wickham striae	Absent	Present
Site of distribution	❖ Upper limbs, genitalia and trunk, sparing oral mucosa.	❖ Wrists, ankles, flexors of the forearms, front of the legs, including oral mucosa.
Pruritus	Uncommon	Very common
Histopathology	❖ Parakeratosis common. ❖ Thin or absent granular layer. ❖ Dermal infiltration containing lymphocytes, epithelioid cells, Langhans' giant cells. ❖ Infiltration localized within 2-3 dermal papillae and appearing claw clutching ball due to hyperplastic rete ridges at the periphery of the lesion.	❖ Parakeratosis uncommon. ❖ Focally increased granular layer. ❖ Lymphocytic infiltration. ❖ Band like infiltration without any limited confinement by the rete ridges.

Features	Lichen spinulosa	Lichen scrofulosorum
Epidemiology	❖ Children are commonly affected. ❖ Adolescents are also affected. ❖ History of atopy, infection and heredity may be present.	❖ Children with nodal or bone tuberculosis are commonly affected. ❖ It may occur following BCG vaccination.
Clinical features	❖ Clusters of grouped skin colored asymptomatic follicular papules with a nutmeg grater like texture. ❖ Each papule is topped with a central keratotic spine. ❖ Size of each group is variable from 2-6 cm. ❖ Lesions are distributed symmetrically. ❖ Neck, extensor arms, abdomen, buttocks and popliteal fossae are the common sites. ❖ Face, hands and feet are spared. ❖ Onset is sudden and lesions undergo a rapid progress for a short period. Then lesions become stable and persist for an indefinite period.	❖ Asymptomatic perifollicular tiny firm lichenoid papules, topped by scale. ❖ Lesions are grouped in clusters. ❖ Trunk is the commonest site. ❖ Lesions may persist for months and heal without scarring.
Mantoux test	Negative	Highly positive
Histopathology	❖ Dilated follicles with follicular plugging.	❖ Superficial granuloma around hair follicles and sweat ducts. ❖ Caseation is little or absent. ❖ AFB negative.

Features	Kimura's disease	Angiolymphoid hyperplasia
Age of onset	Younger	Older
Duration	Longer	Shorter
Morphology & Histopathology	❖ Deep-seated large soft tissue mass with normal overlying skin. ❖ Thin walled blood vessels ❖ Plump of histiocytoid endothelial cells not present ❖ Lymphoid follicles with active germinal center + ❖ Folliculolysis by eosinophils and lymphocytes ++ ❖ Fibrosis +	❖ Multiple soft papular or nodular lesions with normal or ulcerated overlying skin. ❖ Thick walled blood vessels ❖ Plump of histiocytoid endothelial cells present ❖ Lymphoid follicles with active germinal center +/– ❖ Folliculolysis by eosinophils and lymphocytes +/– ❖ Fibrosis –
Peripheral blood eosinophilia	++	±
IgE level	Normal or elevated	Normal

Features	Bowen's disease	Bowenoid papulosis
Chance of malignant transformation	Present	Absent
Association	Chronic arsenicosis	HPV 16 & 18
Number of the lesion	Single	Multiple
Morphology	❖ Scaly or crusted erythematous plaque with irregular surface ❖ Border is well defined but irregular	❖ Hyperpigmented dome shaped papules with smooth surface ❖ Border is well defined and often regular

Features	Pemphigus vulgaris	Bullous pemphigoid	Dermatitis herpetiformis
Age	30-60 years	50-70 years	20-40 years
Pain	++	+/–	–/+
Pruritus	–	+/–	+++
Oral ulcer	+++	+/–	–
Vesicle	+++	++	+/–
Bulla (intact)	+/–	+++	–/+
Papulovesicle	–	+/–	++
Erosion/ulcer	+++	++	+/–
Nikolsky's sign	+	–	–
Bulla spreading sign	+	–	–
Acantholytic cell	+	–	–
Cleft level	Suprabasal	Subepidermal	Subepidermal
Cleft content	Acantholytic cell	Eosinophil	Neutrophil
Immunofluorescence	IgG at intercellular space	IgG & C3 at DEJ	Granular IgA at dermal papillae

Features	*M. leprae*	*M. tuberculosis*
Regeneration time	13 days	20 hours
Acid fastness to	5% H_2SO_4	20% H_2SO_4
Size	Shorter	Longer
State in the tissue	Singly or in bunch	Singly
Cell wall	Two layers	Three layers
Lipid content in the wall	More and having tendency to form foamy macrophage	Less and having no tendency to form foamy macrophage
DNA content	Less, 2.2^9 dalton	More, 2.6^9 dalton

Features	Phrynoderma	Keratosis pilaris
Age of onset	Childhood	Adolescence
Morphology of the lesions	More keratotic	Less keratotic
	Discrete and confluent	Discrete
	Perilesional erythema absent	Present
Commonest sites	Elbows and knees	Outer surface of the arms and anterior surface of the thighs
Response to vitamin A	Excellent	Poor

Features	Lichen spinulosa	Keratosis pilaris
Age of onset	Childhood	Adolescence
Morphology of the lesion	Pin-point size	Pinhead size
	More spiny	Less spiny
	Discrete and confluent	Discrete
	Perilesional erythema absent	Present
Common sites	Widespread, specially trunk	Outer surface of the arms and anterior surface of the thighs

Features	Morphea	Nongenital lichen sclerosus et atrophicus
Morphology	Brownish to whitish indurated and depressed plaque	Hypopigmented to whitish elevated plaque
	Surface may show wrinkling due to epidermal atrophy	Surface shows prominent follicular ostia due to keratin plugging
	Sensory loss may be present	No sensory loss
Histopathology	Epidermal atrophy, homogenization of dermis due to increased collagen	Hyperkeratosis with atrophy of Malpighian layer, basal layer degeneration with lichenoid infiltration, subepidermal edema due to deposition of muco-polysaccharide with papillary dermal homogenization
Response to corticosteroid	Poor	Better

Features	TT	BT	BB	BL	LL
Primary lesion	Macule, patch, papulc or plaque	Patch and plaque	Plaque	Nodule and plaque	Macule, papule, plaque and diffuse infiltration
No. of lesion	1-3	3-10	Many but countable	Many and may not be countable	Numerous
Arrangement of the lesion	Usually unilateral and asymmetrical	May be bilateral but asymmetrical	Bilateral but asymmetrical	Bilateral with a tendency of symmetry	Bilateral and symmetrical
Shape of the lesion	Round and annular	Variable	Round and annular, inverted saucer shaped/ punched out	Round, oval, dome shaped and annular	Macules and papules are round and papules are circumscribed

Contd. to next page

Contd.

Size of the lesion	1-3 cm	3-10 cm may be very large	Variable	Nodules are 0.5-1 cm, but plaques are variable	Macules and papules are 0.3-0.5 cm but others are variable
Margin of lesion	Well defined macule, patch or papule. Annular plaque is having well defined inner and outer margins.	Well to ill defined patch. Annular plaque is having ill defined inner margin and well defined outer margin.	Annular plaque is having well defined inner margin and ill defined outer margin	Nodules are ill defined. Annular plaque is having ill defined both inner and outer margins.	Macules are ill defined. Papules are well defined and having an acute angle between the lesion and skin of the surrounding area
Color of the lesion	Coppery or erythematous	Hypopigmented, coppery or erythematous	Erythematous	Erythematous	Hypopigmented, skin colored or coppery color
Hair loss and sweat loss	+++	++	+	+/–	–
Sensory loss	90-100%	70-80%	50-70%	50%	No loss at early lesions, variable loss at late lesion and presence of gloves and stocking anesthesia at hands and feet
Peripheral nerve thickening	Unlikely	Unilateral or bilateral but asymmetrical	Bilateral but asymmetrical	Bilateral with tendency of symmetry	Bilateral and symmetrical
Special feature	Cutaneous feeding nerve may be present at and around the lesion	Satellite lesion +	Punched out lesion +	Dome-shaped lesion +	Gloves and stocking anesthesia +
Lepromin test	3+	2+	1+	+/–	–
Slit skin smear	+/–	1+	2+/3+	3+/4+	5+/6+
Granuloma	Epithelioid cells ++ Lymphocytes + Circumscribed granuloma No grenz zone AFB +/–	Epithelioid cells ++ Lymphocytes ++ Giant cell +/– Less circumscribed granuloma, Grenz zone +/– AFB 1+	Epithelioid cells + Lymphocytes ++ Diffuse granuloma Grenz zone + AFB 2+/1+	Epithelioid cells +/– Lymphocytes +++ Foamy macrophage +/– Diffuse granuloma Grenz zone + AFB 2+/3+	Foamy macrophage +++ Diffuse granuloma Grenz zone ++ AFB (4-6)+

Features	Psoriasis	Lichen planus	Discoid lupus erythematosus
Symptom	Mild to severe itching	Moderate to severe itching	Burning sensation on sunexposure
Photosensitivity	Absent	Absent	Present
Primary lesion	Scaly papules and plaques	Scaly papules and plaques	Scaly papules and plaques
Number of the lesion	Variable from single, few to numerous	Variable from few to numerous	Variable from single to few, rarely numerous
Distribution	Usually bilateral and symmetrical	Usually bilateral and symmetrical	May be bilateral and symmetrical
Site of involvement	Extensors of limbs, scalp, buttocks and back	Flexors and mucosal surfaces	Photo exposed areas, like face, upper back and upper chest
Scale	Often profuse, loosely adherent and silvery	Variable in amount and adherence	Variable in amount but adherent and thick
Color	Reddish	Violaceous	Reddish, hyperpigmented and depigmented
Initial shape	Round	Polygonal	Round
Initial size	Pea	Pin head to pea	Pea to coin
Special feature	Auspitz sign +	Wickham's striae +	Carpet tack/tin tag sign +
Histopathology	Hyperkeratosis, parakeratosis, Munro's microabscess and regular acanthosis with elephant foot appearance of rete ridges	Orthokeratotic hyperkeratosis with sawtooth appearance, basal layer degeneration, band like lymphocytic infiltration along the basement membrane zone	Hyperkeratosis with/without parakeratosis, follicular plugging, irregular acanthosis, focal basal layer degeneration, patchy lymphocytic infiltration around the vessels and appendages

Features	Telogen effluvium	Chronic telogen effluvium	Diffuse female pattern baldness
Etiology	High fever, parturition or any other physical or mental stress	Unknown	Multifactorial including heredity, hormonal and aging influence
Onset	Abrupt	Abrupt	Gradual
Amount of shedding	Excessive	Profuse and reduced ponytail volume	Minimum
Quality of hair	Diffuse thinning but no miniaturization	Thinning ±, if present, it is diffuse	Central thinning
Bitemporal recession	Absent	Present and common	Present but uncommon
Hair pull test	Positive throughout the scalp	Positive throughout the scalp in active phase	Positive at central part
Trichogram	Reduced anagen and telogen ratio (A:T)	A:T, reduced in active phase	A:T, normal or slightly reduced
Shaft diameter	No variation	No variation	Marked variation
Biopsy	Terminal:vellus hair ratio (T:V), normal 8:1	T:V, normal 8:1	T:V, < 4:1
Prognosis	Self limited and recovered when stress is withdrawn	Prolonged but fluctuating	Slowly progressive

Features	Darier's disease	Benign familial pemphigus
Cleft	Lacunae	Vesicle or bulla
Acantholysis	Less prominent and localized to suprabasal area	Profound, involving whole Malpighian layer
Dyskeratosis	More prominent	Less prominent

Features	Erythema annulare centrifugum	Erythema marginatum
Age	Young and middle aged	Children and young adults
Morphology of the lesions	❖ Annular erythematous plaques. ❖ Lesions start as papules, then flattening of the centers to evolve into annular lesion, scales present at inner margin known as trailing scale. ❖ May enlarge irregularly to form an archiform lesion. ❖ Rarely vesicle, purpura and pigmentation may develop. ❖ Itching may present in some cases. ❖ Lesions last for days, weeks or months. Size become 6-8 cm by 2 weeks.	❖ Annular erythematous lesions, fade within hours to 2-3 days. ❖ Recurrent crops develop at different sites. ❖ Lesions become prominent in the afternoon.
Site of involvement	Buttocks, thighs, upper arms	Trunk, specially abdomen
Histopathology	Perivascular lymphocytic infiltration with tightly cuffed coat sleeve pattern appearance.	Infiltration of polymorphs

Features	Giant cell arteritis	Takayasu's arteritis
Age	> 50 years	< 50 years
Involvement	❖ Major branches of aorta with predilection for extracranial branches of carotid artery.	❖ Major branches of aorta with predilection for retinal artery.
General clinical features	❖ Fever and weight loss, ❖ Polymyalgia rheumatica with aching and morning stiffness of shoulder and pelvic girdle muscle ❖ Localized headache ❖ Facial pain during chewing due to claudication of jaw muscles ❖ Leg claudication ❖ Sudden permanent loss of vision due to occlusion of ocular and orbital arteries ❖ Amaurosis fugax, a transient monocular visual loss	❖ Hypertension and renal dysfunction. ❖ Abdominal pain and bleeding due to ischemia or infarction. ❖ Aortic arch syndrome with arm claudication ❖ Absent radial and brachial pulses
Cutaneous features	❖ Tender, pulseless and nodular artery at temporal or occipital region	❖ Erythema nodosum or induratum like lesion

Contd. to next page

Contd.

Features	Giant cell arteritis	Takayasu's arteritis
Morphology	❖ Tongue ulceration or infarction	❖ Ulcerated subacute nodular lesion ❖ Papulo necrotic eruption ❖ Papular erythematous lesions of hands and fingers ❖ Lump like facial lesion ❖ Panniculitis ❖ Cutaneous necortizing vasculitis
Complications in late stage	❖ Angina, myocardial infarction ❖ Cerebrovascular accident ❖ Neuropsychiatric complication ❖ Bowel angina or infarction	❖ Atherosclerosis and calcification
Histopathology	❖ Lymphocytic and macrophage infiltration of tunica media, followed by intima and adventitia ❖ Fragmented elastic lamina ❖ Concentric intimal thickening ❖ Giant cell, granuloma and fibrinoid necrosis	❖ Inflammatory infiltrate at vasavasorum, followed by panarteritis ❖ Fibrosis, replaces infiltration ❖ Reduction of lumen by fibrosis or by thrombosis
Response to glucocorticoid	Dramatic	❖ Good in early stage but not effective in late stage

AN APPROACH TO DIAGNOSIS

CHAPTER B4

Identification of Skin lesions

* Identification of skin lesions is must to reach a diagnosis and it requires a point by point observation.
* We sometimes misdiagnose one form of lesion as another form due to their clinical mimicry. As an example, an edematous papule may be misdiagnosed as a vesicle, a nodule as a papule or a keratin cyst as a pustule.
* But if we observe carefully, will see surface of the edematous papule may have depressions at hair follicles or a peau-d'-orange appearance and this picture is not expected if it is really a vesicle.
* Similarly in case of a nodule we will get an obtuse angle between the surface of the lesion and surrounding area as the lesion arises from the deeper skin. But in case of a papule the angle is usually acute as it arises mostly from the epidermis or superficial part of the skin.
* In case of a keratin cyst, the color is more white and consistency is firm. In case of a pustule, color is turbid and consistency is soft.

Types of skin lesions

* Primary lesions: Macule, patch, papule, nodule, plaque, vesicle, bulla and pustule.
* Secondary lesions: Erosion, ulcer, fissure, excoriation, sinus, fistula, scar and lichenification.
* Special lesion: Comedone, burrow, milia, telangiectasia, petechiae, purpura, ecchymosis and tumor.

Special structures and changes related to skin lesions

* These are scales, crusts, atrophy, hypertrophy, erythema, induration and lichenification.
* *Though very often scales and crusts are placed under secondary lesions, I feel they are not at all skin lesions.*
* Scales are usually associated with primary lesions.
* Crusts are usually associated with secondary lesions.

Types of primary lesions

- Simple primary lesions: Macule, patch, papule, plaque, nodule, vesicle, bulla, pustule, etc.

- Compound primary lesions: Combination of two or more simple primary lesions, such as maculopapule, papulovesicle, papulopustule, etc.
- Complicated primary lesions: Combination of primary and secondary lesions, such as eroded macule or patch, excoriated or crusted papules, ulcerated plaque or nodule, etc.

Macule

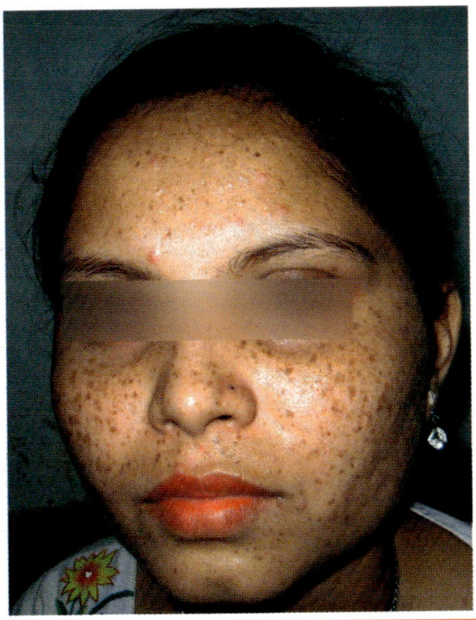

Fig. 1: Multiple hyperpigmented small flat lesions of freckles

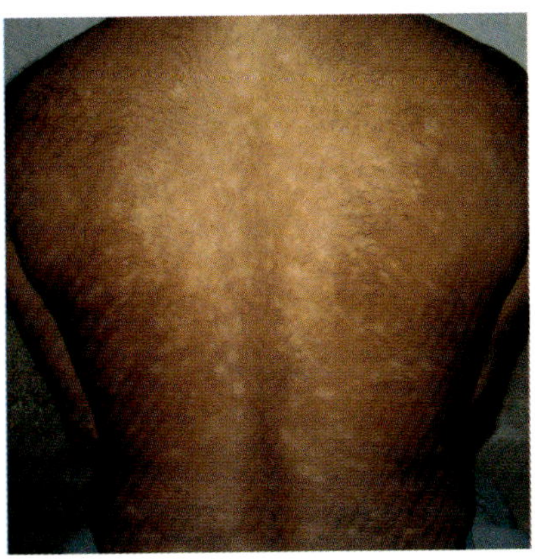

Fig. 2: Multiple ill defined small hypopigmented flat nonelevated lesions in a case of subsiding pityriasis rosea

- The term is used to denote a flat and nonelevated lesion with altered color.
- Many dermatologists like a size barrier for macule as less than 5 mm.
- It mostly occurs due to changes in the epidermis.
- Sometimes dermal changes may produce such lesion as in lichen sclerosus et artrophicus.
- *Along with many others I like to use the term irrespective of size.*
- Classical example is hypopigmented or depigmented flat skin lesion of vitiligo without any other texural change.

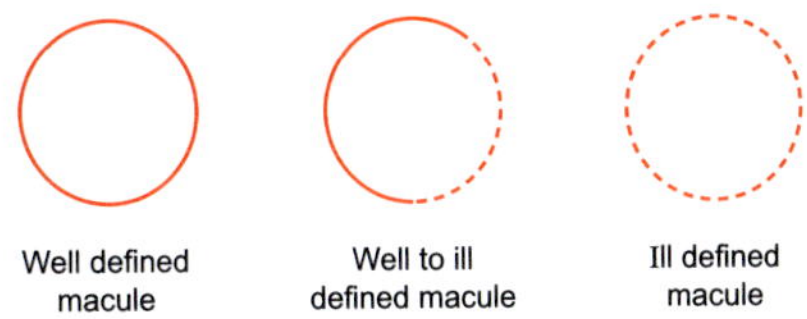

- Variants of macule:
  - Erythematous macule/Purpuric macule: Color is due to underlying dilated dermal vessels or due to extravasated red blood cells.
  - Hyperpigmented macule: Color is due to overproduction of melanin by the melanocytes or from an exogenous or endogenous source.
  - Hypopigmented or depigmented macule: Less production or no production of color by the melanocytes.
  - Well defined macule: When all sides of the margin is well demarcated from the surrounding area.
  - Well to ill defined macule: When most of the margin is well demarcated but some of the part merges with surrounding area or poorly demarcated.
  - Ill defined macule: When all sides of the margin is not possible to make out clearly.

Patch

- The term is used for a flat and nonelevated lesion with altered color, like a macule but size is more than 5 mm.
- It mostly develops due to pathology of the epidermis.

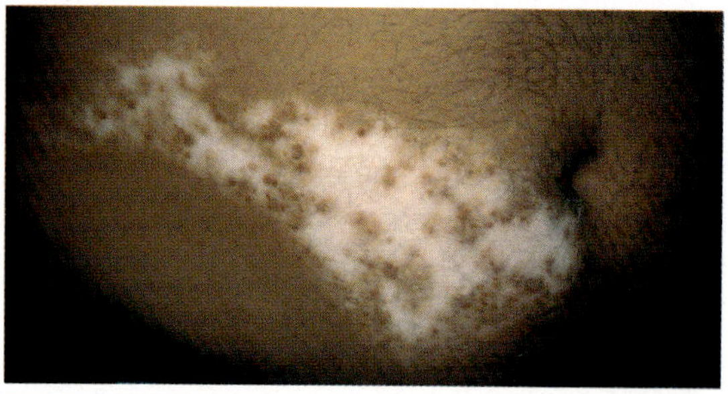

Fig. 3: Irregular flat nonelevated depigmented lesion of segmental vitiligo, studded with repigmented macules

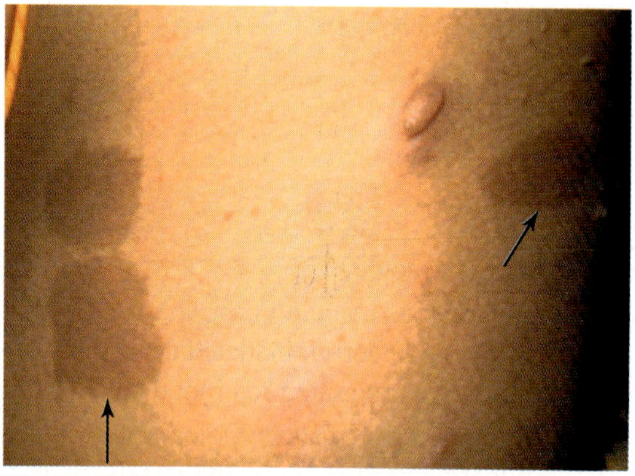

Fig. 4: Well defined hyperpigmented nonelevated flat lesion of Café-au-lait macules in neurofibromatosis

- Sometimes dermal changes may produce such lesion as in morphoea.
- *I like to use the term for a flat nonelevated lesion with some surface changes like wrinkling or scale, etc., irrespective of size.*
- Classical example is hypopigmented or hyperpigmented flat but mild scaly lesions of pityriasis versicolor.
- Sometimes mild elevation (pseudoelevation) may be felt over a patch due to presence of scale.
- Sometimes patch may be depressed due to underlying induration as in morphoea.

Papule and Plaque

- The term 'papule' is used for a superficial, solid, elevated skin lesion with size less than 5 mm and height is more than depth.
- The term 'plaque' is used for a solid elevated skin lesion, having a size more than 5 mm and a plateau-like surface where width is more than height and height is more than depth.

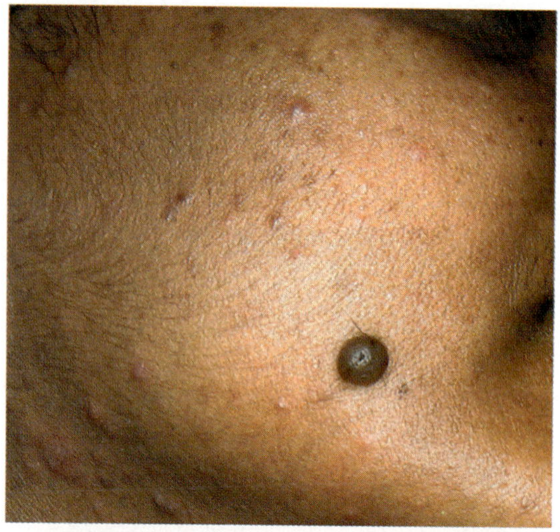

Fig. 5: Single dark colored solid elevated lesions of compound melanocytic nevus and multiple erythematous papules of acne vulgaris

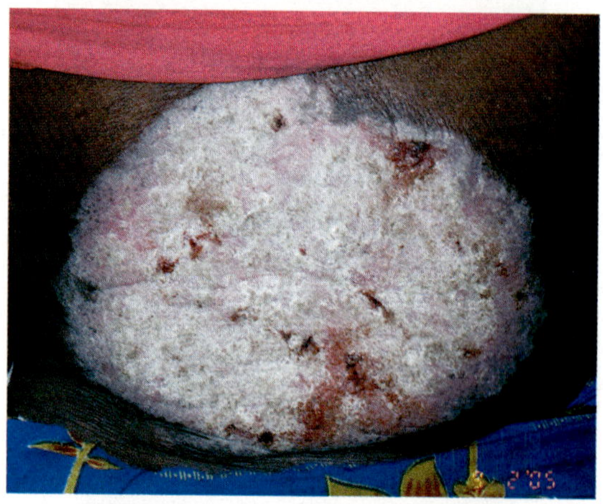

Fig. 6: Well defined scaly plaque of discoid lupus erythematosus

- Pathologically papule/plaque originates from the epidermis.
- Variants of papule and plaque:
  - Surface of the lesion may be smooth/rough/mammilated, atrophic, acuminate, filiform, warty, papillomatous and umbilicated.

- Base of the lesion may be sessile or pedunculated.
- Cosistency of the lesion may be soft, firm, indurated or hard.

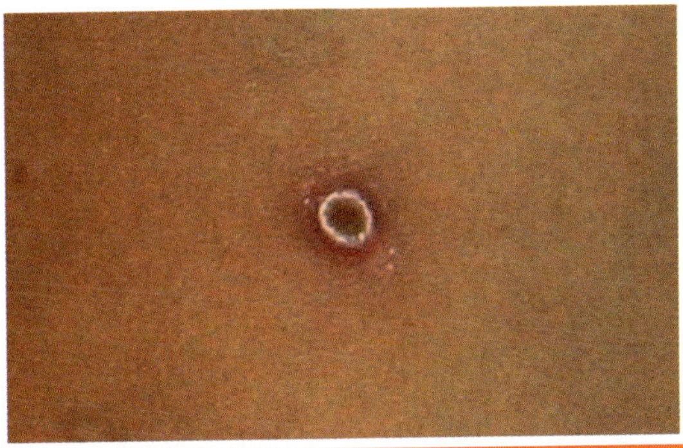

Fig. 7: Umbilicated papule of reactive perforating collagenosis (RPC)

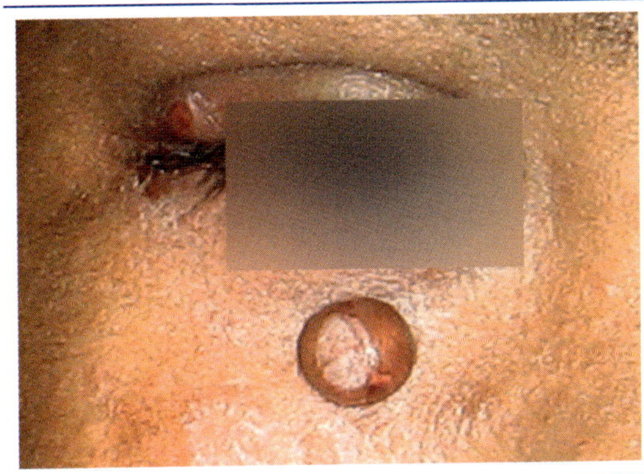

Fig. 8: Umbilicated papule of molluscum contagiosum

Nodule

- The term is used to denote a dome shaped solid lesion, irrespective of size, having a significant depth where depth is more than height.

* Pathologically nodule originates from the dermis and epidermis or only from the dermis or from subcutaneous tissue.
* Variants of nodule:
  - Epidermal: Lesion is localized within or extending upto the epidermis.
  - Dermoepidermal: Lesion is localized at or extending upto the dermoepidermal junction.
  - Dermal: Lesion is localized within or extending upto the dermis.

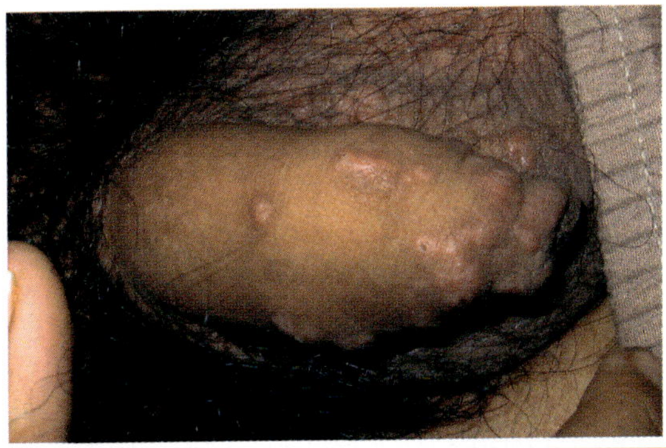

Fig. 9: Dome-shaped round and elongated lesions of genital scabies

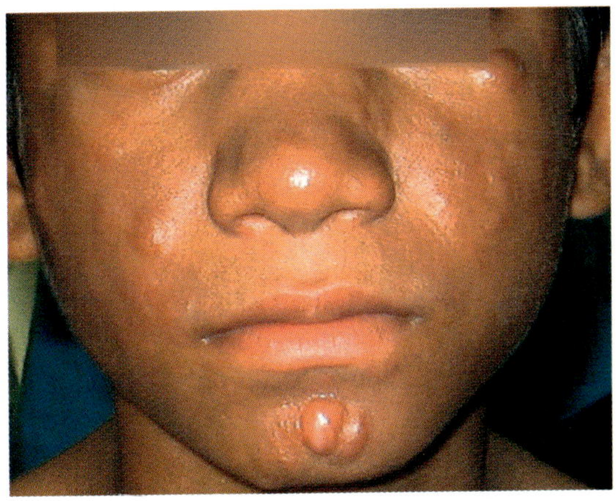

Fig. 10: Dome-shaped solid lesions of BL leprosy

  - Hypodermal/subcutaneous: Lesion is localized within or extending upto the hypodermis or subcutaneous tissue.

* *I like to use the term* ***plaqule*** *to describe the lesion of morphea and morphea- like dermatoses in which poorly circumscribed or diffuse induration of the dermis is more prominent than the changes on the surface.*

Vesicle

* The term is used to denote a fluid filled skin lesion, having a size less than 5 mm in diameter. Fluid content is usually clear but sometimes may be reddish due to presence of blood.
* *I like to use the term hemicle for the lesion containing hemorrhagic fluid.*

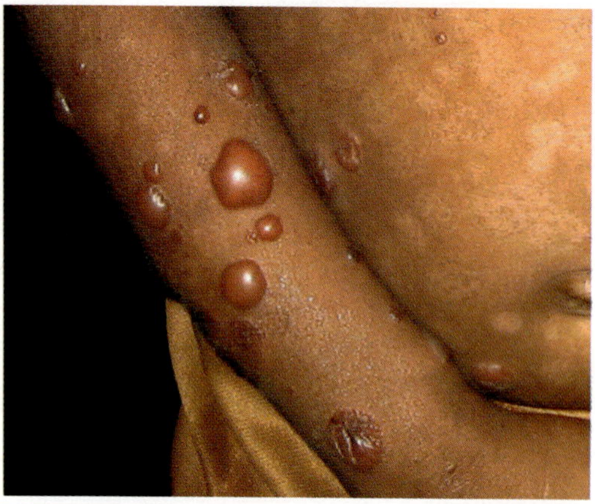

Fig. 11: Vesicles and bullae in case of chronic bullous dermatosis of childhood

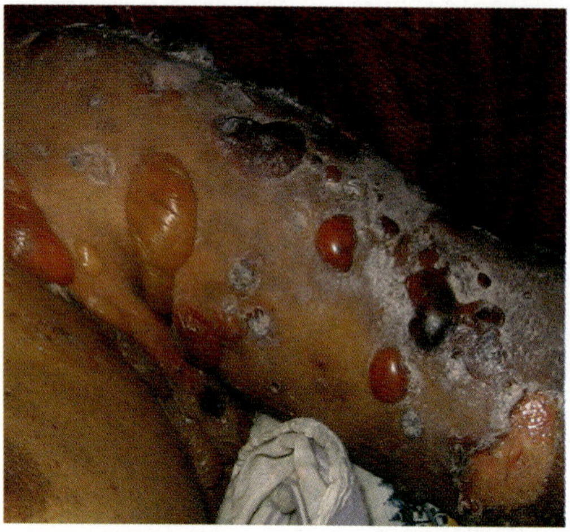

Fig. 12: Vesicles and bullae, some of which contain hemorrhagic fluid, in a case of bullous pemphigoid.

* The term pseudovesicle is used when a solid lesion appears as vesicle. It is due to the profuse edema in the lesion. Lesion of Sweet's syndrome is a classical example.

  Bulla: The term is used for a fluid filled skin lesion, having a size > 5 mm in diameter.

Pustule

* The term is used for a pus filled skin lesion, irrespective of size.
* Commonly seen in
  - Pyoderma
  - Pustular psoriasis
  - Acute generalized exanthematous pustulosis.
  - Drug reaction, eosinophilia and systemic symptoms (DRESS).
  - Subcorneal pustular dermatosis.

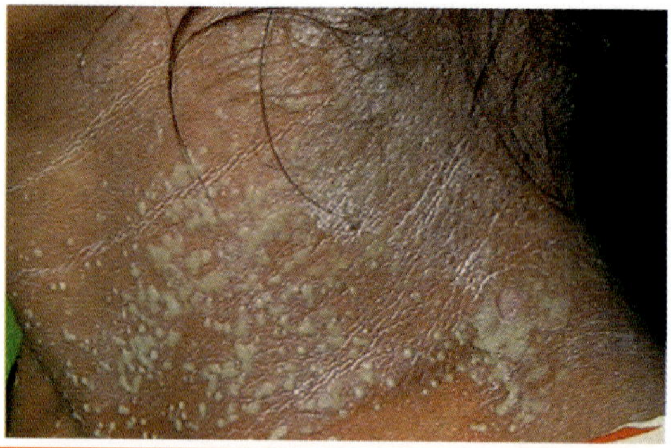

Fig. 13: Multiple pus filled lesions

Scale

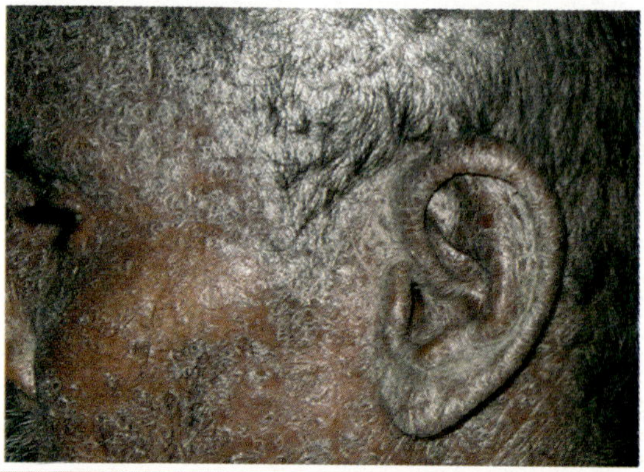

Fig. 14: Silvery scales in a case of psoriatic erythroderma

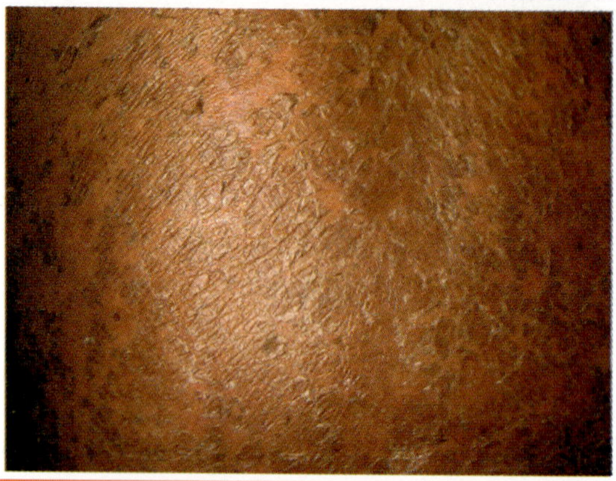

Fig. 15: Moderately adherent skin colored large-sized scales in a case of idiopathic erythroderma

- The term is used for visible peeling of the skin.
- Usually scales are smooth, regular, light colored, shiny, thin and loosely adherent. But there are many exceptions.

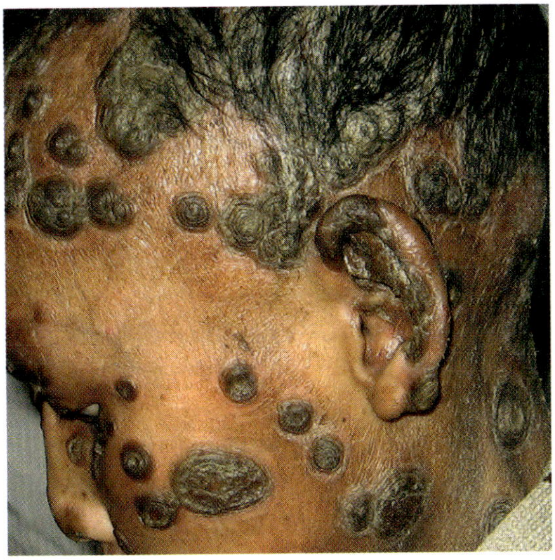

Fig. 16: Crusty scale on the lesions of rupoid psoriasis

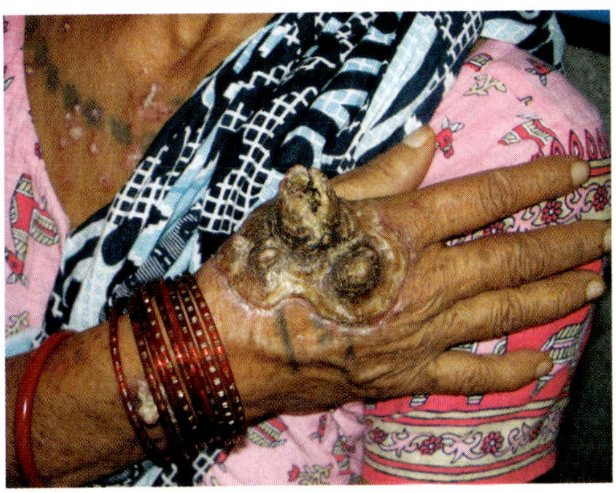

Fig. 17: Heaped up crusty-scale forming cutaneous horn

- Variants of scale:
  - Fine scale, seen in pityriasis alba and pityriasis versicolor.
  - Thick scale, seen in rupoid psoriasis, discoid lupus erythematosus and actinic keratosis.
  - White scale, seen in psoriasis.
  - Hyperpigmented scale, seen in ichthyosis, specially lamellar ichthyosis or in pigmented pityriasis versicolor.
  - Large scale, seen in lamellar ichthyosis and erythroderma.
  - Adherent scale, seen in discoid lupus erythematosus and palmoplantar psoriasis.
  - Double edged scale as seen in ichthyosis linearis circumflexa.
  - Greasy scale, seen in seborrheic dermatitis.
  - Rupoid scale develops due to deposition of scales like column of coins.
  - Horn-like scale develops due to deposition of scales in conical shape like the horn of animals. The structure is known as cutaneous horn.

Crust

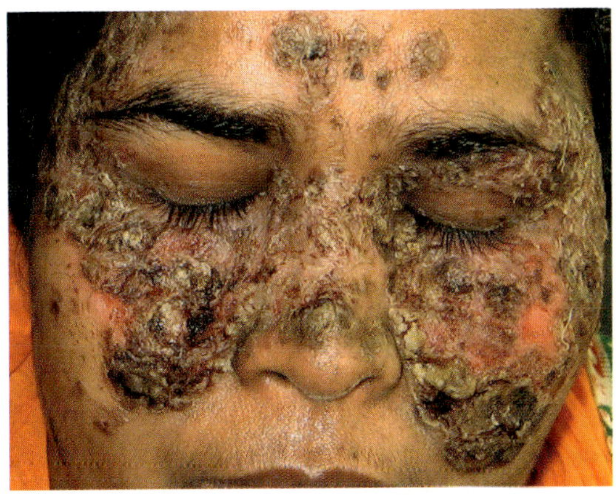

Fig. 18: Crusted erosions of pemphigus foliaceus

- The term is used when a dried mixture of scales and exudate including blood and pus are deposited on the surface of a skin lesion.
- Usually crusts are rough/irregular, dirty, dark colored and well adherent.
- Crusts are seen in exudative condition like subacute dermatitis, impetigo contagiosa, and in healing stage of herpes zoster.
- It usually develops following breakage of vesicle, bulla or pustule.

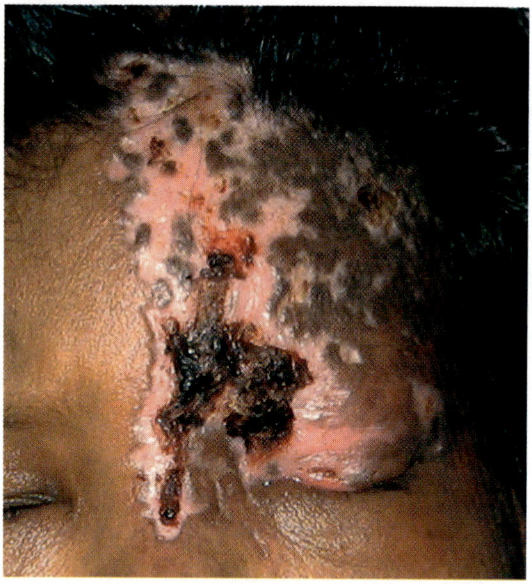

Fig. 19: Hemorrhagic crusts in herpes zoster

Erosion

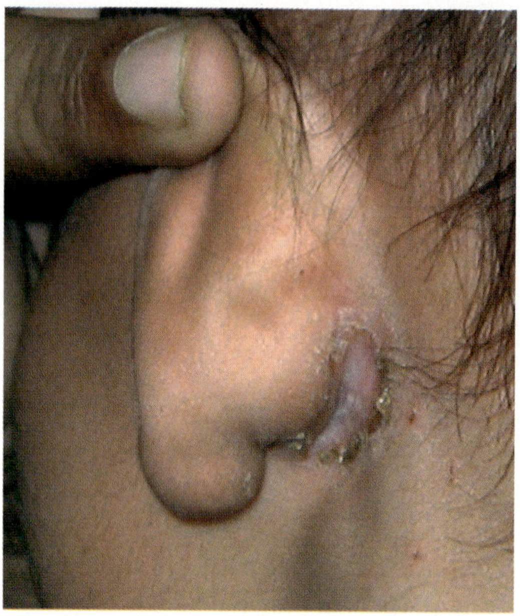

Fig. 20: An erosion of intertrigo with crusted margin

* The term is used for discontinuity of the skin upto the epidermis. It usually heals without any scar formation.

Ulcer

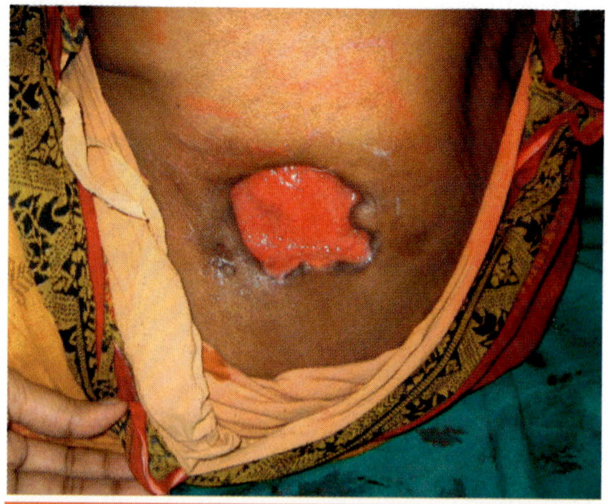

Fig. 21: Tubercular ulcer with undermined edge

* The term is used for discontinuity of the skin beyond epidermis. It usually heals with scar formation.
* Parts of the ulcer:
  - Margin of the ulcer: It is the altered area between the edge of the ulcer and normal skin.
  - Edge of the ulcer: It lies between margin and floor of the ulcer.
  - Floor of the ulcer: It is present at the bottom of the ulcer which is visible from outside.
  - Base of the ulcer: It lies underneath the floor and it is not visible but felt by palpation.
* Variants of ulcer:
  - Punched out ulcer is characterized by sharply cut edge. It is seen in syphilitic chancre.
  - Undermined ulcer in which edge is inclined in such a way that floor of the ulcer becomes broader than opening of the ulcer. It is seen in tuberculosis and pyoderma gangrenosum.
  - Slopping ulcer in which edge is inclined in such a way that opening of the ulcer becomes larger than the floor. Healing ulcers are usually of this type.

- Everted ulcer in which margin of the ulcer comes out and becomes everted, seen in squamous cell carcinoma.
- Rolled ulcer in which margin comes out and becomes rolled, seen in basal cell carcinoma.
- Indurated ulcer in which base is felt firm, seen in syphilitic chancre.
- Tender ulcer is seen in pyoderma gangrenosum, vasculitic ulcer and chancroid.
- Non-tender ulcer is seen in tubercular chancre and syphilitic chancre.
- Painful ulcer is seen in Buerger's disease, orificial tuberculosis and aphthous ulcer.

Fissure: The term is used to denote a linear erosion or ulcer, having definite length and depth but negligible breadth.

Excoriation: The term is used for an erosion or ulcer caused by a scratch.

Sinus

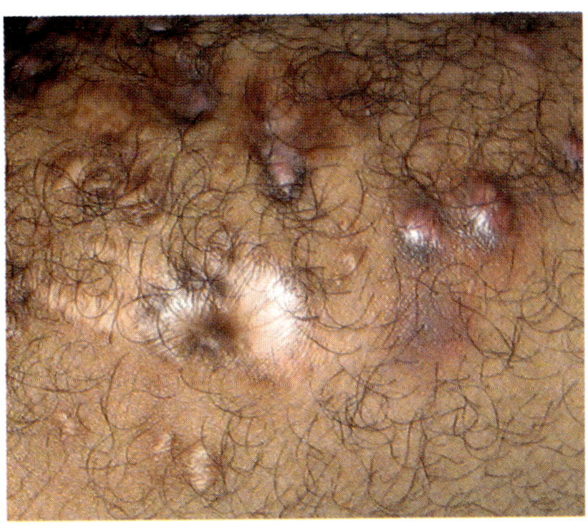

Fig. 22: Multiple sinuses of actinomycetoma.

- It is having an internal blind end and an external open end.

Fistula: It is a channel connecting two hollow organs/structures or one hollow organ with external surface. Basically it connects two epithelial surfaces.

Lichenification

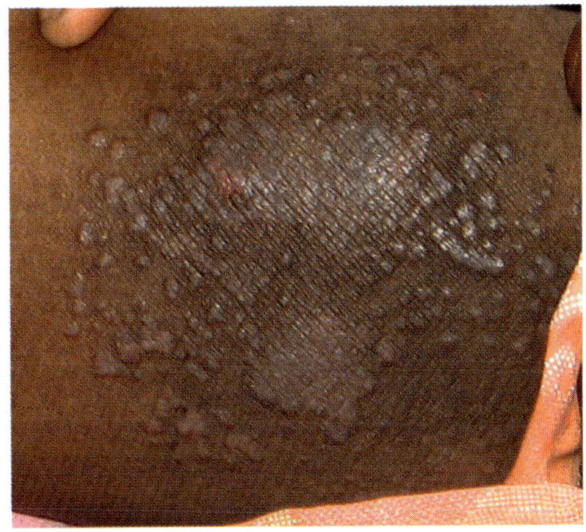

Fig. 23: Lichenified plaque with multiple satellite papules in a case of lichen simplex chronicus

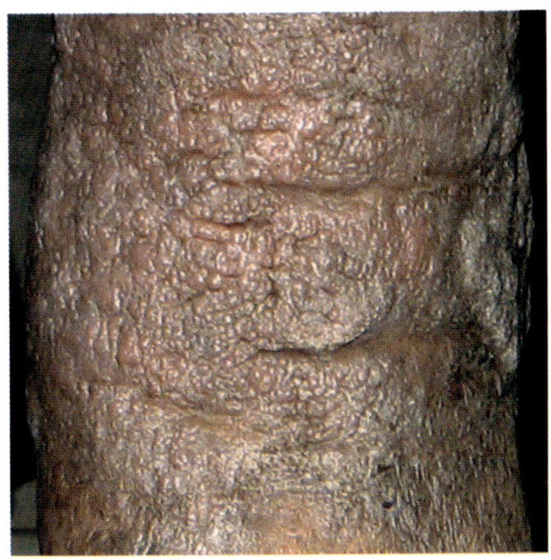

Fig. 24: Lichenified plaque of elephantiasis nostras cutis, studded with minute cystic dilatation of lymphatics, following chronic lymphatic obstruction

- The term is used when a lesion is characterized by hyperpigmentation, thickening and increased skin markings.
  - It is classically seen in chronic lesion of atopic dermatitis and in lichen simplex chronicus.

Induration: The term is used when skin is felt firm and thick, due to dermal thickening.

Atrophy

* The term is used to denote reduction of the mass of the skin.
    - Epidermal atrophy is indicated by wrinkled and shiny appearance of the skin.
    - Dermal and subcutaneous tissue atrophy is indicated by visible depression on the surface.

Scar

* The term is used when a ulcer is healed with connective tissue without overlying epidermis.
* Initially it is thick and pink, and later becomes white and atrophic.
* It may be flat or elevated and elevated scar is known as hypertrophic scar which mimicks keloid.

Types of scar:

- Atrophic scar
- Pitted scar
- Hypertrophic scar
- Varioliform scar
- Cribriform scar, a variant of scar, having multiple well marginated depressions, appearing as a sieve. It is classically seen in pyoderma gangrenosum.

Erythema

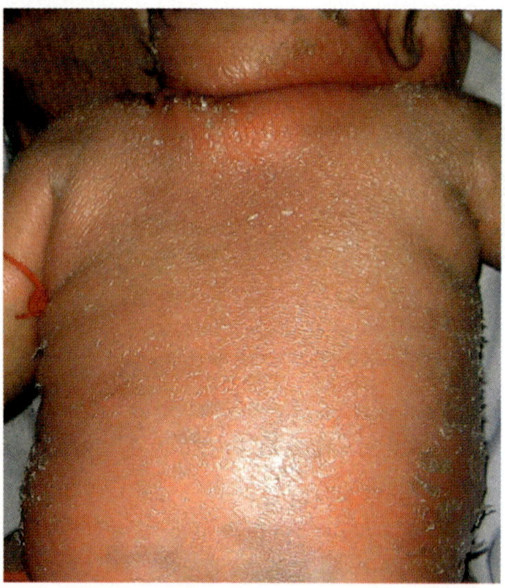

Fig. 25: Generalized erythema in case of infantile erythroderma

* The term is used for redness of the skin due to underlying dilated blood vessels.
    - Non-vasculitic erythema is blanchable.
    - When it is related with vasculitis, it does not blanch.

Burrow

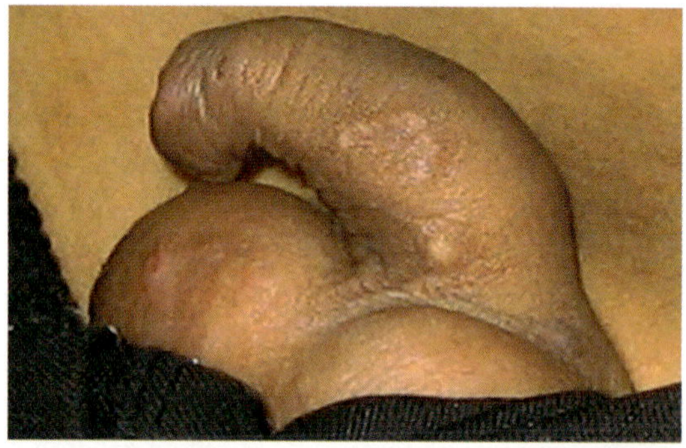

Fig. 26: Curvilinear elevated lesion at shaft of the penis

* The term is used to denote a narrow tortuous tunnel through or just below the stratum corneum, made by *Sarcoptes scabiei*, the causative parasite of scabies. Clinically it is recognized by a linear elevated lesion.
    - It is the pathognomonic sign of scabies.

Comedo (plural, comedones)

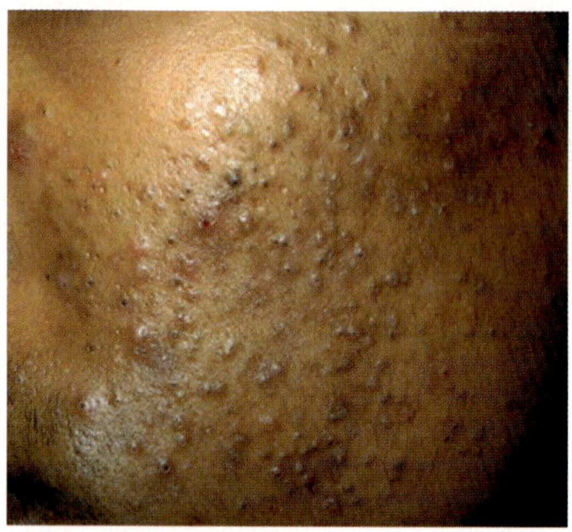

Fig. 27: Multiple comedones with black heads and white heads in acne vulgaris

* The term is used for a papule, originated from the pilosebaceous unit with a central keratinous plug. It is the earliest lesion of acne vulgaris.
* In acne vulgaris, an early lesion appears as a papule with whitish center due to collection of a mixture of sebum and keratin. This lesion is known as white head.
* When the pilosebaceous orifice becomes dilated, the keratin plug is completely or partially lost and the center of the lesion appears as a black pore. This lesion is designated as black head.
* Other than acne these are also seen in nevus comedonicus.

Cyst

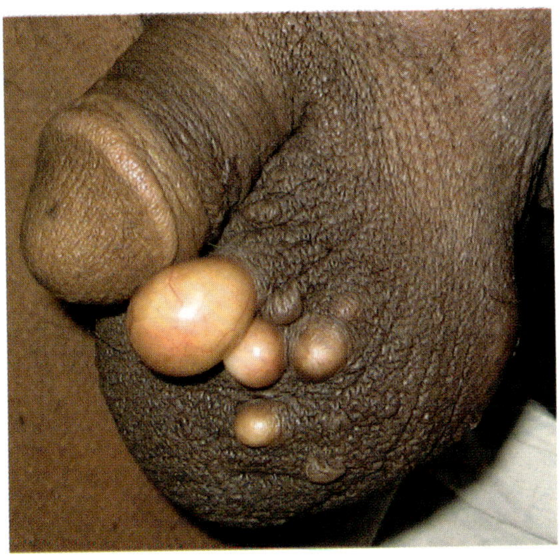

Fig. 28: Multiple lesions of epidermoid cyst

* The term is used to denote a circumscribed lesion, having an epithelial wall and containing fluid or semisolid material.

Tumor

* It is a pathological term and is used to denote a mass of tissue having excessive growth potential.
* It may be benign or malignant.
* In benign tumor, the growth potential is excessive but is under control.
* In malignant tumor, the growth potential is uncontrolled.
* Tumor may appear as papule, plaque, nodule or ulcer.

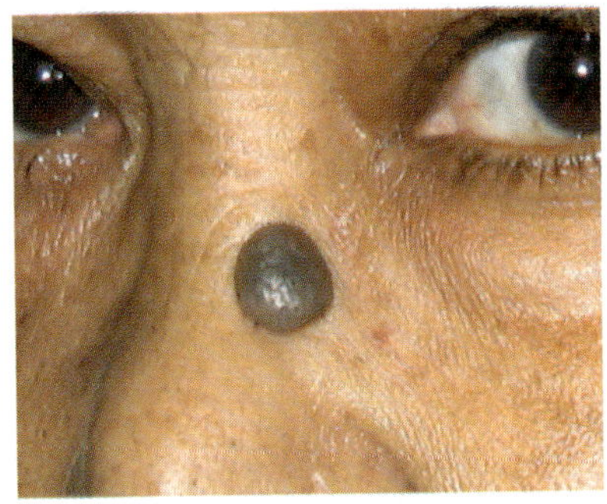

Fig. 29: A pigmented papule of compound melanocytic nevus, one of the common benign tumors

Milia: The term is used to denote tiny superficial keratin filled cyst, without any opening.

Telangiectasia: The term is used for permanent dilatation of cutaneous blood vessels, when they become clinically visible.

- Symmetrically dilated capillaries are seen adjacent to avascular areas (drop out telangiectasia) in systemic scleroderma and dermatomyositis.
- Wandering glomeruloid capillary loops are seen in SLE.

Petechiae/Purpura/Ecchymosis

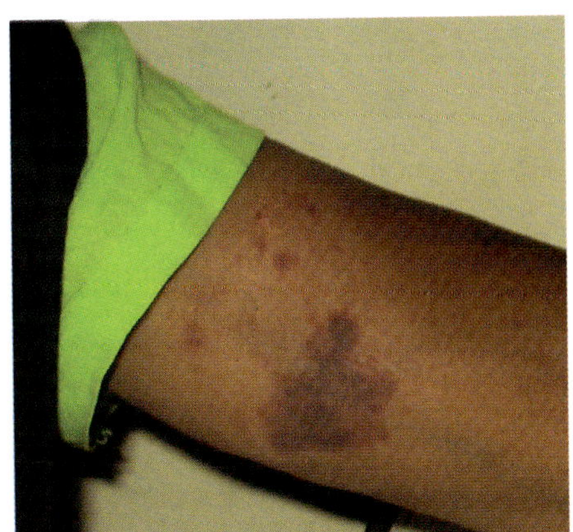

Fig. 30: Lesions of senile purpura and ecchymosis

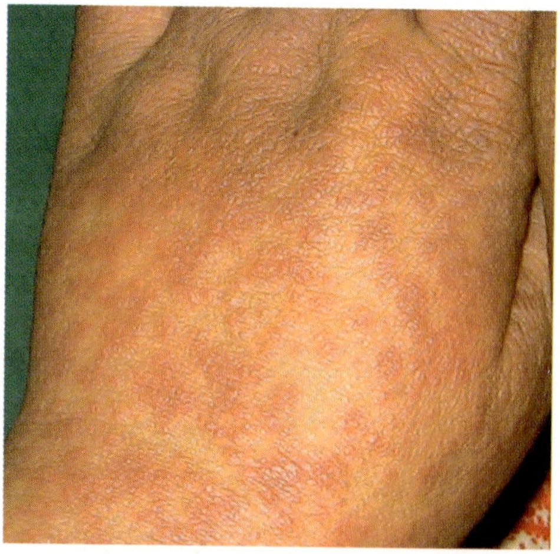

Fig. 31: Lesions of palpable purpura

* These terms are used for reddish pigmentation of the skin due to collection of extravasated blood.
* Different terms are used for different size of the lesion.
    - Petechiae is less than 3 mm.
    - Purpura is 3-10 mm.
    - Ecchymosis is more than 10 mm.
* The term palpable purpura is used when the lesions become elevated and palpable. It is associated with small and small to medium vessel vasculitis.

Annular lesion

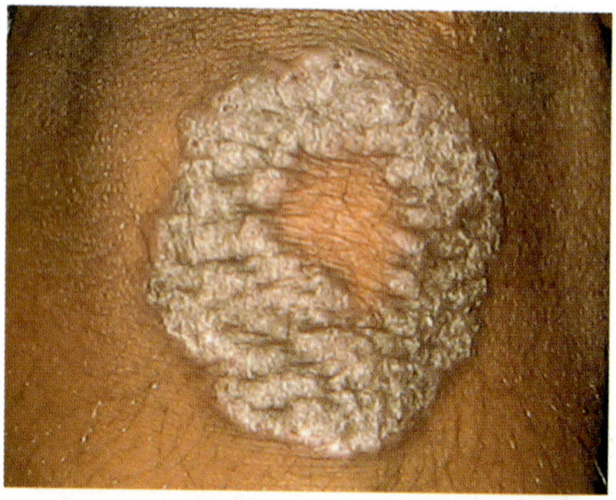

Fig. 32: A verrucous plaque of tuberculosis verrucosa cutis with broad elevated margin and central clearing

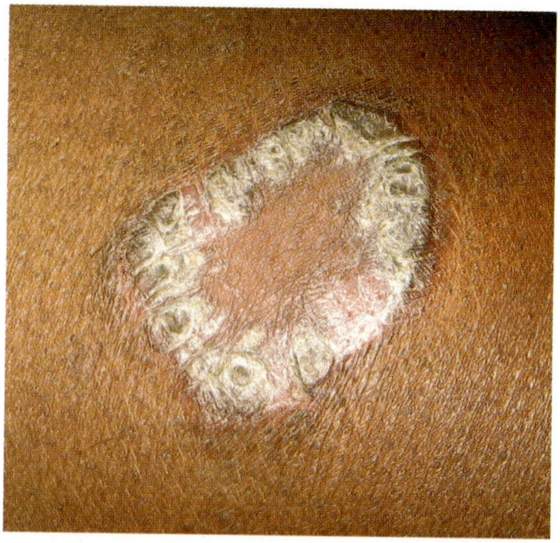

Fig. 33: Annular plaque of psoriasis

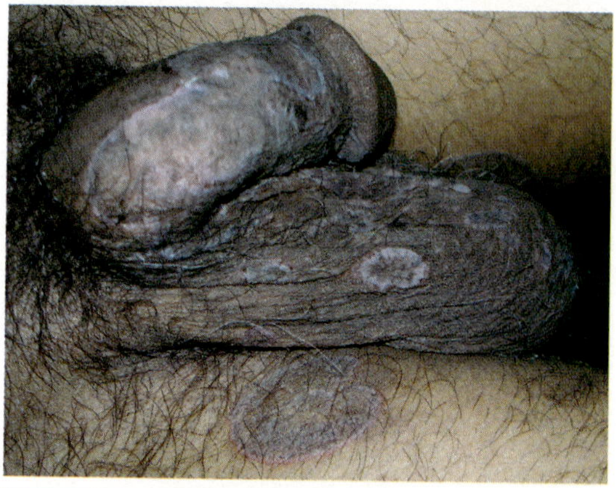

Fig. 34: Annular lichen planus

* The term is used for a circular lesion with elevated or active periphery and relatively depressed or clear center.
* Commonly seen in:
    - Tinea corporis and cutaneous candidiasis.
    - Lupus vulgaris, tuberculosis verrucosa cutis, TT/BT/BB/BL leprosy, and secondary syphilis.
    - Porokeratosis and pityriasis rosea.
    - Granuloma annulare and sarcoidosis.
    - Lichen planus and psoriasis.

- ♦ Erythema annulare centrifugum, erythema marginatum, erythema gyratum repens.
- ♦ Subacute lupus erythematosus and erythema multiforme.
- ♦ Hemangioma and tufted angioma.
- ♦ Marginal zinc deficiency and keloid.

Target lesion: The term is used when a papule or plaque develops with a dusky red central zone, pale edematous middle zone and erythematous peripheral zone.

- ✶ It is classically seen in erythema multiforme.

Arciform/Arcuate lesion

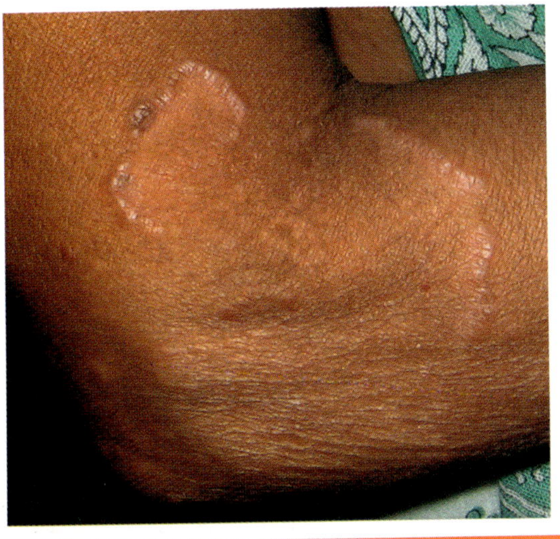

Fig. 35: Arcuate or arciform lesions of granuloma annulare

- ✶ Lesions takes a shape of 1/4 to 3/4 of a circle.
- ✶ Commonly seen in
  - ♦ Urticaria
  - ♦ Mycosis fungoides
  - ♦ Secondary syphilis
  - ♦ Granuloma annulare
  - ♦ Elastosis perforans serpiginosa.

Polycyclic/circinate pattern: Multiple annular lesions coalesce to form a large irregular lesion but maintain the arch of the individual lesion.

- ✶ Commonly seen in:
  - ♦ Tinea corporis/cruris/faciei.
  - ♦ Psoriasis
  - ♦ Subcorneal pustular dermatosis.
  - ♦ Ichthyosis linearis circumflexa.
  - ♦ Circinate balanitis in Reiter's syndrome.

Intracyclic lesion

- ✶ It contains multiple concentric rings or circles.

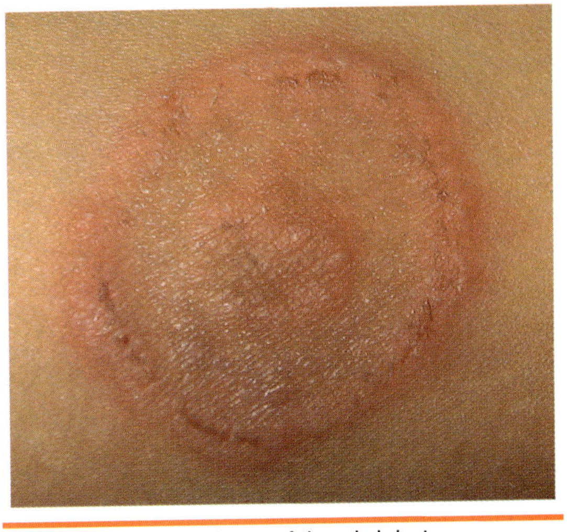

Fig. 36: Intracyclic plaque of tinea imbricata

- ✶ Commonly seen in:
  - ♦ Tinea imbricata, caused by *Trichophyton concentricum*.
  - ♦ Erythema gyratum repens.

Nummular or discoid lesion

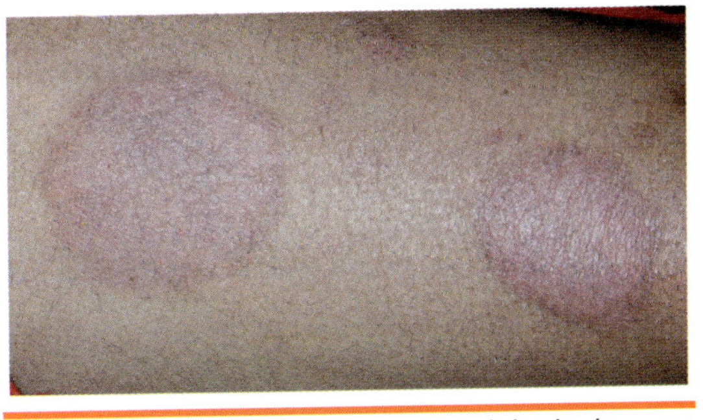

Fig. 37: Round lesion without any central clearing in a case of nummular dermatitis

- ✶ Lesions take a coin like shape without central clearing.

- Commonly seen in:
  - Nummular dermatitis
  - Discoid lupus erythematosus
  - Psoriasis vulgaris

Petaloid lesion

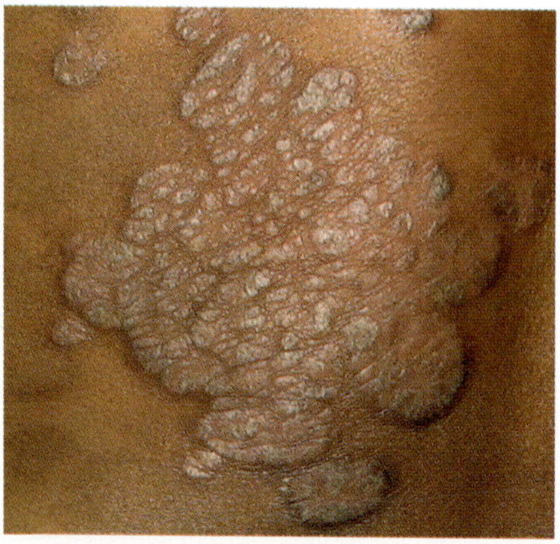

Fig. 38: A petaloid plaque of psoriasis with few satellite lesion

- When multiple nummular lesion coalesce to form a larger lesion, take a petaloid pattern.
- Commonly seen in:
  - Seborrheic dermatitis
  - Psoriasis

Wheal/hive: It is characterized by transient pruritic erythematous and edematous papule or plaque. It develops due to dermal edema following cutaneous vasodilatation.

Verrucous lesion

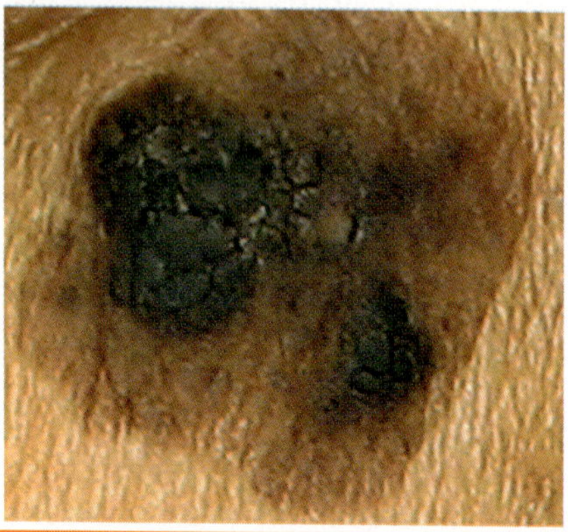

Fig. 39: Verrucous plaque of seborrheic keratosis

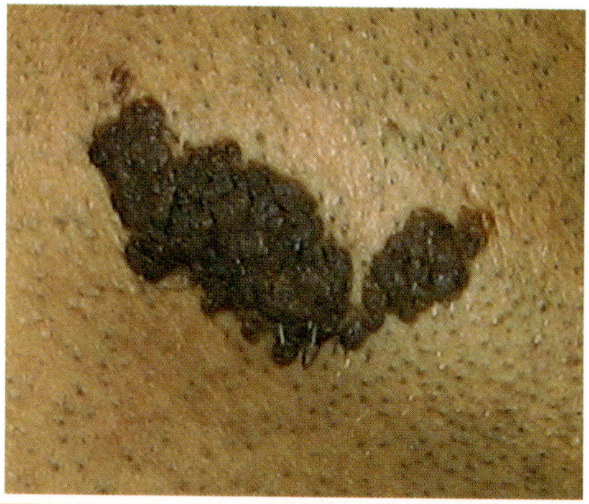

Fig. 40: Lesion of the verrucous epidermal nevus

- The term is used when the surface of a papule or plaque is having finger like projections on the surface.
- Commonly seen in:
  - Verruca vulgaris
  - Tuberculosis verrucosa cutis
  - Seborrheic keratosis
  - Verrucous hemangioma
  - Verrucous epidermal nevus

Satellite lesion

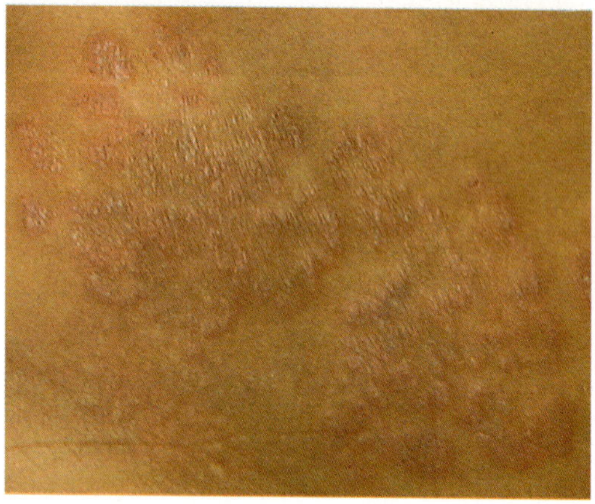

Fig. 41: Few smaller annular lesions around a large mother lesion of tinea corporis

- Smaller lesion surrounding a large lesion is known as satellite lesion.

* Number of the lesion may be single or multiple.
* It is characteristically seen in BT leprosy.

B. Pattern of arrangement of the lesions

Discrete lesions

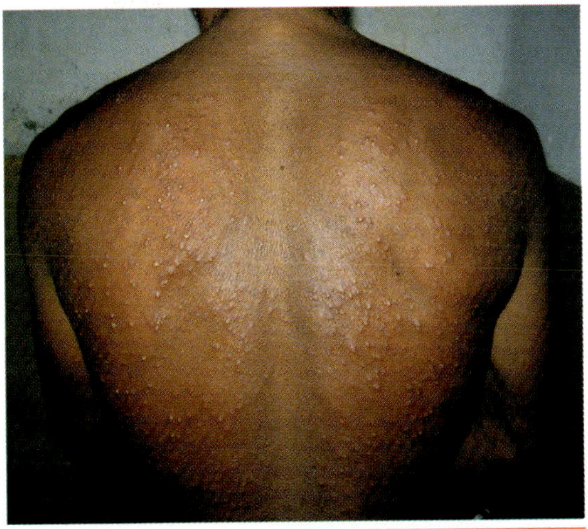

Fig. 42: Discrete lesions of miliaria pustulosa

* Individual lesions remain separated from one to another.

Grouped lesion

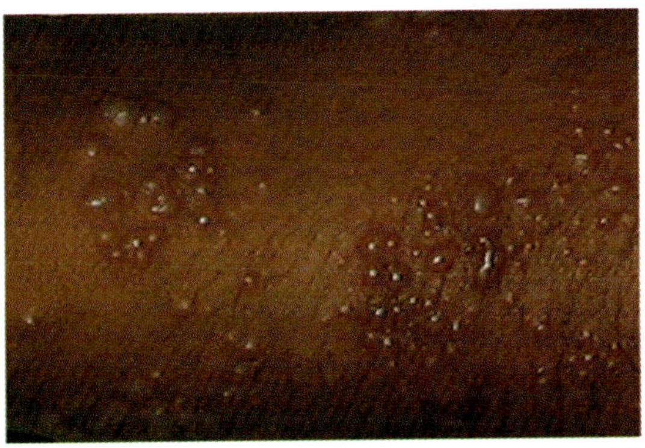

Fig. 43: Grouped vesicular lesion of herpes zoster

* Lesions are arranged in groups but individual lesion remains discrete.
* Commonly seen in:
  - Herpes simplex
  - Herpes zoster
  - Dermatitis herpetiformis

Confluent lesions

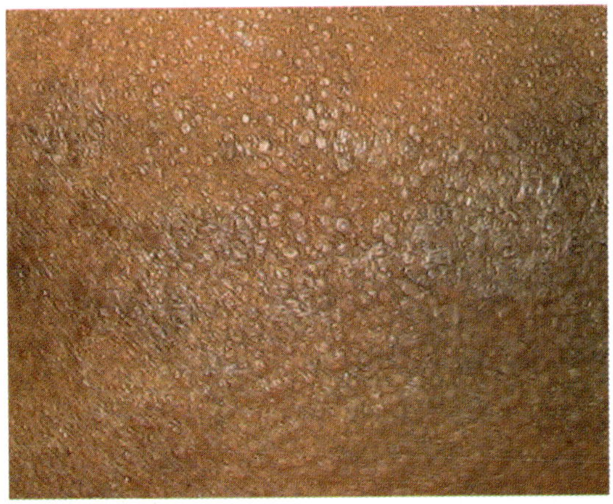

Fig. 44: Confluent papules of allergic contact dermatitis

* Closely set lesions but to some extent maintain their individuality.

Coalesced lesions

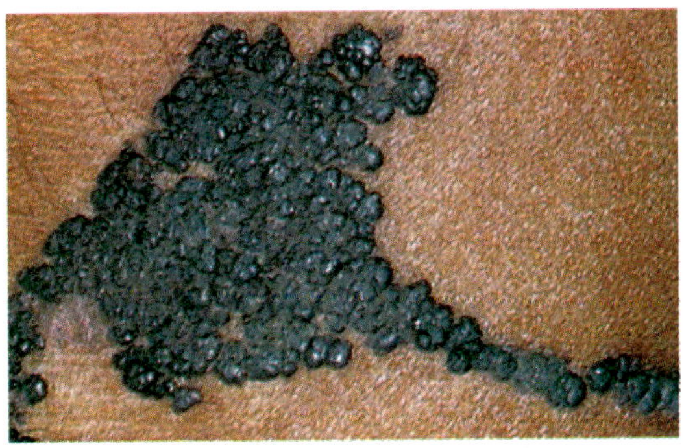

Fig. 45: Hyperpigmented papules of verrucous epidermal nevus, coalesced to form a plaque

* Confluent lesions with loss of individuality.
* Confluent papules when coalesced form an irregular plaque.

Linear lesions

* Lesions are arranged along a line.
* Serpiginous lesion is a form of linear lesions having a wavy pattern.
* Commonly seen in:
  - Lichen striatus, lichen planus, psoriasis and porokeratosis.

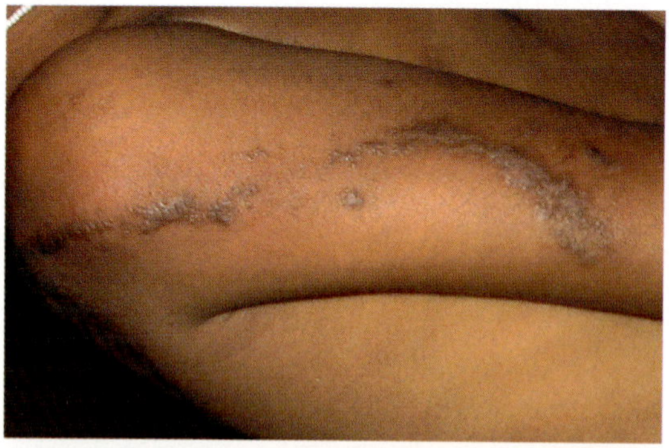

Fig. 46: A linear and serpentine lesion of ILVEN

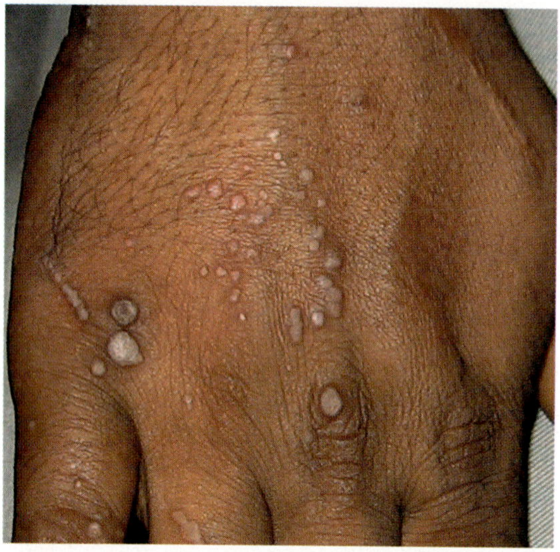

Fig. 47: Lesions of verruca vulgaris along a line of trauma, an example of Koebner phenomenon

- ♦ Linear verrucous epidermal nevus.
- ♦ Inflammatory linear verrucous epidermal nevus (ILVEN).
- ♦ Linear irritant or allergic contact dermatitis.
- ♦ Koebner phenomenon.

Zosteriform lesions

- ∗ The term is used when lesions are distributed along a dermatome.
- ∗ Commonly seen in:
  - ♦ Herpes zoster
  - ♦ Zosteriform herpes simplex
  - ♦ Segmental vitiligo

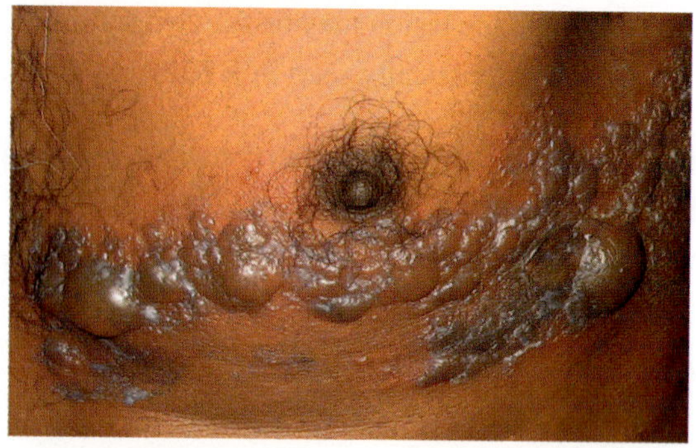

Fig. 48: Lesions of herpes zoster along left sided T7 dermatome

  - ♦ Zosteriform psoriasis
  - ♦ Zosteriform lichen planus.

Reticular/retiform lesions: Lesions are arranged in a net-like fashion.

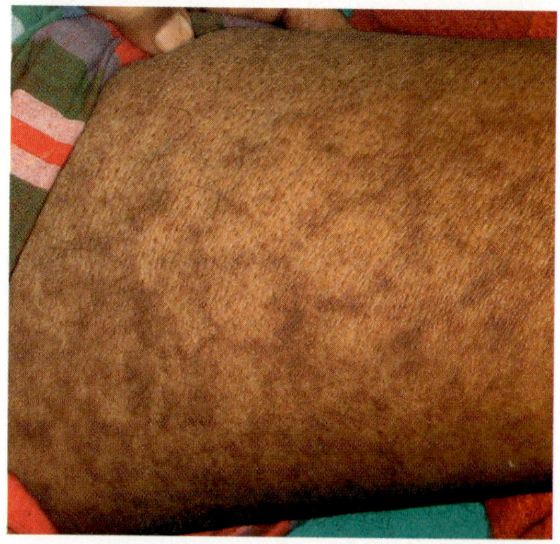

Fig. 49: Retiform purpura in a case of small to medium vessel vasculitis

- ∗ Commonly seen in:
  - ♦ Cutis marmorata and livedo reticularis.
  - ♦ Retiform purpura in medium vessel vasculitis.
  - ♦ Reticular erythematous mucinosis
  - ♦ Reticulate hyperpigmentation.
  - ♦ Retiform parapsoriasis.

Cobble stone lesions

* Closely set papules which make an irregular surface.
* Seen in:
  - Cowden syndrome
  - Crohn's disease
  - Darier's disease.

Leonine lesion

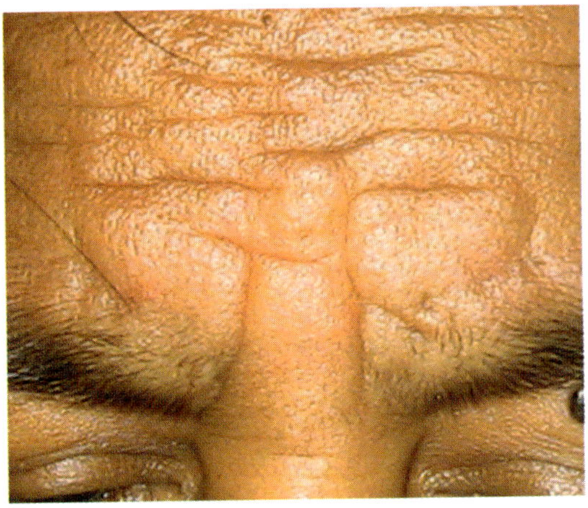

Fig. 50: Leonine lesions in a case of scleromyxedema

* Lesions at forehead when coalesce to form plaques with vertical furrow, appear as lion's face.
* Commonly seen in:
  - Lepromatous leprosy
  - Chronic actinic dermatitis
  - Scleromyxedema
  - Multicentric reticulohistiocytosis.

C. Pattern of distribution of the lesions

Focal/localized: Number of lesions may be single or few and distributed irrespective of any particular site.

Dermatomal

* Lesions are distributed along a dermatome.
* Commonly seen in:
  - Herpes zoster
  - Segmental vitiligo
  - Verrucous epidermal nevus

Unilateral

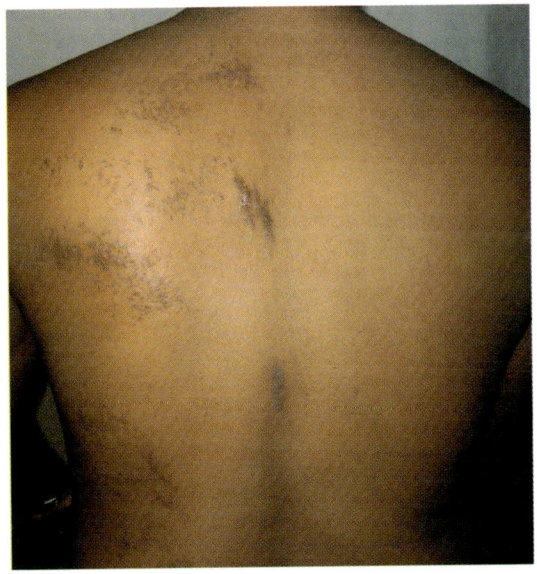

Fig. 51: Extensive but unilateral distribution of lesions of epidermal nevus

* Lesions are distributed at one side of the body.
* This is commonly seen in nevoid conditions.

Bilateral: Lesions are distributed along both sides of the body.

Extensor

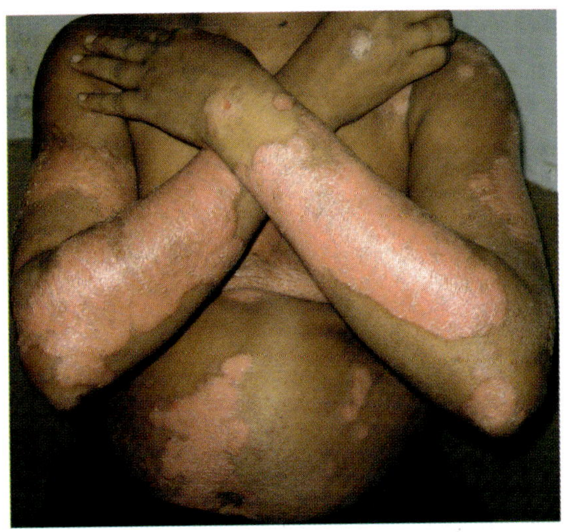

Fig. 52: Lesions of psoriasis, distributed mostly at the extensors of the upper limbs

* Lesions are distributed at extensor sides of the body.
* Commonly seen in psoriasis.

  Flexor: Lesions are distributed at flexor sides of the body.

Flexural

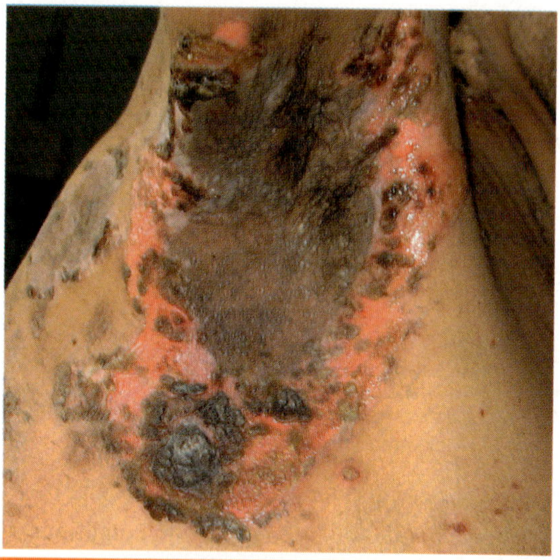

Fig. 53: Crusted erosions of pemphigus vulgaris involving flexural area like axilla

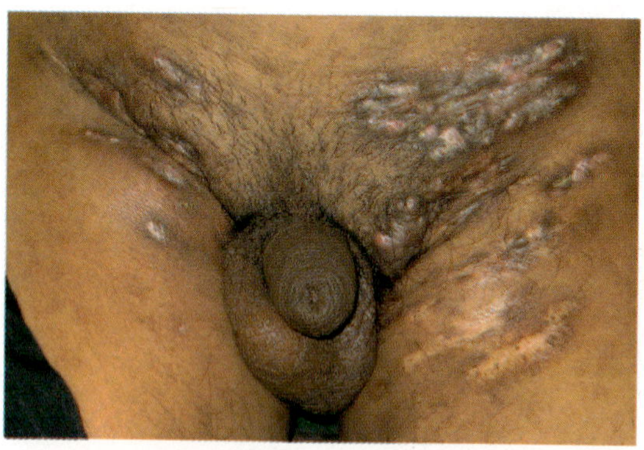

Fig. 54: Multiple interconnected sinuses and linear scars of hidradenitis suppurativa involving groin

* Lesions are distributed at the body folds.

Seborrheic

* Lesions are distributed at areas where sebaceous glands are predominantly present.
* Commonly seen in:
  - Seborrheic dermatitis
  - Darier's disease
  - Pemphigus foliaceus

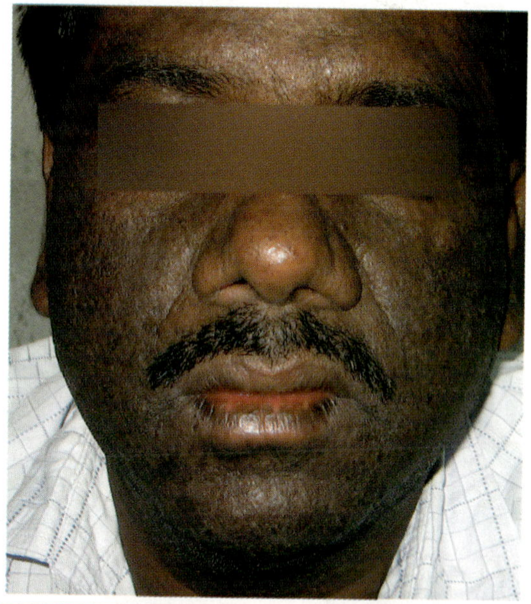

Fig. 55: Lesions of seborrheic dermatitis at seborrheic areas

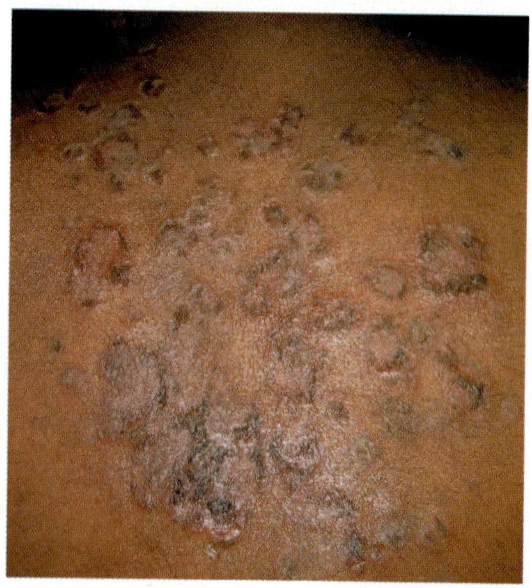

Fig. 56: Crusted erosions of pemphigus foliaceus at seborrheic area of the back

Photodistribution

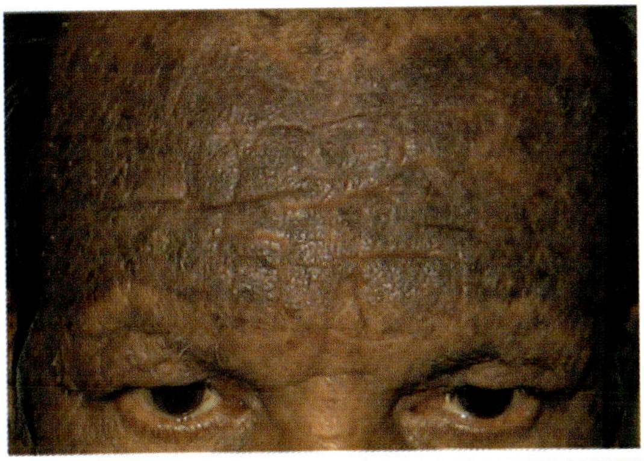

Fig. 57: Lichenified lesions of chronic actinic dermatosis

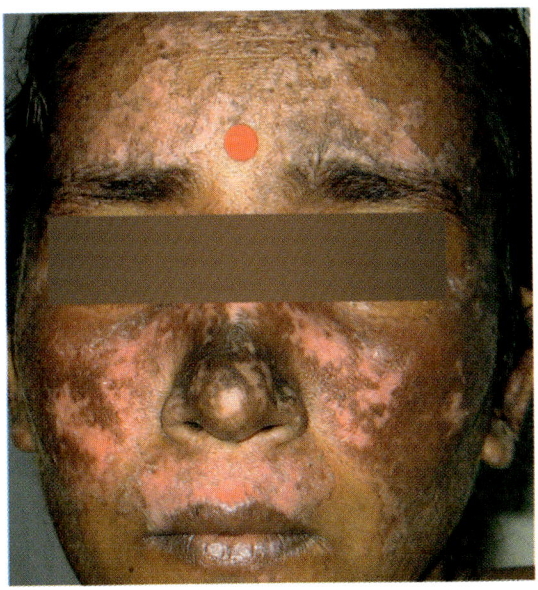

Fig. 58: Lesions of lupus erythematosus at photoexposed areas

* Lesions develop mostly at sun exposed areas.
* Commonly seen in:
  - Polymorphic light eruption
  - Photoallergic/photocontact dermatitis or chronic actinic dermatitis
  - Pellagra
  - Lupus erythematosus
  - Xenodermatoses

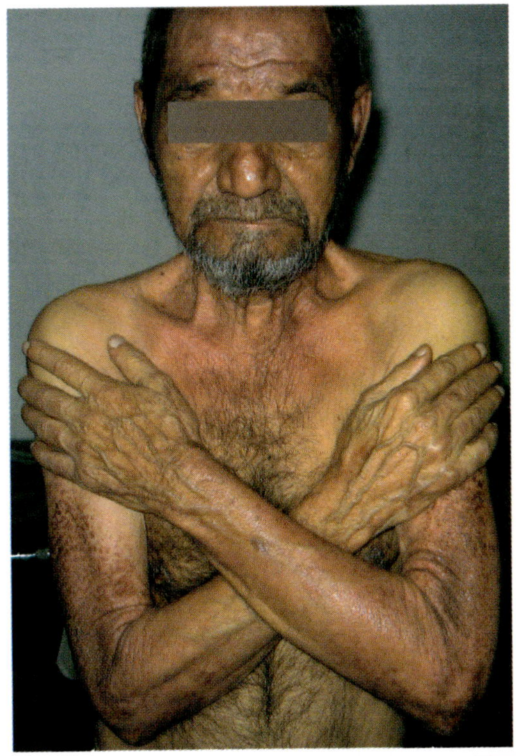

Fig. 59: Classical distribution of lesions of the photoallergic contact dermatitis

Symmetrical: Lesions are distributed at both sides of the body as a mirror image as seen in lepromatosus leprosy.

Tendency of symmetry: Some of the lesions are distributed bilaterally as a mirror image but others are not, as seen in BL leprosy.

Asymmetrical: Lesions are distributed bilaterally but haphazardly as seen in BT leprosy.

Centripetal: Lesions are concentrated within the central parts of the body as seen in small pox.

Centrifugal: Lesions are concentrated at the peripheral parts of the body as seen in chicken pox.

Mucocutaneous

* Lesions are distributed on both cutaneous and mucosal surfaces.
* Commonly seen in:
  - Stevens-Johnson syndrome (SJS)
  - Toxic epidermal necrolysis (TEN)

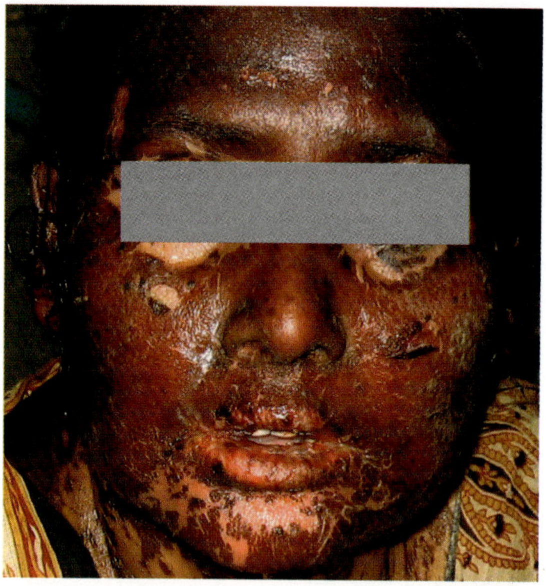

Fig. 60: Epidermal necrosis, involving both skin and mucosa in a case of TEN

- Hand-foot-mouth disease
- Behcet's syndrome
- Systemic lupus erythematosus.

Widespread/diffuse/generalized

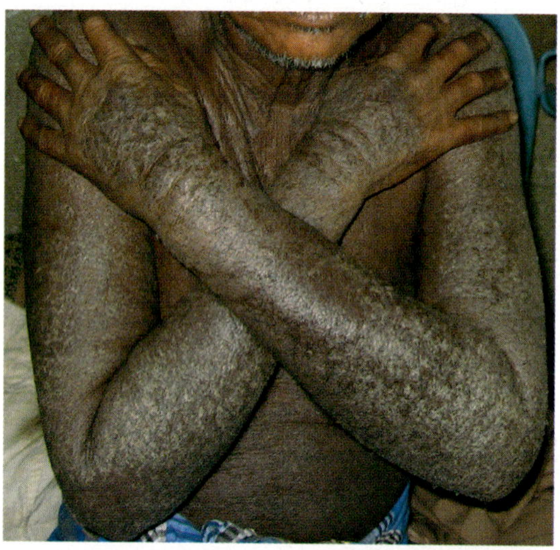

Fig. 61: Lesions of psoriasis distributed widely

* Lesions are distributed all over the body with or without involving mucosal surfaces.

D. Examination of a case

Preparation

* Examination room must be well illuminated.
* Greet the patient to make a warm relation.
* Patient must be observed while entering the examination room. It may show the gait of a patient of Klippel-Trenaunay syndrome or foot deformity of a leprosy patient.
* Patient must be counselled properly to get consent for examination.
* Request the patient to undress as much as possible.
* Presence of female attendant is a must while examining a female patient.
* Have a overall look while asking about the chief complaint.
* Following simple instruments must have during examination:
    - Gloves, torch and measuring tape.
    - Magnifying glass and Wood's lamp.
    - Hot and cold water test tubes, needle and cotton.
    - Glass slides, swab sticks, normal saline, 10-20% KOH solution, Giemsa stain, Gram stain, ZN stain, scalpel blade, spade forceps and light microscope.

History taking

i) Introduction

- Name, age, sex and residence of the patient, to be noted in the case record form.
- These will make a relation between the patient and the dermatologist.
- These informations are important as prevalence of many diseases vary according to age, sex, race and place of residence.

ii) Chief complaint/presenting complaint

* Patient may have many complaints but only those for which the patient was forced to attend the dermatologist, to be noted with duration of respective complaints.

* A psoriasis patient may come with following complaints and those must be described in patient's language.
  - Single/few/multiple reddish, scaly, solid, elevated skin lesions in case of psoriasis vulgaris.
  - Generalized redness and exfoliation in case of erythrodermic psoriasis.
  - Few/multiple/generalized pustules with fever in case of pustular psoriasis.
* A psoriasis patient may suffer from psoriasis for last 40 years which may not be the chief complaint but sudden onset of pustules for last 10 days may be the chief complaint.

iii) History of present illness

* Evolution of present state of the disease and response to treatment.
  - Qualitative and quantitative description of symptoms like itching, pain, anxiety, depression, etc.
  - Description of first lesion and first site with onset whether acute or insidious.
  - Serial description of other lesions according to the development.
  - Details of treatment and response.
* Positive history in favour of provisional diagnosis. Examples:
  - Variation of itching as it aggravates at night, helps to diagnose scabies.
  - Sunlight aggravation as it helps to diagnose lupus erythematosus.
  - Seasonal variation helps to diagnose many diseases as psoriasis flares up in winter.
  - Urticaria may develop after taking of a particular drug or food.
  - Pain during walking and relief on rest, help to diagnose Buerger's disease.
* Negative history to exclude differential diagnosis. Example:
  - Presence of itching almost excludes secondary syphilis.
  - No history of drug intake prior to onset, almost excludes the chance of toxic epidermal necrolysis (TEN).
* Any irrelevant history, narrated by the patient. Example:
  - Genital ulcer following urinating at public toilet.
  - Development of pediculosis capitis while passing by a slum area.
  - Development of acne due to taking of spicy food or due to irregular bowel habit.

iv) History of past illness

* History of previous attack of similar disease.
  - Duration and times of attacks.
  - Treatment details.
  - Outcome of treatment.
* History of any major illness.
  - Diabetes
  - Hypertension
  - Jaundice
  - Tuberculosis
* History of any drug reaction or taking of any immunosuppressive drug.
  - Help to diagnose toxic epidermal necrolysis, fixed drug reaction or erythema multiforme
  - Immunosuppressive drugs dictate treatment plan and prognosis of the disease.
* Irrelevant past illness.
  - History of ligation 20 years back in pruritus vulvae.

v) Personal history

- History of smoking, alcohol, bowel and bladder habit.
- History of anxiety, depression and sleep disturbance.
- Menstrual history.

vi) Family history

- History of similar disease among family members or close relatives.
- History of any unrelated hereditary disease.

General examination

* Patient's level of consciousness and cooperation.
* Examination to find out anemia, cyanosis, clubbing, jaundice, pulse rate, respiratory rate and blood pressure.
* Brief systemic examination including heart sounds, breath sounds, renal tenderness, epigastric tenderness and sternal tenderness.
* Examination of reticuloendothelial system including lymph nodes, liver and spleen.
* Examination for peripheral pulses, pedal edema and varicose veins.

Cutaneous examination

* Identification of primary, secondary and special type of lesions.
* Number, sites of involvement and pattern of distribution of the lesions.
* Description of individual lesion including largest and smallest lesions in cases where lesions are multiple.
    - Size, shape and margin
    - Surface and color
    - Sweat loss and hair loss
    - Tenderness and sensory impairment
* Examination of special areas
    - Scalp
    - Palms and soles
    - Flexural and intertriginous areas
    - Perianal and genital area
    - Orogenital mucosae
* Examination of special structures
    - Hair
    - Nail
    - Peripheral nerves.

Performance of bedside tests

Nikolsky's test

* It should be done at perilesional normal appearing skin and on bony prominence.
* A shearing/tangential pressure is applied with thumb at the selected site.
* If skin is peeled off, the test is positive.
* Positive test is seen in:
    - Pemphigus
    - Toxic epidermal necrolysis
    - Staphylococcal scalded skin syndrome.

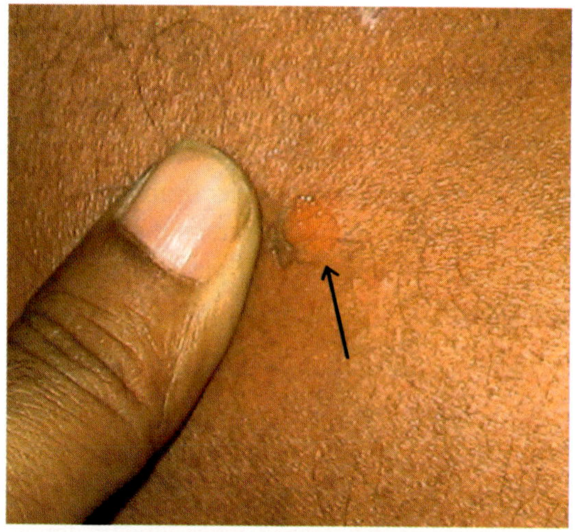

Fig. 62: Normal appearing skin is peeled off by shearing force given by the thumb

Elicitation of bulla spreading sign/Asboe Hansen sign

* A vesicle or bulla is selected and circumference of the lesion is marked with a marker pen.
* A slow but steady and firm pressure is applied at the top of the lesion.
* If the lesion spreads beyond the mark, it is positive.
* Positive test is commonly seen in pemphigus and rarely in bullous pemphigoid.

Grattage test and Auspitz sign

* An erythematous plaque is scraped with the edge of a glass slide. Following removal of all scales, a shiny surface will appear, known as Buckley's membrane and it is removed by further scraping.
* Test is positive if bleeding points appear.
* Procedure of the test is known as Grattage test and positive result is known as Auspitz sign.

* It is commonly positive in psoriasis but rarely may be positive in actinic keratosis and Darier's disease.

Elicitation of Darier's sign and dermatographism

* Selected area of the skin will be rubbed firmly with a blind object like blind end of a pencil or pen.
* Within 2-5 minutes the area may become swollen, erythematous and edematous and the test becomes positive.
* Positive test in mastocytosis is known as *Darier's sign*.
* Positive test in physical urticaria is known as *dermatographism*.

Diascopy

* It is nothing but to see the lesion through a microscopic glass slide or a hand lens by pressing it against the lesion.
* Interpretation:
    - Blanching when capillaries are dilated as in erythema.
    - Nonblanching in purpura due to extravasated RBCs.
    - Apple jelly (yellow brown) colored nodules seen in lupus vulgaris, sarcoidosis, granuloma annulare and necrobiosis lipoidica.

Dermoscopy/Dermatoscopy

* It is a non-invasive, diagnostic tool to visualize certain pattern of changes within and/or on the surface of the skin lesions which are not normally visible with unaided eye.
* Various linkage fluids like water, glycerin, antiseptic solutions, olive oil, and mineral oil are applied on the surface of the skin lesions to improve translucency and thus to improve visibility.
* Glass has refractive index (1.52) similar to skin and so if glass is kept between the skin and lens, the transillumination of the lesion will improve further.
* There are two techniques to examine a lesion.
    - Contact technique: A glass plate of the instrument comes in contact with the linkage fluid applied on surface of the lesion. Use of contact glass is difficult for certain regions like web spaces, flexurals and nail folds. Also these glasses need sterilization.
    - Non-contact technique: A cross polarized lens of the instrument absorbs all scattered rays of the light and allows rays in a single plane to pass through it. So, there is an air-gap which produces decreased illumination and resolution.
* It is most commonly used in white skin to study melanocytic nevi and melanoma.
* It is also useful for diagnosis of other conditions:
    - Basal cell carcinoma and squamous cell carcinoma.
    - Clear cell acanthoma and dermatofibroma
    - Actinic keratosis and seborrheic keratosis.
    - Vascular lesions.
* It may also be used to count follicular density in the donor sample during hair transplantation and monitor adverse reaction to potent topical steroid in psoriasis.

Wood's lamp examination

* It emits ultraviolet light ranging from 320 nm to 420 nm with a peak at 365 nm.
* It has a filter, made of barium silicate with 9% nickel oxide. This filter blocks all light rays, except the desired band.
* When these rays are absorbed by the tissue, it radiates longer wavelength as fluorescent visible light.
* Normal tissue radiates little due to presence of elastin, aromatic aminoacids and melanin.
* Output of Wood's lamp is very low, $< 1 nm/cm^2$.
* Technique:
    - Lamp is allowed to warm for 1 minute.
    - The examination room must be perfectly dark.
    - Light source should be 4-5 inches away from the lesion.

- Washing of the site should be avoided prior to examination as it may dilute the pigmentation. Otherwise it will produce false negative result.
- Topical medicine, soap, etc should not be used, as it may produce false positive result.

* Interpretation:
  - Tinea capitis shows blue-green to dull yellow fluorescence, due to pteridine, produced by all species under *Microsporum* genus. All trichophyton species are non-fluorescent except *T. schoenleinii.*, which shows dull-blue fluorescence.
  - Pityriasis versicolor shows yellow-white or copper-orange fluorescence.
  - Pseudomonas infection shows green fluorescence due to pyoperdin or fluorescein, produced by *Pseudomonas*.
  - Erythrasma shows coral red fluorescence, due to coproporphyrin III, produced by *Corynebacterium minutissimum*.
  - Porphyrins are detected in various tissues like teeth, urine, stool, red blood cells and blister fluid. Addition of hydrochloric acid intensifies the fluorescence as it converts porphyrinogens to porphyrin. Color of the fluorescence depends on the type of porphyria. Usual fluorescence is red-pink.
  - Acne vulgaris: Facial follicular openings show coral red fluorescence due to coproporphyrin, produced by the *Propionibacterium acne*.
  - Hypopigmented lesion in fair skinned person becomes difficult to detect in fairskinned person. Due to lack of melanin, an autofluorescence is produced by dermal collagen and that differentiates the margin sharply demarcated from the normal area. It helps to differentiate early vitiligo from pityriasis alba, indeterminate leprosy and postinflammatory hypopigmentation. It also differentiates hypochromic nevus from nevus anemicus.
  - Hypopigmentation of early vitiligo or hypochromic nevus becomes more prominent under Wood's lamp.
  - Hyperpigmented lesion: Depth of the color of the hyperpigmented lesion may be assessed, specially in melasma. This finding helps to determine the prognosis of melasma and response to therapy.
  - Photodynamic diagnosis: Application of aminolevulinic acid (ALA) on a lesion for 4-6 hours under occlusion and examined under Wood's lamp. Pattern of fluorescence helps to diagnose basal cell carcinoma, squamous cell carcinoma, Bowen's disease, solar keratosis and extramammary Paget's disease.
  - Off level uses:

    #Demonstration of scabitic burrow following application of tetracycline dye or fluorescent dye.

    #Detection of systemically administered drugs like tetracycline or mepacrine in skin and lunulae of the nails.

    #Assessment of protective value of sunscreen.

    #Calculation of circulating time of an intravenously administered fluorescin.

    #Detection of epidermal penetration and turnover through fluorescent tags.

    #Detection of semen on the skin in case of sexual abuse.

    #Light of Wood's lamp can kill *Staphylococcus aureus* and mycobacterium on the skin.

    #Rarely it is used for treatment of childhood wart.

Tests for sensory impairment

- Sensation is compared between affected site and similar contralateral site as well as surrounding normal appearing area.
- It can be done with a wisp of cotton for fine touch, tip of ball pen for crude touch, pin for pain, hot and cold water test tubes for temperature.

Tests for sweating

i. Simple sweat test

- Just compare the temperature of non-erythematous leprotic lesion and surrounding normal area with dorsal surface of fingers.
- In leprotic lesion, normal heat loss by evaporation is impaired due to lack of sweat production and so finger will feel more temperature.
- Positive result indirectly helps to diagnose leprosy, specially of tuberculoid pole.
- It cannot be performed in winter season due to natural lack of sweating.
- False positive result is seen in erythematous lesion.

ii. Iodine-starch test

- An injection of pilocarpine 0.2 ml of 1 in 1000 dilution is given intradermally.
- Injection site is painted with iodine solution and dust with starch powder.
- No need of iodine if quinizarin powder is used instead of starch.
- Sweating causes blue discoloration of powder.
- No color change if there is no sweating.
- The test indirectly helps to diagnose leprosy, specially of tuberculoid pole.

Tests for motor function of peripheral nerves

i. Pen test for abduction of abductor pollicis brevis, supplied by median nerve (nerve roots C5-T1):

- Patient's hand is laid flat and a pen is held slight higher. Then the patient is asked to touch the pen by moving the thumb vertically up (abduction movement).
- Inability to touch the pen indicates loss of abduction and there is an impairment of motor function of median nerve.

ii. Oschner's clasp test/pointing index/Benediction sign for flexion of flexor digitorum superficialis of index finger, supplied by median nerve (Nerve roots C5-T1):

- Patient is asked to clasp the fingers.
- Inability to flex the index finger indicates damage of the median nerve.

iii. Book test/Froment's sign for adduction of 1st palmar interossei, supplied by the deep branch of ulnar nerve.

- Patient is asked to hold a book between thumb and index fingers of both hands and to keep the thumbs straight.
- Flexion of distal interphalangeal joint, indicates damage of the ulnar nerve.

iv. Card test for adduction of palmar interossei, supplied by the deep branch of ulnar nerve.

- A firm paper card is inserted into a finger web and patient is asked to hold it firmly between two fingers while examiner will try to pull it out with same fingers of same hand.
- Inability to hold the card indicates weakess of interossei muscles and damage of the ulnar nerve.

v. Test of the extension of the wrist for long extensor muscles of the hand, supplied by radial nerve.

- Patient is asked to close the fist and to do dorsiflexion of the wrist.
- Inability to do that indicates damage of the radial nerve and at last it is manifested by wrist drop.

vi. Test of the opponens pollicis, supplied by median nerve.

- Patient is asked to touch the tips of other fingers with tip of the thumb.
- Inability to do that indicates damage of the median nerve.

vii. Test of dorsal interossei, supplied by deep branch of ulnar nerve.

- Patient is asked to spread fingers against resistance.

- Inability to do that indicates damage of the ulnar nerve.

viii. Test of 1st and 2nd lumbricals, supplied by median nerve and 3rd and 4th lumbricals supplied by ulnar nerve.
  - Patient is asked to flex the fingers at metacarpophalangeal joints against resistance.
  - Inability to do that indicates damage of median or ulnar nerve respectively.

Pressure test

- This noninvasive test helps to differentiate between a corn and a plantar wart. This differentiation is important because treatment is totally different.
- Examiner will press the lesion directly with the thumb. If patient feels severe pain, then the lesion is a corn, because the corn is having a pointed tip and all force of the pressure accumulates at the tip and so the patient feels severe pain. In case of wart, the force of the pressure is diversed and the patient will not feel so much pain.
- When the examiner presses the lesion from the sides between thumb and index finger, patient feels severe pain in case of wart due to pressure on the nerves endings which are entangled among the projections of the wart. In case of corn patient will not feel pain because force of the pressure is inadequate to produce pain.

Relevant systemic examination

- Joints, lungs and heart examination in systemic lupus erythematosus.
- Muscular system in dermatomyositis.

Differential diagnosis

* All the possible differential diagnosis to be kept in mind.
* Least probable diagnosis to be ruled out one by one through repeating the history and examination.
* At last one to three diagnoses may be impossible to differentiate.

Provisional diagnosis

* Single or two or three most probable diagnoses are stamped as provisional diagnosis.
* If diagnosis is single, laboratory tests may be required for confirmation and if more than one, then laboratory tests are required to rule out others as well as for confirmation of the single diagnosis.

Laboratory examination

i. KOH test for fungal infection

* It is a simple test with tremendous value. I have seen a case of subcorneal pustular dermatosis (SCPD) which was mimicking tinea corporis. But when KOH test was done, it proved that really there was a superficial fungal infection along with SCPD.
* Collection of sample:
  - Scales to be collected by scraping from the lesion, preferably from the active margin.
  - Affected nail is to be clipped and subungual nail debris to be collected.
  - Only 1-2 mm long broken and lusterless hairs to be plucked by spade forceps.
  - Whitish discharge to be collected with swab.
* Preparation:
  - Samples except nail plates are placed on the slide and covered with cover slip.
  - Potassium hydroxide (10-20%) is applied at the edge of the coverslip and allowed to reach to the sample by capillary action.
  - Potassium hydroxide dissolves the intercellular cementing substances without distorting the keratinocytes or fungal hyphae.
  - It will take about 15-30 minutes, but for immediate examination, the sample is gently heated by a low flame and to be pressed, to facilitate separation of epithelial cells.
  - Nails are made of very hard keratin and difficult to separate the cells. So, the sample is to be placed in a watch glass along with several

drops of potassium hydroxide, covered with a petri dish for 24 hours. By this time it will be soft and ready for examination.

- Microscopy:
  - Condenser to be lowered down and dimming of light to make contrast and so hyphae will be seen better.
  - Recognize the hyphae with low power (× 10) after scanning all area under coverslip and confirm with high power (× 40).
- Interpretation:
  - It requires some amount of experience, otherwise there is a chance of mistake.
  - Dermatophytes appear as translucent, branching, bamboo shaped filaments, known as hyphae. These are of uniform width but interrupted lines of separation or septae make irregular appearance.
  - Uniform width, characteristic bending and branching help to distinguish these from hair and other debris.
  - Hyphae may be fragmented into round or polygonal shape.
  - The intersect lines across the cell wall at different planes of epithelial cells, are seen by using the fine adjusting knob.
  - Longitudinal, rod-shaped potassium hydroxide crystals that simulate hyphae may appear if excessive heat is given to the wet mount.
  - Lipid droplets appearing in a single file line between epithelial cells and commonly seen if sample is taken from palms or soles and this is known as mosaic pattern art effect. This is overcome by further heating and pressing which help to separate the cells.

ii. Tzanck test

- Tzanck test is a very simple and rapid technique for cytodiagnosis of pemphigus, herpes, etc.
- Preparation:
  - Sample is collected by scraping from the base of a fresh vesicle after removal of its roof.
  - Collected material is put on the glass slide, air dried and stained usually with Giemsa stain. Other stains are hematoxylin and eosin, Wright, methylene blue, Papanicolaou and toluidine blue. Giemsa stain is composed of methylene blue eosinate/chloride and azure A/B eosinate.
  - The specimen needs an immediate fixation to prevent denaturation, cross-linking of proteins and autolysis of the cells.
  - It is also needed to ensure that the specimen is hardened enough to withstand further staining steps with an intact cellular morphology.
  - Various fixatives are formalin, glutaraldehyde, methanol, ethanol, acetone, acetic acid, chromate, picric acid, etc.
  - For papanicolaou stain, sample should be fixed immediately with alcohol. But alcohol fixation should be used at a low temperature otherwise it may produce distortion or shrinkage of the cells.
- Uses of Tzanck test:
  - Diagnosis of pemphigus, herpes simplex/zoster, varicella, vaccinia, variola, etc.
  - To differentiate between toxic epidermal necrolysis (TEN) and staphylococcus scalded skin syndrome (SSSS).
  - To diagnose or to exclude bullous pemphigoid, Hailey Hailey disease, Darier's disease, vesicular/pustular dematoses in neonates, Stevens-Johnson syndrome and erosive lichen planus.
  - Pustular/bullous superficial fungal infection.
- Interpretation:
  - Tzank smear in pemphigus reveals multiple acantholytic cells/Tzanck cells. An acantholytic cell has a large round nucleus, hazy or absent nucleoli and abundant basophilic cytoplasm. Basophilic stain of the cytoplasm is darker at cell membrane as there is a tendency of the cytoplasm to condense at the periphery and this phenomenon leads to a perinuclear

halo. The term sertoli rosette is used when a ring of leukocytes surrounds an epithelial cell and the term streptocytes is used when an adherent chain of leukocytes is attached.

- In herpes or varicella, acantholytic cell may be multinucleated. The cells appear inflated due to ballooning degeneration, even upto 60-80 μm in diameter. The shape of the giant cells may be tadpole, bipolar, irregular teardrop with a smooth external contour and these may contain 8 or more nuclei. These nuclei are arranged in jigsaw puzzle like fashion.
- In vaccinia or variola, the acantholytic cells contain eosinophilic cytoplasmic inclusions, called Guarnieri body, surrounded by a clear halo.
- In TEN, Tzanck smear shows necrotizing or degenerating basal cells with scattered inflammatory cells and fibroblasts. In SSSS, Tzanck smear shows dyskeratotic cells with very few inflammatory cells.

iii. Slit skin smear test

* It is commonly used to detect lepra bacilli in leprosy and Leishman-Donovan bodies (LD bodies) in cutaneous leishmaniasis or post kala-azar dermal leishmaniasis.
* In leprosy, the aim is to detect bacterial index (BI) and morphological index (MI).
* BI is the quantitative measurement of lepra bacilli which actually indicates the concentration of bacilli in a particular site.
* MI is the qualitative measurement of lepra bacilli which indicates number of solid staining bacilli out of total 100 bacilli.
* Sites:
  - For lepra bacilli: Both earlobes, four active sites and dorsal surfaces of distal parts of the fingers.
  - For LD bodies: Most infiltrated skin lesion.
* Technique:
  - Selected areas, to be cleaned with spirit and dried up.
  - Skin is pinched up with index and thumb, so that blood circulation will be compromised leading to less bleeding during slitting.
  - A 5 mm long and 3 mm depth slit is made with 15 Bard Parker blade and the blade is rotated at 90° to scrape the slit with blunt edge.
  - Scraping is done for several times to collect a little pulp of dermal tissue.
  - If by chance any blood comes, it will be mopped with cotton bud.
  - Material is transferred to glass slide and spread over it with a circular motion to make a smear of 5-7 mm in diameter.
  - Then it is air dried, followed by heating for 5 minutes at 40-50°C with a controlled heating system. But overheating must be avoided. So, easy way to avoid heating the smear is that the smear is kept in formalin fume for 10 minutes.
* Staining for lepra bacilli:
  - The slide is flooded with freshly filtered carbol-fuchsin for 20 minutes at room temperature. This time may be shortened by heating but the quality of stain may be compromised. Heating may be done at 42°C just upto steaming and wait for 15 minutes.
  - Slide is then washed gently under tap water and decolorization is done with acid-alcohol mixture (1% HCl and 70% ethanol).
  - After decolorization, again wash and counterstain with methylene blue for 1 minute and then wash again.
* Staining for LD bodies is done with Giemsa stain.
* Determination of bacillary index:
  - Number of bacilli is calculated on a logarithmic scale, varying from few bacilli (1+) to numerous bacilli (6+).
  - Bacilli are counted under oil immersion (× 1000).
  - For a single site, 25-100 fields are examined and put on logarithmic scale to measure the score.
  - For different sites, total scores is divided by total number of sites.

* Logarithmic scale:
  - >1000 bacilli per field = 6+
  - 100-1000 bacilli per field = 5+
  - 10-100 bacilli per field = 4+
  - 1-10 bacilli per field = 3+
  - 1-10 bacilli per 10 field = 2+
  - 1-10 bacilli per 100 fields = 1+
  - No bacillus per 100 fields = 0
* Determination of Morphological index (MI):
  - MI is the ratio of solid or regular staining bacilli and irregularly staining bacilli.
  - It indicates infectiousness of the patient and response to therapy.
  - Solid or regular staining bacilli means those who are showing uniform and bright stain along their whole length. These are viable bacilli and they are infective.
  - Irregularly stained bacilli means degenerating bacilli and they are not infective.
  - Preferably 100 isolated or non-overlapped bacilli are counted.

iv. Wet mount

* Sample is collected from male urethra or posterior vaginal fornix and mix with few drops of normal saline at body temperature on the glass slide and examined under microscope.
* It helps to demonstrate trichomonas in trichomoniasis and candida in candidiasis.

v. Gram stain

* Specimens
  - Pus/purulent urethral discharge
  - Vaginal discharge
  - Exudate from a discharging sinus or from a pyoderma
* Procedure:
  - Fix the smear with heat.
  - Stain with crystal violet for 1 minute and wash.
  - Stain with Gram's iodine for 1 minute and wash.
  - Decolorize with acetone-ethanol for 10-20 seconds.
  - Counterstain with sofranin or fuchsin for 1 minute and wash.
* Interpretation: Condenser of the microscope should be up and iris diaphragm should be open for maximum light.
  - Gonococci are intracellular gram negative kidney shaped or coffeebean shaped diplococci with size 0.6-0.8 μm. Some bacilli may be present extracellularly.
  - More than 5 polymorphs per high power field (HPF) without any organism in the smear from urethral discharge is suggestive of nongonococcal urethritis.
  - More than 30 polymorphs per high power field (HPF) in cervical smear is suggestive of cervicitis.
  - *Hemophillus ducreyi* are small Gram negative bacilli, grouped in chain as school of fish or rail road track appearance.
  - Vaginal smear shows squamous cells coated with cocco-bacilli, known as clue cells. Clue cells are having indistinct borders and surfaces appear granular or stippled. Normal vaginal discharge may show clue cells upto 20%. More than 20% is suggestive of bacterial vaginosis.
  - *Gardenella vaginalis* are Gram negative small rods with size 1.5-2.5 μm × 0.5 μm. Prevotella/mobilincus spp. are slender and slightly curved rods. They lie singly or in pairs and appear as gull wings.
  - Budding yeasts are Gram positive and appear as figure of 8 and hyphae are also Gram positive.

vi. Acetic acid test

* For clinically inapparent human papilloma virus infection:
  - Acetic acid of 3-5% concentration with a swab stick is applied on the suspected site of human papilloma virus infection.

- After 2-3 minutes infected areas will appear as whitish and thickened papules.

vii. Whip test or Sniff test

- 1-2 drops of 10% KOH solution is mixed with vaginal discharge.
- Enhancement of fishy odor is suggestive of bacterial vaginosis.

viii. Dark ground illumination test (DGI)

* Sample is collected from the lesion of primary, secondary or early congenital syphilis following cleaning with minimum amount of normal saline and by abrading the lesion with dry gauge piece.
* Clear serum is collected by squeezing the lesion and touching the cover slip or slide directly. For deeper lesion it is collected with loop or pipette.
* Seal the edges of the coverslip with petroleum jelly.
* Examination is done with a special set up of microscope, having a dark background and under oil-immersion.

viii. Intradermal tests

- Mantoux test for tuberculosis
- Lepromin test for leprosy

ix. Serological tests

- VDRL and TPHA for syphilis
- ELISA test for HIV infection

x. Immunofluorescence test

* Transport media, like Michel's media or liquid nitrogen is required to transport tissue to the laboratory.
* Direct immunofluorescence test (DIF): It detects the presence of antigen-antibody complex and commonly used in:
  - Pemphigus, bullous pemphigoid, dermatitis herpetiformis
  - Linear IgA bullous dermatosis, epidermolysis bullosa acquisita
  - Henoch-Schonlein purpura
  - Lupus erythematosus
* Indirect immunofluorescence test (IIF): It detects the circulating autoantibodies and commonly used in:
  - Pemphigus
  - Systemic lupus erythematosus

Lupus band test (LBT)

* This is a form of direct immunofluorescence test to detect immunoglobulin and complement in the skin of lupus erythematosus (LE), deposited as a band along the basement membrane zone.
* Immunoreactants are IgG, IgM, IgA and C3.
* When three or more reactants are present at non-lesional skin, specificity is increased highly.
* It is positive in 90-95% cases when sample is taken from lesional skin and in systemic lupus erythematosus, the sensitivity of the test is 95%, but specificity is 87%.
* Staining pattern:
  - Granular in low power.
  - In high power, homogeneous, fibrillar, stippled, shags, lumpy-bumpy, linear or thready.
  - Continous in lupus erythematosus but discontinuous and interrupted in other disorders like actinic keratosis, polymorphic light eruption, rosacea and 80% nonlesional sunexposed skin of lupus erythematosus.
  - Stippled pattern is seen is normal appearing skin of LE.
  - Homogeneous or solid band is seen in chronic atrophic or hypertrophic lesion.
  - Thready or fibrillar pattern is seen in acute LE.
* Uses:
  - It helps to differentiate LE from polymorphic light eruption and Jessner's lymphocytic infiltration.
  - It is very diagnostic of LE when nonlesional photoprotected skin becomes positive for three or more immunoreactants.
  - In systemic LE both lesional and nonlesional photoprotected skin samples are positive but in discoid LE only lesional skin sample is positive.

- So, it has tremendous value to diagnose a case of systemic LE when there is no skin lesion.
- It helps to differentiate LE from other antinuclear antibody positive dermatoses like scleroderma, mixed connective tissue disease, drug induced LE, dermatomyositis, rheumatoid arthritis, etc.
- It also has a prognostic value. Positive result from nonlesional sunprotected skin means prolonged course and indicates chance of renal involvement and result correlates with disease severity.

* False positive result may be seen in:
  - Bullous pemphigoid
  - Porphyria
  - Rosacea
  - Polymorphic light eruption
  - Autofluorescence from dermal collagen and elastin.
  - 20% Cases of healthy individuals.

xi. FNAC

* It is easy to perform but difficult to interprete.
* It gives the result quickly but rarely can confirm the diagnosis.
* It is helpful in getting an idea about a subcutaneous mass, lymph node, bubo, etc.

xii. Histopathology

* It has a crucial value to confirm a diagnosis or to exclude a diagnosis.
* Dermatologists must know to interprete histopathology for better correlation than pathologists.
* So, it has been discussed in detail at separate chapter.

xiii. Immunohistochemistry

xiv. Patch test

* It is the test of choice for allergic contact dermatitis and also helps to detect drug reactions.
* Allergens are usually purchased as readymade or may be prepared according to the relevance.
* Allergens are placed in special wells like Finn chambers, and applied at the back for 48 hours.
* Reading is done at 48 hours and again at 96 hours and at 72 hours for photopatch test.
* Interpretation:
  - Only macular erythema: Doubtful result (+/–)
  - Erythema, infiltration, papule formation: Weak reaction (+)
  - Edema and vesicle formation: Strong reaction (++)
  - Bulla and ulcer formation: Extreme reaction (+++).
  - Irritant reaction: IRR.
  - No response: Negative (–).

xv. LE cell test

- About 5 ml of heparinized blood is stirred with glass beads in a conical test tube for 30 minutes.
- Due to stirring nuclei of some of the neutrophils become naked and are exposed to antinuclear antibodies or serum factor if at all present.
- Blood is incubated for 30 minutes at 37°C, so that these naked nuclei get tagged with antibodies.
- These tagged nuclei are engulfed by the remaining viable neutrophils.
- Blood is centrifuzed to get a buffy-coat.
- A smear is made from the buffy-coat and stained with Giemsa stain.
- Plenty of neutrophils with extra nuclear matrerials (LE cell) are seen in systemic lupus erythematosus (SLE).
- Few LE cells may be seen in scleroderma, discoid lupus erythematosus, rheumatoid arthritis, etc.

Final diagnosis

* It includes usually one diagnosis but may be few due to associated disorders.

* Mixed connective tissue disorder is now considered a single entity but basically it is a combination of at least two connective tissue disorders.
* A systemic lupus erythematosus (SLE) patient may have extensive tinea corporis or crusted scabies.
* In the above case, presenting complaints are to be considered for final diagnosis.
    - If presenting complaint is related to (SLE), then final diagnosis will be SLE with tinea corporis or SLE with crusted scabies.
    - If presenting complaint is related to tinea corporis, then final diagnosis will be tinea corporis in a case of SLE.

PART C

MOST COMMON DERMATOSES FOR UNDERGRAGUATES

CHAPTER C1

PYODERMA

- The term pyoderma is used for bacterial infection of the skin where pus is formed at a stage of the disease.
- It is mostly caused by *Staphylococcus aureus* or *Streptococcus pyogenes*, or by a combination of both.
- Detection of organisms can be done by Gram stain and culture.
- Treatment is mainly topical and systemic antibiotics, covering staphylococcus and streptococcus.

Types of pyoderma

- Primary
- Secondary.

Primary pyoderma

- The term primary pyoderma is used when infection occurs at apparently normal appearing skin.

Secondary pyoderma

- The term secondary pyoderma is used when infection occurs at skin already affected by some other dermatoses.
- It is commonly associated with scabies and dermatitis.

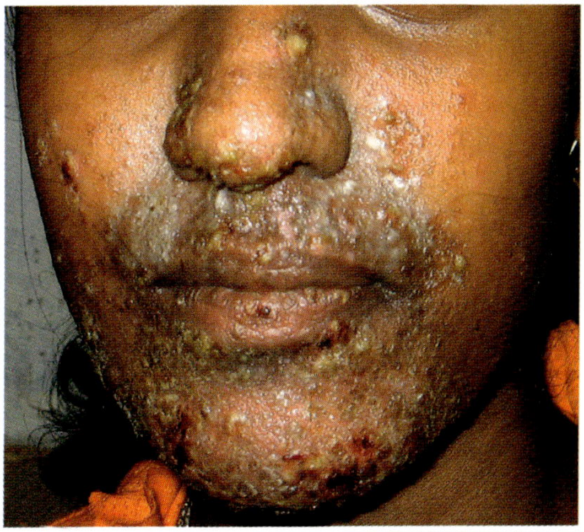

Fig. 1: Pustular lesions, associated with dermatitis

Differential diagnosis

- Infective eczematoid dermatitis.
- Infected dermatitis.

Variants of pyoderma

- Nonfollicular:
  - Bullous impetigo

- ♦ Nonbullous impetigo/impetigo contagiosa
- ♦ Ecthyma
- ♦ Erysipelas
- ♦ Cellulitis

✶ Follicular:

- ♦ Acute superficial folliculitis
- ♦ Chronic deep folliculitis
- ♦ Boil/furuncle
- ♦ Carbuncle

✶ Other:

- ♦ Summer boil/periporitis.

Impetigo

✶ The term impetigo is used for nonfollicular superficial pyogenic infection, manifested as a vesicopustule or pustule.

✶ An epidermolytic toxin is produced by the organisms which causes intraepidermal cleavage.

✶ When the cleavage is just below the corneal layer, the roof ruptures quickly to convert into an erosion and the term is used as non-bullous impetigo. In this form of pyoderma, very often new lesions develop around the old lesions and then the term is used as impetigo contagiosa.

✶ When the cleavage is little deeper i.e., through the spinous layer, it persists for longer time without immediate rupture as in impetigo contagiosa, the term is used as bullous impetigo.

✶ Children in close contact are commonly affected.

✶ Warm, moist climate and poor hygiene are the predisposing factors.

Clinical features of impetigo contagiosa

- ♦ Lesion starts as a superficial blister which ruptures quickly to form a crusted erosion and then spreads peripherally.
- ♦ A few satellite lesions usually develop around an old lesion. These satellite lesions may remain discrete or may enlarge and coalesce to form a polycyclic lesion.
- ♦ After a few days or week when healing start at the center of a lesion it takes an annular configuration, termed as impetigo circinata.
- ♦ Presenting lesions are usually painful erosions, partially covered with honey colored or hemorrhagic crusts and surrounded by varying amount of erythema. Rarely itching or fever is associated.

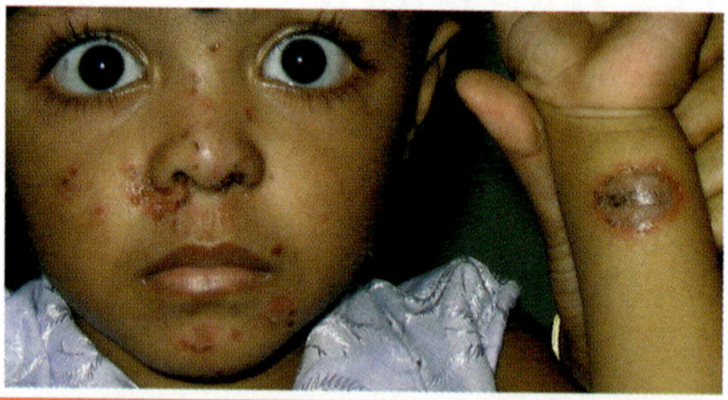

Fig. 2: Multiple erosions with honey colored crusts

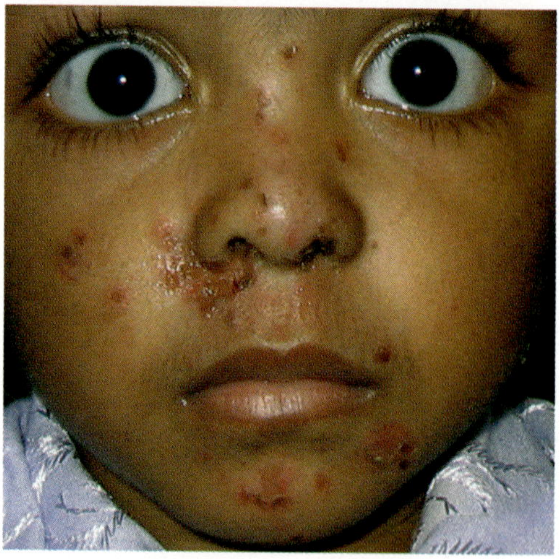

Fig. 3: Impetigo contagiosa in closeup view

- ♦ Lesions may heal spontaneously after several weeks or quickly following treatment.
- ♦ A postinflammatory hypo- or hyperpigmentation may develop following healing of a lesion.
- ♦ It commonly affects face and periorificial areas, specially mouth, nose and ears. But it spares the palms and soles due to very thick stratum corneum.
- ♦ Number of the lesions is variable from single to multiple and size is also variable from few mm to few cm.

- Shape is usually round when the lesions are discrete; but becomes bizarre when lesions coalesce.
- Regional lymphadenopathy is commonly associated.

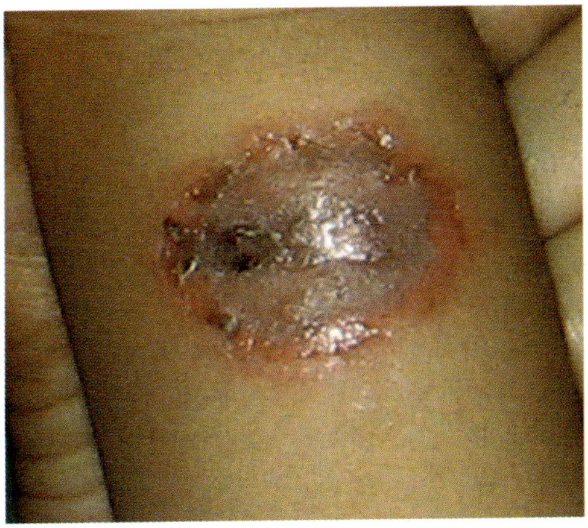

Fig. 4: Impetigo circinata in closeup view

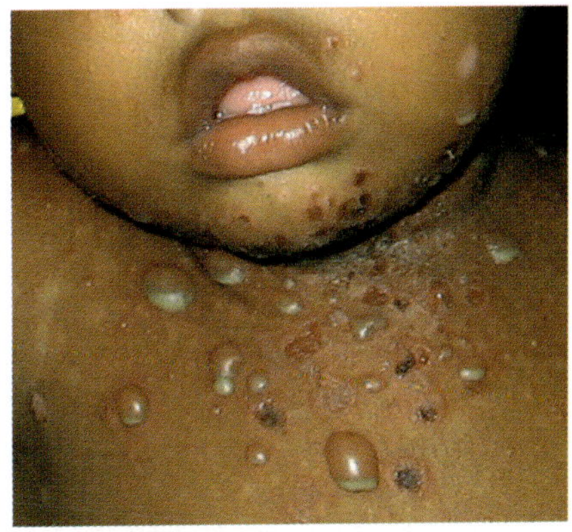

Fig. 5: Multiple bullous lesions at various stages of evolution
Differential diagnosis:
- Chronic bullous dermatosis of childhood
- Porphyria
- Subcorneal pustular dermatosis

Differential diagnosis

- Cutaneous candidiasis
- Tinea corporis

Clinical features of bullous impetigo

- Lesion starts as vesicle or bulla which quickly turns into pustule with varying amount of erythema.
- Sometimes vesicle or bulla may contain hemorrhagic fluid.
- This intact vesicle or bulla persists for days. Gradually the center of the lesion collapses and becomes crusted with a retained peripheral rim of fluid.
- If the crusts are removed, a bright red, moist base is exposed with seropurulent discharge.
- Presenting lesions are single or multiple pustules. They remain discrete in comparison to lesions of impetigo contagiosa which often coalesce.
- Any site but limbs are commonly affected.
- Number of the lesions is variable from single to multiple and size is also variable from 3 mm to 2 cm.

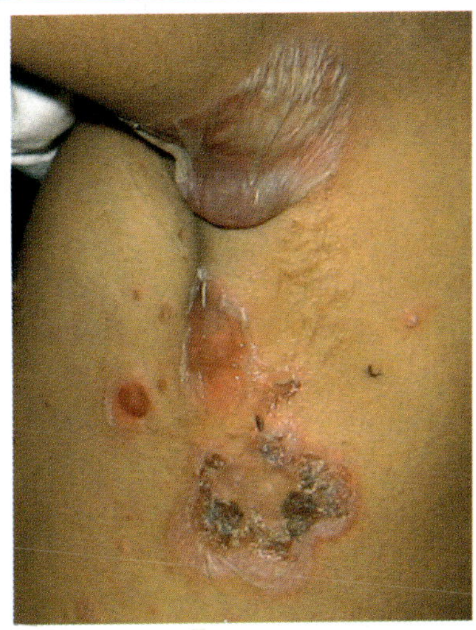

Fig. 6: One flaccid bulla containing hemorrhagic fluid and few other ruptured lesions having crusts at the center and fluid filled rims at the periphery

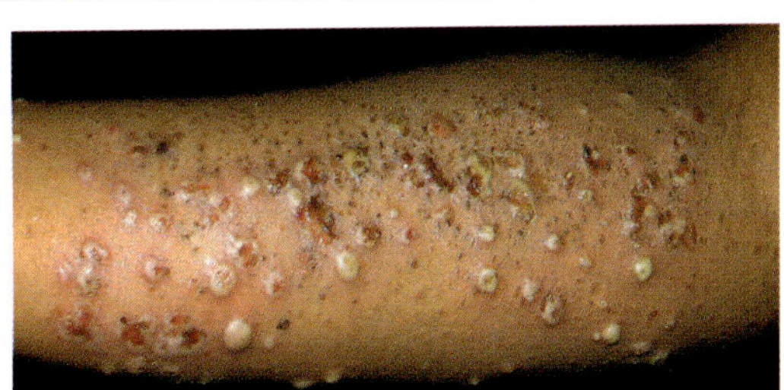

Fig. 7: Multiple pustules of bullous impetigo at the forearm

Differential diagnosis

- Acute superficial folliculitis
- Herpes simplex
- Chicken pox

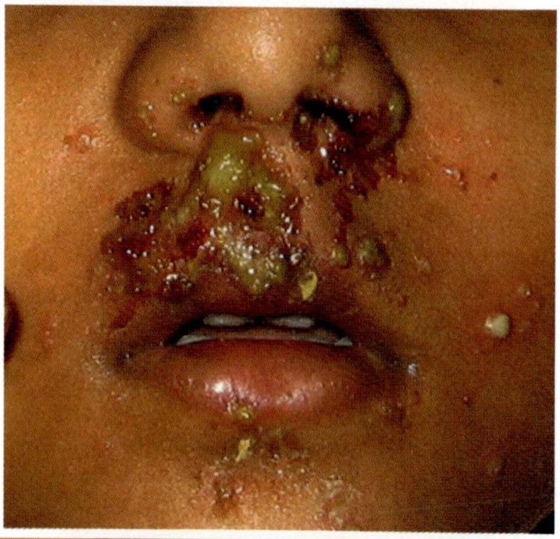

Fig. 8: Dried up deposition of yellowish to honeycolored crusts on the erosions of bullous impetigo

Complications of impetigo

* Poststreptococcal glomerulonephritis may develop following impetigo, caused by streptococcal serotypes 1, 4, 12, 25, 49, but rheumatic fever never develops.
* Acute nephritis
    - It develops 1-3 weeks of acute infection with nephritogenic strains of beta hemolytic streptococci, occurring in 2-5% of all forms of impetigo but varying from 10-25% when it is caused by nephritogenic streptococcus.
    - It commonly affects children between 6-10 years of age and manifests with hematuria in 90% cases, edema of feet and periorbital areas, hypertension, headache, altered conciousness, congestive heart failure and renal failure.
    - Presence of RBC casts in urine is pathognomonic. C3 level is decreased and anti DNase B titer is increased if impetigo lesions are still persisting. Renal biopsy is rarely required for prognosis and therapy.
    - Prognosis is excellent in children. Resolution of edema and hypertension starts within 1-2 weeks. But proteinuria may continue for 6 months and microscopic hematuria for upto 1 year.
* Staphylococcal scalded skin syndrome, characterized by generalized scalding.

Ecthyma

* The term ecthyma is used when bullous impetigo persists for longer time without healing and infection affects deeper layers of epidermis.
* Clinically, it is characterized by wedge-shaped ulcer covered with thick adherent crust.
* Presenting lesions are ulcers, covered with thick and adherent crusts. Sometimes crusts become heaped up and look like oyster shell.
* Usually number is single or few.
* Legs are commonly affected.

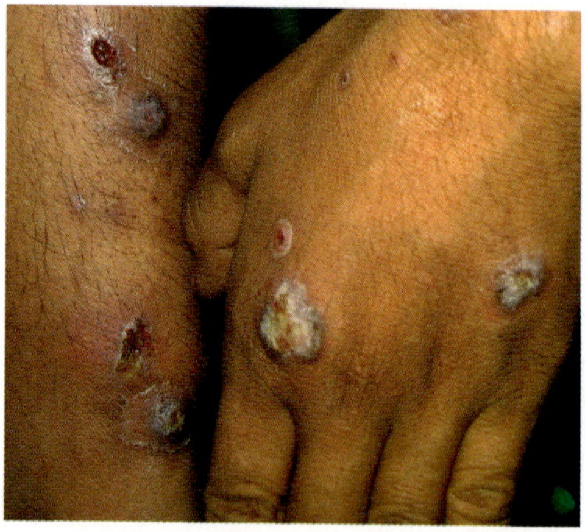

Fig. 9: Crusted ulcers

Treatment of impetigo and ecthyma

- Condy's compress: At least twice daily till oozing is being dried up and crusts are being cleaned up.
- Twice daily application of topical antibiotic as a thin layer till lesions completely healed.
- Oral antibiotics like dicloxacillin, amoxicillin, amoxicillin-clavulanic acid, cephadroxil, etc. for at least seven days.

Erysipelas

- It primarily affects the dermis with significant involvement of the dermal lymphatics.
- It is commonly caused by *Streptococcus pyogenes*.
- In adulthood, women are more affected than men, but in childhood, boys are more affected than girls.
- It occurs more frequently in summer.

Clinical features of erysipelas

- After an incubation period of 2-5 days, there is an abrupt onset of fever, chill, malaise and nausea.
- A few hours to days later, a small plaque of erythema develops and gradually progresses.
- It becomes hot, tense, tender and swollen without pitting.
- Margin is well demarcated at least some places from the uninvolved surrounding skin.
- Painful or burning sensation may be associated.
- Pustule, vesicle, bulla or small area of hemorrhagic necrosis may develop within the plaque.
- Regional lymphadenopathy presents with or without lymphatic streaking.
- Desquamation and postinflammatory hyperpigmentation develop following resolution.
- Previously face was the commonest site but now a days *leg is the commonest site*.

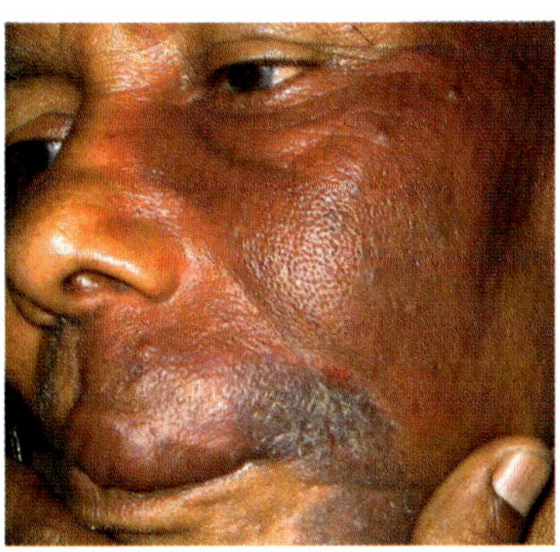

Fig. 10: Well to illdefined eythematous plaque

Differential diagnosis

- Urticaria
- BT leprosy with downgrade type 1 reaction
- Cellulitis

Histopathology of erysipelas

- Diffuse edema of the dermis.
- In early stage neutrophilic infiltration is profound but later it becomes scanty.
- Dermoepidermal separation, dilated lymphatics and foci of suppurative necrosis may be seen.

Treatment of erysipelas

- Penicillin, specially dicloxacillin is the drug of choice and given for 10-14 days by oral, intramuscular or intravenous route according to the severity.

Cellulitis

- It affects deep dermis and subcutaneous tissue and often it is caused by *Staphylococcus aureus* or *Streptococcus pyogenes*.
- Lymphedema, diabetes mellitus, peripheral vascular disease, intravenous drug abuse, and alcoholism are common predisposing factors.

Clinical features of cellulitis

- It is often preceded by fever, chill and malaise.
- Ill defined erythematous, edematous, hot and tender indurated plaque develops at the affected area.
- In severe cases vesicles/bullae, pustules, necrosis and ulceration may develop.
- Gradually infection may affects deeper tissue to produce necrotizing fasciitis.
- In children, head and neck regions are commonly affected but in adults extremities are commonly affected.

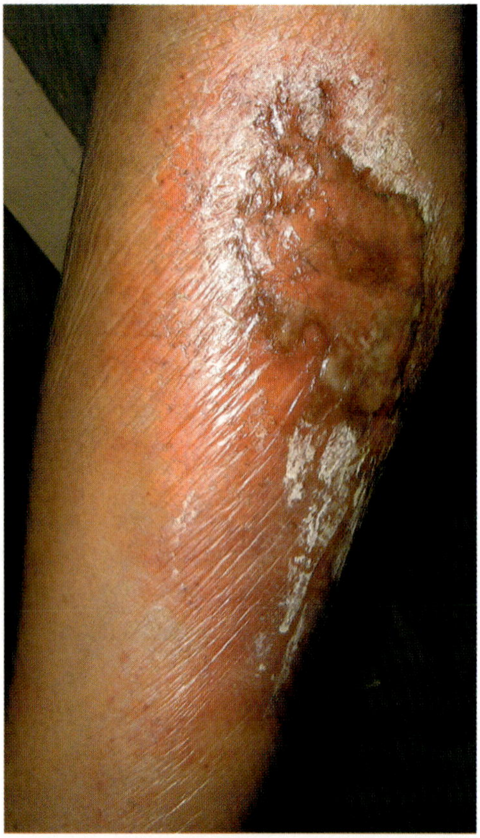

Fig. 11: Ill defined erythematous swelling with eroded surface due to rupture of the blister

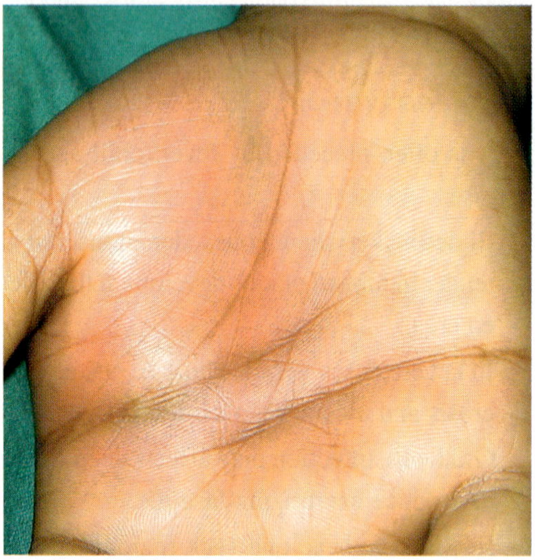

Fig. 12: Ill defined eythematous swelling at the palm with a pus point

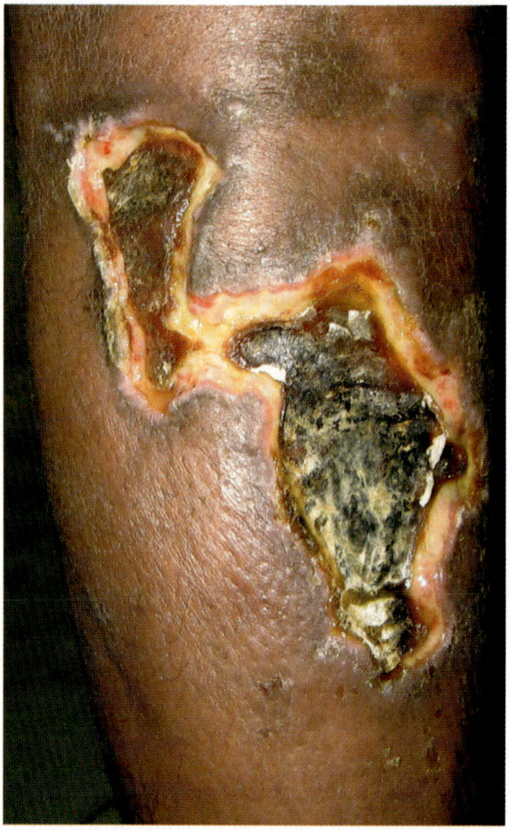

Fig. 13: Necrotic ulcer within an erythematous ill defined swollen area

Folliculitis

* When infection is localized predominantly within the follicle and little around the follicle, the term is used as folliculitis.
* It may be acute and chronic.

Acute folliculitis/Bockhart's impetigo

* The term is used for acute superficial folliculitis.
* Lesions start as folliculitis but appear as impetigo.

Chronic deep folliculitis

* Symptom is itching instead of pain as in other forms of pyoderma.
* Lesions are follicular papules and pustules. Hair may be seen piercing through the lesion in early stage but may not be seen in late stage due to loss of hair.

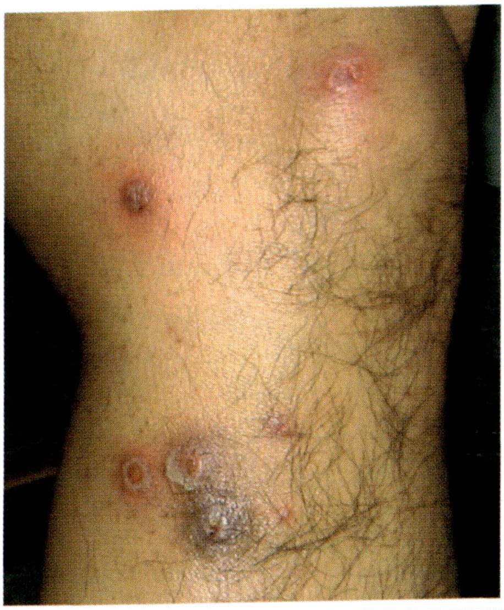

Fig. 14: Follicular erythematous pustules with peripheral impetigo-like crust

- ✶ Intact pustules are often seen in the morning and they rupture at later part of the day due to scratching.
- ✶ When a particular area is affected, active lesions are present at the periphery, as older lesions of the center heal with damage of the follicle.
- ✶ The term sycosis barbae is used when lesions affect mustache and beard areas.
- ✶ When lesions coalesce to form an inflammed plaque and later form scar, then the term is used as lupoid sycosis.

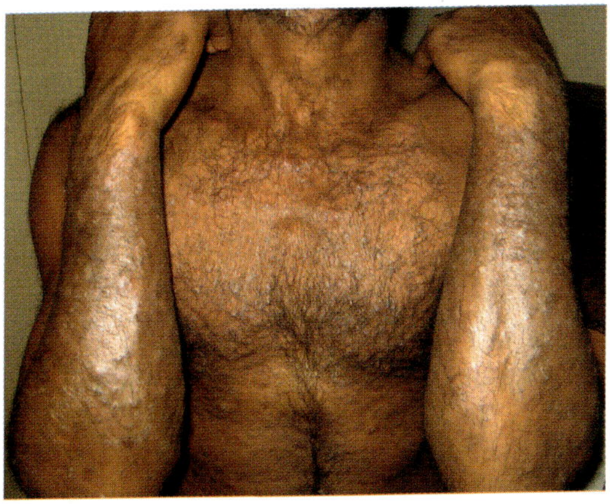

Fig. 15: Multiple follicular pustules

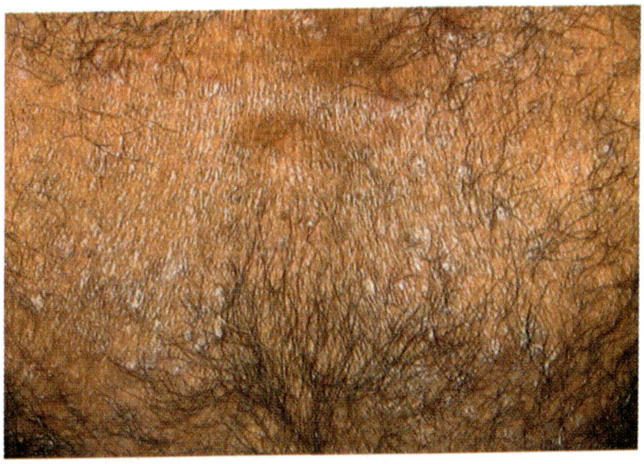

Fig. 16: Multiple follicular pustules with hair loss

- ✶ It commonly occurs in rainy and summer seasons and remains silent during winter.
- ✶ Common sites are beard and mustache area, front and sides of the lower limbs and extensors of the forearms.
- ✶ Recurrence is very common.

Differential diagnosis

- ♦ Seborrheic folliculitis
- ♦ Pustular acne

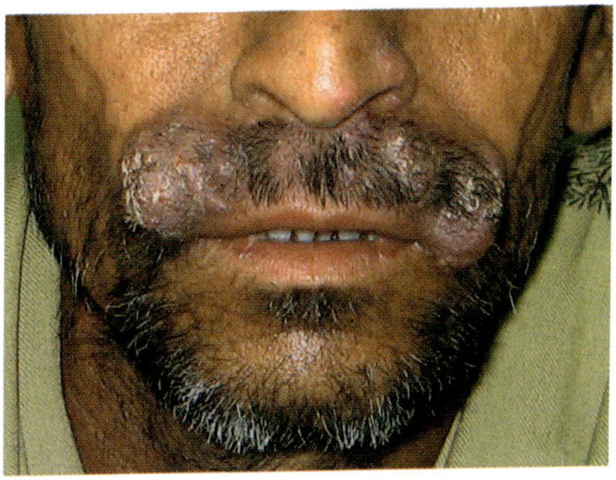

Fig. 17: Erythematous irregular plaque of lupoid sycosis, studded with pustules

Differential diagnosis

- ♦ Tinea barbae

- ✶ Treatment is not very easy. It requires i.m. or i.v. injection of lyncomycin or clindamycin for 1-2 weeks and application of topical mupirocin.

Boil or furuncle

- When infection spreads beyond the follicle along with destruction of the follicle due to intense inflammation, the term is used as boil or furuncle.

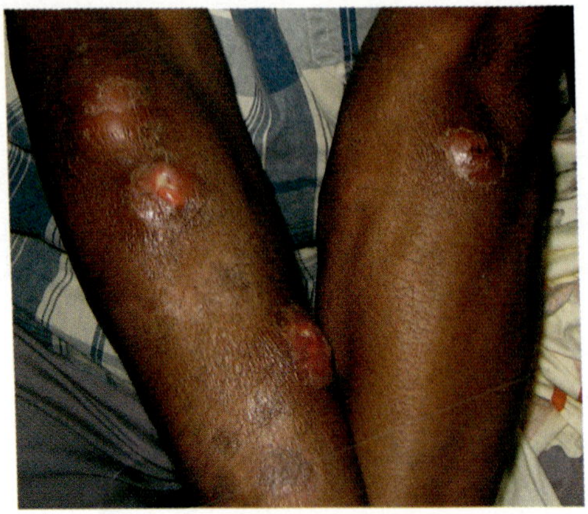

Fig. 18: Multiple tender nodules with central pus points

- Lesions is erythematous, edematous extremely tender nodule and often studded with a pus point at the center, representing the position of the follicle.

Carbuncle

- When adjacent boils are coalesced to form a single inflammed mass, the term is used as carbuncle.
- Lesion is extremely tender.
- It is often associated with diabetes and immunosuppression.
- Treatment is oral, intramuscular or intravenous antibiotics like amoxicillin, amoxicillin-clavulanic acid and dicloxacillin.

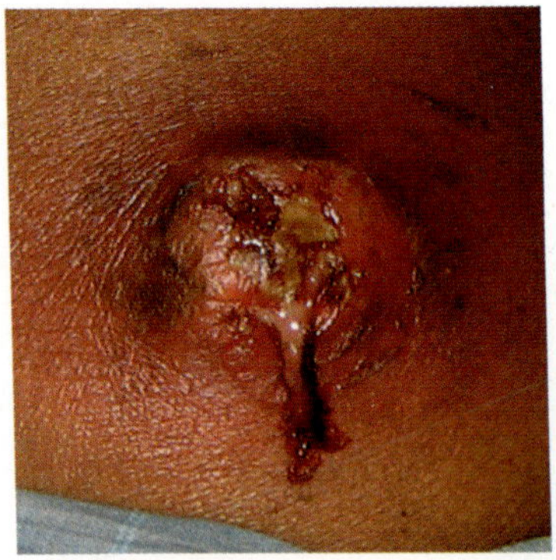

Fig. 19: Single nodular plaque with multiple openings and seropurulent discharge

Periporitis/Summer boil

- The term is used when infection occurs at acrosyringium/epidermal part of the sweat ducts.

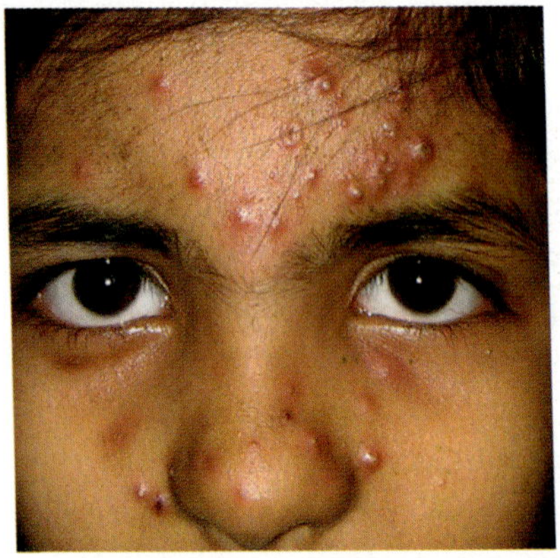

Fig. 20: Multiple cone-shaped erythematous papulonodule with pus point at the top

- Clinically it appears as small cone shaped boil-like nodulo-papule with pus point at the center.

CHAPTER

C2

SUPERFICIAL FUNGAL INFECTIONS

- Superficial fungal infections include fungal infection of the epidermis of the skin, hair follicle, hair shaft, nail and mucosae of the oropharynx and anogenitalia.
- It is the most common among all mucocutaneous infection and commonly caused by following fungi:
  - Dermatophytes
  - Candida spp.
  - Malassezia spp.
  - Trichosporon (yeast)
- These fungi invade the keratinized part of the cutaneous structures.
- Superficial fungal infections are favoured by warm and humid climate, corticosteroid, immunosuppressive therapy, leukemia and HIV infection.
- Candidal infection is common in diabetes mellitus but dermatophytic infections do not increase in it.
- The term dermatophytosis is used when infection is caused by dermatophytes.
- The term epidermomycosis is used when dermatophytes infect the epidermis.
- The term trichomycosis is used when dermatophytes infect hair shaft and hair follicles.
- Onycomycosis is a general term, used for nail infection caused by either dermatophytes or non-dermatophytes including moulds, candida or yeast.
- The term tinea unguium is used when only dermatophytes infect the nail plate.
- Ectothrix infection: Cuticle, the outermost layer of the hair shaft, is affected by the hyphal fragments or arthroconidia leading to the damage of the cuticle. Commonest fungi are:
  - *Microsporum spp.*
  - *Trichophyton mentagrophytes*
  - *Trichophyton schoenleinii*
- Endothrix infection: Infection occurs within the hair shaft without damaging the cuticle. Commonest fungi are:
  - *Trichophyton tonsurans*
  - *Trichophyton violaceum*
  - *Trichophyton schoenleinii*
  - *Trichophyton soudanense*

* Kerion is commonly caused by following fungi:
  - *Trichophyton verrucosum*
  - *Trichophyton mentagrophytes var. mentagrophytes.*
  - Geophilic species
* Favus is commonly caused by:
  - *Trichophyton schoenleinii*
  - *Trichophyton violaceum*
  - *Microsporum gypseum*

Diagnosis of superficial fungal infection

- It is mainly done by clinical examination and confirmed by direct demonstration of fungal spore or hyphae with KOH test and culture in Sabouraud's dextrose agar media.
- Wood's lamp examination shows fluorescence when tinea capitis is caused by *trichophyton rubrum*.

Treatment of superficial fungal infection

- Topical or only systemic or both, depending on the type of the fungal infection, age of the patient and presence of precipitating factors.

Commonest dermatophytes

- *Trichophyton rubrum*, commonly causes tinea faciei, having a tendency to be chronic and to form arthroconidia. It cannot be viable for long time in scale.
- *Epidermophyton floccosum* is commonly associated with epidemic tinea cruris in the set up of locker rooms or dormitories. It has no tendency of chronicity, no tendency of extension beyond the groin, and formation of arthroconidia. It can be viable for long time in scale.
- *Trichophyton mentagrophytes var. mentagrophytes*, produces more severe and chronic form with intense inflammation and pustulation.

Types of superficial fungal infection

* Dermatophytic infection
  - Tinea corporis
  - Tinea capitis
  - Tinea faciei
  - Tinea barbae
  - Tinea cruris
  - Tinea manuum
  - Tinea pedis
  - Tinea unguium
  - Tinea imbricata
  - Tinea incognito
  - Dermatitic tinea
* Non-dermatophytic infection
  - Candidiasis
  - Tinea versicolor/pityriasis versicolor
  - Tinea nigra.

Tinea corporis

* The term tinea corporis is used when dermatophytic infection affects any part of the skin except scalp (tinea capitis), non hairy part of the face (tinea faciei), hairy part of the face (tinea barbae), groin (tinea cruris), palms (tinea manuum) and soles (tinea pedis).

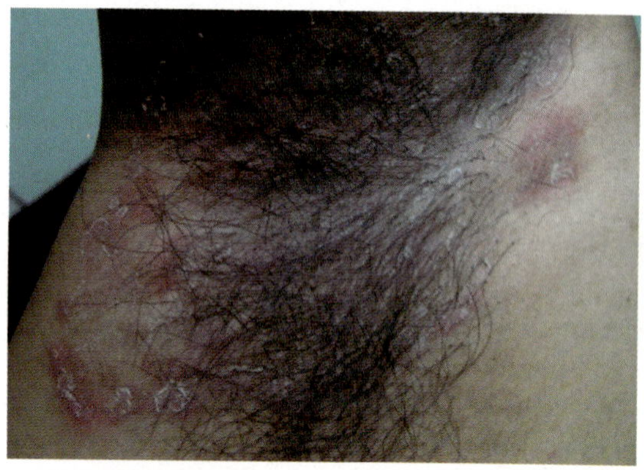

Fig. 1: Polycyclic patch at the axilla with erythematous scaly active border and relatively clear center

Differential diagnosis

- Cutaneous candidiasis
- Granuloma annulare
- Erythema annulare centrifugum.

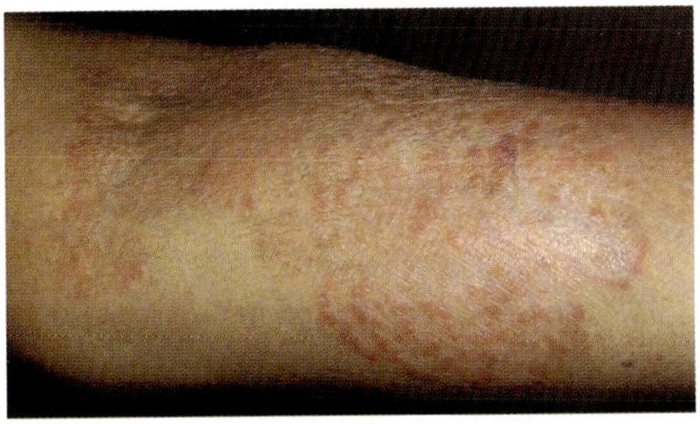

Fig. 2: Polycyclic irregular patch at the forearm, studded with numerous erythematous papules and minimum scale

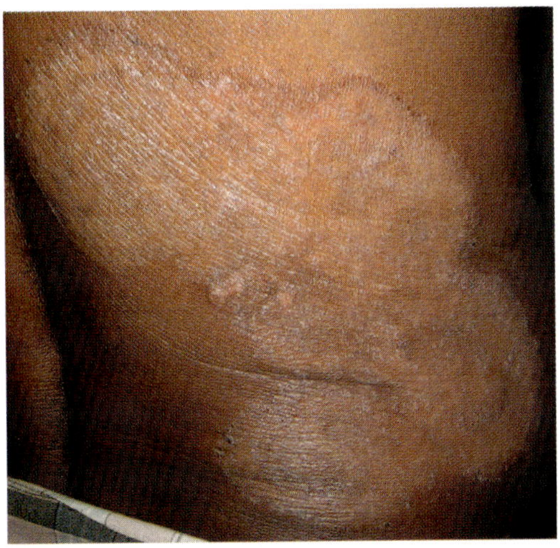

Fig. 3: Well defined erythematous scaly patch at the flank with crusted papules at the margin

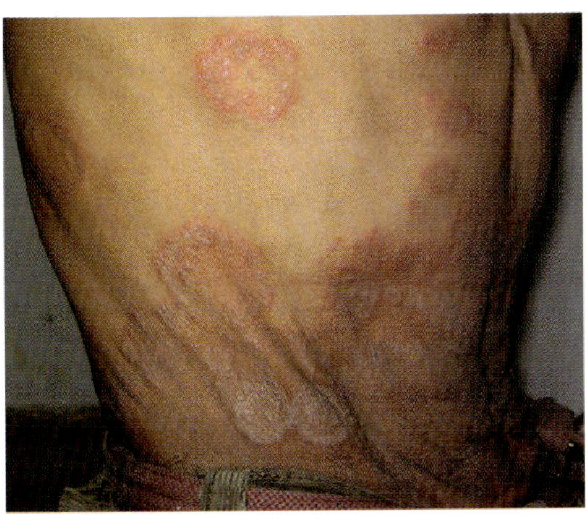

Fig. 4: Annular patches, few are discrete and few are coalesced, presenting at the flank

Differential diagnosis:

- Nummular dermatitis.

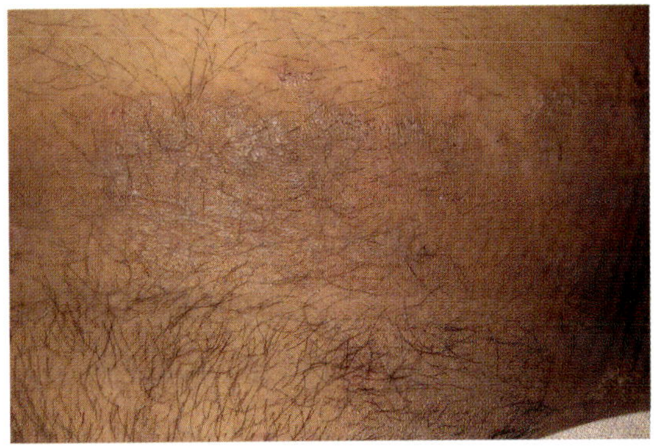

Fig. 5: Well to ill defined polycyclic patch at the flank, studded with scaly and crusted papules without clear cut center, mimicking allergic contact dermatitis

Differential diagnosis:

- Allergic contact dermatitis.

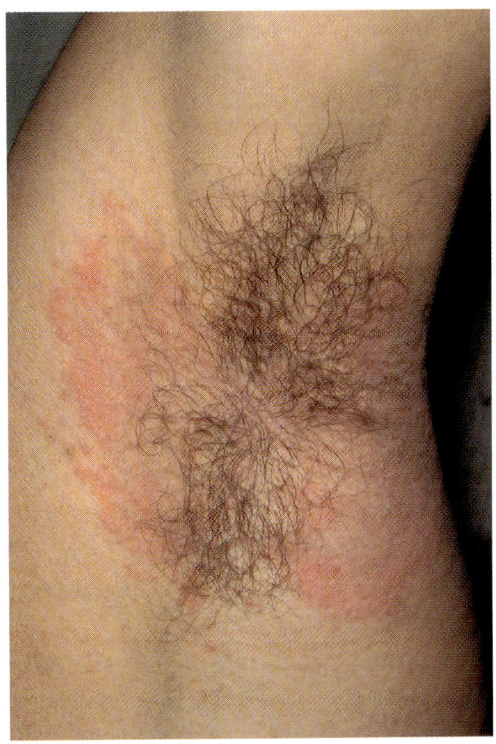

Fig. 6: Polycyclic patch, studded with minute papulopustules and intense erythema but no scale

Differential diagnosis:

- Irritant reaction.

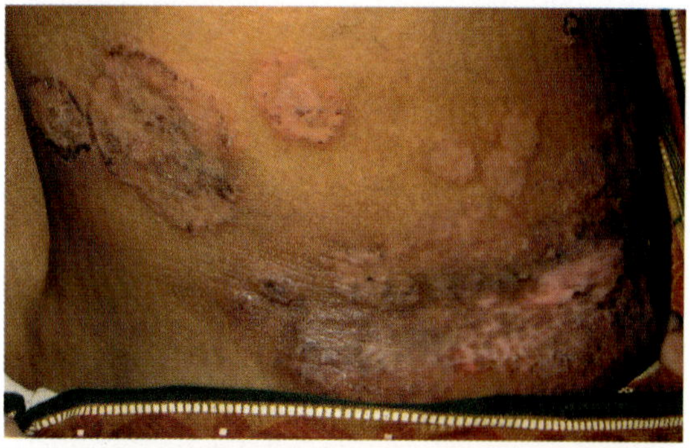

Fig. 7: Annular patches with prominent crusts at the border and few pustules

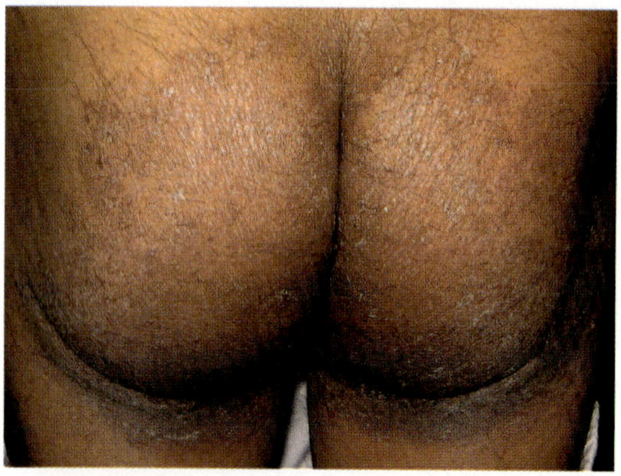

Fig. 8: Polycyclic patch involving both buttocks with mild scales and no central clearing

Differential diagnosis:

- Pityriasis versicolor.

Clinical features of tinea corporis

- It is variable from season to season, i.e., more aggressive in summer and rainy seasons but to some extent silent during winter season.
- Pruritus is the main symptom, but severity is variable.
- The early lesion usually presents as a sharply defined scaly plaque of 1-2 cm in size. It gradually enlarges towards the periphery with a relatively clear and flat center, and prominent or elevated margin. So, it takes an annular shape and for this, it is also commonly called as ring worm.
- Margin of the plaque contains either only scales or in combination with papules, papulovesicles, vesicles, pustules, crusts or excoriations. Color of the margin is often erythematous during hot and humid climate, but becomes less erythematous during winter season.
- Center of the lesion often contains scattered scales, papules, pustules or papulovesicles.
- Color of the lesion is variable from red to brown.
- Number of the lesion is variable from single to multiple and distributed asymmetrically.
- When lesions are multiple and individual lesion enlarges, nearby lesions often coalesce to form bizzare shaped polycyclic lesions.
- Though the starting shape of the lesion is annular, gradually it changes into oval, circinate or any uncharacteristic form.
- Though the initial size is 1-2 cm, but it is variable from few to several cm to involvement of the entire body. When > 90% body skin is involved it mimicks erythroderma.

Treatment

* Duration of treatment ranges from 2-4 weeks.
* Topical antifungals:
  - Miconazole, clotrimazole, ketoconazole
  - Terbinafine, amorolphine, ciclopirox olamine
  - Sertaconazole.
* Systemic antigungals
  - Terbinafine – 250 mg/day
  - Fluconazole – 150 mg/week
  - Itraconazole – 200 mg/day
  - Ketoconazole – 200 mg/day
  - Griseofulvine: Dose of micronized form is 15 mg/kg/day and maximum 500 mg/day and dose of ultramicronized form is 10 mg/kg/day. Taking of the drug with fatty meal helps in better absorption.

Tinea cruris (jock itch)

- It one of the very common superficial fungal infection, affecting the groin and upper thighs, occurring in adults and adolescents.
- Males are more affected than females and hot and humid climate favour development.
- It commonly occurs in obese person due to their moist groin and close apposition of lower abdomen and thighs as well as in vigorous outdoor workers wearing tight underwears.

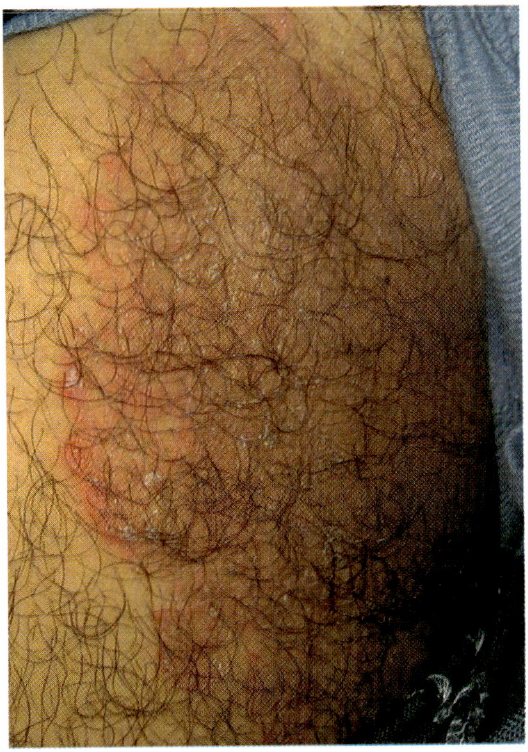

Fig. 9: Polycyclic patch with active and erythematous border, extending from the groin

Differential diagnosis

- Candidiasis: Presence of fissuring and satellite papulopustules.
- Seborrheic dermatitis: Prominent scales, aggravation in winter, absence of papules or pustules.
- Lichen simplex chronicus: Starting at the inner side of the thigh and extending to the groin, unilateral involvement, prominent thickening, pigmentation and increased skin markings, but minimum scaling, presence of satellite papules but absence of pustule, and no seasonal variation.
- Flexual psoriasis: Well defined flat scaly plaque with prominent erythema, extending from groin to intergluteal fold.

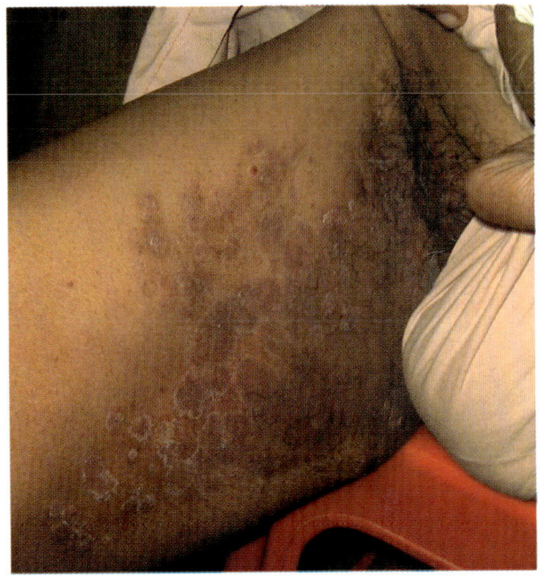

Fig. 10: Large irregular scaly patch with multiple satellite lesions

- Clinical features of tinea cruris are same as tinea corporis with following special features:
  - In chronic lesion, margin may not be prominent or well defined and center may not have any papule, papulovesicle or pustule, but it may be thickened and slight scaly, i.e., lichenified.
  - It usually affects bilaterally and symmetrically.
  - Lesions may extend to the buttocks and suprapubic area.
  - Scrotum and labia majora are usually spared. But they are commonly involved in candidiasis.
  - Tinea pedis is commonly associated with it.

Treatment

- It is same as tinea corporis.
- Prophylactic use of clotrimazole powder may be helpful.

Tinea capitis

* It is the most common dermatophytosis in childhood and commonest victims are children of age between 3-7 years.
* Boys are more affected than girls.
* Causative fungi affect the skin of the scalp, part of the hair shaft near the scalp and keratinized part of the hair follicle.

Types of tinea capitis

- Gray patch type
- Black dot type
- Kerion
- Favus

* Clinical features of gray patch type/small spored ectothrix tinea capitis:
  - Lesion starts as small circular or irregular patch with partial alopecia.
  - Few small patches may coalesce to form a larger patch.

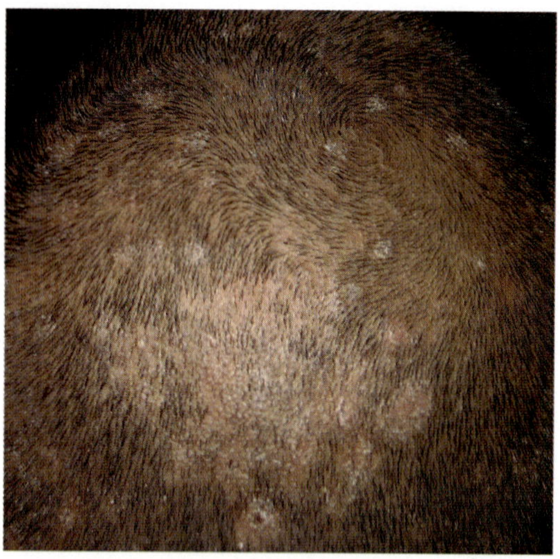

Fig. 11: Scaly patches of the scalp with prominent hair loss in gray patch tinea capitis

  - Hairs become brittle and breakage of the shafts occur at or slightly above the scalp.
  - Each patch contains numerous broken hairs which are dull gray in color due to coating with arthrospores.
  - Inflammatory response is minimum but scaling is prominent.
  - If lesions are many, they are distributed randomly.

Differential diagnosis:

- Seborrheic capitis
- Alopecia areata

* Clinical features of black dot tinea capitis/Endothrix tinea capitis:
  - Lesion starts as small circular or irregular patch with partial alopecia.
  - Initial patch tends to enlarge in a irregular fashion and to become poorly circumscribed.
  - Surface of the lesions contains lots of dots which are nothing but broken-off hairs at surface level of the scalp.
  - Folliculitis may be present in some cases.
  - Onychomycosis may be associated in 2-3% cases.
* Clinical features of kerion:
  - It is characterized by extremely painful boggy swelling in the form of nodule or plaque, studded with purulent discharge.
  - Pus discharges from multiple follicular openings.
  - Hair does not break-off but come out easily with minimum force and hair pull does not produce any pain.
  - Adjacent hairs within the lesion become matted due to thick crust.
  - Number of the lesion is usually single but it may be multiple and even may involve the entire scalp.
  - Lesion heals with scarring alopecia.
  - Regional lymphadenopathy is often associated.

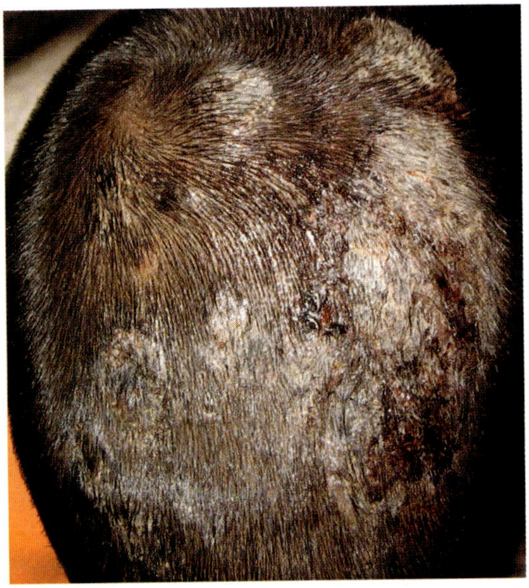

Fig. 12: Irregular plaques with scales and crusted ulcers

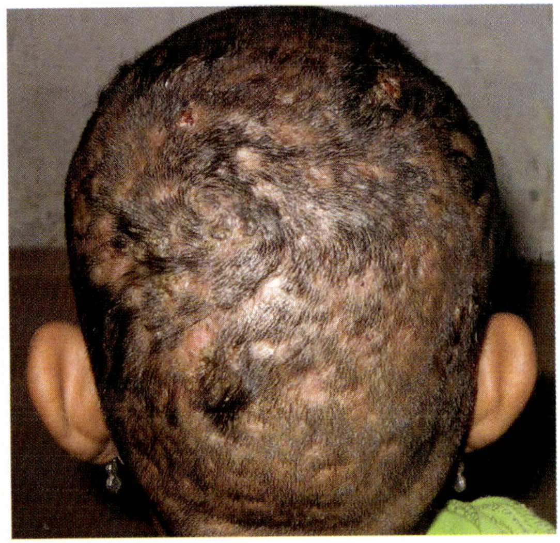

Fig. 13: Multiple depressed scar with few crusted ulcers of favus

Differential diagnosis:

- Infective eczematoid dermatitis
- Pyoderma
- Infected dermatitis

* Clinical features of favus:
  - Lesions start as perifollicular erythema and matting of hair, followed by development of thick yellow crusts which are cup-shaped, known as scutula.
  - Scutula is formed by skin debris and fungal hyphae and these are pierced by remaining hair shafts.
  - Lesion is characterized by foul smell.
  - At the end, scarring alopecia develops.
  - Lesions often mimick impetigo, ecthyma and crusted boils.

Differential diagnosis

- Secondary scarring alopecia due to pyoderma.
- Pseudopelade

Treatment of tinea capitis

* There in no role of topical antifungal.
* Duration of treatment is longer than tinea corporis and usually ranges from 4-8 weeks.
* Systemic drugs:
  - Griseofulvin is the drug of choice.
  - Terbinafine (5 mg/kg/day), itraconazole, ketoconazole, fluconazole (6 mg/kg/day) may be given.
* Adjunctive therapy:
  - Prednisone 1 mg/kg/day for two weeks in children with severe painful kerion.
  - Systemic antibiotics like erythromycin, dicloxacillin, amoxycillin-clavulanic acid may be given along with antifungal in case of kerion or favus.
  - Ketoconazloe/selenium sulfide shampoo is enough for close contacts or asymptomatic carriers.

Tinea faciei

* Morphology of the lesion is more or less like tinea corporis.
* It may affect cheeks, eyelids, eyebrows and forehead.
* History of photosensitivity is a special feature.
* Tinea barbae may be associated.

Differential diagnosis

- Seborrheic dermatitis

- Rosacea
- Perioral dermatitis
- Allergic contact dermatitis
- Granuloma multiforme
- Granuloma annulare
- Erythema annulare centrifugum.

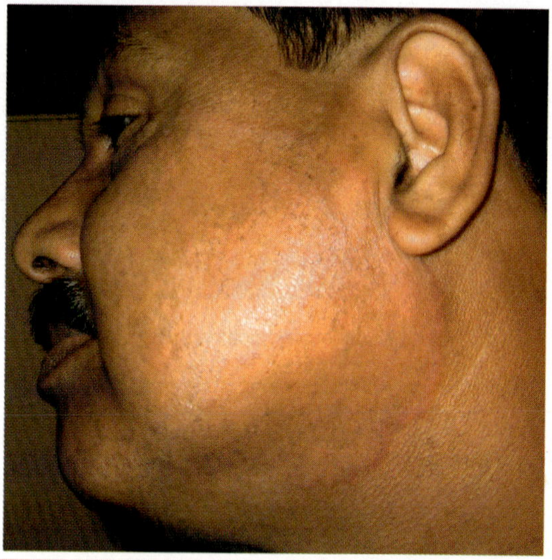

Fig. 14: Well defined mild scaly patch with very much active erythematous round border

Clinical features of tinea barbae

- Lesions start as erythematous follicular papules which gradually turn into pustules, and affect beared and mustache areas. Rarely eyelashes and eyebrows are affected.
- Amount of exudate and crusting depends on inflammation.
- Affected hairs become loose and easily pluckable.
- Affected follicles may coalesce to form erythematous plaque, studded with pustules.
- When this plaque becomes very much inflammed, it becomes boggy studded with purulent nodules as in kerion.

Tinea manuum

- It is characterized by well demarcated, hyperkeratotic and scaly patches with relative central clearing and fissuring, affecting the palms.
- Lesions often extend on the dorsal surfaces of the palms and may have follicular papules, nodules and pustules.
- Dyshidrotic form is characterized by vesicles and bullae on the palms and lateral sides of the fingers. But these are rarely seen at the margin of the lesion.
- Diffuse hyperkeratosis with pronounced involvement of creases is another presentation.
- Sometimes patient may present with patchy scaling of the dorsum of the hand and sides of the fingers.
- Unilateral involvement is seen in 50% cases and often associated with tinea pedis, tinea cruris or tinea unguium.

Differential diagnosis of tinea manuum

- Palmar psoriasis
- Dyshidrosiform dermatitis

Treatment

- It is more or less same as tinea corporis, but needs longer period.

Tinea pedis

- Infection is precipitated by hot and humid weather, excessive sweating and using of tight foot wear.
- Clinically it may be of following types:
  - Interdigital type
  - Moccasin type
  - Bullous type
  - Ulcerative type
- Interdigital type
  - It is characterized by erosive lesions which may be either dry and scaly or moist, macerated, scaly and fissured.
  - Space between the 4th and 5th toes is commonly affected.
- Moccasin type
  - Well demarcated fine scaly patches with or without minute papules on the margin affect heels, soles and lateral borders of the feet.
  - Bilateral involvement is common.

- Diffuse hyperkeratotic type of involvement also may occur.

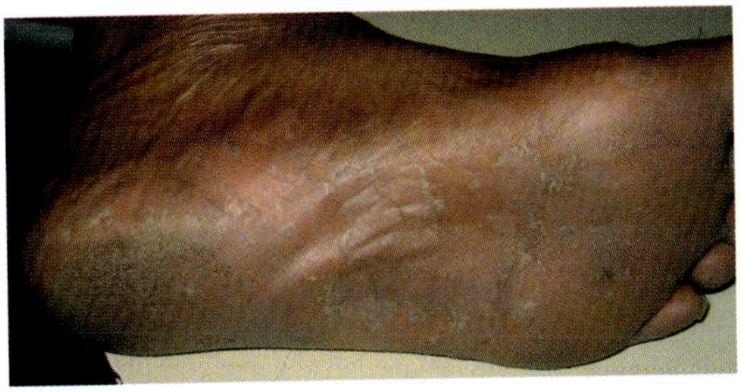

Fig. 15: Scaly patch with an erythematous background.

Differential diagnosis

- Hyperkeratotic dermatitis
- Plantar psoriasis

* Bullous type
  - Vesicles and bullae develop which rupture to form erosions with ragged ring like border.
  - Pustule may form due to secondary infection.
  - Insteps of the soles are commonly affected. It may be associated with id eruption.

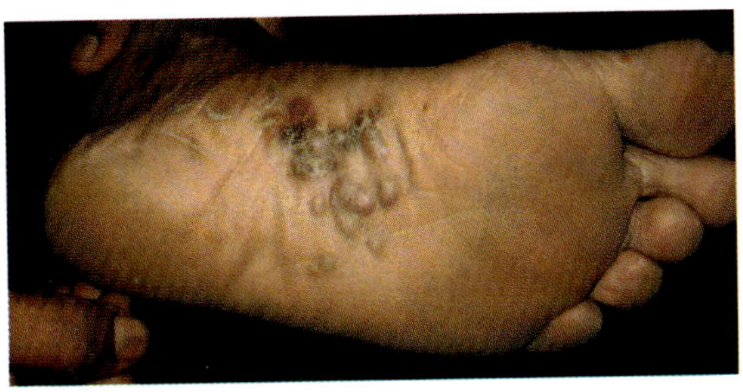

Fig. 16: Vesiculobullous lesions at sole

Differential diagnosis

- Pompholyx
- Dyshidrosiform dermatitis

* Ulcerative type

- Extension of the interdigital type into dorsal or plantar surface and complicated by secondary infection.

Treatment

- It is same as in tinea manuum.

Differential diagnosis of tinea pedis

- Soft corn and inverse plantar psoriasis for interdigital type.
- Pompholyx and pustular psoriasis for bullous or ulcerative form.
- Juvenile plantar dermatosis and dyshidrosiform dermatitis for moccasin type.

Tinea unguium/dermatophytic onychomycosis

* Males are commonly affected than females.
* Toe nails are commonly involved than finger nails.
* When toe nails are affected, tinea pedis is frequently associated.
* Single nail may be involved but often multiple nails of one or both sided finger or toe nails are involved.
* Subungual hyperkeratosis is developed when hyponychium is invaded, followed by development of discoloration and onycholysis.
* Eventually whole nail plate is affected to form total dystrophic pattern.
* Cellulitis may develop as a serious complication.
* According to the site of nail involvement it may be of following patterns.
  - Distal/lateral subungual
  - White superficial
  - Proximal subungual
  - Dystrophic.

Distal/lateral subungual

- It is the most common pattern, affecting the distal or lateral margin of the nail plate.

White superficial

- It is due to direct invasion into the superficial nail plate, usually caused by *Trichophyton mentagrophytes*.

Treatment

- Terbinafine 250 mg daily for 3-6 months for finger nails and 6-9 months for toe nails.
- Itraconazole 200 mg twice daily for 7 days in a month for 3-6 months.

Candidiasis

* Occlusive dressing and moist environment help the infection.

Types

- Intertriginous type/intertrigo
- Follicular type
- Nonfollicular nonintertriginous type

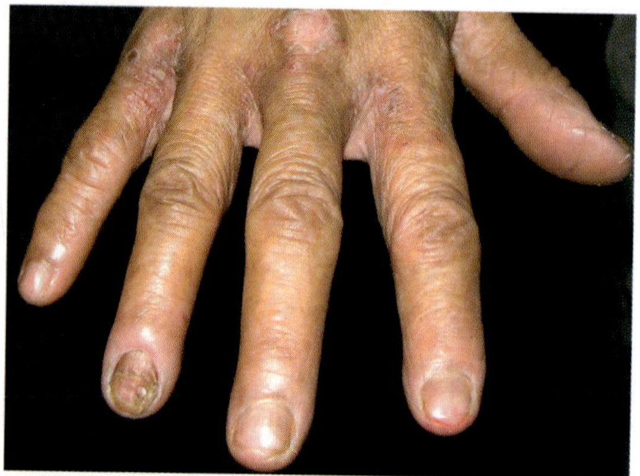

Fig. 17: Erosions at webs as well as at dorsum of the middle finger

Clinical features of candidal intertrigo

- It is characterized by erythematous, moist, erosion bordered with macerated epidermis appearing as collarette of scales.
- Common sites affected are webs of the fingers and toes, retroauricular folds, arm pits, groins, intergluteal regions, undersurface of large pendular breast, abdominal folds or neck folds and umbilicus.
- In the groin, it resembles tinea cruris but it is having less scale, more fissuring and tiny superficial pustules at adjacent area appearing as satellite lesions. It gradually becomes lichenified due to persistent pruritus.

Interdigital/erosion interdigitalis blastomycetica is a variant, characterized by erosion or fissuring, surrounded by thickened and white skin, affecting spaces between 3rd and 4th fingers or toes, often associated with onychomycosis or paronychia.

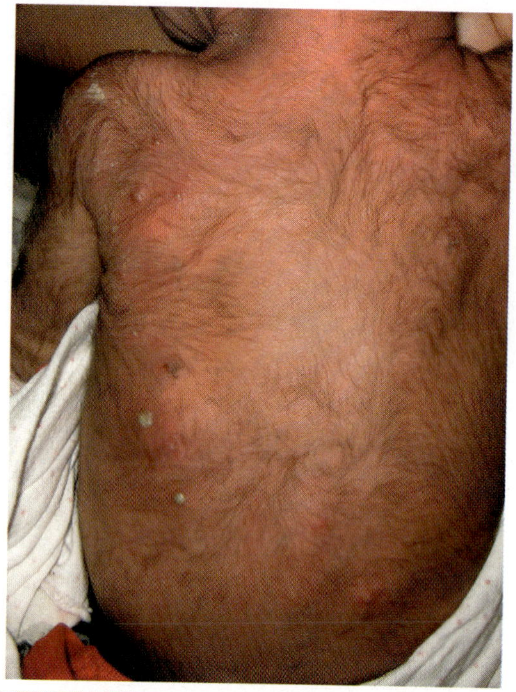

Fig. 18: Few papules and pustules of systemic candidiasis

Clinical features of follicular type

- Small, discrete pustules at openings of the follicles.

Clinical features of nonfollicular, nonintertriginous type

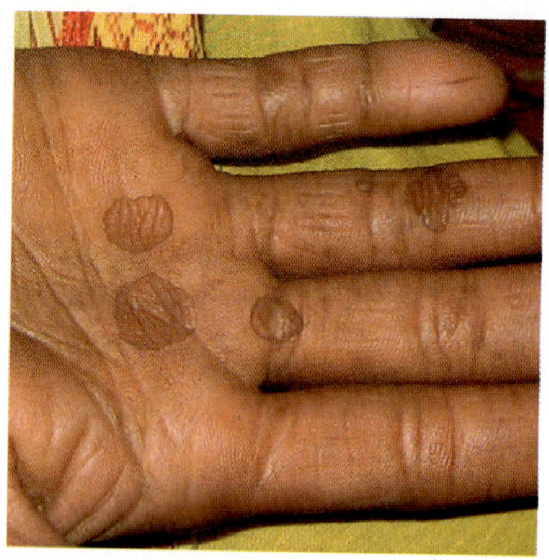

Fig. 19: Well defined erosion with dry floor

- Lesions start as macular erosions and gradually enlarge in size as well as they coalesce to form larger lesions.
- Lesions are having well defined margin and nonscaly dry floor when the palms and soles are involved.
- Though the lesions on the palms and soles donot have any scale or crust, lesions on the dorsa of the hands and feet usually have crusts like tinea corporis or circinate impetigo.
- Lesions of the palms and soles may extend upto the dorsal surfaces after involving the web spaces.
- Sometimes isolated erosions may develop on dorsal surfaces of fingers and toes or hand and feet.

Chronic paronychia

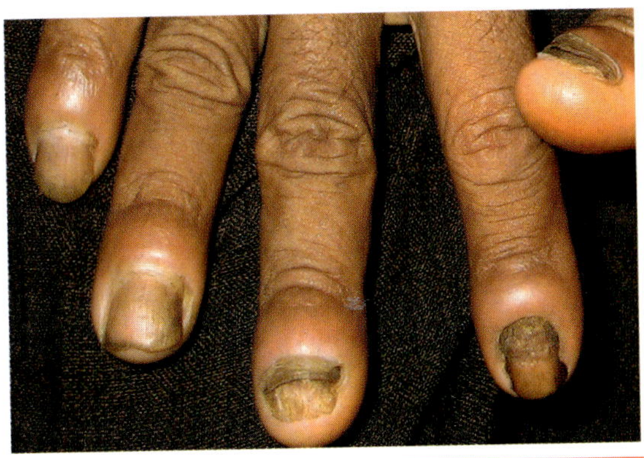

Fig. 20: Swollen proximal nail folds with onycholysis at middle finger and dystrophic proximal nail of index finger in chronic paronychia

- Paronychia is the inflammation of nail folds, caused by infections, allergic or irritant contact dermatitis and housewifes are commonly affected. It may be acute, chronic and acute in chronic. Frequent soaking of water is the predisposing factor.
- Acute paronychia is often caused by Gram-positive and Gram-negative organisms. It is characterized by sudden onset of extremely painful and tender erythematous swelling of the nail folds. After few hours pus is formed. Treatment includes incision and drainage and antibiotics.
- Chronic paronychia is often caused by candidal infection. But may be caused by dermatitis also. It is characterized by erythematous swelling with mild pain and tenderness. Cuticle remains intact when it is caused by candida. Cuticle becomes distorted when it is caused by dermatitis. Development of granuloma pyogenicum is a complication and frequently occurs at great toe nails. Treatment includes topical and systemic antifungals for 2-6 months when the cause is candida and topical and systemic corticosteriods when the cause is dermatitis.

Pityriasis versicolor/Tinea versicolor

- It is a chronic superficial epidermomycosis, caused by hyphal form of *Malassezia furfur*.
- These fungi are lipophilic and so, the disease commonly affects young adults in summer season when sebum production is highest.
- Hot and humid environment, hereditary factors, oily skin, application of oil, hyperhidrosis, glucocorticoid therapy and immunodeficiency favour the infection.
- In favourable condition, fungi converted from blastospore form to mycelial form following infection and produce dicarboxylic acid which inhibits tyrosinase enzyme and thus hypopigmentation develops. Hyperpigmentation is due to hyperkeratosis.
- 20% KOH mount shows combination of short and thin filamentous hyphae and spores. This is known as spaghetti and meatballs appearance.

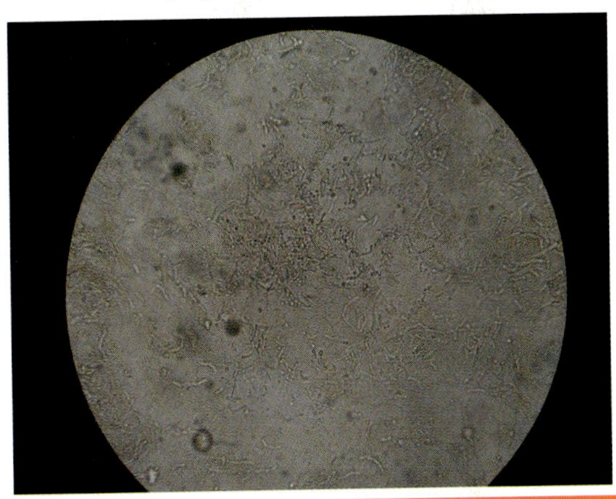

Fig. 21: Short septate hyphae with spores

- Wood's lamp examination elicits blue-green fluorescence of the scales.
- Infection may persist for years and hypopigmentation may persist for months even after successful treatment.

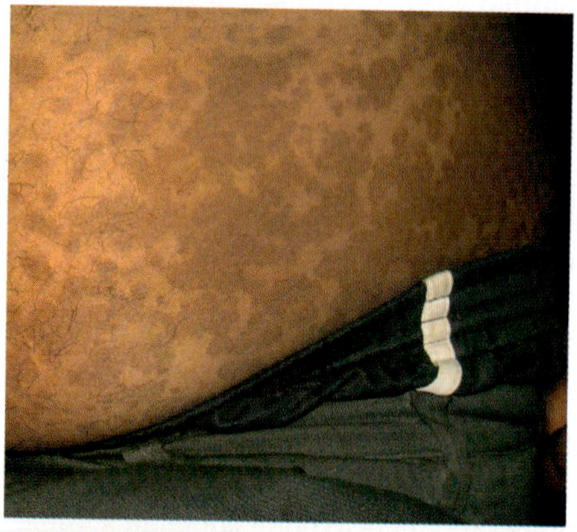

Fig. 22: Pigmented lesions

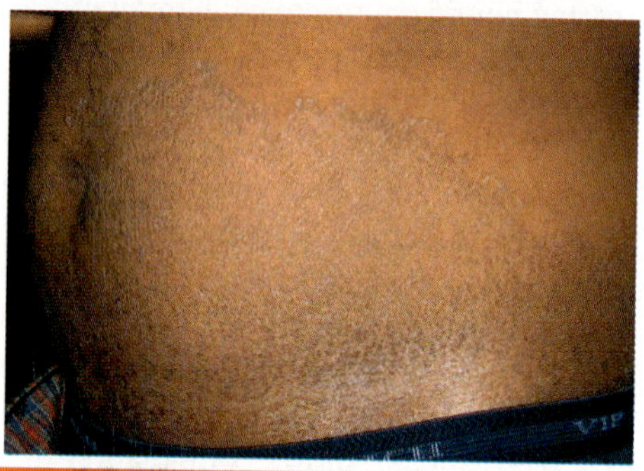

Fig. 23: Well defined hyperpigmented scaly patch, mimicking tinea corporis

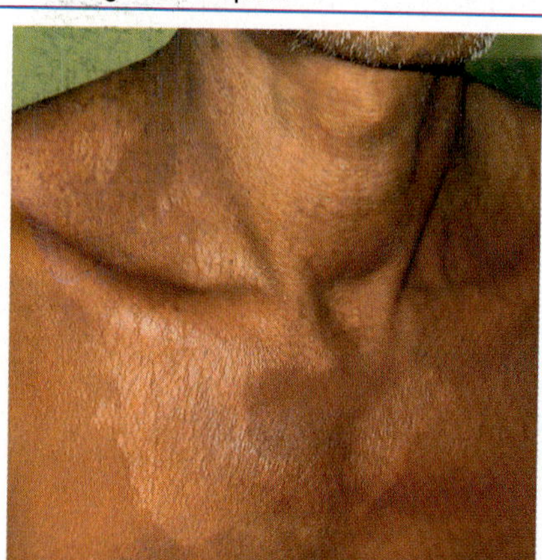

Fig. 24: Hypopigmented mild scaly geographic patch

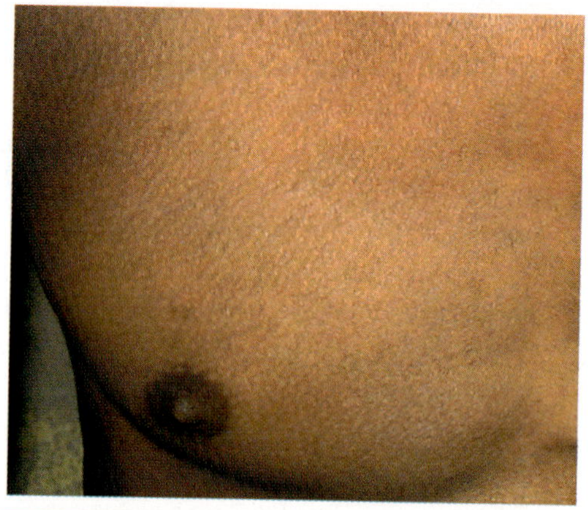

Fig. 25: Confluent scaly hypopigmented macules

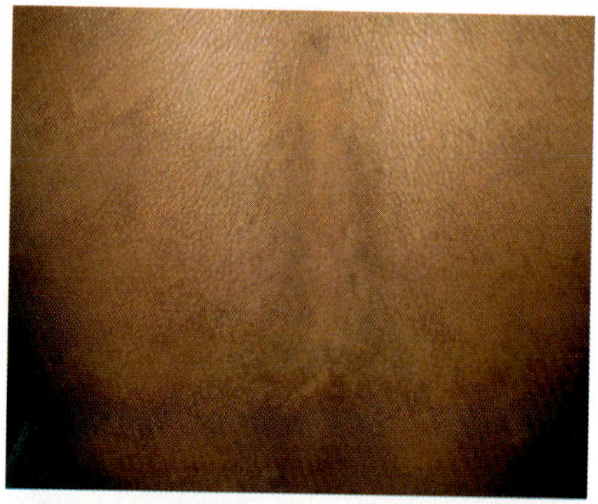

Fig. 26: Confluent scaly and hypopigmented follicular macules

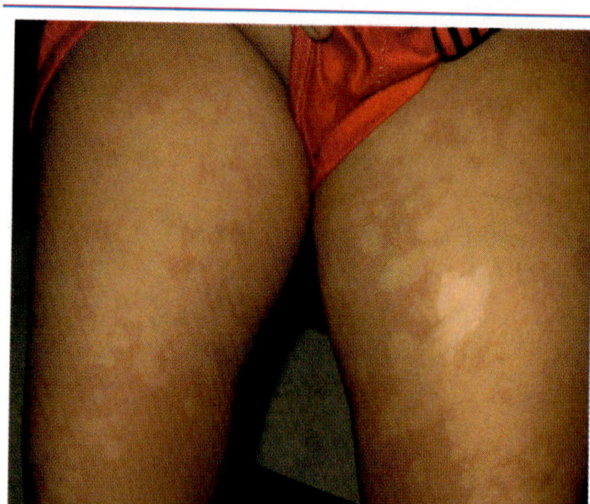

Fig. 27: Irregular hypopigmented patches with fine scales at both the thighs

Clinical features of pityriasis versicolor

- Primary lesions are macules and patches studded with fine scales. When scales are profuse, lesions may be mild elevated.
- Lesions start as well defined macules around the follicles and gradually coalesce to form patches of various shapes and sizes and often take a geographic shape. But sometimes lesions remain as discrete perifollicular macules.
- Scales are best appreciated by abrading with finger nail or edge of the glass slide or no.15 scalpel blade.
- Color of the lesion is variable from hypopigmentation to light brown to dark brown.
- Rarely color may be red. So far I have seen only one of such a case.
- Commonly involved sites are upper trunk, arms, neck, axillae, face, groins, thighs and external genitalia.

Treatment

- Selenium sulfide (2.5%) lotion, to be applied daily for 10-15 minutes for 7 days.
- Ketoconazole (1% or 2%) lotion, to be applied for 5 minutes daily for 7 days.
- Ketoconazole, econazole, miconazole, clotrimazole in cream forms, to be applied once daily for 2 weeks.
- Oral ketoconazole, itraconazole or fluconazole, any of these may be given 400 mg as single dose.
- Prophylactic therapy may be given with ketoconazole lotion once or twice in a week or oral fluconazole 400 mg once per month for one year.

Differential diagnosis of pityriasis versicolor

- Hypopigmented lesion
  - Vitiligo
  - Pityriasis alba
  - Seborrheic dermatitis
  - Postinflammatory hypopigmentation, specially pityriasis rosea.
  - Hypopigmented tuberculoid leprosy.
  - Post Kala-azar dermal leishmaniasis.
- Hyperpigmented lesion
  - Tinea corporis, specially in winter season.
  - Pityriasis rosea
  - Irritant contact dermatitis.

PARASITIC INFESTATIONS

CHAPTER C3

Scabies

* It is an intensely pruritic and highly contagious dermatosis, caused by mite, *Sarcoptes scabiei*.

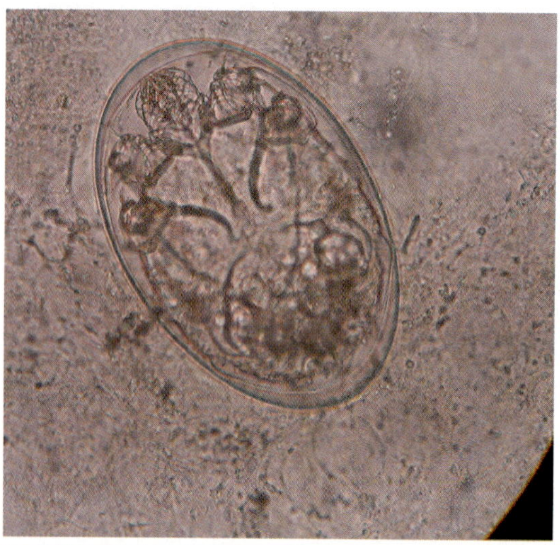

Fig. 1: Microscopic view of the larva of the mite

* In some population, it occurs in a cyclical pattern at every 15-20 years interval.
* Scabies should be suspected in any person having generalized pruritus or dermatitis or impetigo.

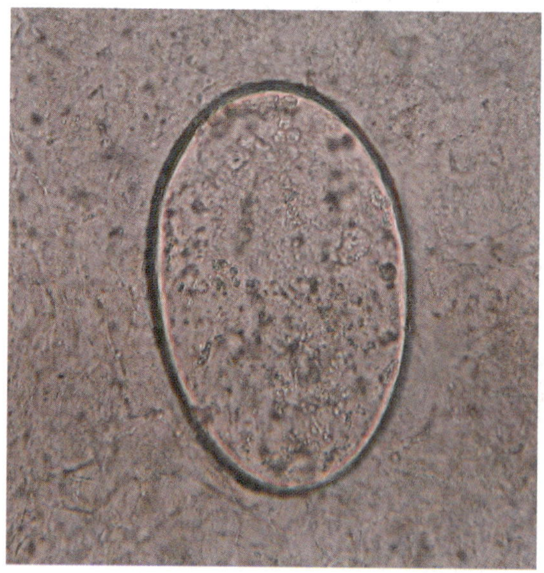

Fig. 2: Microscopic view of the egg of the mite

* Number of mite in a case of ordinary scabies is about 12-15, but in Norwegian or crusted scabies this may be more than a thousand.
* It occurs in all ages and sexes but commonly children are affected.

* Presence of immune suppression, specially due to long term systemic steroid, psychological problem leading to loss of insight, neurological or metabolic disorders, are predisposing factors to develop more severe form of scabies known as Norwegian or crusted scabies.
* It spreads from person to person through direct contact. But rarely transfer may occur from clothes and beddings, when they are contaminated from an infested person.
* Infestation occurs when a female mite burrows into the skin and lays eggs. After 2-3 days, larvae emerge and dig new burrow where they mature and female mites copulate to become pregnant. Thus the cycle goes on and each cycle takes about two weeks to be complete.
* Presence of itching among the close family members is almost a pathognomonic feature. But absence of such family history does not exclude scabies. It is a vivid experience that when we enquire about it, the answer is negative. Only repeated asking may find out the positive result.
* Pruritus is due to delayed hypersensitivity reaction to mites and their products.
* Pruritus is the hallmark of scabies which is aggravated at night, just after going to bed. This is due the immunological reaction to eggs and fecal materials of the mites as the eggs are laid at night when body temperature remains at higher level.

Clinical features

- Clinical manifestations start 2-6 weeks after initial infestation but reinfection manifests quickly even within 48 hours.
- Presenting lesions are papules, vesicle, papulovesicles, pustules and crusted erosions or ulceration.
- Nodular lesions are seen at penile and scrotal skin of the male and areolar or nipple skin of the females. This pruritic nodular lesion in male genitalia is almost pathognomonic.

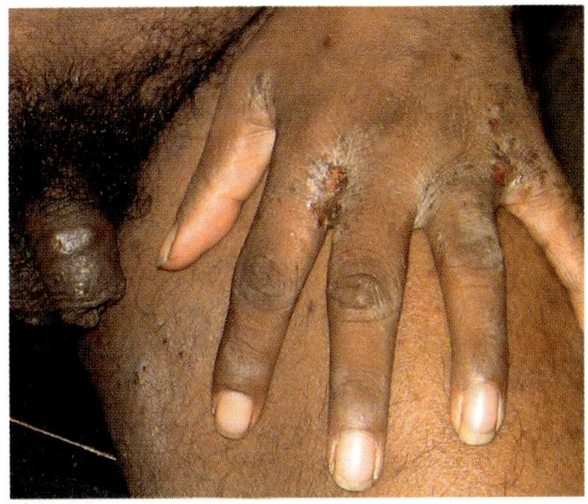

Fig. 3: Crusted papules and erosions at finger webs and at the shaft of the penis

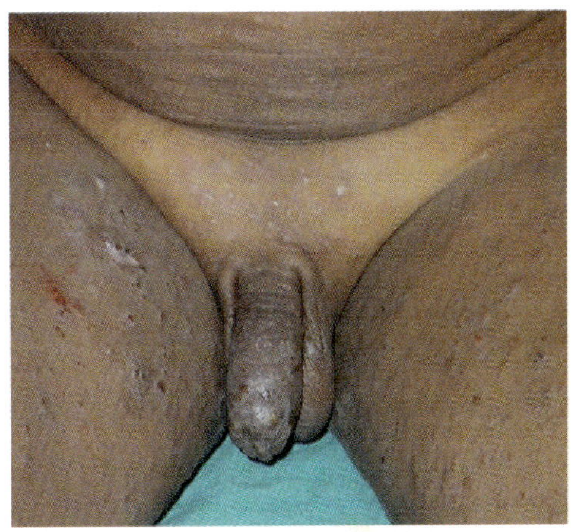

Fig. 4: Excoriated and crusted papules involving lower abdomen, inner sides of thighs and genitalia

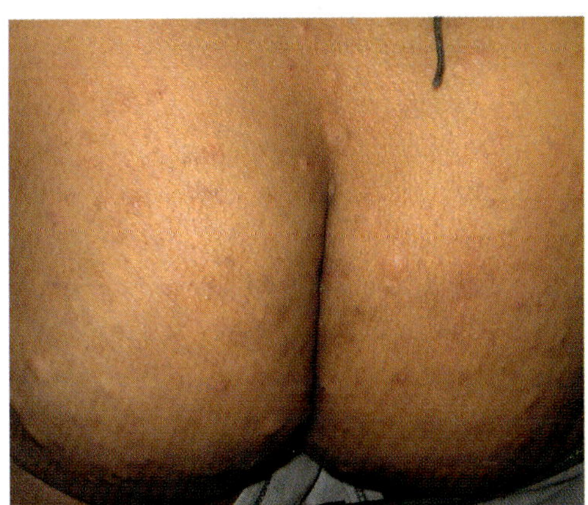

Fig. 5: Papular lesions at buttocks

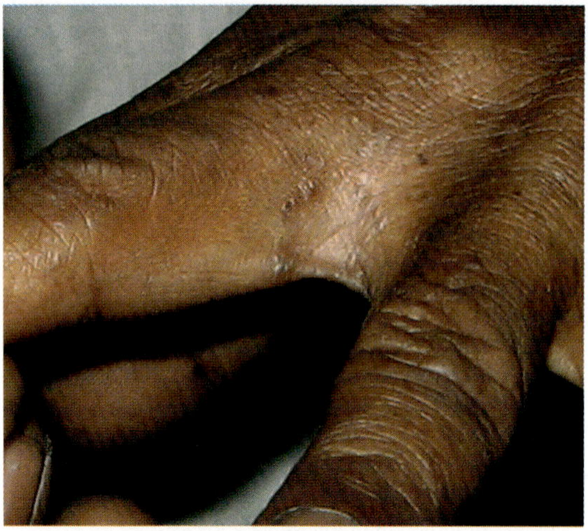

Fig. 6: A crusted linear lesion of burrow

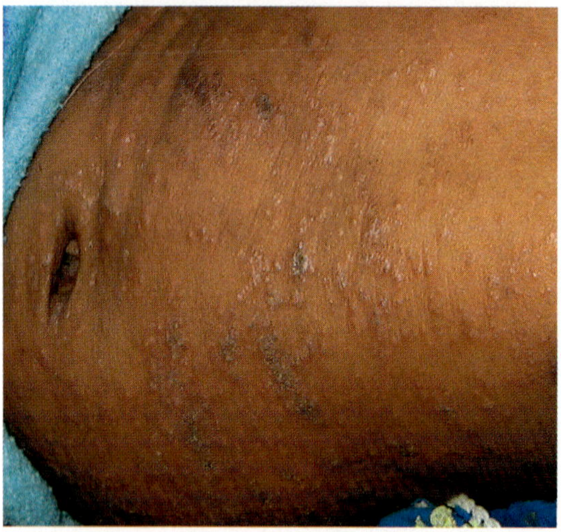

Fig. 7: Generalized dermatitis in scabies (scabid)

- Papules and vesicopustules are common in children and lesions often become generalized irrespective of any site of predilection.
- In very young babies who may not scratch but may have poor feeding, show characteristic pinkish-brown nodules at their trunks.
- Burrow is the pathognomonic sign of scabies. It is a short, wavy, scaly grayline on the skin surface. These are commonly seen at web spaces, thenar and hypothenar eminences, innerside of the wrist and penile skin. They are often missed due to vigorous scatching and secondary infection or eczematization.
- Development of dermatitis and pyoderma are very common.
- Dermatitis may be present prior to onset of scabies or may develop following scabies. But both of them complicate each other.
- Development of impetigo occurs mostly in children and produces pain.
- Common sites of involvement in both sexes and all ages, are web spaces of fingers and toes, innersides of the wrists, extensors of elbows and ankles, anterior axillary folds, periumbilical region and innerside of the thighs. Combination of all sites from neck to feet of both sides of the body make a circle which is known as Hebra's circle.
- Head and neck are not affected in adult probably due to presence of excess amount of sebum.
- Male genitalia and areolar skin of female breasts are commonly affected.
- Head, face, neck, palms and soles are also affected in neonates and infants.

Diagnosis of scabies

- History of itching at night or in the evening and affection of family members.
- Demonstration of mites by light microscopy from the sample, collecting by scraping the burrow or a papule or crusts in Norwegian scabies.

Norwegian or crusted scabies

* It occurs due to impaired immune response as associated with HIV infection or systemic steroid therapy, due to lack of pruritus or due to patient's physical inability to scratch.

Clinical features

- Pruritus may be absent but may be severe in some cases.
- It is one of the common cause of institutional outbreaks of scabies.

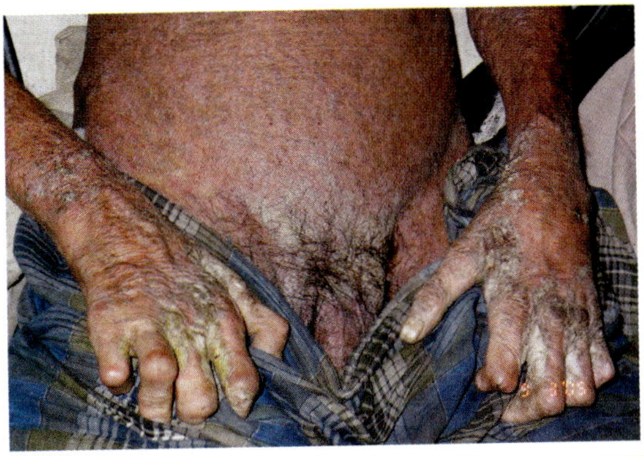

Fig. 8: Crusted lesions at suprapubic area and finger-webs in person having neurological deformities of both hands.
Differential diagnosis
- Hand dermatitis
- Psoriasis

- Clinically characterized by marked thickening and crusting of the skin, specially affecting hands, face and scalp.

Treatment of scabies

- Among the antiscabitic preparations, permethrin is drug of choice in many countries like UK, USA and Australia.
- It is applied at whole body, except head and neck in adults, once in a week for consecutive two weeks and patient should take bath after 12 hours of application.
- In children upto age of 2 years and immunocompromised adults, application should be extended to the scalp, neck, face and ears.
- Hand of infant should be covered to prevent sucking.
- Any alcoholic preparations should be avoided in children for their stinging sensation.
- Only one oral antiscabitic available is ivermectin, which is given at a dose of 200 μg/kg as a single dose for total two doses at 2 weeks interval. It is not recommended in children having body weight less than 15 kg.

Precautions for treatment of scabies

- Proper application antiscabitic preparations.
- Treatment of close family members.
- Cleaning of clothes and beddings at above 50°C.
- Taking of antipruritic drugs.
- Treatment of complications like pyoderma or dermatitis.
- Even after proper treatment itching may persists upto 6 weeks.
- Itching persisting more than 6 weeks demands retreatment.

Treatment failure in scabies

- May be due to reinfestation
- May due to sucking of the drug by the infants or washing of the drug by the adults.
- May be due to escaping treatment due to fear of harm by the drug in pregnancy.

Treatment of scabies in pregnancy

- Permethrin is the treatment of choice in pregnancy as very little amount is absorbed and detoxified readily without any retention in the body.

Differential diagnosis of scabies

* Papular urticaria
  - History of insect bite and exclusively occurring in young children.
  - Negative history of involvement of family members.
  - Classical distribution of the lesions at extensors of the limbs, and dorsa of the hands and feet.
  - Sparing of the web spaces and innerside of the wrists.
* Prurigo simplex
  - It is also an extremely pruritic dermatosis, occurring in adults, and having a history of insomnia, anxiety or depression.
  - Past history of papular urticaria and hypersensitivity to insect bite may be present.
  - Classical distribution of the lesions mostly at extensors of upper limbs and other easily approachable areas.
  - When new bites occur, old lesions reappear.

Pediculosis/Louse infestation

* It is caused by three obligate ectoparasites
  - *Pediculus humanus capitis* (head louse), causing pediculosis capitis
  - *Pediculus humanus humanus* (body louse), causing pediculosis corporis.
  - *Pthirus pubis (crab louse)*, causing pediculosis pubis.
* Louse are wingless, six legged insect and 1-2 mm in length with translucent gray white color.
* Transmission occurs commonly by direct contact from person to person or indirectly by contact with infested bedding, clothing or comb.
* Head louse does not act as vector for any other infective disease.

Pediculosis capitis

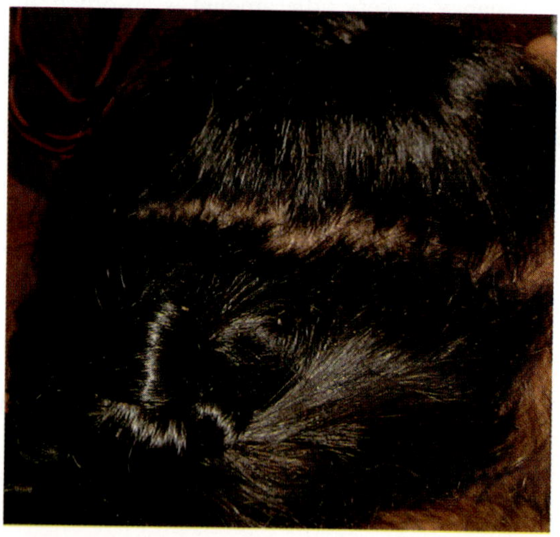

Fig. 9: Lots of nits at scalp hair

* It commonly occurs in girls of 4-12 years of age. But may occur at any age and in any sex.
* Most of the sufferers have only < 10 lice at their scalp and they like to live at occipital and postauricular region. Rarely headlice infest beard or other hairy areas.
* Nits within 4-5 mm of scalp is suggestive of active infestation.
* When eyelashes are infested with headlice, it is called pediculosis palpebrarum.
* Nits are nothing but the minute (1 mm) oval grayish egg-capsules, firmly cemented to the hair shafts and lie near the scalp and go away along the growth of the hair. Their number is variable from few to thousands.
* Viable eggs are creamy yellow in color.
* Lice, nits or eggs are readily detectable by naked eye but better visible with hand lens.
* Wood's lamp examination shows pearly fluorescence from the live eggs but not from the nits.

Clinical features of pediculosis capitis

- Pruritus presents at the back and sides of the scalp.
- Bite reactions may present at the nape of the neck as wheals, papules, excoriations, acute subacute and chronic dermatitis.
- Excoriations following scratching often produce secondary pyoderma with occipital and cervical lymphadenopathy.
- In severe cases, a purulent mass of matted hair develops with crusts and exudates.
- Pediculid is a form of hypersensitivity reaction, presented with viral exanthem like rashes.

Treatment

- Avoidance of contact with infested person or infested materials.
- Application of permethrin (1%) for only 10 minutes and to be repeated within 7-14 days.
- Application of malathion (0.5%) for 8-12 hours.
- Application of gammabenzene hexachloride (1%) for 4 minutes and to be repeated within 7-14 days. It is not indicated in pregnant and lactating women.
- Oral ivermectin 200μg/kg may be given as single dose and to be repeated on 10th day.

* Differential diagnosis
  - Seborrheic capitis.

Pediculosis corporis

* The louse is larger than head louse, about 2-4 mm in size and lives in seams of clothings and grab the body hair to feed.
* Lice and nits are seen in cloth seams.
* It occurs in poor socioeconomic condition when regular cleaning of the clothes is not done.
* Body lice transmit many infectious diseases during their feeding.
    - *Bartonella quintana*, causing trench fever.
    - *Rickettsia prowazekii*, causing epidemic typhus and Brill-Zinsser disease/louse-borne relapsing fever.

Clinical features

- Excoriated and crusted papules present which may be complicated with secondary pyoderma and eczematization.
- When lesions heal postinflammatory hypo/ hyperpigmented scars.
- Clothing may be stained with blood.

Treatment

- Cleaning of the body, bedding and clothing.
- Rarely permethrin/malathion is required to apply for 8-24 hours.

Differential diagnosis

- Scabies
- Pulicosis, caused by flea Pulex irritans.

Pediculosis pubis/Pthiriasis

* It commonly occurs in young adults and more extensively in males.
* It occurs at areas having coarse hairs, specially pubic, thighs, axillae, chest and upper eyelashes.
* The louse likes humid environment and is having less tendency to wander. It appears as 1-2 mm brownish-gray specks, grasping a hair at both sides with its claws.
* Transmission occurs through close contact, specially sexual contact and sharing of clothes/bed.

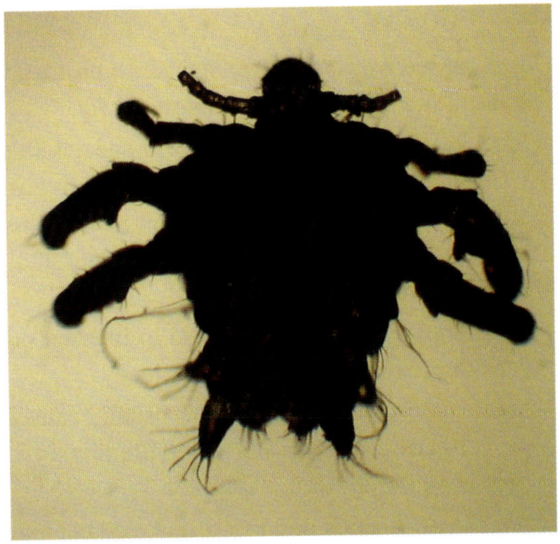

Fig. 10: Microscopic view of *Pthirus pubis*

Clinical features

- Varying amount of pruritus is the symptom.
- Feeling of nodularity at the root of the hair during scratching and patients are able to pick up the lice immediately.
- Excoriation, secondary pyoderma and regional lymphadenopathy may develop.
- Papular urticaria like lesions develop at the sites of feeding.
- Maculae ceruleae (taches bleuatres) are bluish gray or slate gray macules, 0.5-1 cm in diameter, irregular and nonblanching. Pigmentation is probably due to breakdown of heme by the louse saliva.
- When eyelashes involved, serous crusts may be formed along with the lice and nits.

Treatment

- Application of permethrin (1%) for 10 minutes or gamma benzene hexachloride (1%) for 5 minutes only. It may be repeated after 7-10 days.
- For eyelashes involvement, permethrin (1%) for 10 minutes or thick application of any harmless eye ointment or vaseline may be helpful.
- Sexual partner must be treated.

Leishmaniasis

* It is caused by *Leishmania* species, a protozoa, transmitted to human by female sand fly.
* Skin lesions caused by Old world species like L.tropica and L.major are either exudative or crusted and lesions caused by new world species like L.mexicana, are multiple chronic small ulcers or single large ulcer.
* Cutaneous infection may spread to internal organs in presence of immunodeficiency.
* Mucocutaneous leishmaniasis is usually caused by L.brasiliensis. Visceral leishmaniasis is caused by L.donovani.
* Average incubation period is 2-4 weeks; but may be months to years.
* PKDL occurs in 20% cases of Indian visceral leishmaniasis. But in some cases history of kala-azar may not be present.
* Leishmanin test is negative in Indian PKDL; but positive in African PKDL.

Variants

- Leishmaniasis recidivans
- Disseminated cutaneous leishmaniasis.
- Post-kala-azar dermal leishmaniasis (PKDL).

Types

- Visceral leishmaniasis (Kala-azar)
- Mucocutaneous leishmaniasis
- Cutaneous leishmaniasis

Clinical features of cutaneous leishmaniasis

- Lesions start as small red papules or nodules with or without pain and pruritus.
- They gradually ulcerate with heaped up margin and granulomatous floor.
- They usually heal spontaneously with atrophic scars.
- Leishmaniasis recidivans is characterized by serpiginous lupoid nodules with granulomatous papules at the margin and central healing, and has a chronic course.
- Disseminated cutaneous leishmaniasis is characterized by widespread nodular lesions mimicking lepromatous leprosy.
- Mucocutaneous leishmaniasis is characterized by presence of single or multiple painful papules and nodules at mucocutaneous junctions of nose and mouth. Gradually lesions increase in size as well as coalesce and affect the mucosal surfaces as ulcerative growth. Central facial destruction is the last episode. This form must be differentiated from midline granuloma, histoplasmosis, paracoccoidiomycosis, rhinosporodiosis and neoplasm.

Clinical features of PKDL

- Primary lesions are hypopigmented macules or patches, mostly affecting the trunk and face.
- Few or multiple infiltrated papules and plaques are present at cheeks, chin, ears, buttocks, limbs and even genitalia.

Clinical features of disseminated visceral leishmaniasis

- Fever, cachexia, hepatosplenomegaly, pancytopenia and features of hypergamma globulinemia.
- Brown to gray discoloration of the skin.

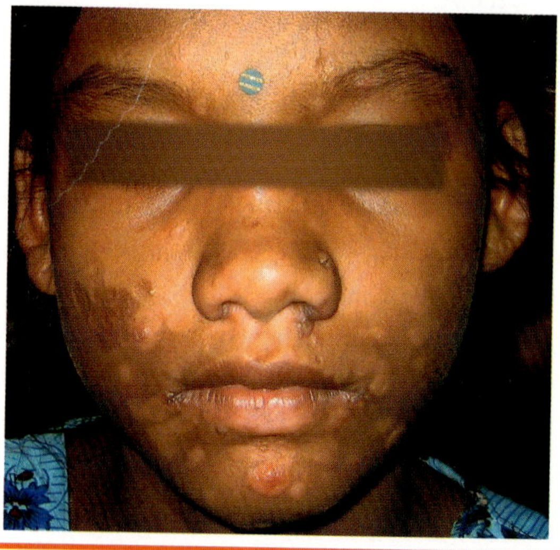

Fig. 11: Hypopigmented patches with infiltrated papules and nodules

- Development of macules, papules, plaques, nodules and ulcers.
- Some cases present like psoriasis, dermatomyositis or erythroderma.

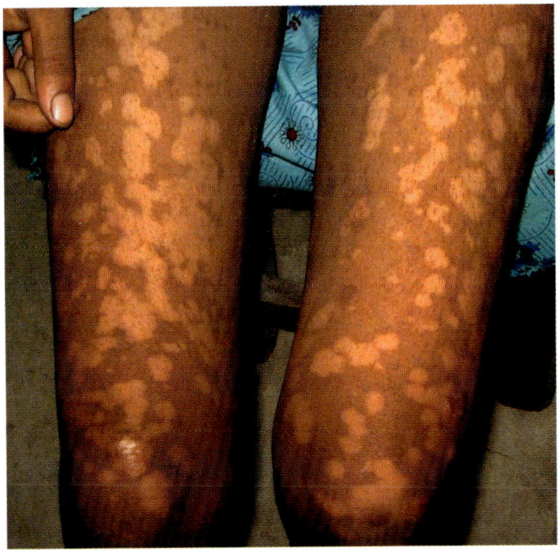

Fig. 12: Multiple well defined hypopigmented macules and patches

Diagnosis

- Direct demonstration 1-5 μm intracellular LD bodies within the macrophages in tissue smear or in histopathology. Useful stains are Giemsa, hematoxylin and eosin, or Brown-Hopps stains.
- Culture in Novy-McNeal-Nicole media.
- Antibody detection.
- Antigen detection by PCR.
- Estimation of serum IL_{10}.

Treatment

* Topical therapy for localized lesions:
  - Intralesional stibogluconate, given 1-2 weeks interval for 2-4 times. It is diluted with local anesthesia as 1:3 dilution.
  - Cryotherapy or surgical excision.
  - Topical paromomycin (15%) twice daily.
* Systemic therapy for leishmaniasis recidivans type, disseminated type and PKDL.
  - Pentavalent antimonial, 20 mg/kg/day for 3-4 weeks or more for PKDL.
  - Liposomal amphotericin B.
  - Miltefosine.
  - Sitamiquine.
  - Paromomycin.
  - Pentamidine.

CHAPTER C4

VIRAL INFECTIONS

Molluscum contagiosum (MC)

* It is a contagious and common cutaneous viral infection, caused by *Molluscum contagiosum virus* (MCV), a DNA virus under Molluscipox genus. The virus has 4 major viral types: MCV1, MCV1a, MCV2 and MCV3.
* The infection spreads by direct skin to skin contact, through fomites or by autoinoculation.
* Incubation period is 2-8 weeks.
* It can affect any age but mostly affects young children, sexually active adults or immunocompromised persons.
* A disseminated form in HIV infected person indicates an advanced immunodeficiency state.
* The natural course of the disease is spontaneous clearance within 2-4 years from the onset. But immunocompromised patients never achieve enough immunity to be cleared spontaneously.

Clinical features of molluscum contagiosum

- Lesions appear as a small 1-2 mm pearly white or flesh colored and umbilicated papules. But umbilication may not be apparent at an early stage.
- Number of the lesions is variable from 11-20 to hundreds. Any site may be affected, specially face and trunk.
- Secondary bacterial infection produces purulent discharge, erythema and crusting or an infective eczematoid dermatitis.
- Rarely the lesion may be larger or giant size, specially in AIDS.

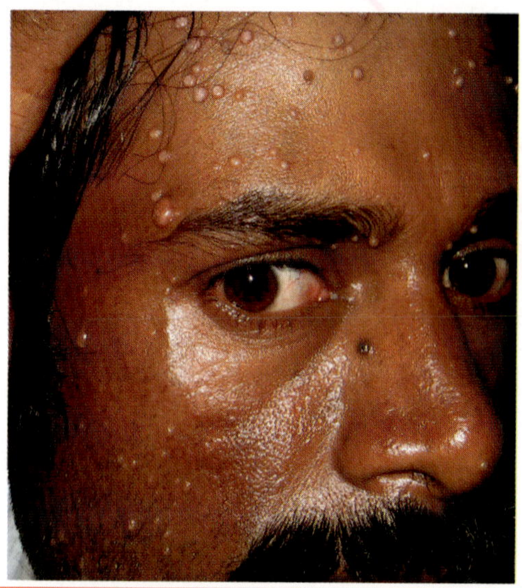

Fig. 1: Multiple papules with whitish centers in an adult

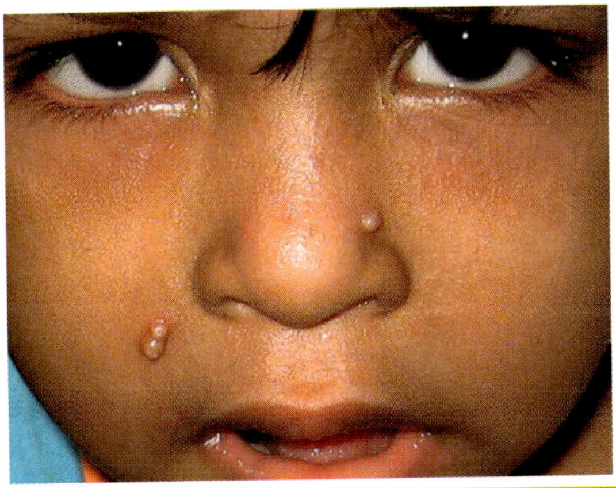

Fig. 2: Whitish umbilicated papules in a child

Differential diagnosis

- Milia
- Sebaceous hyperplasia
- Comedone

Histopathology

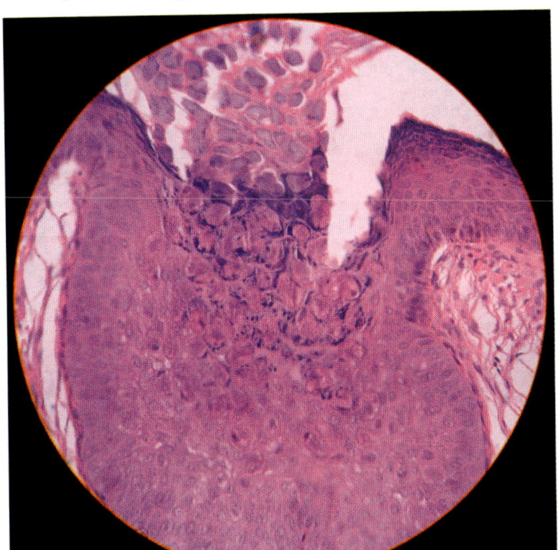

Fig. 3: Bluish to eosinophic mollucum bodies, embedded within keratinocytes

- Epidermal hyperplasia at the periphery and atrophy at the center.
- Many keratinocytes contain intracytoplasmic inclusion bodies, known as molluscum bodies.
- These bodies first appear at the lower part of the spinous layer. One to two cell layers above the basal layer their color is eosinophilic.
- When these invaded keratinocytes go up, molluscum bodies increase in size and the nuclei of the keratinocytes get compressed to become thin crescent and lie at the periphery of the cell.
- When they reach at the level of the granular layer, staining reaction is changed from eosinophilic to basophilic.
- At the corneal layer the size of molluscum body becomes 35 μm in diameter. These bodies are known as Henderson-Paterson bodies.
- Little or no dermal reaction is seen except when the lesion ruptures and content is discharged into dermis.
- Electron microscopy shows that molluscum body contains large number of molluscum viruses embedded in a protein matrix.

Treatment

- No treatment is essential for periocular site as individual lesion tends to persist for few weeks only.
- Avoid sharing of towel/bath tub to prevent spread.
- Presence of dermatitis or infection is to be treated prior to treatment proper.
- Following modalities are useful:
  - Application of 10% KOH solution, silver nitrate solution, cidofovir (3%) for recalcitrant cases as in HIV.
  - Extirpation and cryosurgery.

Varicella–Zoster virus (VZV)/HHV-3 infection

- This viral infection causes following two different diseases:
  - Varicella (Chicken pox)
  - Herpes zoster
- Varicella occurs through inhalation of the droplets, containg the organisms or by direct contact with vesicular fluid, containing the organisms.

* The disease starts to develop after an incubation period of 11-20 days. But herpes zoster occurs after an uncertain period of primary episode of varicella, due to reactivation of VZV. But in 20% cases, there may not be any past history of chicken pox. In such cases, a family history of chicken pox may be present.
* Varicella may develop following direct contact with vesicular fluid of herpes zoster but herpes zoster does not develop from contact with herpes zoster.
* An attack of chicken pox does not confer lifetime immunity but very unusual to have two or three episodes in whole life.
* Histopathology of vesicular lesion of varicella or herpes zoster shows ballooning degeneration of the epidermis with intraepidermal cleft formation. Cleft often contains multinucleated keratnocytes or Tzanck cell.
* Tzanck test also demonstrates multinucleated keratinocytes.

Varicella/Chicken pox

* It is a self-limiting disease with a good prognosis. Development of pock-like scars is the commonest cosmetic problem after the recovery.
* Infectivity of the disease starts 5 days before the rash and 7 days after the rash or till the lesions become crusted.

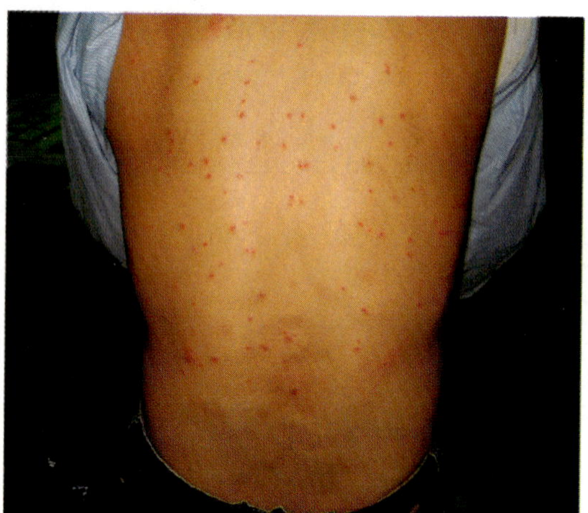

Fig. 4: Multiple erythematous papulovesicles

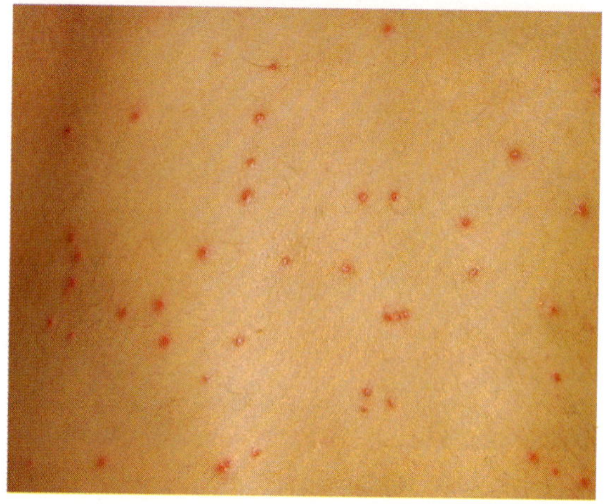

Fig. 5: Multiple erythematous papulovesicles

Characteristic features of chicken pox

- It starts with a prodromal symptoms like mild fever, malaise, myalgia, sore throat, etc., followed by mild pruritic maculopapular skin rash.
- After 12-14 hours, these papular lesions evolve into vesicles which are 1-3 mm in size and at the same time new lesions continue to appear.
- So, the initial lesions contain clear fluid with persisting perilesional reddish hallow, appearing as a dew drop on rose petal. But sometimes vesicles may contain hemorrhagic fluid, specially in presence of immunosupression. Gradually vesicles are turned into pustules and they collapse at their centers to become crusted.
- Lesions spread from face, scalp and trunk to extremities. Number of the lesion is variable from few to hundreds.
- As new lesions continue to appear, lesions are seen at various stages of evolution and for this, lesions are described as pleomorphic.
- An uneventful healing occurs by two weeks and results in depressed or hypertrophic scars.
- Secondary bacterial infection is the commonest cause of scar formation.

- Other rare complications are pneumonia, myocarditis, hepatitis, vasculitis, keratitis, encephalitis, etc.
- When it occurs at 1st or 2nd trimester of pregnancy, fetus may suffer from congenital varicella syndrome, resulting in birth defect and fetal death. When it occurs 5 days before or 2 days after the delivery, baby may suffer from severe form of chicken pox.

Herpes zoster

- This is also a self-limiting disorder with commonest complication of post herpetic neuralgia.
- Following an attack of chicken pox, varicella-zoster virus remain dormant within dorsal root ganglia and due to an unknown mechanism, they become activated resulting in herpes zoster.
- Virus reactivation occurs once in a lifetime but second attack may occur in less than 5% cases.
- Pain in zoster or zoster associated pain (ZAP) is due to injury of the peripheral nerves and altered central nervous system signal processing.
- Neural changes:
  - Lower activation threshold
  - Exaggerated response to stimuli
  - Spontaneous discharge from the peripheral neurons.
  - Axonal regrowth producing nerve sprouts is also responsible for unprovoked discharge.

Factors helping in reactivation

- Increase incidence with age as T cell immunity gradually decreases.
- Immunosuppressive drug therapy.
- Zoster may be the earliest clinical sign of AIDS.
- Lymphoma.
- Radiation therapy.
- Fatigue.
- Emotional upset.

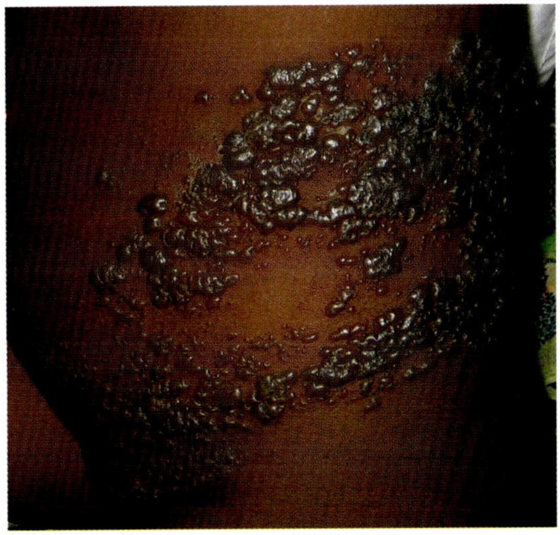

Fig. 6: Grouped vesiculo-bullous lesions along left sided T11 dermatome

Characteristic features of herpes zoster

- Patient starts to feel pain or burning sensation or sometimes itching at particular dermatomal segment of the skin.
- Constitutional features like fever, malaise, headache, etc. may be associated which are usually absent in children.
- After 4-5 days, suddenly a group of fluid filled skin lesions with reddish background appear.
- Earliest lesions are erythematous papules which rapidly turn into vesicles.
- But rarely skin eruptions do not appear following pain which is called "zoster sine herpete" i.e., zoster without rash.
- Sometime skin eruptions develop without any symptom.
- Within another 3-4 days vesicles become cloudy and successive crops of lesions continue to appear for few days. Initial vesicles appear in group or herpetiform pattern, latter when number of lesions increase, they become diffuse and lose their herpetiform pattern.
- Subsequently, centers of the lesions collapse to become umbilicated or rupture to become crusted erosions or ulcers.

- Crusts usually fall off within 2-3 weeks and lesions heal by scar formation.
- Lesions are distributed unilaterally and along a dermatome. But rarely may be bilateral and occasionally few vesicles may appear across the midline.
- Usually 1-3 adjacent dermatomes may be affected.
- In elderly or debilitated person lesions may become more reddish, oozy, ulcerated, hemorrhagic, necrotic, infected with pyogenic bacteria, followed by extensive scarring. Later these scars normalize, may become hypertrophic or may turn into keloid.
- In 50% cases of uncomplicated herpes zoster, a viremia develops with upto 20 vesicles, scattered outside the affected dermatome. But when these scattered lesions are more than 20, it is known as disseminated zoster.
- Regional lymphadenopathy may be present.
- Ophthalmic zoster: It involves any branch of the ophthalmic division of the trigeminal nerve. The branches are frontal, lacrimal and nasociliary nerves. It occurs in 10-15% of all zoster cases and involvement of ophthalmic division is 5 times more common than mandibular or maxillary division.
- Post-herpetic neuralgia: It occurs following healing of the lesions and may persist for weeks, months or even years. Incidence increases with age as 80% cases occur above 80 years of age.
- Hutchinson sign: It is the presence of vesicle at the tip or sides of the nose due to involvement of nasociliary nerve.
- Ramsay-Hunt syndrome: It occurs following reactivation of VZV of the geniculate ganglion.

* Features of Ramsay Hunt syndrome
  - Vesicles at ear canal, tongue, and hard palate.
  - Pain at the ear, loss of taste sensation at the anterior two-thirds of the tongue with dry mouth and tongue.
  - Acute facial nerve paralysis.
* Other systemic complications are retention of urine and stool, motor paresis, encephalitis, etc.

Differential diagnosis

- Acute irritant contact dermatitis
- Zosteriform herpes simplex.

Herpes simplex virus infection

* It is a common infective dermatosis, caused by Herpes simplex virus 1 & 2.
* Nongenital infection is commonly caused by HSV1.
* It is often associated with immune suppression.
* Herpetic infection at perioral region is commonly associated with HSV1.
* Herpetic whitlow is the severe painful paronychia and digital infection mimicking cellulitis.

Clinical features of herpes simplex virus infection

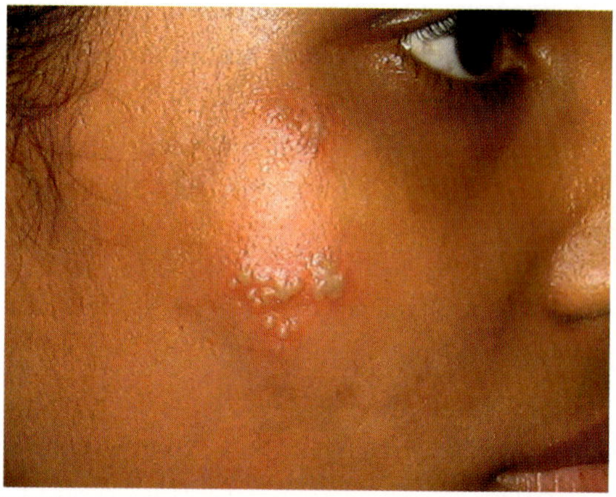

Fig. 7: Grouped vesicles with erythematous background

- Primary lesions are erythematous papulovesicles which quickly turn into vesicles and then pustules. Within hours to day these lesions collapse at their center to become umbilicated and ultimately become necrotic.

- Lesions are arranged in groups; but rarely have a dermatomal pattern like zoster.

Histopathology

- Ballooning degeneration followed by reticular degeneration of the epidermis.
- Vascular dilatation and perivascular infiltration and damage of the superficial vessels.

Common Wart/verruca vulgaris

- This is primarily an asymptomatic cutaneous infection of human papilloma virus (HPV).
- Various serotypes affect various sites of the body as well as morphology of the lesions also vary according to infective serotypes.

Disease pattern and serotypes

- Verruca vulgaris: 1, 2, 4, 7, 49
- Verruca plana: 3, 10, 28, 49
- Palmoplantar wart: 1, 2, 3, 4, 27, 29, 57
- Butcher's wart: 7
- Giant condyloma acuminata of Buschke and Lowenstein: 6

- It is often self limited as in 60% cases lesions disappear within 2 years.
- It affects all ages and sexes.

Characteristic features of wart

- Lesion starts as hyperkeratotic papule with rough surface. Gradually number of the lesion may increase and nearby lesions coalesce to form a verrucous plaque.
- Color of the lesion is usually skin colored but may be of flesh colored, specially when mucosal surfaces are affected.
- Sometimes black dots may be seen due to thrombosed vessels and these are wrongly designated as seeds of the lesion.
- Very commonly lesions are seen at dorsa of the hands, feet, forearms and legs. But any area including mucosal surfaces may be affected.
- Some lesions may be of filiform pattern, having spike like projections and these are usually seen at face, mucous membrane and hair-bearing areas.
- Symptom like pain occurs when lesions develop at pressure bearing areas of the palms and soles. This is a secondary phenomenon as the lesions are as such painless.
- Flat warts are smaller in size, about 2-4 mm. They are flat-topped and reddish-brown in color. Their surfaces are less verrucous. Face is the commonest site.
- When genital and perianal areas are affected, lesions are called condyloma acuminata. These are more flesh colored, vegetative and moist.

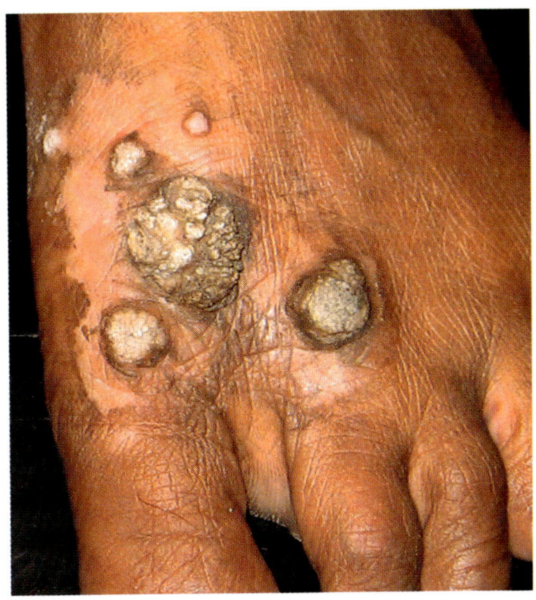

Fig. 8: Few verrucous papules and plaques with hypopigmented background due to application of kerotolytic agent

Differential diagnosis

- Tuberculosis verrucosa cutis
- Callosity.

Histopathology

- Hyperkeratosis, papillomatosis and acanthosis.
- Elongated rete ridges with inward projecton of peripheral rete ridges towards the center, known as arborization.
- Presence of parakeratotic column of epithelium, foci of vacuolated keratinocytes or koilocytes and foci of clumped keratohyaline granules.
- Koilocytes are having small, round, deeply basophilic nuclei with perinuclear halo and pale staining cytoplasm. They are completely or partially, lacking keratohyaline granules even though present at granular layer.
- Vertical tiers of parakeratotic column is often present at the crests of papillomatous elevations of the epidermis overlying the foci of koilocytes.
- Nuclei of parakeratotic keratinocytes are larger and deeply basophilic. Most of them are round rather than elongated in other parakeratotic disorders like psoriasis.
- No granular layer is present at the papillomatous crests but this layer is prominent at the valley area i.e. area between two crests. This area contains heavy and irregular clumps of keratohyaline granules.

Treatment

- Physical destruction with electrosurgery, cryosurgery or laser surgery.
- Trichloroacetic acid (80-90%) or phenol (88%) for plane wart.
- Podophyllin (25%) for condyloma acuminata.

Hand-Foot-Mouth disease (HFMD)

- Hand-foot-mouth disease (HFMD) is a self-limiting and nonfatal disease of viral etiology.
- It commonly affects children below 10 years of age and is often presented with features like fever, sore in the mouth and vesicular skin rash.
- Due to painful oral lesions, the affected children become reluctant to take food and the parents become anxious. So, they are forced to visit general physicians or pediatricians.
- At the point if the physicians are not very confident to say that *this is a simple disease with good prognosis*, the anxiety of the parents will not stop till the disease subsides.
- HFMD, commonly occurs among age below 10 years. Male are little more affected than females.
- It is caused by non-polio enteroviruses, commonly coxsackie A16 and enterovirus 71. It is transmitted via feco-oral route and rarely through inhalation.
- Incubation period is short, about 3-6 days only but viral shedding may persists for upto 5 weeks.
- There is a high transmission rate among household contact. It commonly occurs in summer and rainy seasons.
- The disease is world wide distributed with a chance of sporadic or epidemic outbreak. The largest recorded outbreak was in Taiwan in 1998, affecting more than 1,20,000 people and causing 78 deaths.

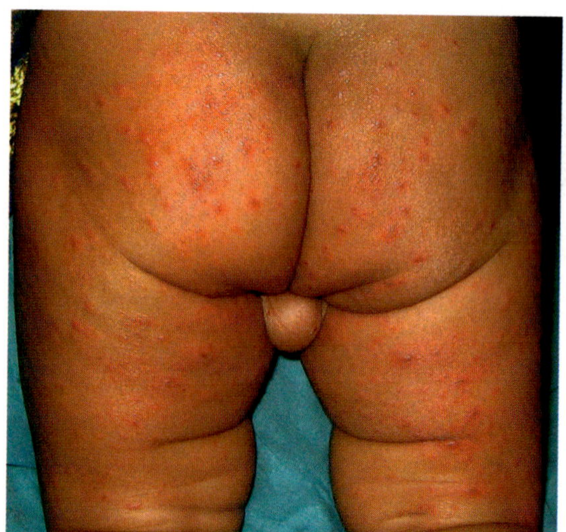

Fig. 9: Numerous erythematous papulovesicles.

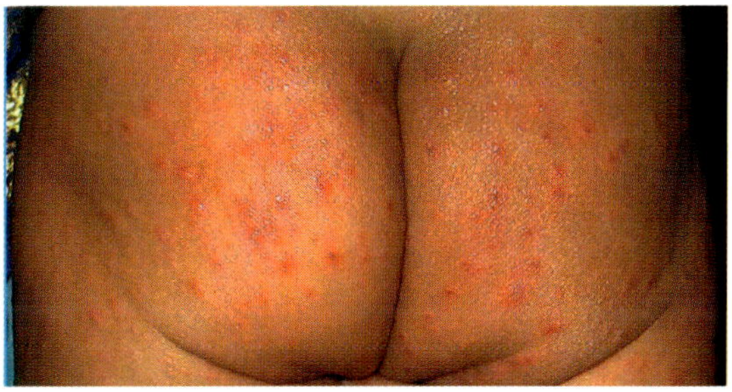

Fig. 10: Numerous erythematous papulovesicles.

Clinical features

- Patient may present with a complaint of low grade fever, pain abdomen, sore throat, sore mouth or skin rash.
- Fever lasts for only one or two days. Nearly all cases have a few painful oral lesions which start as bright red papules, then turn into vesicles and rupture to form erosions.
- Tongue, buccal mucosa, hard palate and oropharynx are affected. Cervical and mandibular lymphadenopathy may develop.
- Cutaneous lesions appear in 2/3rd cases, soon after oral lesions. These start as reddish macules which turn into vesicles of varying shapes like oval, elliptical (American football) or triangular.
- Commonest sites are palms, soles, sides of hands and feet, buttocks, knees, elbows, face, legs and external genitalia. Number of the lesions may be few or numerous.
- Gradually vesicles become crusted and heal within 7-10 days.

Complications

- Lesions may be severe if patient is already having some chronic dermatitis like atopic dermatitis and this is known as eczema herpeticum or Kaposi's varicelliform eruption.
- Very rare complications are aseptic meningitis, encephalitis, polio-like syndrome, myocarditis, pulmonary edema or hemorrhage and death.

Differential diagnosis

- Aphthous stomatitis: Only oral lesions, not associated with fever are present and recurrence is very common.
- Chicken pox: Only skin lesions are present, distributed at central parts of the body like face and trunk.
- Drug eruption/erythema multiforme: It is often difficult to differentiate if HFMD becomes very extensive or these two become localized. Only experience can help in such a situation.
- Herpangina: Another viral infection, associated with oral ulcers affecting the tonsillar pillars.
- Herpetic gingivostomatits: Painful ulcers with history of recurrence.

Investigation

- Nothing is required. PCR can detect the virus.

Treatment

- No treatment is required for usual cases. Complications will be treated accordingly.

Prognosis

- It is a benign, self-limiting disease. Occasionally, it is associated with prolonged fever, diarrhea and joint pain. Though I got a case with severe itching, so far it was not mentioned in standard text books.

Prevention

- Universal precaution
- Discourage to attend school
- Isolation, if possible upto 5 weeks.

Measles/Rubeola

- It is caused by a RNA virus of paramyxoviridae family.
- Virus is transmitted through inhalation of droplets or direct contact.
- Nasopharyngeal mucosa is first affected, sometimes conjunctivae, followed by affection of reticuloendothelial system.
- Measles antibodies are responsible for protection from future infection or reinfection.

- Preschool children are most commonly affected.
- Modified measles: When it occurs in vaccinated person. It is characterized by mild prodrome, short duration and absent Koplik spots.
- Atypical measles: When natural measles occurs in a person vaccinated with killed measles vaccine. It is characterized by high fever, headache, myalgia, hemorrhagic exanthem, Koplik spots, delayed neurodegenerative disease, seizure, coma and even death.

Clinical features

- Prodromal features are cough, coryza and conjunctivitis and fever.
- An exanthem, known as Koplik spots, appear during prodromal period. These are punctate gray-white to erythematous papules at buccal mucosa.
- Exanthem appears within 2-4 days of prodrome. These lesions are erythematous to purple-red macules and papules. Lesions show a tendency to become confluent.
- Lesions start to appear at forehead, hairline, behind the ears and spread in a cephalocaudal direction.
- Lesions subside by following same direction of appearance.
- Postinflammatory coppery macules and exfoliation are left behind following subsidence.
- Complications are pneumonia, bronchitis, otitis, gastroenteritis, myocarditis and encephalitis.

Rubella/German measles

- It is caused by a RNA virus of Togaviridae family.
- Virus is transmitted from infected human direct contact with nasopharyngeal secretion or through droplets inhalation.
- Incubation period is 14-23 days.
- Generalized lymphadenopathy is usually present, specially involving suboccipital, postauricular and cervical groups.
- Anemia, neutropenia and thrombocytopenia may be associated.

Clinical features

- Prodromal features are low-grade fever, sore throat, rhinorrhea, cough, headache, malaise, eye pain, arthralgia and arthritis.
- Prodromal features last for 2-5 days before development of exanthem.
- Exanthem consists of erythematous to rosepink macules and papules.
- Lesions have a tendency to become confluent.
- In severe cases flaky exfoliation may be seen in some areas.
- Face and trunk are commonly affected.
- A characteristic enanthem develops as erythematous and petechial macules at soft palate. This is known as Forchheimer's spots.
- Lesions spread in a cephalocaudal direction and after 1-3 days when they start to involute, follow the same direction.
- Commonly affected joints are those of the fingers, wrists and knees.
- Other complications are encephalitis, myocarditis, pericarditis and hepatitis.

HIV/AIDS

- It is caused by Human immunodeficiency virus 1 or 2.
- The virus is a single stranded RNA virus, under the group of retroviruses and having reverse transcriptase.
- AIDS is the advanced stage of the infection and stands for acquired immunodeficiency syndrome, first time termed in 1981.
- HIV2 infection was first documented in Africa in 1980s and spread to India in 1990.

Modes of transmission

- Unprotected sexual intercourse.
- Perinatal
- Blood transfusion and inoculation.
- Needle sharing by drug abusers.
- Organ transplantation
- Direct contact with tissue fluid in professionals

Clinical category

A. Documented HIV infection, without features of B and C.
- Asymptomatic HIV infection
- Acute primary HIV infection, consisting of fever, malaise, lymphadenopathy and truncal exanthem.
- Persistent generalized lymphadenopathy, lasting more than 3 months and at least two inguinal regions.

B. Neither A nor C but presence of documented HIV infection.
- Constitutional symptoms, fever > 38.5°C or diarrhea > 1 month.
- Oral hairy leukoplakia.
- Oropharyngeal candidiasis.
- Persistent or recalcitrant vulvovaginal candidiasis.
- Pelvic inflammatory disease.
- Recurrent or multidermatomal zoster.
- Listeriosis.
- Idiopathic thrombocytopenic purpura.
- Bacillary angiomatosis.
- Cervical dysplasia or carcinoma in situ.
- Peripheral neuropathy.

Relation with CD4 cell count
- A1/B1/C1: CD4 > 500/μL.
- A2/B2/C2: CD4 between 200-500/μL
- A3/B3/C3: CD4 < 200μL.

C. AIDS defining illness
- Esophageal candidiasis.
- Candidiasis of bronchi, trachea or lungs.
- Invasive cervical carcinoma.
- Disseminated or extrapulmonary coccidioidomycosis.
- Extrapulmonary cryptococcosis.
- Cryptosporidiosis.

Cutaneous manifestations

A. Infective

* Bacterial
  - Pyoderma and staphylococcal acneiform eruptions.
  - Mycobacterial infection, specially Mycobacterium avium-intracellulare.
  - Bacillary angiomatosis, caused by Bartonella.
  - Other sexually transmitted infections, like syphilis, gonorrhea, chancroid, etc.
* Viral
  - Persistent ulcerated herpes, specially at perianal site.
  - Recurring zoster in younger age.
  - Widespread and recalcitrant condyloma acuminata.
  - Widespread and recalcitrant plane and common warts.
  - Numerous and occasionally giant molluscum contagiosum.
* Fungal
  - Ulcerative or recalcitrant candidal infection.
  - Onychomycosis, specially proximal white onychomycosis.
  - Cutaneous cryptococcosis.
* Parasitic and protozoal
  - Leishmaniasis.
  - Scabies.

B. Noninfective and nonmalignant

- Pruritus
- Alopecia and elongated eyelashes
- Yellow nail syndrome, leukonychia and splinter hemorrhage.
- Linear nail pigmentation due to antiretroviral therapy.

- Xerosis or ichthyosis
- Psoriasis
- Pityriasis rubra pilaris
- Reiter's disease
- Seborrheic dermatitis
- Atopic dermatitis
- Eosinophilic folliculitis
- Papular dermatitis of AIDS
- Drug reactions
- Leucocytoclastic vasculitis and idiopathic thrombocytopenic purpura
- Telangiectasia and cherry angioma
- Oral hairy leukoplakia.
- Aphthous stomatitis.

LEPROSY

CHAPTER C5

- Leprosy is a slowly progressive immunologically mediated disease, caused by *Mycobacterium leprae*, mainly affecting the skin and peripheral nerves.
- *Mycobacterium leprae*, an acid fast bacillus, prefers cooler areas of the body to grow and that is why internal organs, hairy scalp, axillae, groins, scrotum are less affected.

Mycobacterium leprae bacilli

Morphology

- These are nonmotile, nonsporing, slender, straight or slightly curved rod shaped bacilli, having parallel sides with rounded ends.
- Size: 1-8 μm in length and 0.3 μm in breadth.

Cell wall

- The bacillus contains cell wall and cytoplasm.
- Cell wall is 15-20 nm in thickness.
- Cell wall contains lipids like pthiocerol dimycocerosate and phenolic glycolipid 1 (PGL1) in the outer layer and proteins like peptidoglycan-arabinogalactan-mycolic acid complex in the inner layer.
- These lipids are responsible for the foamy macrophages in lepromatous leprosy.
- Lipid layer also protects the bacteria from the toxic effects of lysosomal enzymes and reactive oxygen or nitrogen intermediators.

Antigen

- Serologically important antigens are phenolic glycolipid 1 (PGL1) and lipoarabinomannan (LAM).

Staining

- Bacilli are acid fast as well as alcohol fast. Their acid fastness is due to presence of mycolic acid in cell wall. Pyridine treatment can remove the acid fastness but not their Gram positivity.

Culture

- They are microaerophilic, obligate intracellular and not culturable in artificial media.
- But they may be regrown in mouse foot pad or in 9-banded armadillo. In animal models, they divide by binary fission and take 11-13 days to regenerate. Optimum temperature re-

quired for growth is 27-30°C. The minimum infective dose is 1-10 bacilli.

- They are viable 7-10 days at 4°C.

Classical types of leprosy

- Indeterminate leprosy
- Pure neuritic leprosy
- Tuberculoid leprosy (TT)
- Boderline tuberculoid leprosy (BT)
- Boderline borderline leprosy (BB)
- Boderline lepromatous leprosy (BL)
- Lepromatous leprosy.

Atypical types of leprosy

- Ulcerative BT
- Leprosy tenosynovitis
- Single lesion BL
- Histoid leprosy
- Lucio leprosy
- Ulcerative LL

Field classification for treatment

* Paucibacillary (PB) leprosy: Slit skin smear is usually negative or mildly positive (Bacterial index, 0-1+) and it includes:
    - Indeterminate leprosy
    - TT leprosy
    - BT leprosy, having </=5 lesions
    - Pure neuritic leprosy, having <2 peripheral nerve trunk involvement.
* Multibacillary (MB) leprosy: Slit skin smear for lepra bacilli is usually positive (Bacterial index, 2-6+) and it includes:
    - BT leprosy, having >5 lesions
    - BB, BL, LL and histoid leprosy
    - Pure neuritic leprosy, having =/>2 peripheral nerve trunks.

Cardinal signs in leprosy

* There are three cardinal signs, any of which if present, is enough to establish the diagnosis a case of leprosy.
    - Anesthetic skin lesion: It is having a complete or partial loss of sensation of temperature either to cold or to hot, pain to pin-prick and light touch with wisp of cotton or to head of a ball pen.
    - Thickened peripheral nerve: In endemic area of leprosy like in India, if a patient presents with a thickened peripheral nerve, the first diagnosis is leprosy, the second diagnosis is leprosy and even the third diagnosis is leprosy.
    - Demonstration of *M.leprae*: It is demonstrated by slit skin smear from the skin lesion or nasal mucous membrane.

Indeterminate leprosy

* It usually occurs in children or rarely in adult, in whom immunity is unable to determine the course of the disease.
* It may undergo spontaneous healing or remain as such for several years or convert to other form of leprosy.
* Slit skin smear is negative.

Clinical features of indeterminate leprosy

- Primary lesion is characterized by ill-defined hypopigmented patch with a vague sensory impairment. It may be mild scaly and faintly hypopigmented.
- Size is usually 1-3 cm.
- No sweat or hair loss is present within the lesion and no peripheral nerve becomes thickened.
- Number of the lesion is usually single but may be few.
- Common sites are face, buttocks, trunk and proximal parts of the extremities.

Histopathology

- Perineural and periappendageal nonspecific lymphohistiocytic infiltration, not amounting to form a granuloma.
- Rarely Fite's stain may detect bacilli within a nerve section.

Differential diagnosis

- Pityriasis alba
- Seborrheic dermatitis
- Early vitiligo
- Postinflammatory hypopigmented patch.

Tuberculoid leprosy (TT)

- It occurs at any age when immunity is enough to have a fight with the bacilli.
- Lepromin test is highly positive.
- Slit skin smear is expected to yield negative result.

Clinical features of TT leprosy

- Primary lesion is characterized by hypopigmented or coppery color, well defined patch or plaque, having dry or xerotic surface.
- Loss of hair, sweat and sensation are predominant. Sensation loss is almost complete except light touch which may not be lost fully, specially in facial lesion.
- Untreated patch gradually may turn into an infiltrating plaque.
- Plaque often takes an annular shape, having sharply cut both outer and inner margins.
- Regional peripheral nerve may be thickened with thickening of small nerve twig passing through the lesion, known as feeding nerve.
- Number of lesion is usually 1-3 but may be more than that and lesions are distributed asymmetrically. Size of the lesion is variable from 1-5 cm or even more.
- Common sites are face, dorsal aspects of extremities and trunk.

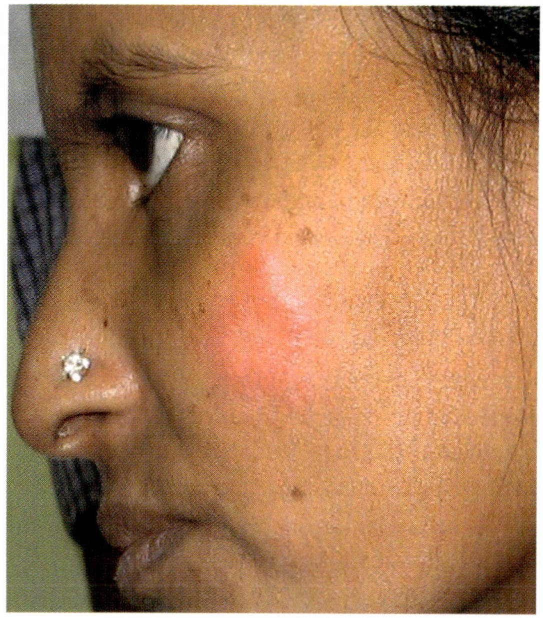

Fig. 1: Well defined annular plaque

Differential diagnosis

- Morphea
- Granuloma annulare
- Sarcoidosis
- Lupus vulgaris

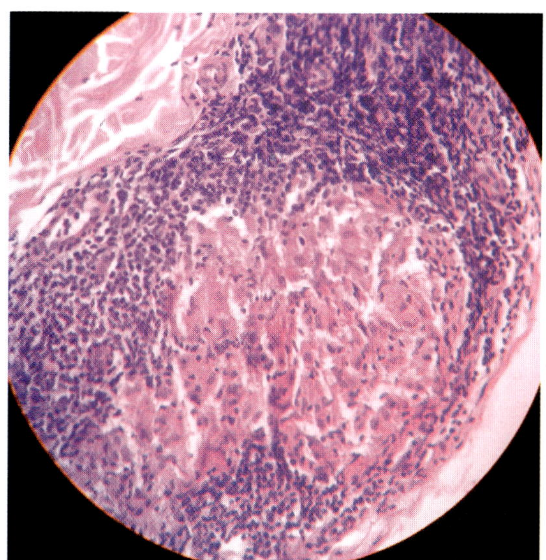

Fig. 2: Well circumscribed granuloma

Histopathology

- Epidermal atrophy and absence of grenz zone.
- Well formed localized epithelioid granuloma, invading the epidermis and typical absence of Langhans' giant cell
- Destruction of nerve by the granuloma
- Usually Fite's stain is negative for lepra bacilli.

Borderline leprosy

- It constitutes of three forms, such as borderline tuberculoid (BT), mid borderline (BB) or lepromatous (BL).
- These occur at any age.
- Patients are immunologically unstable and prone to develop lepra reaction.
- Primary lesions vary during type 1 upgrade or downgrade reaction and annular plaques always show a dimorphic pattern.

BT leprosy

- It is the commonest form of leprosy.
- Lepromin test is moderately positive.
- Slit skin smear is rarely positive for lepra bacilli.

Clinical features of BT leprosy

- Primary lesions are well to ill-defined patches or plaque or both. Very often characteristically a large lesion is surrounded by one or few small lesions, known as satellite lesions.
- Plaque often takes an partial annular shape and is having sharply cut outer margin but flattened inner margin.
- Hair loss, sweat loss and sensory impairment are less prominent than tuberculoid (TT) leprosy.
- Lesions may be bilateral but definitely asymmetrical.
- Number of lesion is usually 3-10, but may be single or even upto hundred.
- Patches are hypopigmented but plaques are coppery color.
- Size of the lesions is very much variable from few cm to several cm and even may involve a whole limb.
- Shape of the lesion is also variable.
- A long standing large plaque may show pseudopodia like outward extension from the margin or this may be due to coalescence of satellites lesions with the large lesion.
- Peripheral nerves often enlarge but usually do not correlate with corresponding site of a skin lesion.

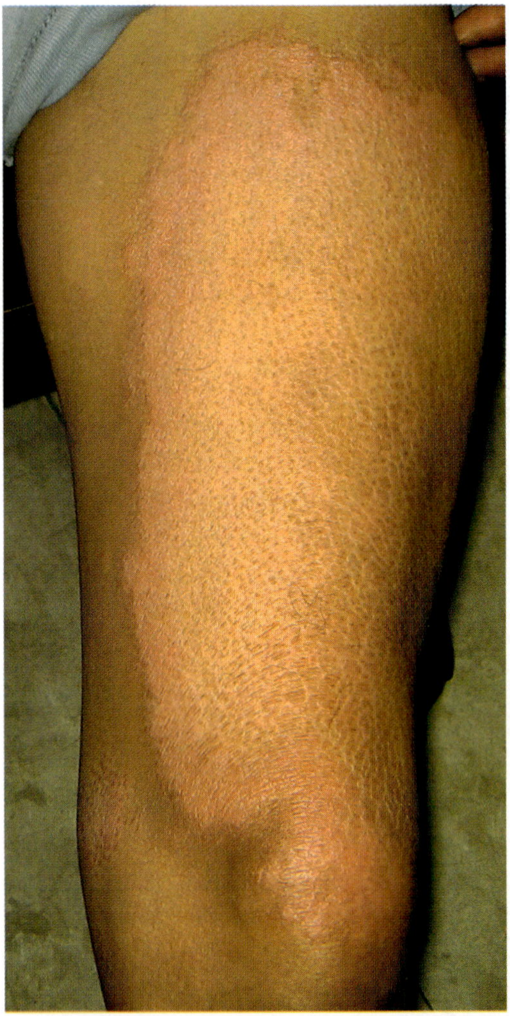

Fig. 3: Well defined erythematous annular plaque with sharp outer margin and inner slopping margin, a satellite lesion is visible at inner side of lower end and pseudopodia at places

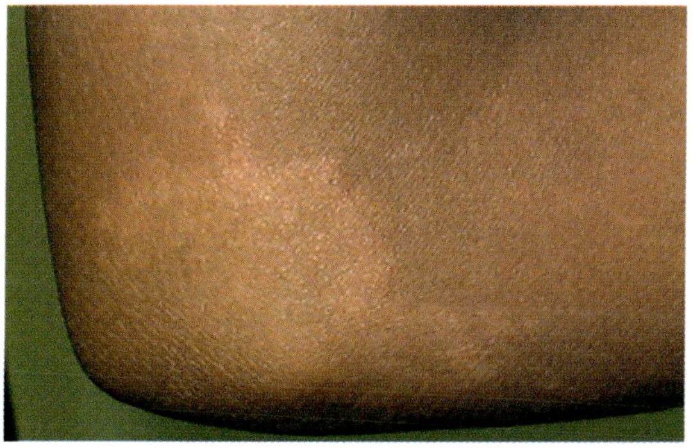

Fig. 4: Hypopigmented patch with well to ill defined irregular border, surrounded by characteristic satellite lesions

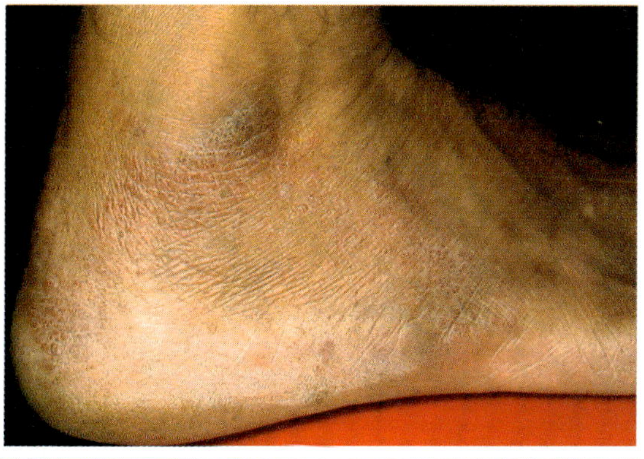

Fig. 5: Well to ill defined icthyotic coppery color plaque at dorsolateral surface of right foot

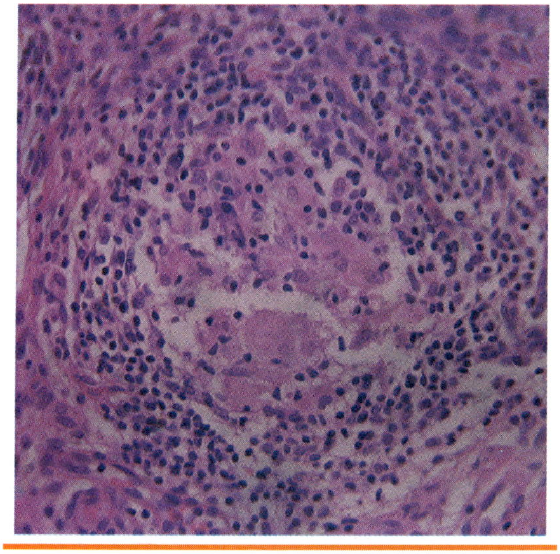

Fig. 6: Granuloma containing central epithelioid cells and peripheral rim of lymphocytes.

Histopathology

- Epidermal atrophy and thin poorly defined grenz zone.
- Circumscribed granuloma containing less epithelioid cells and predominant lymphocytes. Langhans' giant cells may be present but if present, they are few in number and smaller in size.
- Granuloma invades the dermal nerves and destroys them.

BB leprosy

* It is the most unstable form of borderline leprosy.
* Lepromin test is weakly positive.
* Slit skin smear is moderately positive.

Clinical features of BB leprosy

- Characteristic primary lesions is a punched out plaque, revealing a sharply defined inner border which indicates tuberculoid pole and outer ill defined border which indicates lepromatous pole.
- But other uncharacteristic papules and bizarre shaped plaques may be present.
- Number of the lesions may be few or multiple and they are distributed asymmetrically.
- Size and shape are variable.

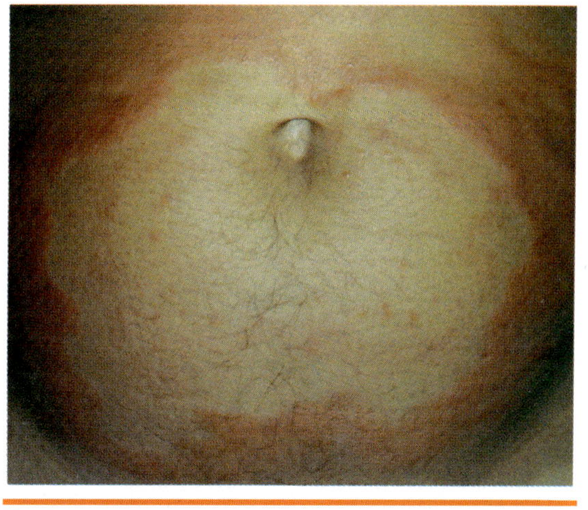

Fig. 7: Erythematous large annular plaque with sharply cut inner border and slopped outer border

- Color of the lesion is coppery.
- Hair loss, sweat loss and sensory impairment are less prominent.
- Peripheral nerves enlarge but asymmetrically.

Histopathology

- Epidermal atrophy and more defined grenz zone.
- Less circumscribed dermal granuloma with predominant epithelioid cells, scanty lymphocytes and no giant cell.
- Dermal edema may be present.
- Perineural infiltration may be present.
- Fite's stain for lepra bacilli mild to moderately positive.

BL leprosy

- It is the borderline leprosy closest to lepromatous pole.
- Lepromin test is usually negative.
- Slit skin smear is moderately positive.

Clinical features of BL leprosy

- Characteristic lesions are dome-shaped papules and nodules, having a slopping margin which imperceptibly merge with normal skin.
- Another characteristic lesion is an annular plaque in which the elevated peripheral rim is having slopped inner and outer margin and both of them imperceptibly merge with normal skin.
- Surface is smooth, erythematous and shiny and shape is usually round.
- Number of lesions is variable from multiple to numerous and bilaterally distributed with a tendency of symmetry.
- Hair loss, sweat loss and sensory loss are not remarkable.
- Peripheral nerves enlarge bilaterally but asymmetrically.

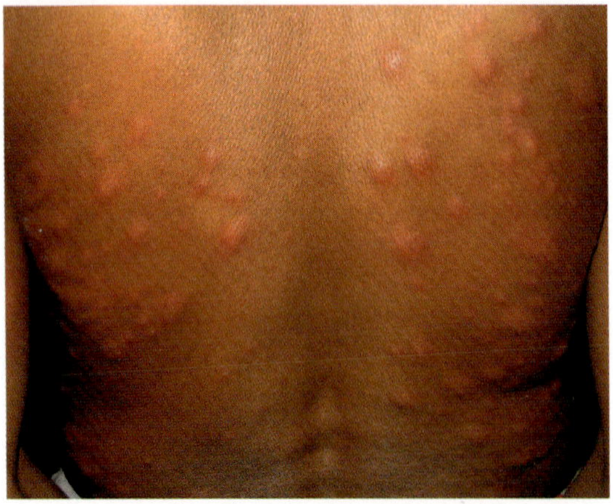

Fig. 8: Multiple nodules with a tendency of symmetry

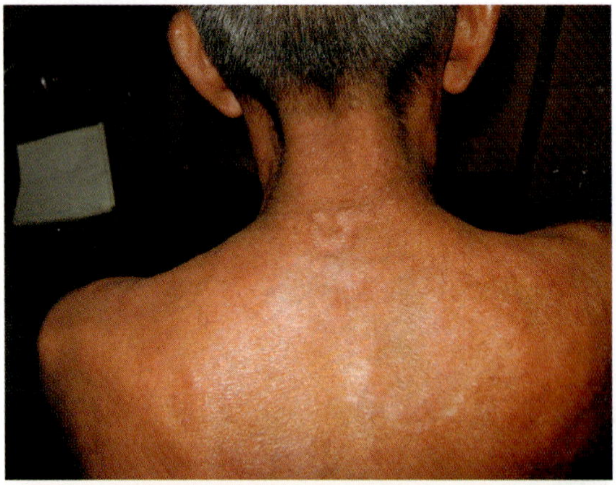

Fig. 9: Annular plaque with rolled margin and borders are having slopping at both inner and outer sides

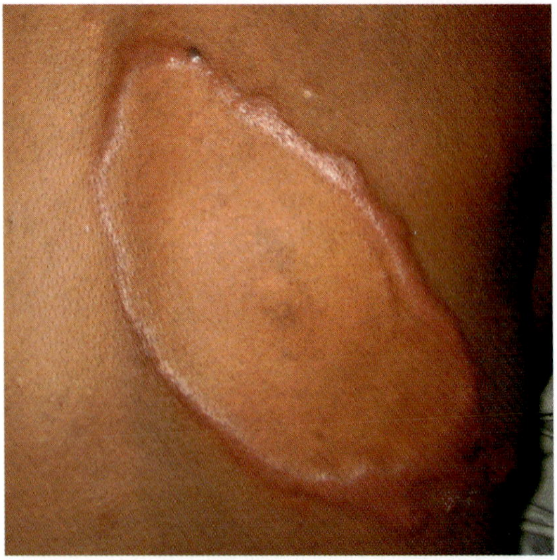

Fig. 10: Annular plaque of BL leprosy, having rolled border with slopping at both inner and outer sides.

Histopathology

- ♦ Epidermal atrophy and well formed grenz zone.
- ♦ Diffuse granuloma containing histiocytes, lymphocytes and sparse foamy macrophages
- ♦ Proliferation of perineural fibroblasts appearing as onion peel in cross section.
- ♦ Fite's stain for lepra bacilli moderately positive, bacillary index (BI) 4-5, but no globi.

Clinical features of LL leprosy

- ✶ Characteristic lesions are macules, papules, nodules, plaques and diffuse infiltration.
- ✶ Number of the lesion is numerous, distributed widely and symmetrically.
- ✶ Macules are ill defined, hypopigmented or mild erythematous and shiny.
- ✶ Hair loss, sweat loss and sensation loss are not present within the macules in early stage but may present in late stage in a mild degree.
- ✶ Papules are more circumscribed than a papule of BL leprosy.
- ✶ Plaques are having pebbled surface and having depth like a nodule.
- ✶ Nodules are uncharacteristic but having a depth more than nodule of BL leprosy.
- ✶ Diffuse infiltration is characterized by shiny and edematous surface with prominent perifollicular swelling, appearing as peau d' orange or orange peel. Skin creases also become prominent.
- ✶ Peripheral nerves enlarge at late stage, bilaterally and symmetrically.
- ✶ Other features
  - ♦ Gloves and stocking anesthesia of hands and feet, and slipping of chappal during walking.
  - ♦ Edema of hands and feet.
  - ♦ Loss of eyebrows, known as superciliary madarosis and loss of eyelashes, known as cillary madarosis.
  - ♦ Nasal stuffiness and even blood stained discharge from the nose.
  - ♦ Hoarseness of voice due to laryngeal involvement.

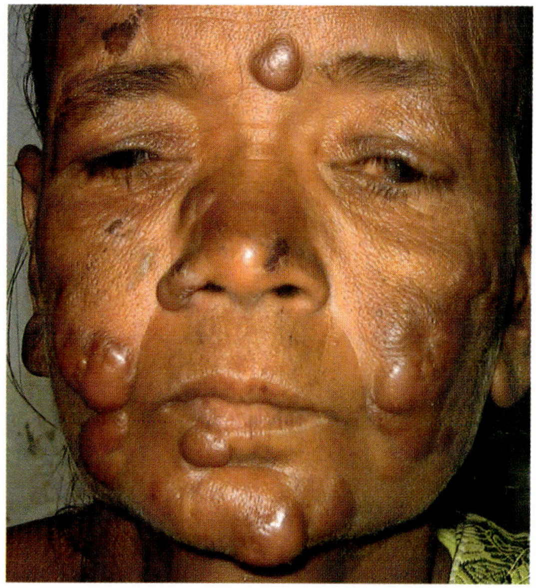

Fig. 11: Well circumscribed nodules and plaques

  - ♦ Facies leprosa is characterized by collapse of the nasal bridge due to destruction of nasal spine, flattening of cheeks due to destruction of zygomatic processes and loss of upper incisor teeth due to destruction of maxillae.
  - ♦ Eye changes include lagophthalmos, reduced corneal sensation, iris pearl due to deposition of lepra bacilli at margin of iris and complications like iritis and iridocyclitis due to reaction.

Histopathology

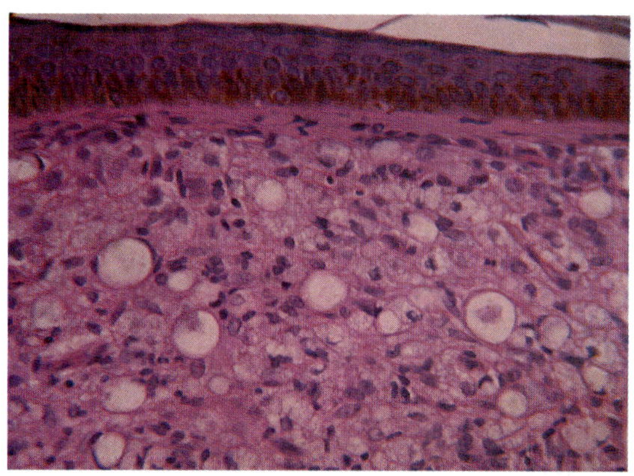

Fig. 12: Diffuse granuloma containing foamy macrophages

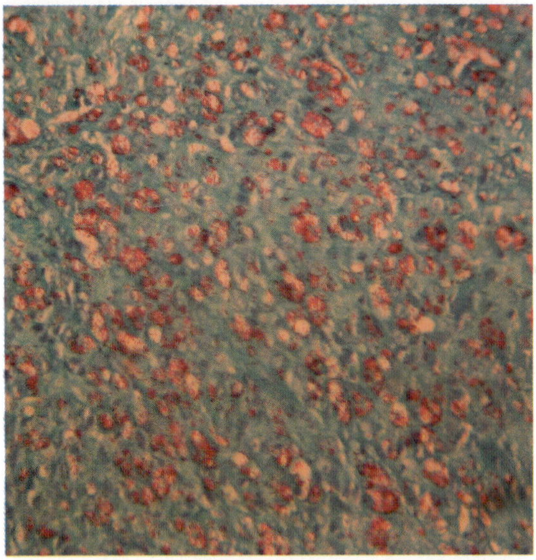

Fig. 13: Fite's stain shows foamy macrophages are filled up with lepra bacilli

- Epidermal atrophy, flattened rete ridges and well formed grenz zone.
- Diffuse granuloma extends upto subcutaneous fat.
- Granuloma contains profuse foamy macrophages, plasma cells, scanty lymphocytes and no epithelioid cells.
- Macrophages have abundant eosinophilic cytoplasm, containing mixed population of solid and fragmented bacilli.
- Solid bacilli are packed like bunch of cigar, known as globi.
- Large foamy macrophages containing bacilli, known as lepra cell or Virchow cell.
- Endothelial cells also contain lepra bacilli.
- Preservation of nerve in early stages but fibrosis in late stages.
- Destruction of appendages is seen in late stage.
- Fite's stain for lepra bacilli is highly positive.

Histoid leprosy

- It is often associated with long back dapsone monotherapy; but may occur as de novo.
- Slit smear for AFB is highly positive and bacilli are large and lie in bunch.

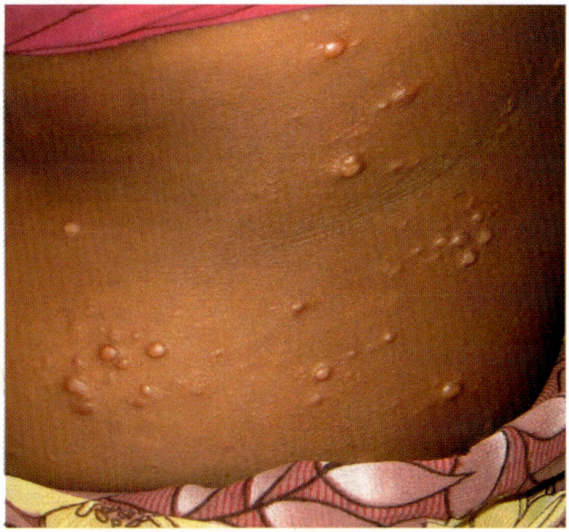

Fig. 14: Multiple shiny coppery colored papules at flank

Clinical features of histoid leprosy

- Asymptomatic skin colored well circumscribed papules and nodules.
- Trunk and limbs are commonly affected.
- Size of the lesions is usually less than 5 mm.
- Number of lesions is usually countable and does not exceed 150.

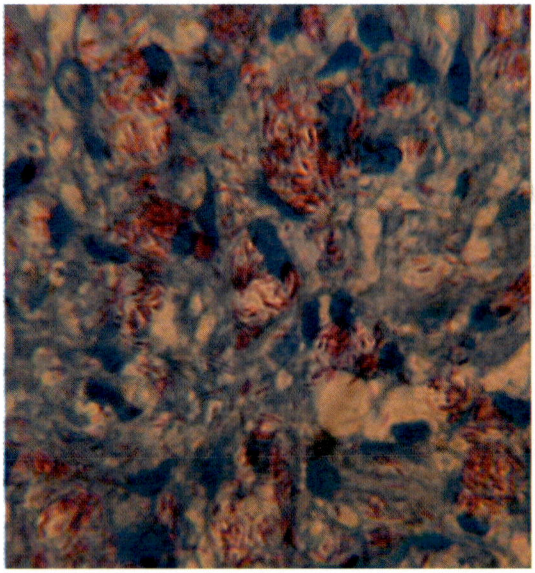

Fig. 15: Lot of large and stout lepra bacilli in magnified view

Histopathology

- Dermis contains profuse spindle shaped macrophage infiltration, mimicking dermatofibroma.
- Fite's stain is highly positive.

Lepra reaction

- It is the development of different sets of clinical manifestations other than existing leprosy lesions or sudden changes of existing lesions, due to hypersensitivity reactions.
- It usually occurs in presence of active disease and treatment.
- But it may occur without any antileprotic treatment and even after discontinuation of treatment.

Types of lepra reactions

- Type 1 lepra reaction is caused by type IV hypersensitivity reaction (delayed hypersensitivity reaction).
- Type 2 lepra reaction, is caused by type III hypersensitivity reaction (immune complex mediated hypersensitivity reaction).

Types of severity of lepra reaction

- Mild degree: It is characterized by few skin lesion without any neuritis.
- Moderate degree: It is characterized by skin lesions without ulceration and neuritis without palsy.
- Severe degree: It is characterized by skin lesions with pustulation, vesiculation, or ulceration and neuritis with frank palsy or impending palsy.

Precipitating factors in reaction

- Older age, pregnancy.
- Antileprotic treatment except clofazimine.
- Presence of HIV infection.

Type 1 lepra reaction

- It occurs in all forms of borderline leprosy (BT, BB and BL).
- Patients having disseminated skin lesions or nerve involvement are more prone to develop this reaction.
- When the patient regains immunity following treatment or spontaneously, type 1 reaction becomes more aggressive, it is designated as reversal reaction.
- When patient loses immunity further, reactive features become less aggressive, it is designated as downgrade reaction.
- Sometimes features of both types of reactions may present in same patient in same time.
- Usually reversal reaction occurs during first 6 months of antileprotic therapy in BT and BB but later in case of BL.
- Reversal reaction occurs in 33% cases within first 6 months of therapy, in 16% cases between 7-12 months of therapy and in 10% cases after release from treatment.
- Late reversal reaction occurs in 3-9% cases of all BT, BB and BL cases in combination.

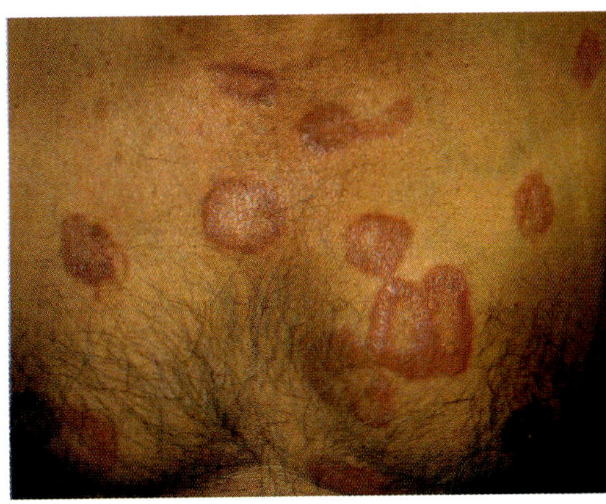

Fig. 16: Numerous well defined erythematous plaques of BT leprosy in reaction.

Features of reversal reaction

- Most of the patients present with involvement of both skin and peripheral nerves. But in some cases either skin or nerve becomes predominant.

- Existing skin lesions become tender, erythematous, edematous, and scaly mimicking psoriasis.
- Some lesion may ulcerate and development of new lesion is unusual.
- General symptoms are absent except few such as tenderness at palms and soles and edema of the hands and feet.
- Peripheral nerves become swollen and tender with increment of anesthesia or occurrence of palsy of the limbs.
- Slit skin smear for Lepra bacilli usually negative.

Histopathology

- Hyperkeratosis, epidermal atrophy or sometimes mild acanthosis.
- Dermal edema, disorganization of granuloma and invasion of the epidermis by the granuloma.
- Dispersed granuloma may contain many larger size giant cells.
- Caseation necrosis of the granuloma and dermal nerves.
- Fibrinoid necrosis within the peripheral nerves.
- Bacilli are not seen in Fite's stain.

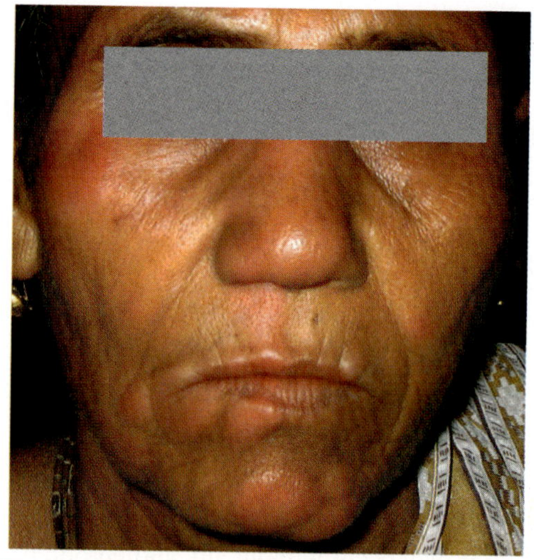

Fig. 17: Erythematous, edematous and shiny plaques, a result of downgrade reaction from initial BT leprosy

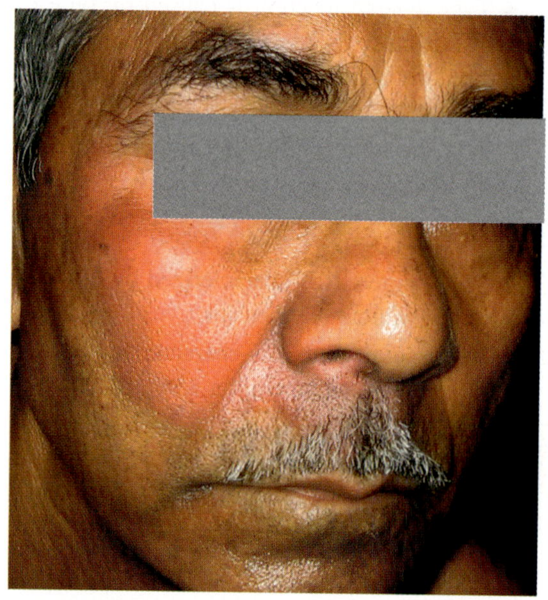

Fig. 18: Shiny nonscaly erythematous and edematous plaque

Features of downgrade reaction

- Multiple or few shiny erythematous, edematous, indurated and tender new lesions develop.
- Existing old lesions are usually remain unaltered.
- Edema of hands, feet, face and nasal mucosa may develop.
- New peripheral nerves become swollen and tender.
- Lepra bacilli may be present in slit skin smear.
- Course is more prolonged and may lead to change of the disease spectrum towards lepromatous pole.

Histopathology

- Epidermal atrophy and dermal edema.
- Disorganized granuloma contains more foamy macrophages.
- Bacilli may present in Fite's stain.

- No necrosis within the granuloma or dermal nerves is seen.

Type 2 lepra reaction

- It occurs in BL and LL, with high bacterial index, > 4+ and seen in more than 50% cases of LL and 25% cases of BL.
- Late type 2 reaction is seen in 3% of BL and LL in combination.

Clinical features

- It is characterized by prominent general features including fever, arthritis, lymphadenitis, edema of the limbs or face.
- Sudden onset of crops of tender, erythematous nodules, known as erythema nodosum leprosum (ENL) or erythema multiforme like lesions.
- Lesions may turn into transient vesicle, followed by pustulation and necrosis or ulceration.
- Most of the lesion appear in the evening due to low physiological steroid level.
- Each lesion persists for 2-3 days and gradually subsides with residual hyperpigmentation or scarring.
- Size of the lesion is variable from 0.5-3 cm.
- Common sites are face, distal upper limbs and proximal lower limbs.
- Recurrence is very common and it usually happens within 3 months of previous attack.
- Other associations include iridocyclitis, epididymo-orchitis, etc.

Histopathology

- Variable dermal edema
- Increased dermal vascularity with dilated vessels.
- Influx of polymorphs, invasion vessel walls by the polymorphs and leukocytoclasia.
- Sometimes occurrence of complete obliteration of vascular lumen due to swelling of the endothelial cells.
- Presence of fragmented and granular lepra bacilli.

Relapse in leprosy

- It is seen in inactive leprosy.
- It occurs insidiously, often after 1-2 years of termination of treatment.
- Smear for lepra bacilli may be positive.
- It does not respond to steroid but to antileprotic therapy.

Clinical features

- Area of the old lesion extends with increased thickening due to infiltration.
- New lesion may appear.
- Disease spectrum may be changed.
- Fresh nerve may be involved.

Treatment of leprosy

- For PB leprosy, treatment is given for 6 months and drugs include:
  - Dapsone 2 mg/kg/day or 100 mg/day in adult.
  - Rifampicin 10 mg/kg body weight in child or 450-600 mg in adult per month.
- For MB leprosy, treatment is given for 12 months and drugs include:
  - Dapsone 2 mg/kg/day or 100 mg/day in adult.
  - Rifampicin 10 mg/kg body weight in child or 450-600 mg in adult per month.
  - Clofazimine 300 mg per month as well as 50 mg/day in adult.
- Alternative regimen in case of drug resistance or intolerable adverse effect, observed following standard therapy.
  - ROM therapy, given monthly, but total duration of therapy is yet to be standardized and it includes, Rifampicin 600 mg, Ofloxacin 400 mg and Minocycline 100 mg in adult.
  - Ofloxacin may be in place of dapsone when later one is intolerable.
- Treatment of reaction includes systemic steroids, clofazimine, thalidomide, chloroquine/hydroxy-

chloroquine and nonsteroidal antiinflammatory drugs.

- Systemic corticosteroid is indicated for both type 1 and type 2 reactions but definite indications are:
  - (a) Severe neuritis, not responding to conventional analgesic.
  - (b) Impending nerve palsy or recent nerve palsy.
  - (c) Presence of iritis, iridocycliis or orchitis.
  - (d) Presence of vesiculo-pustular lesions, erythema multiforme like lesions or ulcerative lesions.
- Thalidomide is only effective in type 2 reaction.
- Clofazimine in high doses (300-400 mg/day) is given in type 2 reaction.

* Treatment of DDS and rifampicin both resistant multibacillary leprosy:
  - Clofazimine 50 mg daily.
  - Any of two drugs daily for 6 months
    #Ofloxacin 400 mg
    #Minocycline 100 mg
    #Clarithromycin 500 mg
  - Anyone of the drugs for next 18 months
    #Ofloxacin 400 mg
    #Minocycline 100

Lucio phenomenon

* It is associated with diffuse form of non-nodular lepromatous leprosy or Lucio leprosy and mostly encountered by Mexicans.
* It is due to massive invasion of endothelial cells of the arterioles by profuse number of lepra bacilli.
* Initially, it was named as lepra manchada.

Clinical features

- Painful and tender erythematous patches, specially at extremities in early stage.
- Gradually center of the individual lesion becomes purpuric, necrotic, ulcerated and crusted.
- The brown to black crust or eschar is sloughed out within few days and forms superficial atrophic scar.
- Commonly affected sites are legs, thighs, forearms and buttocks. Trunk or face is usually spared.

Histopathology

- Ischemic epidermal necrosis.
- Necrotizing vasculitis at upper dermis.
- Neutrophilic abscess may be formed.
- Panniculitis may be present.

Complications in leprosy

* Due to nerve damage:
  - Trophic ulcer at pressure points of the foot and burn-ulcers at working hand.
  - Facial deformities including Bell's palsy, sadal nose and loss of teeth.
  - Limb deformities including clawing of the fingers and toes, wrist drop and foot drop.
  - Bony deformities including osteomyelitis, resorption or shortening of the digits.
  - Eye complications including madarosis, exposure keratitis, iritis and iridocyclitis.
  - Exfoliative and other forms of drug reactions.
* Due to reaction:
  - Eye complications
  - Limb deformities
  - Edema of hands and feet
* Due to drugs:
  - Reactions in leprosy and adverse effects of the drugs.

Types of trophic ulcer

- Acute ulcer
- Chronic ulcer
- Recurrent ulcer
- Complicated ulcer, associated with osteomyelitis, malignancy, etc.

Stages of trophic ulcer

- Concealed ulcer, characterized by focal erythema and tenderness on deep pressure.
- Threatened ulcer, characterized by focal erythema and soft consistency.
- Overt ulcer, characterized by frank ulcer.

Pathogenesis of trophic ulcers at foot

- Pressure of the body weight.
- Shearing and frictional pressure during walking at forefoot.
- Atrophy of foot pad due wasting of muscles.
- Disproportionate pressure due to loss of arch of the foot. Fissuring due to loss of sweat and secondary infection through cracks.
- Repeated injury to insensitive foot with soft tissue damage.

Frequency of sites of trophic ulcers at foot

- Forefoot: 70-90%
- Base of the big toe: 30-50%
- Heel and mid lateral border: 5-10%
- Tips of the toes: 1-5%.

Stages of nerve involvement in leprosy

- Stage of parasitization.
- Stage of host response.
- Stage of clinical involvement.
- Stage of nerve damage.
- Stage of nerve destruction.

Onset and progress of nerve damage

- Insidious onset and gradual progress
- Episodic onset and saltatory progress
- Catastrophic onset and catastrophic progress
- Late onset and silent progress

Residual signs of leprosy for which no treatment is required

- Post inflammatory wrinkling, hypo-/hyperpigmentation, scar, etc.
- Persisting or even increment of anesthesia due to silent fibrosis of nerve trunk.
- Thickened nerve without tenderness.
- Presence of deformities.

Signs of active disease for which further treatment is required

- Erythematous thickened lesion.
- Active lesions at eye, ear and nose.
- Increasing size and number of the lesion.
- Thickened tender peripheral nerve.
- Presence of solid staining bacilli in slit skin smear.

Signs of subsiding lesion in response to treatment

- Reduction of all points of activity.

Pathogenesis of bone changes

- Disuse atrophy of the bones.
- Osteomyelitis due to complicated trophic ulcers.
- Impaired blood supply due to endarteritis.
- Leprous osteitis.
- Osteoporotic changes due to lack of testosterone when testicles are affected.

Dimorphic lesions in leprosy

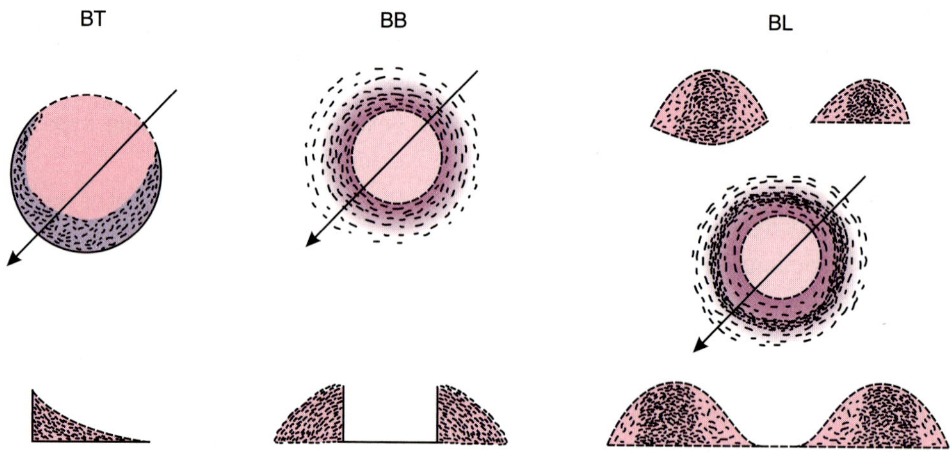

Lesion	Outer margin	Inner margin
BT	Well defined	Ill defined
BB	Ill defined	Well defined
BL	Ill defined	Ill defined

CUTANEOUS TUBERCULOSIS

CHAPTER C6

Classification of cutaneous tuberculosis

(i) Exogenous

- Tubercular chancre
- Tuberculosis verrucosa cutis
- BCG vaccination induced tuberculosis

(ii) Exogenous/endogenous

- Lupus vulgaris
- Orificial tuberculosis

(iii) Endogenous

- Scrofuloderma
- Tubercular gumma
- Miliary tuberculosis

(iv) Tuberculid

- Micropapular: Lichen scrofulosorum
- Papular: Papulonecrotic tuberculid
- Nodular:
  #Erythema induratum of Bazin
  #Erythema nodosum

* Causative agents
  - Classical *mycobacterium tuberculosis*
  - Atypical mycobacterium
* Mode of infection
  - Exogenous
  - Endogenous

Lupus vulgaris

* It develops when the organisms enter the skin through hematogenous route or directly.
* The host is having moderate degree of immunological response to the organisms.
* It is the commonest form of cutaneous tuberculosis and the bacilli entered the site either by direct inoculation or via blood circulation.
* Mantoux test is usually moderately positive (10-15 mm).

Clinical features

- It starts as soft to firm papule which gradually enlarges or few new lesions develop and coalesce to form larger plaque.

- On diascopy apple jelly colored nodules are seen at the periphery.
- After a variable period in many cases, healing with scar may be seen either from one side of the lesion or from the center of the lesion, but the disease progresses from other sides.
- Some lesions may be hyperkeratotic, ulcerative or mutilating.
- Number of the lesion is usually single but rarely may be multiple.
- Common sites are head, neck, buttocks, elbows and knees.

Clinical variants

- Papular type: It is associated with disseminated lupus.
- Plaque type: Extension occurs with little or no central scarring. When scales are prominent it mimicks psoriasis.
- Nodular or tumor-like: Deeply infiltrated nodules which may be huge and soft myxomatous or reddish yellow tumor-like. Scaling and scarring are absent. Lymphedema and vascular dilatation may be marked in s3.ome cases.
- Ulcerovegetative type: Tendency of rapid ulceration with crusting appears as vegetative growth. It mimicks pyoderma gangrenosum.
- Ulceromutilating type: Ulcer becomes deeper to destroy underlying tissue like cartilage and leads to deformities.

Differential diagnosis

- Sarcoidosis
- Lymphocytoma
- Discoid lupus erythematosus
- Hypertrophic lichen planus
- Sporotrichosis
- BT/BL leprosy
- Lupoid leishmaniasis
- Lupoid sycosis

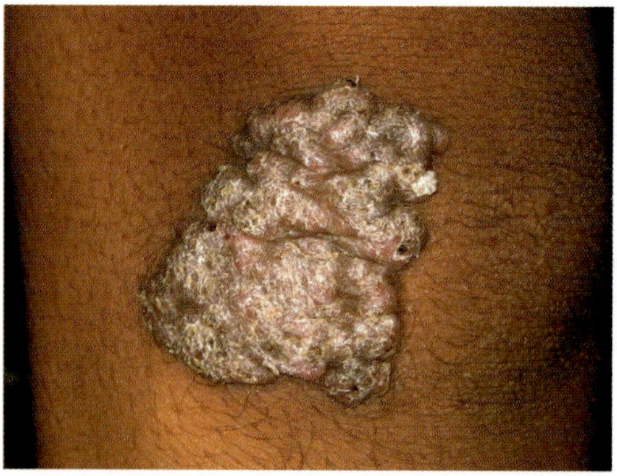

Fig. 1: Well defined irregular erythematous and crusted plaque at left knee

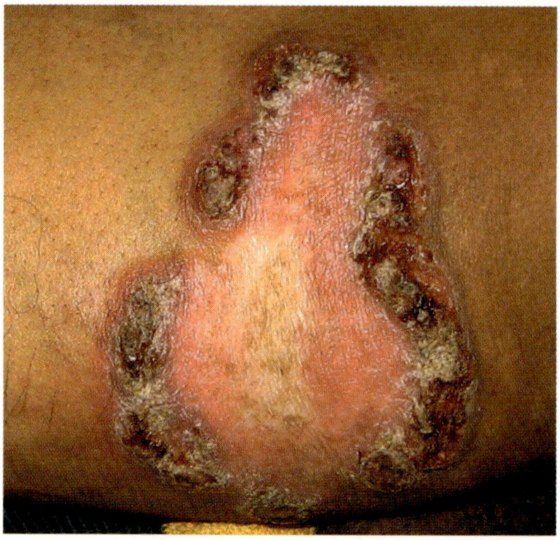

Fig. 2: An annular erythematous and crusted ulcerovegetative plaque at back of the thigh

Histopathology

- Hyperkeratosis, papillomatosis and irregular acanthosis.
- Secondary epidermal changes including atrophy and ulceration.
- Pseudoepitheliomatous hyperplasia at the margin of the ulcer.
- Chronic inflammatory infiltration at papillary dermis, invading the epidermis and downward extension upto subcutaneous tissue.
- Tuberculoid granuloma may be obscured by a profuse chronic inflammatory infiltrates.

- Granuloma often contains mostly Langhans' giant cell but foreign body type also may be present.
- Destruction of appendages by the granuloma and extensive fibrosis during healing.

Tuberculosis verrucosa cutis

- It occurs solely, due to direct inoculation of the bacilli.
- Mantoux test is highly positive as 15-20 mm in an average.

Clinical features

- It starts as firm warty papule which gradually enlarges to form an irregular plaque.
- Purulent discharge may come out on deep pressure.
- Sometimes, it may heal from the center to form an annular plaque.
- Common sites are dorsa of hands and feet including fingers and toes, buttocks, etc.

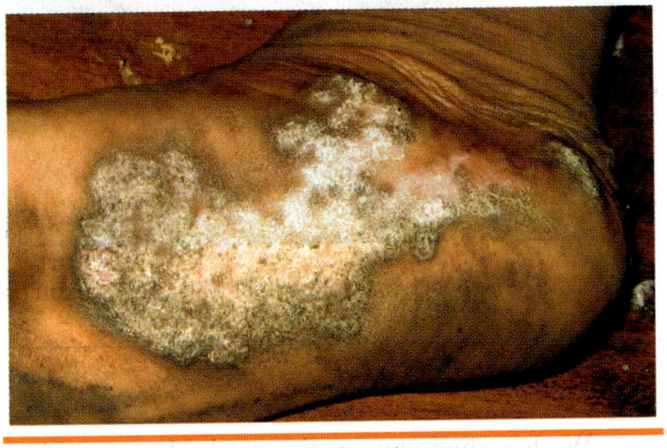

Fig. 3: An irregular verrucous plaque

Differential diagnosis

- Wart
- Hyperkerotic lupus vulgaris
- Chromoblastomycosis

Histopathology

- Hyperkeratosis and acanthosis.
- Pseudoepitheliomatous hyperplasia.
- Acute inflammatory infiltration at papillary dermis.
- Formation of abscesses at papillary dermis or within the expanded rete ridges.
- Tuberculoid granuloma with moderate amount of caseation at mid dermis.
- Caseating granuloma in the upper or lower dermis.
- Neutrophilic abscess formation at papillary dermis or within lower epidermis.

Scrofuloderma

- It occurs when the organisms first invade some underlying tissue specially lymph nodes or bones via hematogenous route and then spread to the overlying skin.
- Mantoux test is moderately positive.

Clinical features

- Lesion starts as movable firm subcutaneous nodule.
- Gradually it becomes soft and doughy. Then nearby nodes become matted to form an irregular and adherent mass.
- This non-tender mass becomes fluctuant and ruptures to form ulcer and discharging sinus.
- Ulcer may be linear, serpiginous or irregular in shape.
- Discharge may be pus or caseous material.
- Edge of the ulcer is undermined, inverted and dissecting through alternating areas of fluctuating abscess and bridging scars.
- Common sites are cervical, parotidal, submandibular, subclavicular and inguinal regions.

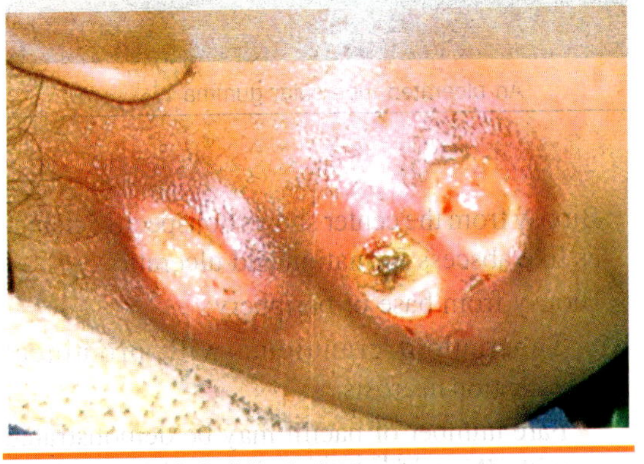

Fig. 4: Multiple boil like lesions

Differential diagnosis

- Boil
- Hidradenitis suppurativa
- Pyoderma gangrenosum

Histopathology

- Massive neutrophilic infiltration like pyogenic abscess.
- Tubercular granuloma may be found at the wall of the sinus.

Tuberculous gumma/metastatic tuberculous abscess

* It is a form of hematogenous tuberculosis.

Clinical features

- Lesion starts as firm subcutaneous nodule which gradually softens to become ill defined soft and fluctuant swelling. Then overlying skin breaks down to form undermined ulcer.
- Extremities are more involved than trunk.

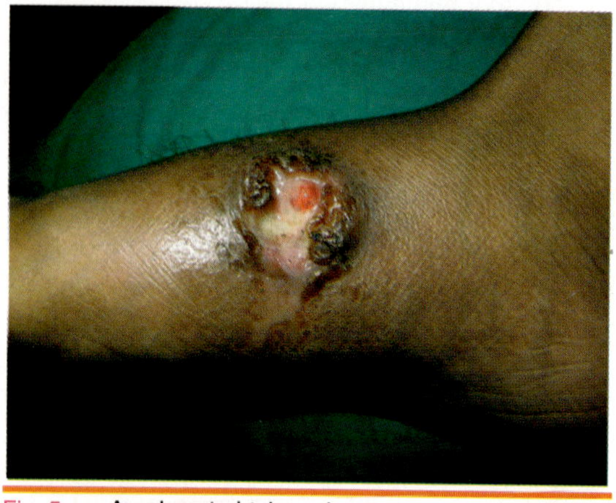

Fig. 5: An ulcerated tubercular gumma

Histopathology

* Biopsy from the center shows nonspecific changes like abscess formation and ulceration.
* Biopsy from base or periphery:
    - Tuberculoid granuloma with prominent caseation necrosis.
    - Fare number of bacilli may be demonstrated with ZN stain in comparison to lupus vulgaris and tuberculosis verrucosa cutis.

Papulonecrotic tuberculid

* It is a reactive form of cutaneous tuberculosis and so no organism can be demonstrated from the lesion.
* In some cases pulmonary or extrapulmonary tuberculosis may be associated.
* It commonly occurs in children and young adults.
* Obliteration of dermal vessels due to thrombosis and vasculitis leads to necrosis.
* Mantoux test is highly positive.

Clinical features

- Necrotic papules appear symmetrically in crops and heal spontaneously with pitted scars.
- Papules are livid or dusky red, having central depression with adherent crusts.
- Common sites are extremities, buttock, glans penis and lower trunk

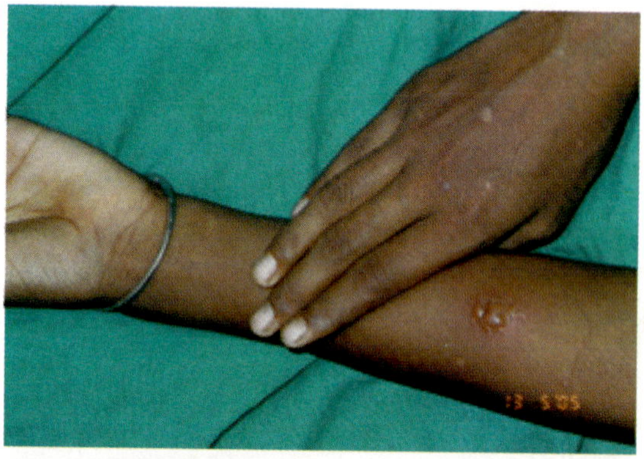

Fig. 6: Highly positive Mantoux test with minute papules and few scar marks

Histopathology

- Wedge-shaped necrotic area in the upper dermis, extending into the epidermis.
- Mixed inflammatory infiltrates around the necrosis which may be granulomatous.
- Partial or complete obliteration of dermal vessels due to vasculitis and thrombosis.

Treatment

* Following 4 drugs for first 2 months and then first 2 drugs for last 4 months. All drugs are taken daily in an empty stomach.
    - Rifampicin: 10 mg/kg
    - Isoniazide: 5 mg/kg
    - Pyrazinamide: 30 mg/kg
    - Ethambutol/streptomycin: 15 mg/kg.

SEXUALLY TRANSMITTED INFECTIONS (STIs)

CHAPTER C7

Classification of STI

* Major
  * Syphilis
  * Chancroid
  * Granuloma venereum
  * Lymphogranuloma venereum
  * Gonorrhoea
  * Herpes genitalis
* Minor:
  * Condyloma acuminata
  * Candidiasis
  * Trichomoniasis
  * Bacterial vaginosis
  * Molluscum contagiosum
  * Scabies
* Others, usually don't have any direct genital lesions
  * HIV infection
  * Hepatitis B

Syphilis

* It is caused by *Treponema pallidum*, a thin delicate spirocheta, having 6-14 spirals.
* It transmits through sexual contact, from mother to fetus or through contact with infected blood products.
* Incubation period is variable from 9-90 days and average is 1 month.

Types

* Primary syphilis
* Secondary syphilis
* Tertiary syphilis

* The spirochetes transmit through the intact or microabraded mucous surface and enter the lymphatics and blood before developing the primary lesion. Primary lesion develops at the site of inoculation due to local proliferation of the spirochetes and host immunological response. Cell mediated immunity of TH1 pathway is responsible for spontaneous healing of the primary disease. Later circulatory spirochetes invade the blood vessels to produce endarteritis and thus development of secondary syphilis occurs.
* Secondary syphilis develops 2-6 months after infection or 2-10 weeks after development of primary syphilis.

* In some cases lesions of primary and secondary syphilis may coexist.
* Even without treatment, chancre heals completely by 4-6 weeks period and infection either leads into early latent syphilis, having no clinical feature or into secondary syphilis.
* Lesions of the secondary syphilis also may heal spontaneously without treatment but may recur with maculopapular eruptions or with papular eruptions and 20% of them have 3-4 such reccurences over a period of 1 year. Then the infection turns into late latent phase. One-third of latent syphilis turns into tertiary syphilis.
* Early and late latent syphilis also defined as duration of infection less or more than 1 year respectively without any clinical manifestation.
* If syphilis remains untreated for > 4 years, it rarely remains communicable except in pregnancy where mother can transmit the disease to the fetus irrespective of the duration of the disease.

Clinical features of primary syphilis

- Primary lesion starts as a button-like papule which turns into an ulcer, known as chancre. The ulcer is classically painless and having a raised border, indurated base and mild serous exudative floor.
- Extragenital ulcer, specially at finger is painful and genital ulcer may be painful due to secondary infection.
- Number of the lesion is usually single, may be few or even multiple.
- Common sites in males are inner prepuce, coronal sulcus, shaft and base of the penis. In females common sites are clitoris, vulva, vagina and cervix.
- Extragenital sites are anus, rectum, mouth, lips, tongue, tonsils, breasts, nipples, fingers and toes.
- Regional lymphadenopathy develops within 7 days of infection. Nodes are discrete, firm, rubbery and nontender. These are usually unilateral and persist for months.

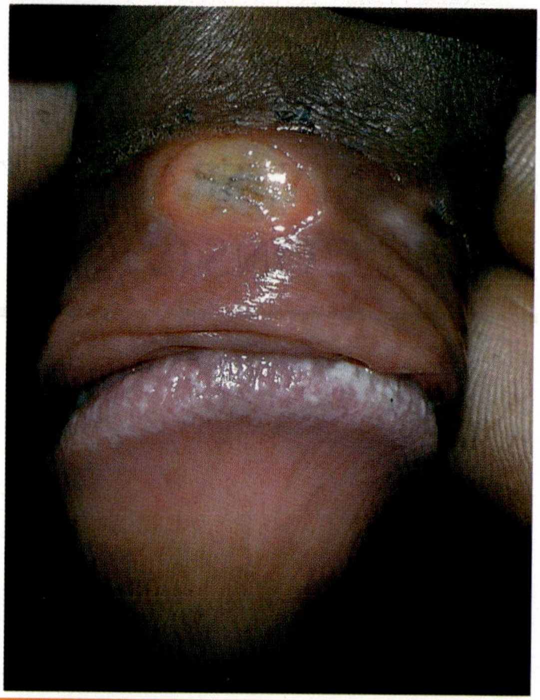

Fig. 1: Painless punched out ulcer at the corona of 1 week duration along with candidal balanoposthitis (Courtesy: Dr. Piyush Kumar, PGT)

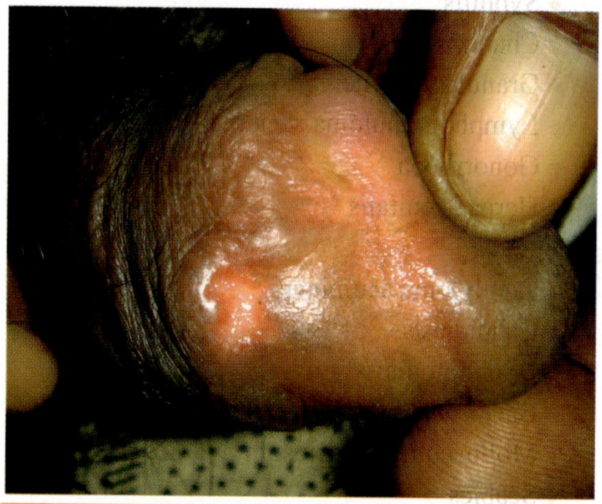

Fig. 2: Painless punched out ulcer at the corona of 2 weeks duration (Courtesy: Dr. Piyush Kumar, PGT)

Clinical features of secondary syphilis

- There is a dictum that in secondary syphilis all forms of primary skin lesions develop except vesiculobullous which may be seen at palms and soles in congenital syphilis.

- Primary lesions are macules, papules, pustules or acneiform eruptions.
- Earliest lesions are faint macules and lesions which develop later are more papulosquamous.
- Papules are firm but mucosal or intertriginous papules, known as **condyloma lata**, are soft in consistency and are having moist surface.
- Macules and papules are round or oval in shape and plaques may be annular or polycyclic.
- Arciform plaques are usually seen in relapsing secondary syphilis.
- Lesions are scattered and discrete with a tendency of symmetric distribution.
- Special sites are hairline, nasolabial fold, scalp, neck, palms and soles.
- Other than condylomata lata mucous patches are seen at oral and genital mucosae as well as split papules at angle of the mouth. These patches are asymptomatic, small, round or oval, mild elevated, flat-topped and are covered by grayish membrane.
- Scalp hairs may be diffusely lost including temporal and parietal region or patchy moth-eaten alopecia and loss of eyelashes or lateral third of eyebrows.
- Generalized lymphadenopathy including cervical, suboccipital, epitrochlear, inguinal and axillary groups, associated with splenomegaly are often present.
- Fever, arthralgia, nocturnal tibial pain due to periostitis, iritis, uveitis, optic neuritis, pharyngitis, gastritis, hepatitis, proctitis, cystitis, prostitis, nephritic syndrome or glomerulonephritis are seen in some cases.

Investigation

- **Dark-field microscopic** examination of the serous fluid collected from the lesion for direct demonstration of the spirochetes. These are recognized as corkscrew like organisms, 5-20 μm in length and showing rotatory contractile movements.

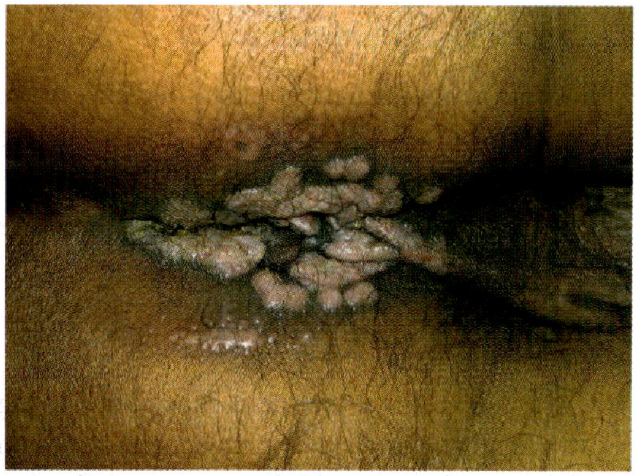

Fig. 3: Flat-topped moist confluent papules around the anus

- **Direct fluorescent Treponema pallidum antibody test** to detect the spirochetes within the exudates.
- PCR may be used for direct demonstration of treponema pallidum antigen.
- Rapid plasma reagin test (RPR) and VDRL test are nontreponemal antibody detection tests. These tests may be negative when antibody is in very high concentration, known as **prozone phenomenon**.
- FTA-Abs test and MHA-TP test are treponemal antibody detection test.
- Histopathology of the lesion shows ulceration in chancre and psoriasiform hyperplasia of lesion of secondary syphilis with lymphocytic and plasmacytic dermal infiltration, proliferation of capillaries and lymphocytic endarteritis.

Treatment of primary, secondary and early latent syphilis

- Benzathine penicillin G 2.4 million units is given intramuscularly as 1.2 million units in each buttock.
- In case of penicillin sensitivity, doxycycline 100 mg twice daily for 2 weeks.

- In case of penicillin sensitivity with pregnancy, desensitization to be done and then penicillin to be given.

Chancroid/soft chancre

- It is an acute sexually transmitted infection, caused by *Hemophilus ducreyi*, a gram-negative streptobacillus.
- It is mostly transmitted during sexual intercourse and it acts as cofactor for transmission of HIV infection.
- Incubation period is 4-7 days.
- Disease develops at the site of inoculation along with regional lymphadenopathy due to initiation of delayed hypersensitivity reaction following accumulation of CD4+ and CD8+ T lymphocytes and macrophages.
- With treatment ulcer heals within 7-14 days.
- Sexual partner should be examined and to be treated accordingly.

Clinical features

- Primary lesion starts as a tender papule with an erythematous halo which gradually turns into a transient pustule followed by formation of an ulcer.
- Ulcer is painful and tender with undermined edge and sharp border.
- Floor of the ulcer contains friable granulation tissue and gray yellow exudates and base is not indurated.
- Edema of the prepuce is commonly associated when male genitalia is affected.
- Shape of the ulcer is usually round but may be irregular or serpiginous.
- Number of the ulcer is usually single but may be multiple.
- Common sites in male are prepuce, frenulum, coronal sulcus, glans penis, and shaft, and in female are fourchette, labia, vestibule, clitoris, vaginal wall, introitus, cervix and perianal area.
- Extragenital sites are breast, fingers, oral mucosa and thighs.
- In 50% cases, painful inguinal lymphadenopathy develops after 1 to 3 weeks of primary lesion. Gradually inflamed lymph node turns into unilocular abscess or bubo. It may burst and drain spontaneously. Sometimes bubo forms after spontaneous healing of the ulcer.

- Detection of the organism may be done by gram stain, culture or PCR, but all these are not very easy.

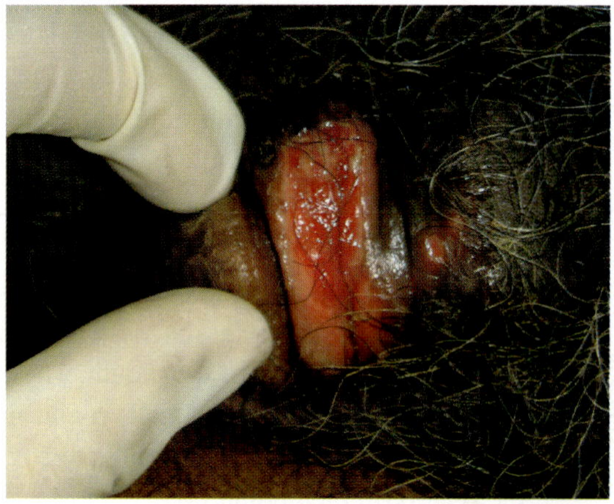

Fig. 4: One large ulcer at inner prepuce and two small ulcers at shaft of the penis (Courtesy: Dr. Piyush Kumar, PGT)

Histopathology

- It shows three different zones of infiltration.
  - Outer zone contains neutrophilic infiltration.
  - Middle zone contains lymphocytic infiltration around the vessels.
  - Deeper zone contains fibrotic changes.

Treatment

- Any of the followings:
  - Azithromycin 1 g orally a single dose.
  - Ceftriaxone 250 mg intramuscularly as a single dose.
  - Erythromycin 500 mg orally bid for 7 days.
  - Ciprofloxacin 500 mg orally bid for 3 days.

Gonorrhoea

- It is also an acute sexually transmitted infection, caused by *Neisseria gonorrhoeae* (gonococcus) a gram-negative diplococcus. In upto 40% cases, it is coinfected with *Chlamydia trachomatis* infection.
- It is mostly transmitted through sexual intercourse.
- Incubation period is 3-5 days in male but little more in female.
- Gonococcus has affinity for columnar epithelium and stratified or squamous epithelium are more resistant to this infection.

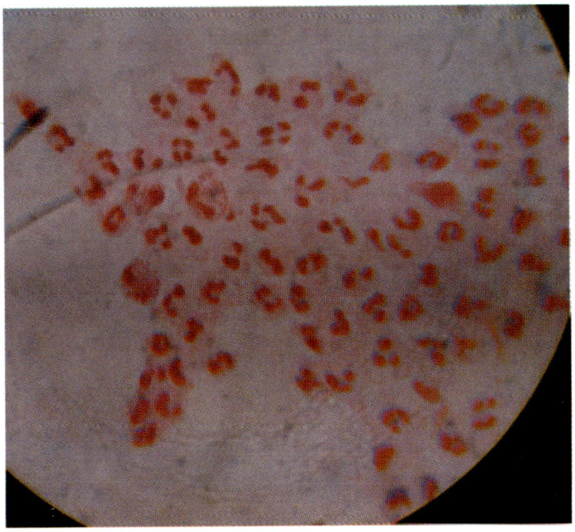

Fig. 5: Intracellular gram negative diplococci

Clinical features

- Male patients usually present with purulent urethral discharge and dysuria. Amount of discharge is variable from scanty to profuse and quality of discharge is variable from copius to clear.
- It is often associated with edema of the meatus, prepuce and glans. In uncircumscribed men often have a balanoposthitis with accumulation of subprepucial discharge and in circumcised men have only balanitis.
- Deeper structures may be involved and produce prostatitis, epididymitis, vesiculitis and cystitis.
- Folliculitis or cellulitis may develop at thighs or lower abdomen in both males and females.
- Female patients often present with dysuria and purulent urethral discharge due to urethritis and deep pelvic or lumbar pain due to cervicitis. Deeper structures may be involved and produce peritonitis, endocervicitis, endosalpingitis, endometritis and all these are termed as pelvic inflammatory disease (PID).
- Vagina is not affected due to squamous cell guard.
- Anorectal involvement produces tenesmus, burning or stinging pain during defecation, blood stained stool and purulent discharge.
- Pharyngeal involvement produces mild sore throat with erythema due to pharyngitis.
- Eye involvement produces profuse purulent discharge, conjunctivitis, corneal ulceration, severe hyperemia, chemosis, swollen eyelids. During delivery eyes of the newborn may be affected, known as ophthalmia neonatorum.
- Acral hemorrhagic pustules may develop in disseminated gonococcal infection.

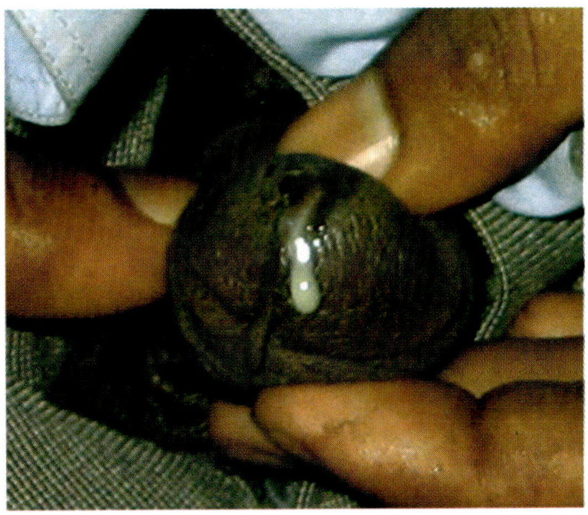

Fig. 6: Purulent discharge from the urethral meatus

- Diagnosis can be confirmed by Gram stain which demonstrates gram-negative intracellular diplococci and by culture.

Treatment

- Ceftriaxone, 125 mg/250 mg intramuscularly, as a single dose.
- Doxycycline 100 mg bid for 7 days.

Trichomoniasis

- It is caused by a protozoa, *Trichomonus vaginalis*.
- Incubation period is 4-28 days.
- Vaginal pH is > 4.5.
- In females vaginitis and cervicitis develop.
- In males urethritis develops.
- Protozoa can be demonstrated directly under microscope as a motile organism.
- Gold standard to confirm the diagnosis in cases where direct microscopy failed, is culture in Diamond media, in modified Diamond media or in Feinberg-Whittington media.

Clinical features

- In females:
  - Profuse homogeneous malodorous vaginal discharge.
  - Color of the discharge is yellowish white or greenish yellow.
  - Cervix shows punctate hemorrhage, often called as strawberry cervix.
  - Abdominal pain may be a presenting feature of severe vaginitis or cervicitis.
- In males:
  - Dysuria, urgency and postcoital burning sensation.

Treatment

- Tab Metronidazole 2 g as a single dose.

Bacterial vaginosis

- It is a common disorder presented with vaginal discharge.
- It develops following aberration of normal vaginal flora. Basically non-pathogenic lactobacilli are replaced by other pathogenic organisms.
- Commonest organisms are *Gardenella vaginalis* in 50% cases, *Mycoplasma hominis*, and *Mobiluncus spp*.
- As pathologically no inflammation occurs at vaginal wall, the term vaginosis is used instead of vaginitis.
- It is commonly seen in middle aged females aged between 20-40 years of age with a peak at 30 years.
- Vaginal pH is > 4.5.
- Fishy odor is produced when few drops of 10% KOH is mixed with discharge. This test is known as Amine test or Whiff test.
- Demonstration of clue cells in vaginal discharge helps in diagnosis.
- Clue cells are nothing but vaginal epithelial cells, studded with causative organisms.
- Nugent score > 30 is diagnostic.
- Nugent score is based on presence of Lactobacillus as large Gram positive organisms, Gram negative or Gram variable organisms and Gram negative curved organisms.
- Score is counted according to the presence of bacilli per oil immersion field (OIF).
- Score is variable from 4+ to 1+ if lactobacilli are present ranging from no bacilli to > 30 per OIF.
- Score is variable from 1+ to 4+ if other organisms are present ranging from no bacilli to > 30 per OIF.

Clinical features

- Non-viscous, malodorous vaginal discharge which is uniformly adherent at the wall.

Treatment

- Intravaginal clindamycin 100g daily for 3 days, specially in pregnancy.
- Metronidazole 400 mg twice daily for 7 days.

Lymphogranuloma venereum

- It is a sexually transmitted disease, caused by *Chlamydia trachomatis*, serotype L1, L2 and L3 and primarily lymphatics and lymph nodes are affected.

- Incubation period is 2-12 days for primary phase and 10-30 days for secondary phase.
- Affection of lymphatics and lymph nodes depends on site of primary inoculation:
  - Inguinal group of lymph nodes are affected when inoculation sites are penis, vulva, anus and anterior urethra.
  - Perirectal or deep iliac groups of lymph nodes are affected when primary inoculation sites are posterior urethra, vagina, cervix and rectum.

Clinical features

- Primary phase is transient and observed only in 1/3rd of cases in males and rarely seen in females. Lesion starts as a painless small papule, vesicle or grouped vesicles (herpetiform) or ulcer at the site of inoculation, such as penis, labia, posterior vagina or fourchette. This lesion heals quickly within few days.
- Secondary phase starts with painful swelling of inguinal lymph nodes, the most common presentation, after 2-6 weeks of sexual exposure. Unilateral lymph nodes are involved in 2/3rd cases. Initially nodes are discrete, but gradually become matted due to progressive periadenitis and turn into a single suppurative and fluctuant multilocular abscess or bubo.
- Overlying skin becomes thin and it ruptures in 1/3rd cases to form multiple sinuses.
- When lymph nodes above and below the inguinal ligaments, i.e., inguinal and femoral lymph nodes respectively, both are involved, a groove is formed in between, known as groove sign. But this sign is nonspecific. In 75% cases deep iliac nodes are involved and present as pelvic mass which rarely suppurate.
- Sometimes in male patient, a cordlike lymphangitis along the dorsal surface of the penis may be seen or lymphangeal nodule may be formed. This nodule is known as bubonulus. Gradually it may rupture to form multiple discharging sinuses and fistulas, connecting the urethra.
- In case of anal intercourse, hemorrhagic proctitis develops and regional lymphadentitis, such as intestinal and perirectal lymphatics are involved. Overgrowth of lymphatic tissue presents like hemorrhoids or perianal condylomata. This may be complicated by formation of perirectal abscess and ischiorectal, anal and rectovaginal fistulas, followed by formation of rectal stricture.
- After 1-20 years of primary infection, specially in females, elephantiasis of genitalia may develop with multiple ulceration, known as esthiomene.
- Erythema nodosum like lesions develop in 10% cases.

Treatment

- Doxycycline 100 mg twice daily or erythromycin 500 mg 6 hourly for 3 weeks.

Differential diagnosis of bubo

- Pseudobubo
- Chancroid
- Scrofuloderma
- Pyogenic adenopathy
- Carbuncle.

Granuloma venereum/Donovanosis

- It is a rare sexually transmitted disease, caused by *Calymmatobacterium granulomatis/donovani*. These are encapsulated, gram-negative, intracellular rods.
- Touch or crushed smear is made from punch biopsy specimen of the lesion and organisms are demonstrated as safetypin like Donovan bodies within the cytoplasm of the macrophages.
- Incubation period is variable from 8-80 days and average is 30 days.

Clinical features

- Lesion starts as button like papule or subcutaneous nodule which gradually ulcerates within few days.

- Common sites are prepuce, glans, shaft of the penis or scrotum in males and labia minora, mons veneris or fourchette in females. Extragenital sites are face, lips and mouth.
- Ulcer is sharply defined but irregular in shape.
- It is having a beefy-red surface due to granulation tissue with a tendency to bleed on touch.
- Though the ulcer is painless but due to secondary anerobic infection, it often produces pain and foul smell.
- Large subcutaneous nodular lesion mimicks swollen lymph node, designated as pseudobubo.
- Clinical variants are ulcerovegetative, nodular, hypertrophic and cicatricial/sclerotic.

Treatment

- Trimethoprim-sulfamethoxazole (double strength) or doxycycline 100 mg twice daily for at least 3 weeks.

Differential diagnosis

- Chancroid
- Herpes genitalis
- Squamous cell carcinoma

Genital candidiasis

- It is caused by *Candida albicans*, one of the common normal inhabitant of vagina.
- It is often associated with pregnancy, diabetes mellitus, antibiotics and drugs like tamoxifen.
- Male partner of an affected female may suffer from candidal balanoposthitis.
- KOH test shows pseudohyphae and fungal culture confirms the diagnosis.

Clinical features

- Commonest symptoms are pruritus and burning sensation.
- Labia, prepuce and glans become erythematous, moist and macerated or fissured.
- Vagina contains white discharge.
- Cervix becomes hyperemic, edematous and eroded.
- Cervix may be studded with tiny vesicles.
- Quality and quantity of vaginal discharge vary from mild to profuse and from watery to whitish or curdlike.

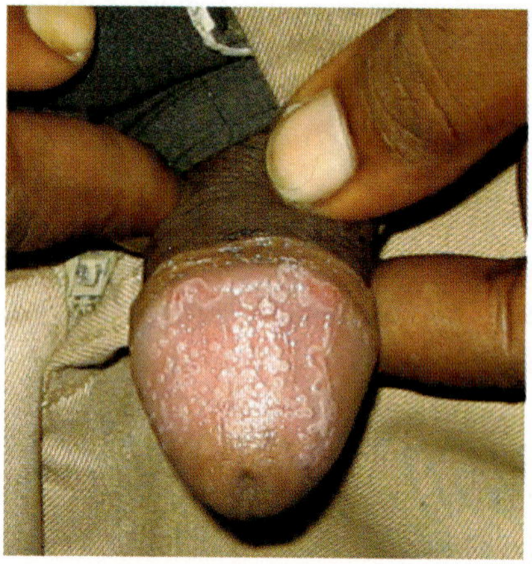

Fig. 7: Multiple discrete tiny erosions covered with whitish membrane

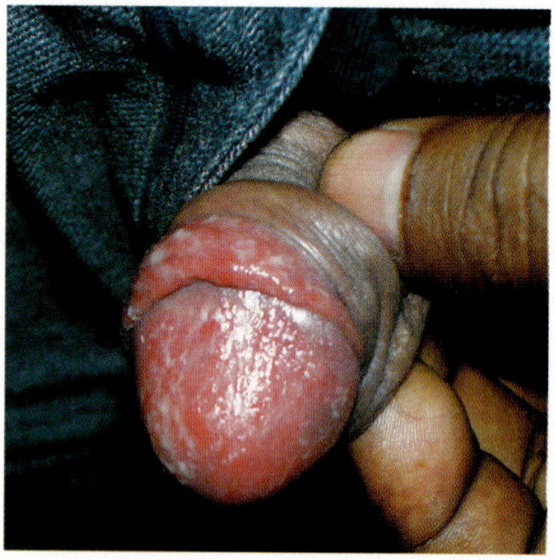

Fig. 8: Confluence of tiny erosions with curdy discharge (Courtesy: Dr. Piyush Kumar, PGT)

Treatment

- Single dose of oral fluconazole 150 mg.
- In resistant cases, fluconazole 100-200 mg per day or itraconazole 100-200 mg per day for 5-10 days.

- Topical nystatin, miconazole and terconazole may be given.

Herpes genitalis

- It is an acute, chronic and recurrent sexually transmitted infection, caused by herpes simplex virus (HSV).
- HSV2 infection is more common than HSV1.
- It mostly transmits through sexual intercourse.
- Incubation period is 5-7 days, ranging from 2-20 days.
- Prior HSV1 infection may provide some amount of protection against HSV2 infection.
- Primary lesions develop at the site of inoculation. After this primary infection, HSV ascends along the peripheral sensory nerves and enters the sensory or autonomic nerve root ganglia. Then remains there as a latent phase. Later it recurs in a favourable time.
- Infection is mostly asymptomatic as in 90% cases and symptomatic only in 10% cases.
- Anorectal herpes is often caused by HSV1.
- Tzanck smear prepared from the floor of the vesicle, may demonstrate multinucleated giant keratinocytes.
- Diagnosis may be confirmed by viral culture or direct fluorescent antibody test or serological test.

Clinical features of primary infection

- General symptoms are fever, headache, malaise and myalgia, occurring within 3-4 days of infection and resolving by 3-4 days of onset of the lesions.
- Localized symptoms like pain, itching, dysuria and lumbar radiculitis develop depending on the sites of involvement.
- Primary lesions are grouped vesicle with an erythematous background. These may turn into transient pustule, followed by formation of erosions or ulcers.
- Erosions or ulcers are sharply defined and tender. They may remain discrete or coalesce to form a larger ulcer.
- Ulcers or erosions heal within 2-4 weeks with hypo-/hyperpigmentation and rarely with scarring.
- Tender inguinal lymphadenopathy may develop within 2-3 weeks. Deep pelvic pain may be present due to deep inguinal lymph node involvement.
- Lymph nodes become tender and firm.
- Vaginal or urethral discharge may be associated in some cases.
- Common sites of involvement are glans, prepuce, shaft, sulcus, scrotum, thigh and buttocks in males and labia majora/minora, perineum and inner thighs in females.

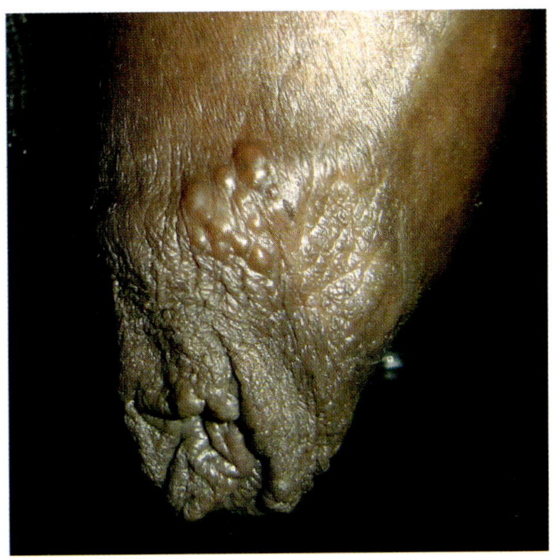

Fig. 9: Grouped vesicles (Courtesy: Dr. Piyush Kumar, PGT)

Clinical features of recurrent herpes genitalis

- Common symptoms are itching, burning, irritation prior to onset.
- Primary lesions are same but less severe.
- Erosions or ulcers heal more quickly within 1-2 weeks.

Clinical features of anorectal herpes

- ♦ Tenesmus, anal pain, proctitis, discharge and ulceration are the common features.
- ♦ Lesions may develop as far as 10 cm into the anal canal.

Clinical features in association with HIV infection

- ♦ Anorectal herpes is common.
- ♦ Lesions are larger in size, persist for longer time and heal with scarring.

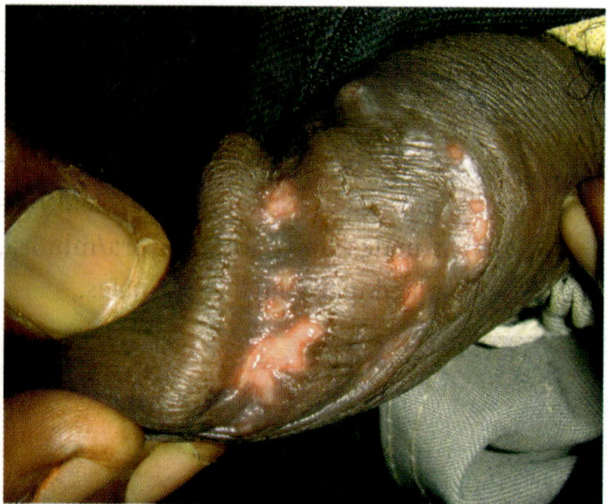

Fig. 10: Multiple round, oval and irregular ulcers in a HIV infected patient (Courtesy: Dr. Piyush Kumar, PGT)

- ✶ Histopathology shows intraepidermal as well as subepidermal vesicle with characteristic **ballooning degeneration.**

Treatment of primary infection

- ♦ Acyclovir 400 mg thrice or valacyclovir 1000 mg twice or pencyclovir 250 mg twice daily for 7-10 days or until clinical resolution occurs.
- ♦ To reduce the frequency of recurrence, acyclovir 400 mg twice daily may be given for 1 year.

Condyloma acuminanata

- ✶ It is nothing but verruca vulgaris or wart, affecting the anogenital area and it is caused by *Human papilloma virus* (HPV). It is highly infectious.
- ✶ It is mostly transmitted through sexual intercourse.
- ✶ Incubation period is variable from weeks to months to years such as 3 weeks to 8 months.
- ✶ There are more than 20 types of HPV affecting the genitalia.
  - ♦ Most common serotypes-6, 11
  - ♦ Serotypes associated with dysplasia and carcinoma-16, 18, 31, 33, 35.
- ✶ The DNA virion of HPV enters the basal layer and proliferates along with basal cell divisions to produce a hyperkeratotic epidermal growth.
- ✶ In benign lesion, virion acts as a plasmid in cellular cytoplasm and replicating extrachromosomally. But in malignant or dysplastic lesion, virion integrates into host chromosome and E1 and E2 regions of the virion become dysregulated, resulting in malignant transformation.
- ✶ HPV infection may remain in a dormant state for years and becomes infectious intermittently.
- ✶ Exophytic lesions are more infective than subclinical infection.
- ✶ Immunosuppressed state favours to produce extensive lesions and makes them recalcitrant for treatment.
- ✶ Spontaneous regression occurs in 10-30% cases within 3 months but even after such regression subclinical infection may persist for whole life.
- ✶ Recurrence more commonly occurs from subclinical infection rather than reinfection.

Clinical features

- ♦ Lesions are asymptomatic but rarely associated with itching, burning, bleeding, vaginal or urethral discharge and dyspareunia.
- ♦ Primary lesions may be small papules, flat-topped papules or plaques, vary much keratotic and cauliflower like plaques. Flat-topped lesions are commonly seen at cervix.
- ♦ Color of the lesion is also variable from skin color to pink, red, tan and brown.
- ♦ Lesions may be solitary, few or confluent mass. Lesion becomes huge in immunosuppressed state.

- Application of acetic acid makes the lesions more visible.

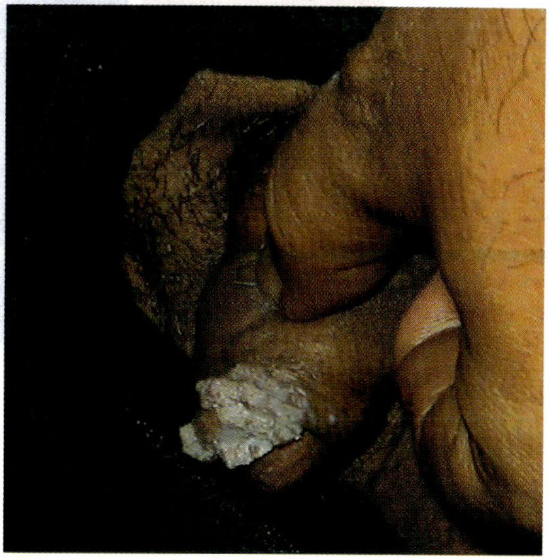

Fig. 11: Verrucous plaque at prepuce.

- Common sites in males are frenulum, corona, glans, prepuce, specially at junction of inner and outer prepuce, shaft and scrotum, and in females labia, clitoris, periurethral area, perineum, vagina and cervix.
- In both sexes, perianal, anal canal, rectal, urethral meatus, urethra, bladder and oropharynx also may be affected.

Differential diagnosis

- Tuberculosis verrucosa cutis
- Verrucous carcinoma
- Chromoblastomycosis

Histopathology

- Hyperkeratosis
- Tier of parakeratosis
- Papillomatosis and acanthosis
- Presence of koilocytes
- Bending of peripheral rete ridges towards the center, known as arborization.

Treatment

- Application of 5% imiquimod or 25% podophyllin or 80-90% trichloroacetic acid.
- Electro/cryo-/laser surgery.
- In pregnancy, trichloroacetic acid or cryosurgery is the best choice.

CHAPTER C8

DERMATITIS/ECZEMA

Dermatitis

- The term eczema or dermatitis is often used interchangeably.
- It is clinically manifested with a wide range of polymorphous eruptions due to a variable reaction pattern in both epidermis and dermis.

Types

- According to etiology:
  - Exogenous
  - Endogenous
- According to clinical stage
  - Acute
  - Subacute
  - Chronic
- According to severity
  - Mild: <20% body surface area involvement.
  - Moderate: 20-50% body surface area involvement.
  - Severe: >50% body surface area involvement.

Exogenous subtypes

- Irritant contact dermatitis
- Allergic contact dermatitis
- Combined allergic-irritant contact dermatitis

Endogenous subtypes

- Atopic dermatitis
- Seborrheic dermatitis
- Pompholyx
- Nummular/discoid dermatitis
- Asteatotic dermatitis
- Stasis dermatitis
- Id eruption
- Miscellaneous

  #Pityriasis alba

  #Fingertip dermatitis

  #Forefoot dermatitis

  #Hyperkeratotic dermatitis

  #Lichen simplex chronicus

Allergic contact dermatitis

- It is a classical example of delayed cell-mediated hypersensitivity reaction.
- Allergen is taken up and processed by the Langerhans cell and then presented to the T cells within the regional lymph nodes with the help of MHC class II molecules. In response, T cells proliferate and reach to the home site of the skin from the lymph nodes through the circulation to

face the rechallenge. During the rechallenge with similar type of antigens, inflammatory cytokines are released from the sensitized T cells, keratinocytes and Langerhans cells. This results in dermatitis.

* The eruption starts in a sensitized person usually within 48 hours or sometimes days after contact with allergens.
* Initially lesions are localized to the sites of contact, such as earlobe in case of contact with earring and dorsum of the foot in case of contact with shoe. But gradually it extends to become generalized.
* So initially area of the lesion may maintain the pattern of the contact but gradually that pattern is lost.
* Initially lesions remain confined within the area of contact and gradually that localization is lost.
* Lesions are confluent and prominent at the center and are mild and discrete at the periphery.
* Irritant contact dermatitis is the most common form of occupational dermatitis, occurring in 80% cases.
* Secondary infection often complicates dermatitis and produces infected dermatitis.

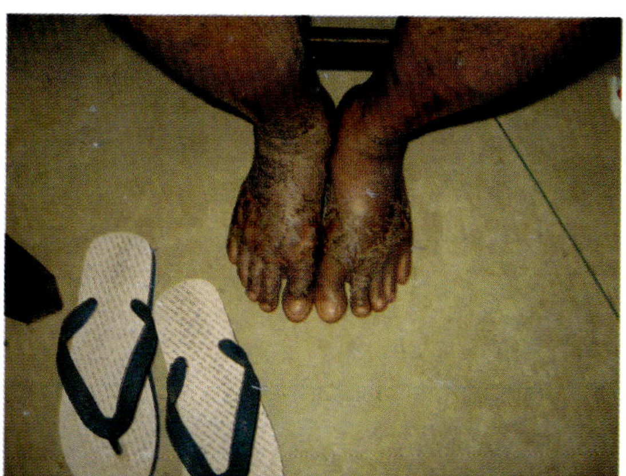

Fig. 1: Lesions confined within contact area of the shoes, a hall mark of contact dermatitis. Lesions at right side spread beyond the site of contact

* Sometimes dermatitis develops following superficial pyogenic infection, designated as infective eczematoid dermatitis.
* Duration and severity is variable and gets worse following continuation of contact with allergen. Some cases may resolve by 1-2 weeks.

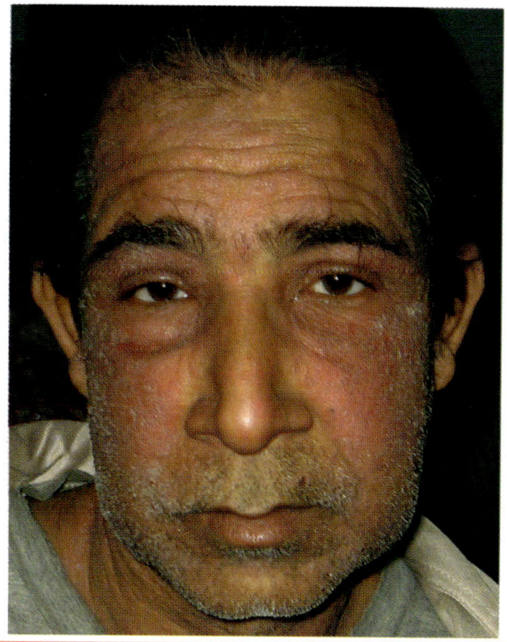

Fig. 2: Erythematous papular lesions due to contact with hair dye

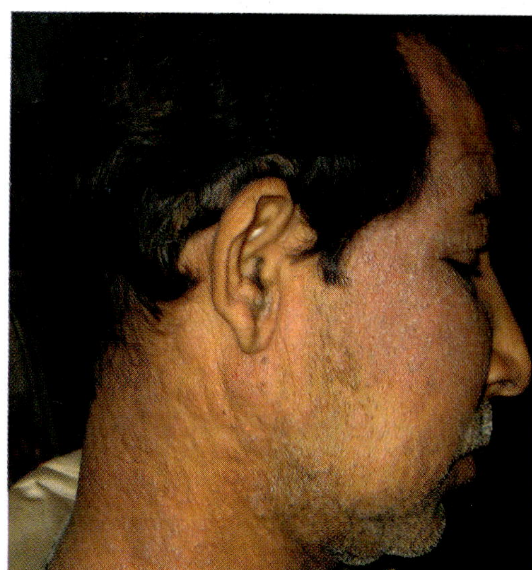

Fig. 3: Erythematous mild scaly and papular eruption of contact dermatitis at face and neck

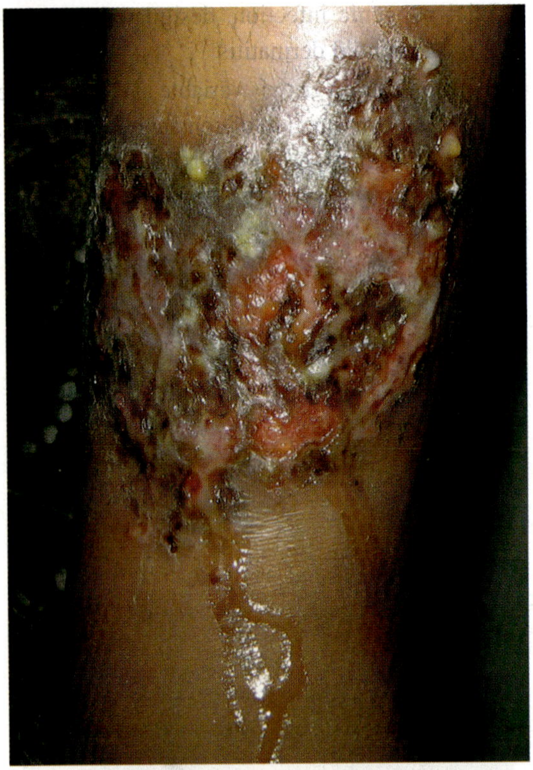

Fig. 4: Ulceration, oozing and crusting and presence of secondary infection in acute dermatitis

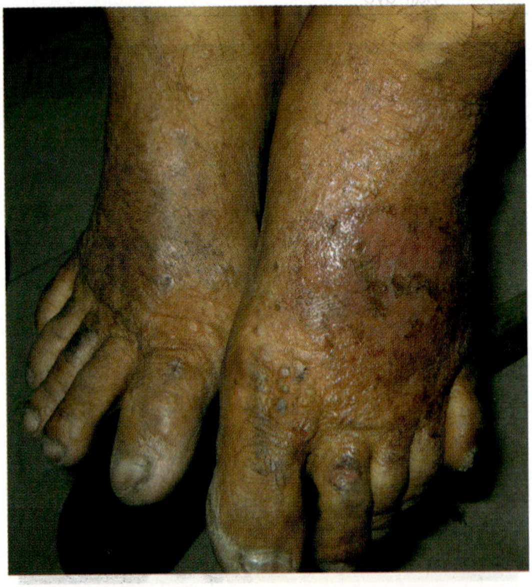

Fig. 5: Crusted erosion at the center with discrete papules at the periphery in subacute dermatitis

Clinical features of acute ACD

- Onset of pruritic papules, papulovesicles, non-umbilicated vesicles with a background of erythema and edema is the earliest feature. In severe cases, bullae, erosions or ulceration, oozing and crusting also develop.
- Discharge may be purulent or hemorrhagic due to secondary infection.

Clinical features of subacute ACD

- Lesions are mild erythematous and minimally oozy but mostly crusted. Sometimes these are associated with firm erythematous and crusted papules.

Clinical features of chronic ACD

- Lichenified plaques and satellite papules with variable amount of scaling are the main features.
- Lesions become hyperpigmented, thickened with exaggerated skin markings.

Patch test

- It helps to detect the allergen.
- It should not be done in presence of active disease.
- Patient should be disease free for at least 2 weeks prior to patch testing.
- Patch should be applied only on the previously unaffected skin, preferably at the back.

Histopathology of acute dermatitis

- Epidermal atrophy in severe form.
- Intraepidermal intercellular edema, known as spongiosis and lymphocytic and eosinophilic exocytosis.
- Lymphohistiocytic infiltration in the dermis with dermal edema.

Histopathology of subacute dermatitis

- Hyperkeratosis and mild to moderate acanthosis.
- Mild spongiosis with lymphocytic infiltration in the epidermis (exocytosis).
- Lymphohistiocytic infiltration in the dermis.

Histopathology of chronic dermatitis

- Hyperkeratosis, acanthosis and rarely spongiosis.
- Mild dermal lymphocytic infiltration.

Treatment for acute or subacute dermatitis

- Avoidance of the allergens.
- Application of Condy's compress or Burrow's solution for oozing, followed by application of calamine lotion for widespread lesions or moderately potent corticosteroid gel for focal lesion.
- Systemic antibiotic for presence of infection, i.e., in presence of purulent discharge.
- Systemic corticosteroid in a dose of 30-40 mg prednisolone/day for 1-2 weeks, when lesions are extensive or no improvement after 1 week of conventional therapy.

Treatment for chronic dermatitis

- Avoidance of friction or rubbing or scatching.
- Administration of sedative antihistaminic for itching.
- Application of potent topical corticosteroid, like clobetasol propionate or halobetasol or steroid-salicylic acid combination.

Variants of allergic contact dermatitis (ACD)

- Photoallergic contact dermatitis
- Follicular ACD
- Pustular ACD
- Purpuric ACD
- Ichthyotic ACD
- Leukodermic ACD
- Dermal ACD
- Granulomatous ACD
- Lymphomatoid ACD

Irritant contact dermatitis (ICD)

* It is the result of acute or chronic irritation of the skin, caused by chemical or physical agents.

Factors modifying the clinical manifestations

- Potency of the irritant agents.
- Duration and repetition of contact.
- Site of exposure.
- Pre-existing condition of thc skin.
- Environmental factors.

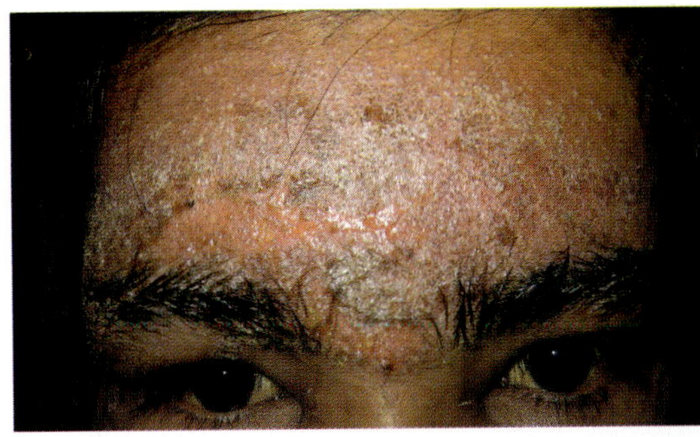

Fig. 6: Erythematous patch with crusting, pustules and erosion

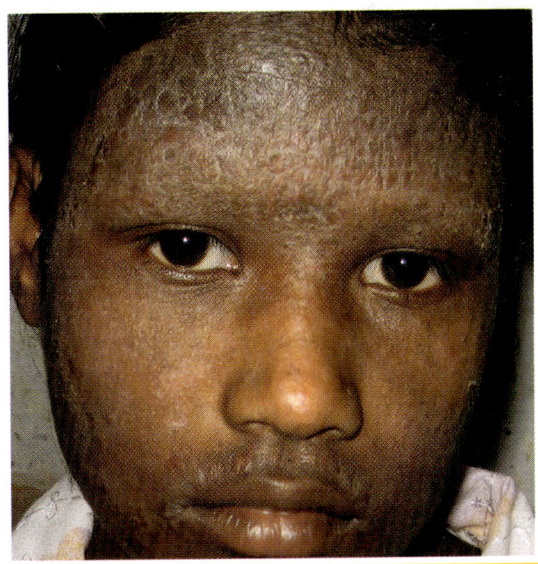

Fig. 7: Profuse crusting following application of adapalene

Time for initiation of subjective symptoms

- Start within seconds after contact with acids, chloroform, methanol, etc.
- Starts within 1-2 minutes, peaks after 5-10 minutes and fades after 30 minutes following contact with aluminium chloride, phenol, propylene glycol, etc.

- Starts within 8-24 hours following contact with anthralin, ethylene oxide, benzalconium chloride, etc. In this case itching is more prominent than burning sensation.
- Subjective symptoms are burning, stinging, and smarting pain sensations. Itching may present in late stage.
- In comparison to ACD, papules do not develop in ICD.

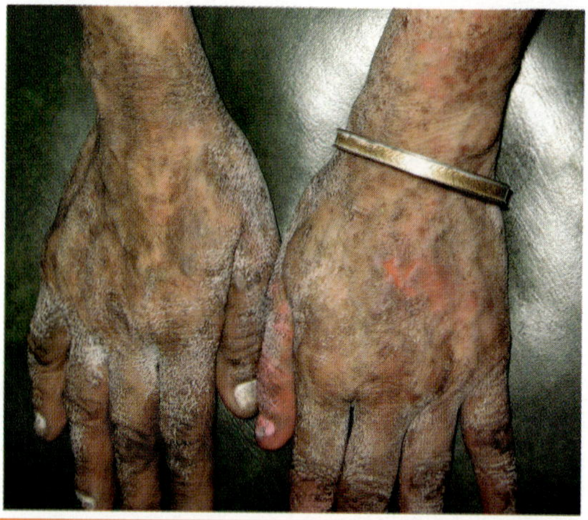

Fig. 8: Xerotic skin with scaling, crusting and erosion due to frequent washing of the hand with raw washing powder

Clinical features of acute ICD

- Lesions start as intense erythema at the contact area, followed by vesiculation, erosion or ulceration or even necrosis, oozing and crusting depending on the potency of the irritant substance.
- Affected area is usually well demarcated.
- Lesions may heal with hyper-/hypo-depigmentation and with or without scarring.

Clinical features of chronic ICD

- Lesions start as mild erythema, xerosis or dryness, chapping or fissuring and scaling or mild crusting.
- Affected area is usually not sharply demarcated.

Treatment

- Avoidance of irritant substance.
- Application of Condy's compress or Burrow's solution for oozing, followed by application of calamine lotion.
- Systemic antibiotics for presence of secondary infection.
- Systemic corticosteroid is rarely prescribed for recalcitrant cases just to reduce inflammation rapidly.
- Chronic cases require frequent application of emollient.

Variants of irritant contact dermatitis (ICD)

- Acute ICD
- Delayed acute ICD
- Irritant reaction
- Cummulative ICD
- Acneiform/pustular ICD
- Asteatotic ICD
- Airborne ICD
- Frictional ICD
- Traumatic ICD
- Non-erythematous ICD
- Sensory ICD.

Atopic dermatitis (AD)

- It is a chronic and relapsing dermatitis, occuring mostly in infancy and having intense pruritus with dry skin.
- In 60% cases develop between 2 months to 1 year of age, 30% cases develop between 1-5 years of age and only 10% cases develop between 5 years to 20 years of age.
- Serum IgE level is often raised.
- Exact etiology is still unclear. It is due to a complex interaction between genetic, environmental and immunological responses. Following facts are associated:
  - In 80% children develop AD when both the parents had AD.
  - House dust mites and pollens are commonly associated with exacerbation of AD.
  - It usually flare in winter and improve in summer.

- Woollen cloths aggravate the pruritus.
- Egg, milk, fish, peanuts, soyabeans, beans, etc. also aggravate the disease.
- Disrupted barrier function of the skin due to reduced ceramide level, is responsible for easy entry of various allergens.
- Exotoxins of *Staphylococcus aureus* may act as superantigens which stimulate T cells and macrophages.
- Autoallergen from damaged tissue may trigger the formation of IgE antibody which helps to maintain the inflammation.
- There is a biphasic T cell response. In acute stage T cells produce interleukin 4 and interleukin 13, but in chronic stage, they produce interleukin 5, interleukin 12, interferon γ and granulocyte-monocyte colony stimulating factor (GM-CSF).

Clinical features

- Pruritus and dry skin or xerosis are consistent features of AD.
- White dermatographism is a unique feature of AD. It is elicited by stroking the skin which gives rise to blanching instead of redness as in case of normal skin.
- Morphology of the lesions varies from acute to chronic stage.

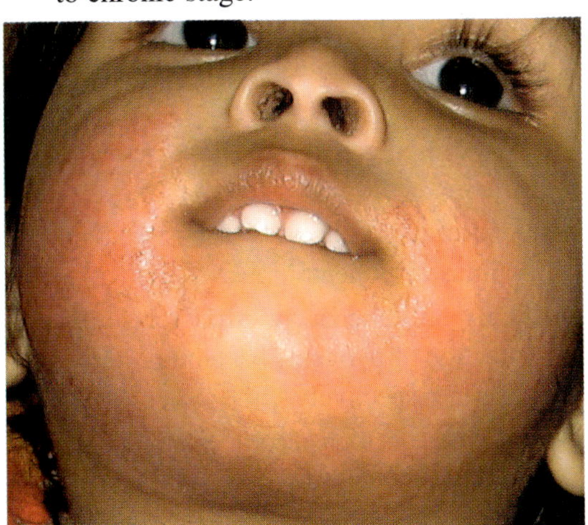

Fig. 9: Erythematous confluent and coalesced papules without any scale

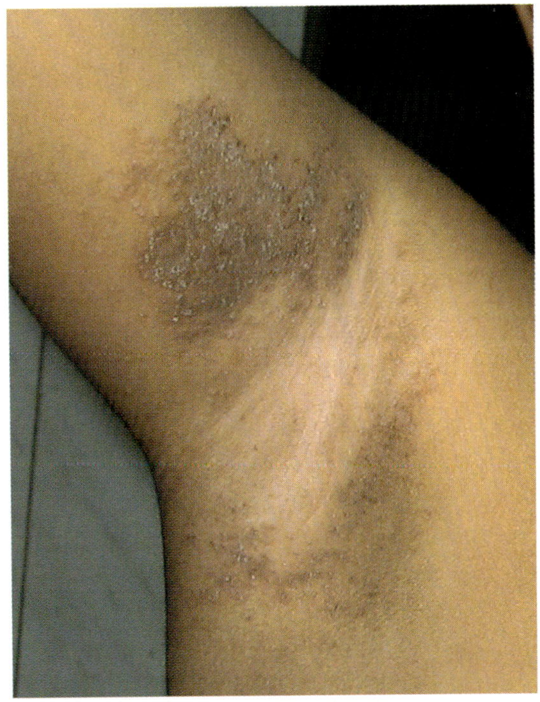

Fig. 10: Recurrent development of scaly papules

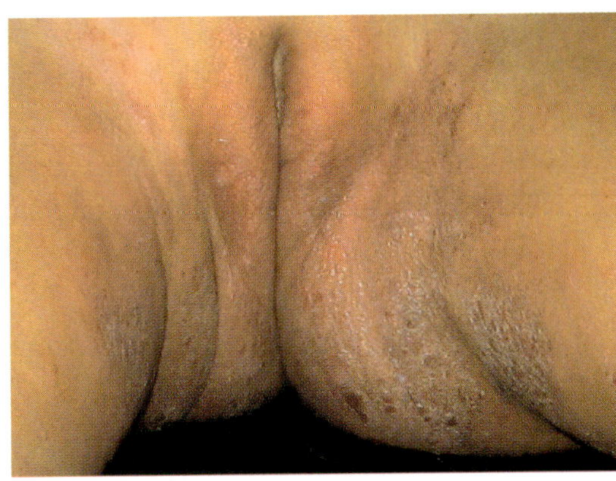

Fig. 11: Lichenoid papules with a background of erythema

Acute stage

- Lesions start as poorly defined erythematous patches studded with papules or papulovesicles. These papules or papulovesicles gradually become confluent and then coalesce to form plaques (Fig. 9).
- Skin in and around the lesions becomes puffy and edematous.

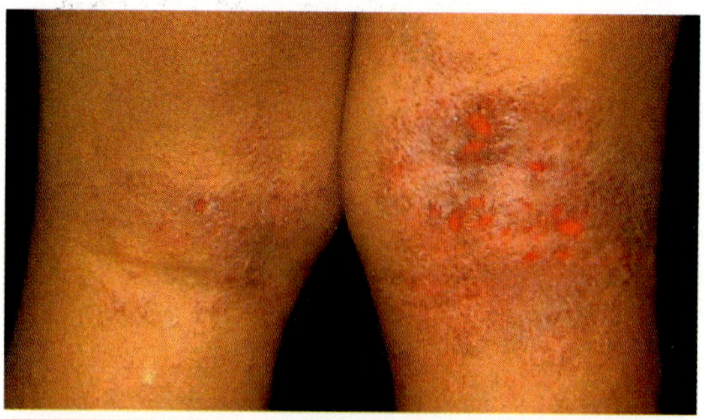

Fig. 12: Ill defined lichenified plaques, studded with papules, crust and erosions at popliteal fossae

- Linear or punctate erosions may be present due to vigorous scratching.
- Oozing and crusting may develop and may further be complicated by secondary infection such as pyoderma and Kaposi's varicelliform eruption.

Chronic stage

- Lesions become lichenified due to repeated rubbing and scratching with or without scaling and crusting.
- Brown and black person often develop lichenified follicular papules.
- In black people, a special form of discrete follicular papules develop, affecting all follicles of the involved site. This is known as follicular dermatitis.
- Alopecia of the lateral third of the eyebrows is known as Hertoghe's sign.
- Deepened infraorbital fold, known as Dennie-Morgan fold/sign, is also a characteristic feature.
- Periorbital pigmentation may be associated due to repeated rubbing.

Age related distribution

- Lesions may be localized or generalized but to some extent variable according to the age of the patient.
- In infancy: Commonly affected sites are scalp, cheeks and extensors of limbs.
- In childhood and adult: Flexor areas of elbows, knees, ankles, wrists, neck, dorsa of the hands and feet, eyelids and perioral region.

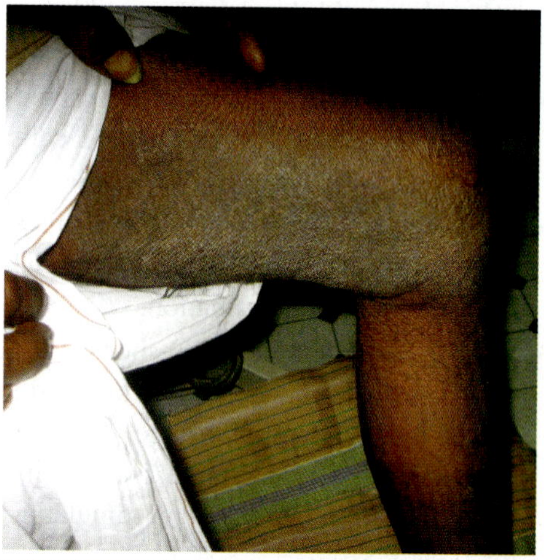

Fig. 13: Lichenified plaque with scaling and crusting

Histopathology

- Features depend on the morphology of the lesion; but the main feature is spongiotic dermatitis.

Treatment

- Avoidance of aggravating factors.
- Application of emollient containing antipruritic agents like camphor or menthol.
- Oral sedative antihistaminic such as hydroxyzine.
- Wet dressing with potasium permanganate solution or Burrow's solution in oozy state.
- Application of topical corticosteroid and tacrolimus or pimecrolimus.
- Oral antibiotic or antiviral for superadded infection of pyogenic bacteria or herpetic infection respectively.
- Use of potent topical corticosteroid for lichenified lesions.
- For recalcitrant cases systemic corticosteroid, cyclosporin, PUVA therapy, azathioprine and mycophenolate mofetil may be used.

Seborrheic dermatitis

- It is also one of the common and chronic endogenous dermatitis, having greasy scales at seborrheic areas where sebaceous glands are most active.
- Seborrheic areas are scalp, face, presternal area, interscapular area, axillae, groin and pubic region.
- It commonly occurs in infancy, puberty, between 20-50 years of age and even in older age.
- A hereditary diathesis is commonly associated with immunocompetent patient.
- Incidence is more in HIV infection and intractable seborrheic dermatitis often warrants to suspect HIV infection.
- Malassezia furfur may play a role in pathogenesis.
- Role of immunosuppression due to other causes than HIV, association of zinc and pyridoxine deficiency and association with Parkinson's disease are yet to be determined.
- Onset is slow and in some patients, it becomes worse in winter and improves in summer.

Clinical features

- Pruritus of variable amount is the main symptom.
- Common sites from above downwards are scalp, eyebrows, eyelashes, bearded area, forehead, butterfly area of the face, nasolabial folds, glabella, retroauricular spaces, external auditory meatus, axillae, suprasternal area, interscapular area, submammary regions, umbilicus, pubic area, groin and scrotum. It never involves palms and soles.
- Scaly macules, patches and papules are the main primary lesions.
- Quality and quantity of scales are very much variable. Scales are usually moist but may be dry in mild cases. These mild dry scales when develop on the scalp, is known as dandruff/ pityriasis sicca. It is sometimes associated with alopecia in severe cases.
- When forehead is affected, it is known as corona seborroica.
- Prominent hyperpigmentation and mild seborrheic dermatitis at seborrheic areas of the face is known as seborrheic melanosis.
- When scales on the patches become sticky to form crusts, lesions are also turned into well defined plaques. When these occur on infantile scalp, it is known as craddle cap. When these occur at trunk of infant or adult, the lesions may be of various forms like pityriasiform, petaloid form and nummular form.
- When lesions are localized at follicles, it is known as follicular seborrheic dermatitis and it is notoriously pruritic. It commonly occurs at beared area of face, axillae and pubic regions. Photosensitivity may be associated with facial lesion and in such cases it is often misdiagnosed as other photosensitive dermatoses.
- When lesions are mostly papular, it is known as papular seborrheic dermatitis. It commonly occurs at cheeks, back and chest.
- When it affects eyelid margins, it is known as seborrheic blepharitis.
- Lesions of the axillae, groin, submammary regions and umbilicus are sharply marginated and brightly erythematous. It is commonly associated with erosion and fissuring. These lesions are often be confused with candidiasis.
- In severe cases patient may turn into erythroderma.

Histopathology

- Hyperkeratosis with focal parakeratosis and intercellular edema (spongiosis).
- Collection of neutophils in the stratum corneum at the tips of the dilated follicles.

Treatment

- Regular use of shampoo containing selenium sulfide, ketoconazole, zinc pyrithione and tar for hairy areas.
- Application of mild potent topical corticosteroid like hydrocotisone and desonide for

nonhairy areas as well as severe involvement of hairy areas.

- In recalcitrant and severe cases systemic therapies are given including oral retinoids, doxycycline, minocycline and fluconazole.
- For cradle cap, application of warm oil, followed by shampoo and application of mild topical corticosteroid are required.
- For seborrheic blepharitis, corticosteroid containing eye ointment may be used.

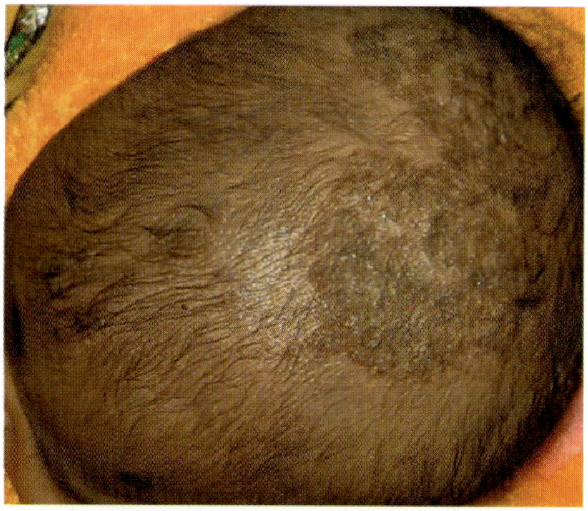

Fig. 14: Well defined plaque with creamy scales and crusts

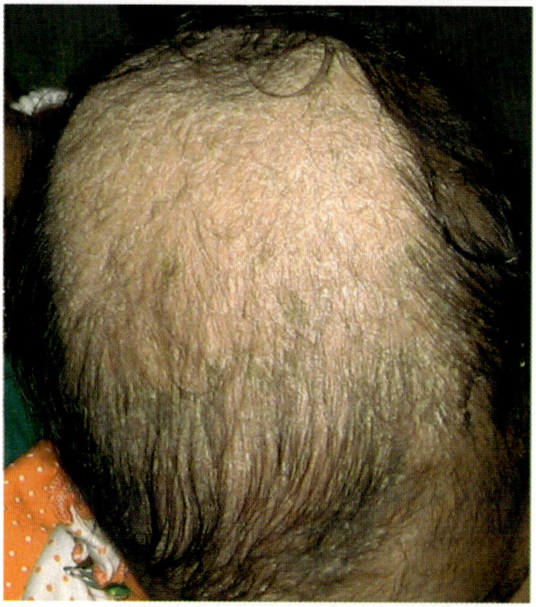

Fig. 15: Moist creamy scales on the scalp

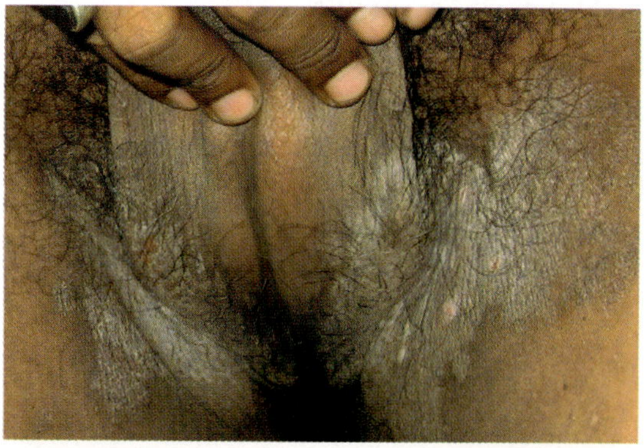

Fig. 16: Lichenified plaque of adult seborrheic dermatitis

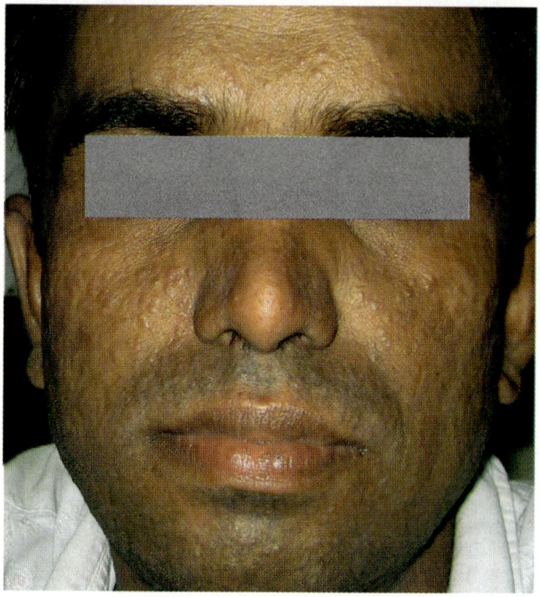

Fig. 17: Papular eruption of adult seborrheic dermatitis

Pompholyx/dyshidrosiform dermatitis/ vesicular palmar eczema

- It is an acute, chronic and recurrent vesicular eruptions of hands and feet.
- Recurrence is the rule and spontaneous healing occurs within 2-3 weeks.
- Interval between attacks is variable from weeks to months.

Clinical features

- Sudden onset of many deep seated vesicles or bullae, preceded by intense pruritus.

- It affects palms, soles, sides of the finger and toes, sides of the hands and feet, and rarely dorsa of the hands, feet, fingers and toes.
- Gradually fluid filled lesions are healed leaving by scales, fissures and thickening of the skin, leading to hyperkeratotic dermatitis.
- Secondary infection may form pustules, crusts, cellulitis, lymphangitis, painful lymphadenopathy and even disability.

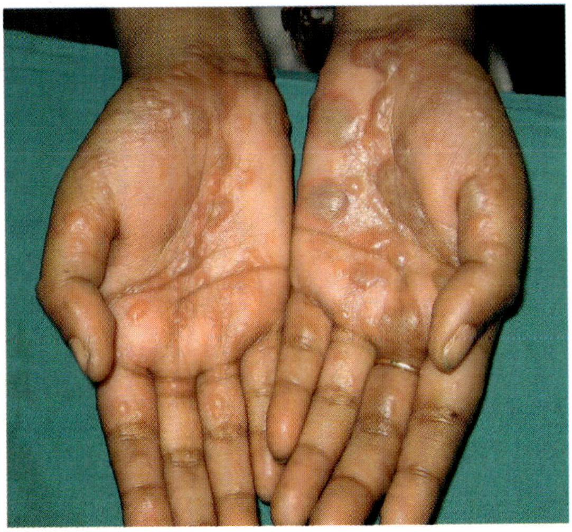

Fig. 18: Multiple vesicles and bullae at plams

Histopathology

- Hyperkeratosis with parakeratosis.
- Acanthosis with spongiosis.
- Intraepidermal spongiform vesicle.

Treatment

* For an acute attack:
  - Short course of systemic corticosteroid as oral prednisolone 40 mg/day for 7 days.
  - Systemic antibiotic for secondary infection.
  - Condy's compress for oozy condition.
* To prevent recurrence:
  - Application of potent topical corticosteroid.
  - PUVA therapy.
  - Methotrexate 7.5 mg/week.

Nummular dermatitis/Discoid eczema

* It commonly occurs in children and older persons in winter season.

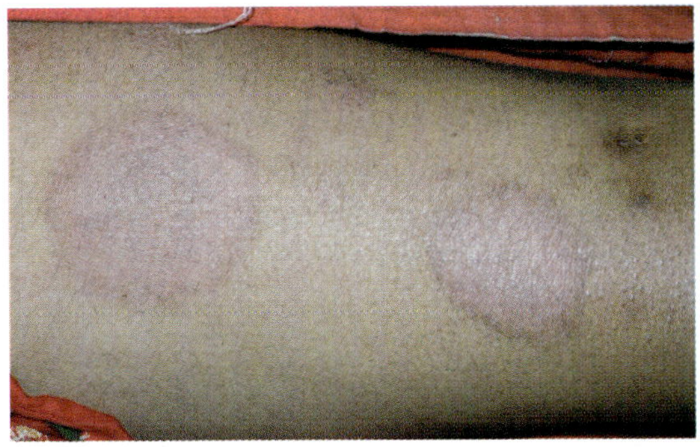

Fig. 19: Erythematous and crusted coin shaped plaques at the thigh

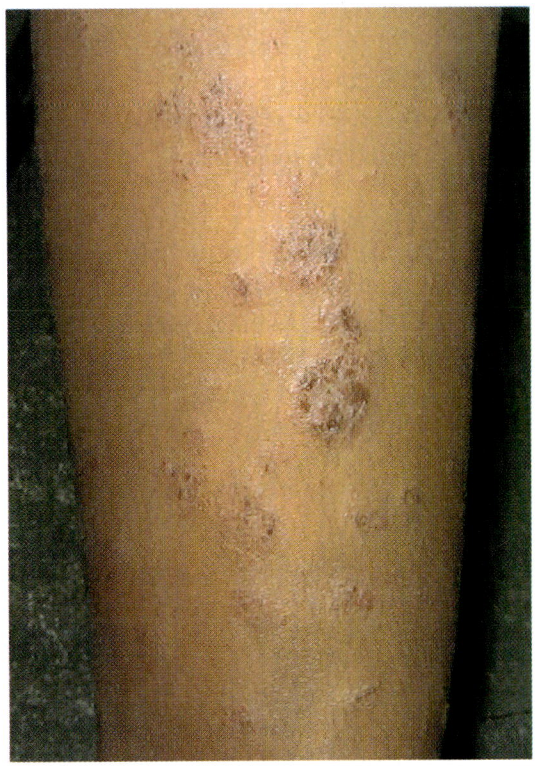

Fig. 20: Discoid and crusted lesions at thigh

Clinical features

- Pruritus is the commonest symptom.
- Lesions start as grouped papulovesicles which coalesce to form crusted plaques. Though it

is classically a subacute dermatitis but sometimes lesion may be exudative, dry and lichenified. It may be complicated by excoriation and secondary infection.

- Margin of the lesion is well dermarcated. But sometimes margin may be prominent than the center like an annular lesion.
- Shape may be round, nummular or coin shaped.
- Size is variable from 1 cm to 5 cm or even more.
- Lesions may be localized or generalized.
- Common sites are lower legs and trunk; but any site may be affected.

Differential diagnosis

- Psoriasis with crusting
- Tinea corporis

Histopathology

- Hyperkeratosis with parakeratosis
- Acanthosis with spongiosis

Treatment

- Application of emollient and moderately potent topical coricosteroid in cream form.
- Systemic corticosteroid is required for recalcitrant and generalized cases. Prednisolone 40 mg/day for 2 weeks and then to be tapered and stopped by another 2 weeks.

Asteatotic dermatitis/Eczema craquele

* It classically occurs in older person in winter season with low relative humidity.

Clinical features

- Continuous pruritus is the commonest symptom.
- Skin of the affected areas becomes dry and fissured superficially with scaling or mild crusting.
- Common sites are legs, arms, hands and trunk.

Treatment

- Frequent application of emollient and avoidance of bath with soap.
- Moderately potent topical corticosteroid may be required for areas where inflammation is more.
- Systemic corticosteroid is required for recalcitrant and severe cases.

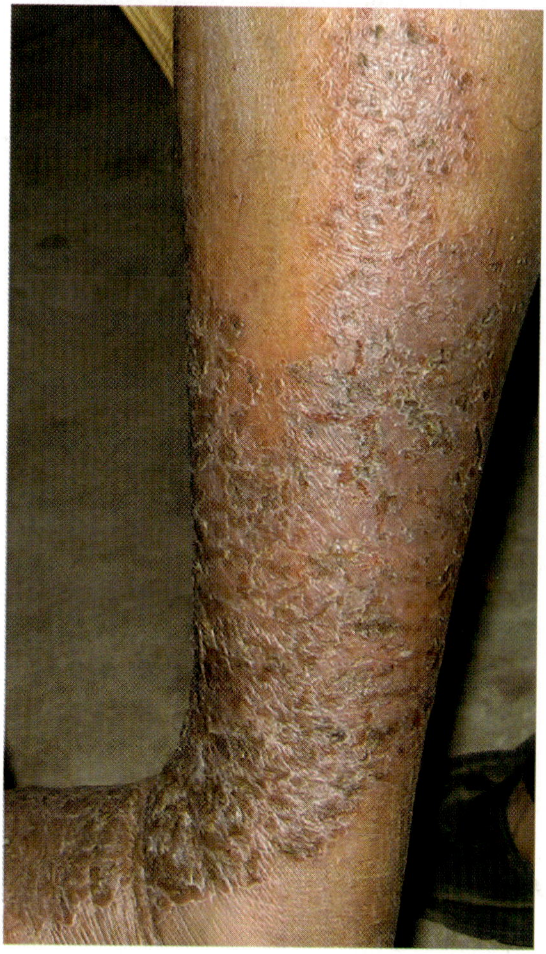

Fig. 21: Crusted plaque with intervening fissures

Stasis dermatitis

* It is a chronic endogenous dermatitis occurring at lower legs due to failure of immediate return of deoxygenated blood to the heart leading to skin changes.
* Normal blood flows from the superficial veins to deep veins through the perforators. When valves of deep veins or perforators become in-

competent, blood flows backwards and increases pressure within the capillaries.

* Due to this back pressure, superficial veins become tortuous and dilated as well as the capillaries also become dilated. The spaces between the endothelial cells enlarge and through these fenestrations contents of blood come out. The extravascular blood-contents get deposited along the capillary walls which further prevents diffusion of oxygen and other nutrients.
* Thus skin becomes malnourished and devitalized leading to develop edema and dermatitis. Also this malnourished skin becomes ulcerated easily by minor trauma.

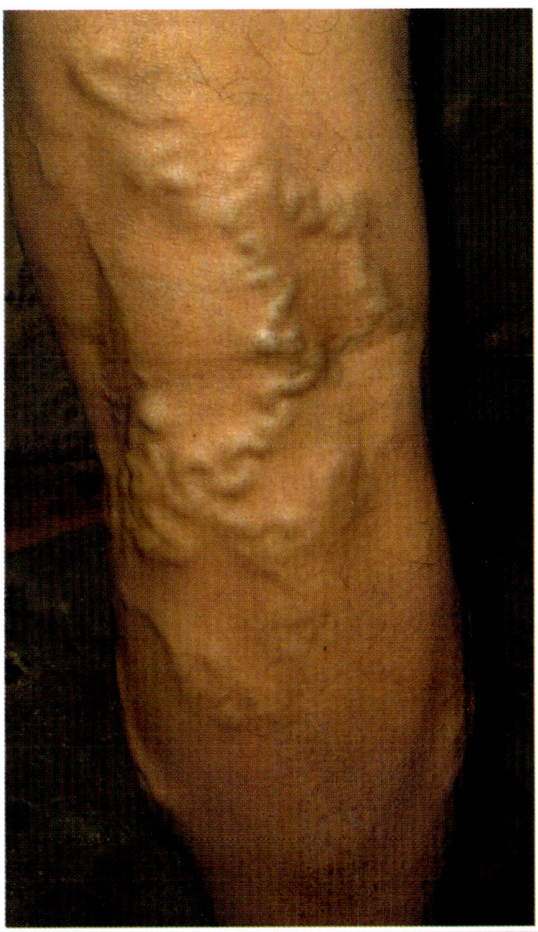

Fig. 22: Tortuous and dilated superficial veins, a marker of venous hypertension due to incompetent valves of deep veins

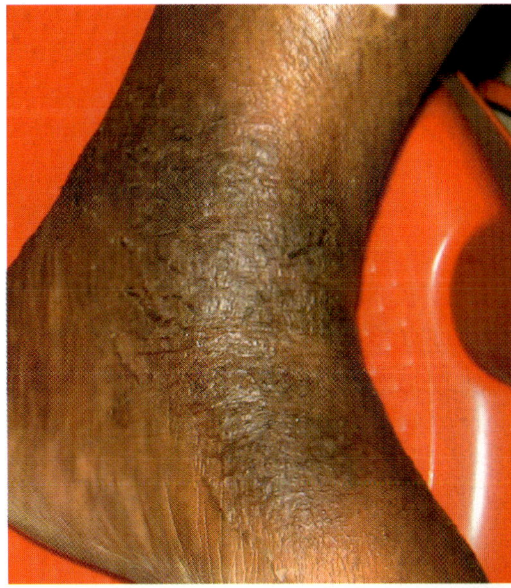

Fig. 23: Ill defined plaque of early stasis dermatitis

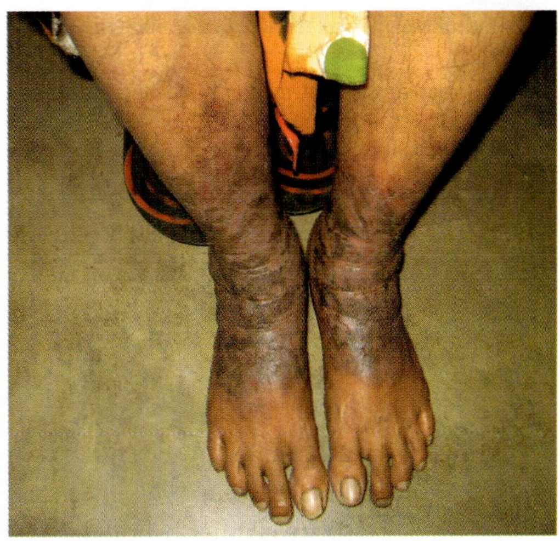

Fig. 24: Crusted lesions at both lower legs

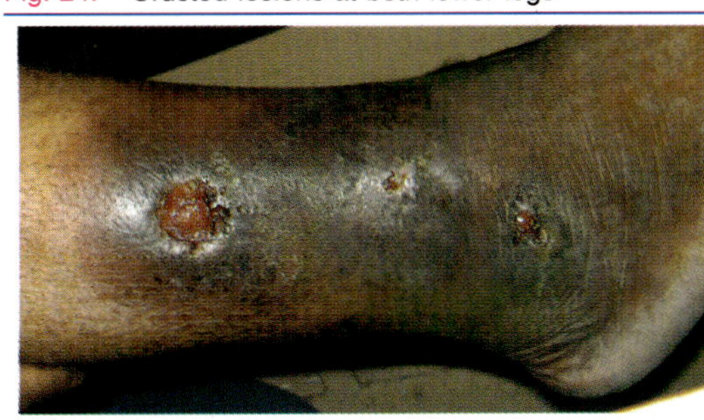

Fig. 25: Multiple ulcers on the background of erythema and hyperpigmentation

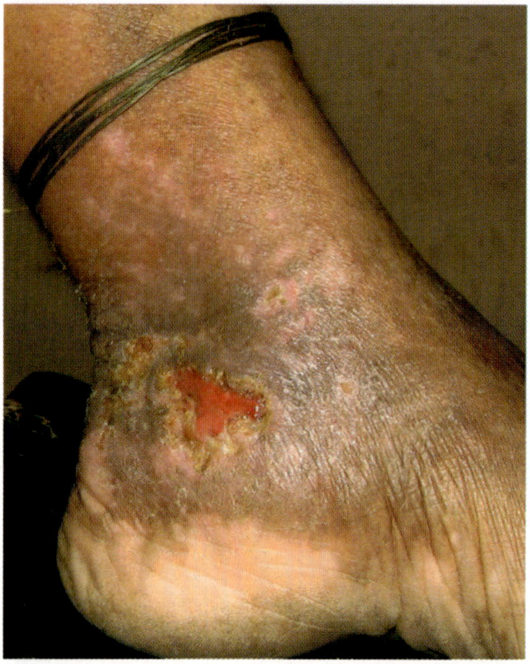

Fig. 26: Irregular ulcer at medial malleolus, surrounded by crust, erythema and dyspigmentation. Herbal plants are commonly compassed above the ulcer as a common practice in Indian villages

- It commonly occurs in persons who do their work in standing position like barbers, bus conductors, security professionals, etc. and persons who are overweight.

Clinical features

- Edema of the affected leg is the earliest sign. Initially it occurs following prolonged standing which is improved after overnight rest at horizontal position. It affects dorsum of the foot, ankle and lower third of the leg.
- Gradually papules papulovesicles, oozing and crusting develop at lower leg and ankle.
- This dermatitis is often complicated by secondary infection and allergic contact or irritant contact dermatitis following application of various medications including herbal products.
- Ulceration develops due to infection or following a trauma.
- Dermatitis may disseminate at other parts of the body due to autosensitization, known as id eruption.

Treatment

- Leg end elevation during sleep as well as for 30 minutes at 3-4 hours interval during work.
- Systemic antibiotic for infection, Condy's compress for oozing and application soothing agent like calamine lotion in acute stage.
- Systemic corticosteroid for recalcitrant dermatitis and for id eruption.

Lichen simplex chronicus

- It is a chronic dermatosis of unknown etiology but emotional stress often precipitate the disease.
- Patients are used to develop a habit to rub and scratch the lesion to counteract an irresistable feeling of itching. Repeated rubbing and scratching produce thickening, pigmentation and increased skin markings in the lesion.
- Patients often feel pleasure by scratching. They usually scratch unconciously and the habit of rubbing becomes automatic or reflexive. There is no itching during an enjoyable work but it becomes severe during the work of boredom or during the time of leisure.
- It usually occurs in person older than 20 years of age.
- It commonly develops at easily approachable sites.

Clinical features

- Pruritus is the commonest symptom, often in paroxysms.
- Lesions start as few papules which gradually increase in number and coalesce to form plaque.
- The plaque is slowly going on increasing in size, thickness, deepening of creases and pigmentation, unless and until there is stoppage of rubbing.
- Scale is minimum but excoriation is often obvious.

- Plaque is sharply defined with a slopping from the center to periphery.
- Number of the lesion is usually solitary but may be few and scattered at various sites.
- Common sites are nape of the neck, inner sides of the thighs and vulva in females, scrotum in males, around the natal cleft, ankles, dorsa of the hands or fingers, scalp and extensors of forearms and legs.

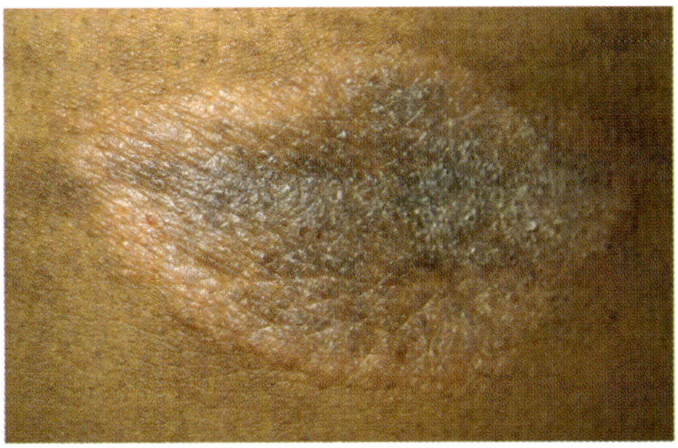

Fig. 27: Well defined thickened, pigmented plaque with increased skin creases

Histopathology

- Hyperkeratosis and parakeratosis.
- Psoriasiform hyperplasia of the epidermis.
- Vertical orientation of dermal collagen within the papillae.
- Thickened dermal nerves.

Treatment

- Complete restriction of rubbing.
- Application of potent topical corticosteroid with salicylic acid (6%) ointment. Ointment should apply softly without rubbing on the lesion.

Pityriasis alba

* It is a form of endogenous dermatitis, often associated with atopic dermatitis.
* It commonly occurs in children and adolescents and manifests with hypopigmented patch.
* It presents vividly in dark colored skin.
* The cause of hypopigmention is not clear. But ultrastructurally there is a reduction of melanosome within melanocyte and melanin within keratinocyte.
* Hypopigmentation may persist for months or years but finally it resolves spontaneously.

Clinical features

- Lesion starts as an erythematous macule with well defined margin but gradually the color fades to become a ill defined hypopigmented mild scaly patch.
- Sometimes the lesion may be surrounded by hyperpigmentation.
- Number of the lesion is usually solitary but may be multiple and symmetrically distributed.
- Size is variable from 0.5 to 2 cm.
- It primarily affects the face but other areas may be affected.

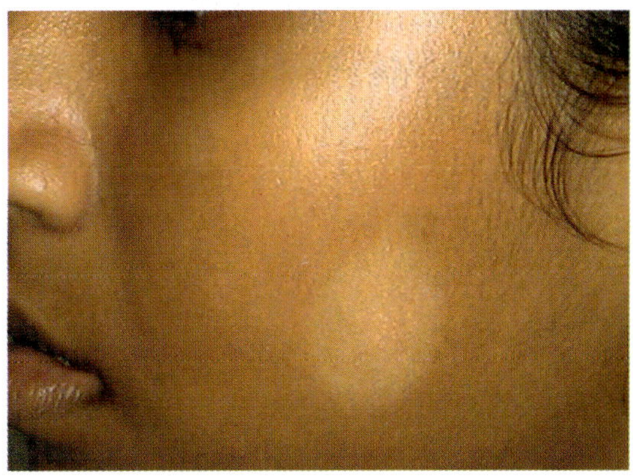

Fig. 28: Well to ill defined mild scaly hypopigmented patch

Differential diagnosis

- Pityriasis versicolor: Presence of well defined hypopigmented scaly perifollicular macules.
- Seborrheic dermatitis: Onset at puberty, prominent scales, coalescence of the lesions and affection of other seborrheic areas.
- Early vitiligo: Non scaly.
- Indeterminate leprosy: Presence of mild epidermal atrophy and sensory impairment.

Treatment

- Only reassurance as it resolves spontaneously.
- Application of mild potent topical coticosteroid (hydrocortisone/desonide) or just emollient is enough to counteract the anxiety of the parents.

Juvenile plantar dermatosis/Forefoot dermatitis

- It is an endogenous dermatitis, often associated with atopy and many other external factors.
- Prepubertal children are commonly affected, starting from age of 3 years.
- External factors are shoes made of plastic and rubber and humid environment causing maceration of the stratum corneum during prolong use.
- Dry skin of atopics and relatively thinner stratum corneum in prepubertal skin help to develop the disease.

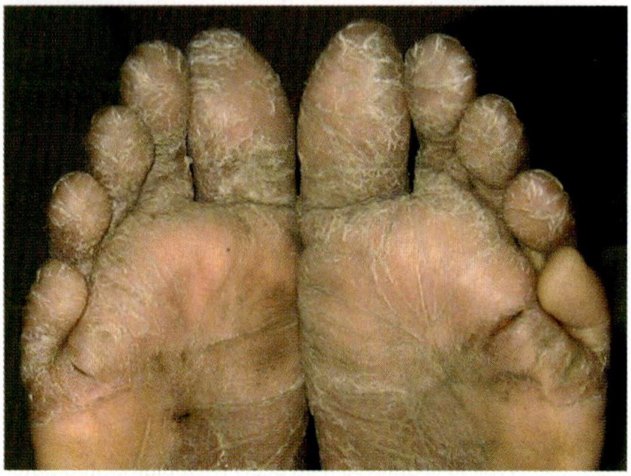

Fig. 29: Scaly and fissured keratotic skin at forefeet

Clinical features

- Symptom is the pain due to presence of fissuring.
- Skin becomes erythematous, dry, scaly, glazed and fissured.
- Commonest site is the plantar surfaces of the forefeet.
- Specially balls of the feet and toepads are symmetrically affected.

Differential diagnosis

- Plantar psoriasis
- Allergic contact dermatitis
- Tinea pedis: Unilateral involvement, moist and nonerythematous background.

Treatment

- Frequent application of moisturizing agents.
- Avoidance of sudden change of socks.

Nipple dermatitis

- This is a form of endogenous dermatitis commonly occurring in young females.
- Itching and oozing are commonly associated.

Clinical features

- Well circumscribed crusted plaques involving the nipples and areolae.
- Lesions may be at acute or subacute stage.

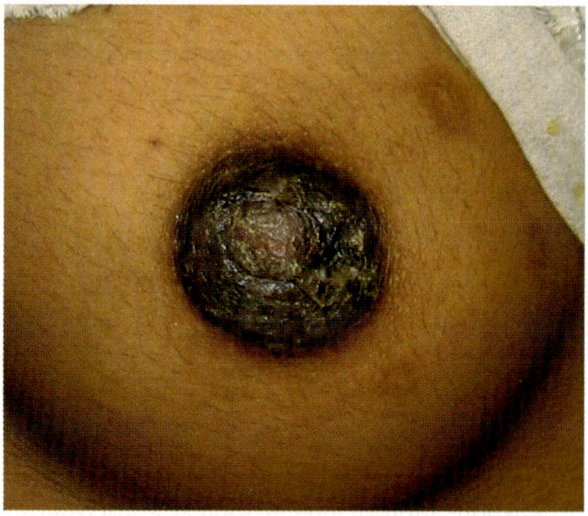

Fig. 30: Crusted plaque with distorted nipple

Differential diagnosis

- Paget's disease.

Treatment

- Condy's compress twice daily till oozing persists.
- Moderately potent topical corticosteroid to be applied.
- Systemic corticosteroid in recalcitrant cases.

Diaper dermatitis

- One of the most common dermatosis in infancy and it typically occurs between 6-12 months of age.
- It develops at diaper-occluded area and infrequent diaper changing creates overhydration and maceration. Thus the skin becomes more sensitive to friction and ultimate result is impairment of normal barrier function.
- Impaired barrier function leads the skin vulnerable to various irritants like digestive stool enzymes (trypsin/lipases) as hydration and alkaline pH increase the activity of these enzymes.
- Aggravating factors are poor skin care, growth of microorganisms, diarrhea, use of broad spectrum antibiotics and urinary tract abnormality.
- Its clinical features are flaky skin with a background of erythema at convex surfaces sparing the folds.
- Sometimes more aggressive lesions may develop with erosion (Jacquet's form), psoriasiform and vesiculobullous lesions due to candidal or bacterial infections.

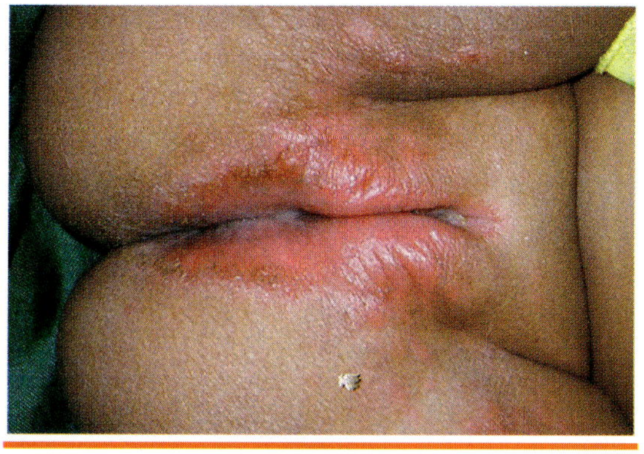

Fig. 31: Erythematous and eroded skin at vulvae and inner thighs

- Treatment includes proper skin care, frequent changing of diaper, use of barrier cream (zinc oxide ointment/paste), and antifungal/antibacterial if necessary.

Lip-licking dermatitis

- It is a mild form of allergic-irritant contact dermatitis.

Clinical features

- It is characterized by hyperpigmented, dry and erythematous patches, studded with tiny papules and scaling.
- Perioral area reachable to the tongue is affected.

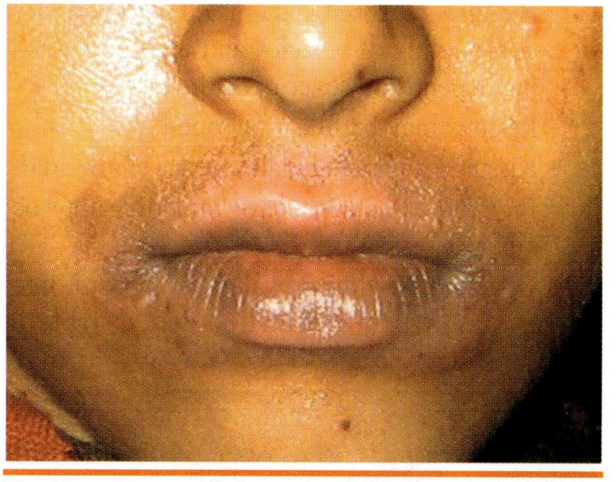

Fig. 32: Chapped lips, surrounded by papular eruptions

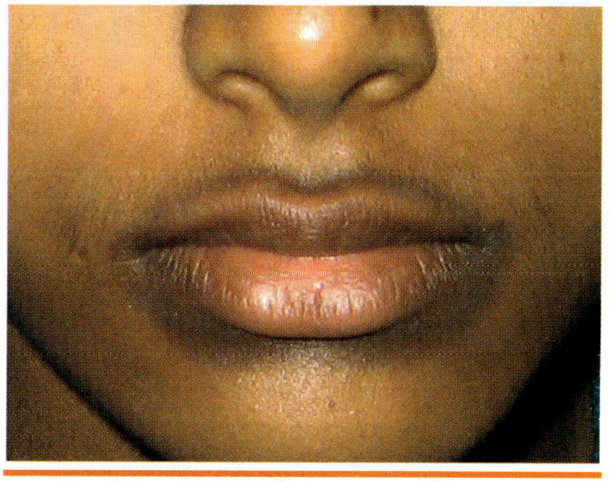

Fig. 33: Chapping of the lips

Pederus dermatitis

- This is a very common seasonal irritant contact dermatitis due to crush of pederus insect on the skin.
- The insect contains pederin, an irritant chemical.
- Affected person usually moves on vehicle and the insect becomes crushed. This leads to release of the irritant substance and subsequently disease develops.
- This also occurs during high speed blowing of the wind.

Clinical features

- Severe burning sensation is the earliest and unique symptom.
- Site of contact becomes erythematous and blister develops within minutes to hours.
- Gradually center or site of maximum contact becomes necrosed and crusted with peripheral spreading of vesicles and erythema. Oozing depends on severity of the disease.
- Lesions may be linear or round.
- Kissing lesions are usually seen at elbow-folds.
- In some cases secondary infection may occur.
- Lesions heal within few days with postinflammatory hyperpigmentation and scarring in some severe cases.

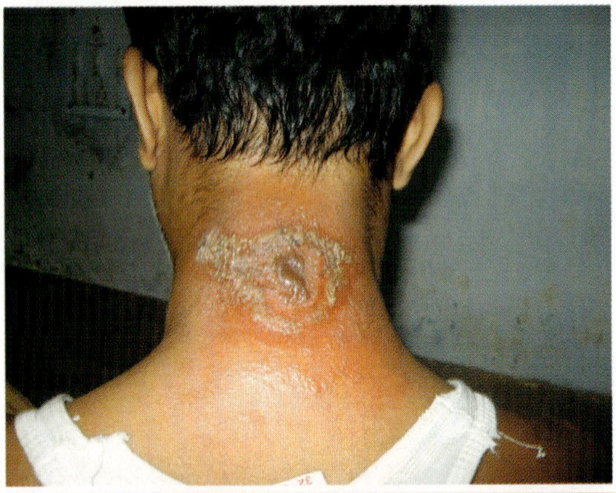

Fig. 34: Erythematous patch, studded with central bulla and peripheral pustulation and vesiculation

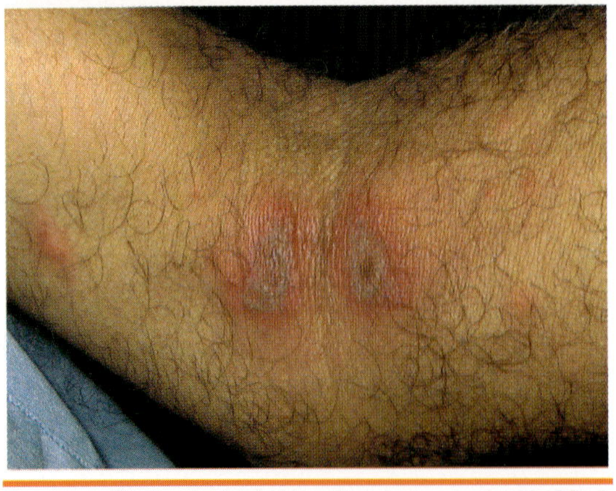

Fig. 35: Kissing lesions at junctional area, a classical finding in pederus dermatitis

Treatment

- Condy's compress if oozing present.
- Antibiotic for secondary infection.
- Application of calamine lotion.
- Short course of systemic corticosteroid for rapid improvement.

Prurigo simplex and prurigo nodularis

- It is one of the common chronic and recurrent pruritic dermatosis of adult.
- Exact etiology is not clear; but mental stress is probably the sole cause.
- History of atopy may be present.
- Prurigo simplex usually occurs in young adult and middle aged persons and prurigo nodularis in elderly.
- Males and females both are affected.
- Prurigo simplex is commonly seen in females.

Clinical features

- Primary lesions are extremely pruritic papules. They become excoriated quickly due to scratching. This stage is known as prurigo simplex.
- Gradually lesions tend to become hypertrophic and take a nodular shape. This stage is known as prurigo nodularis.
- Secondary infection is very commonly seen.
- Lesions may develop dyspigmentation.

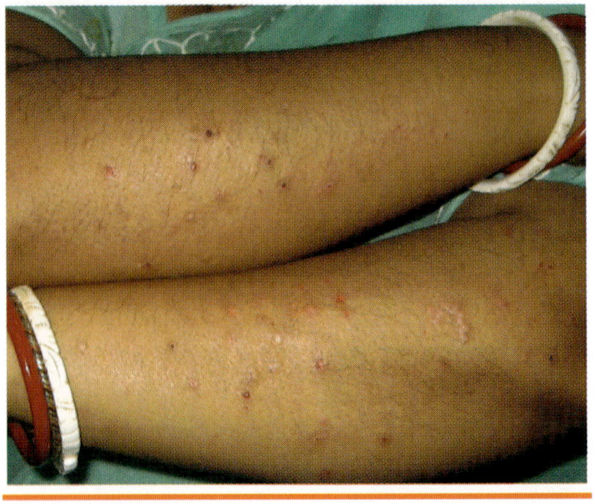

Fig. 36: Excoriated papules at extensors of upper limbs

Treatment

- Avoidance of scratching.

- Potent topical corticosteroid.
- Intralesional triamcinolone is specially required for recalcitrant prurigo nodularis.

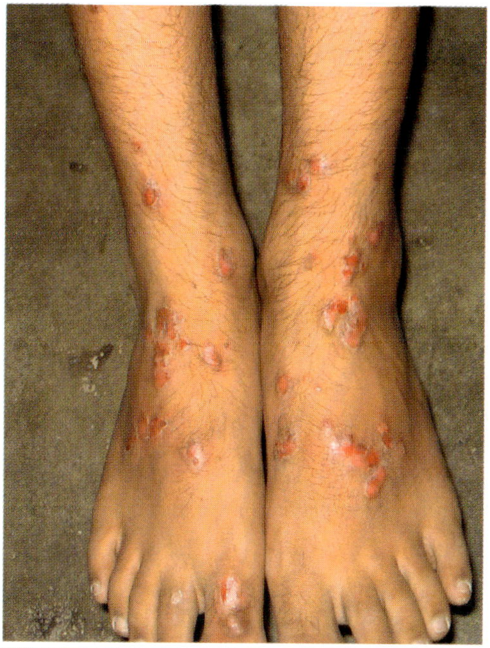

Fig. 37: Excoriated papules of prurigo simplex turning into prurigo nodularis at lower limbs

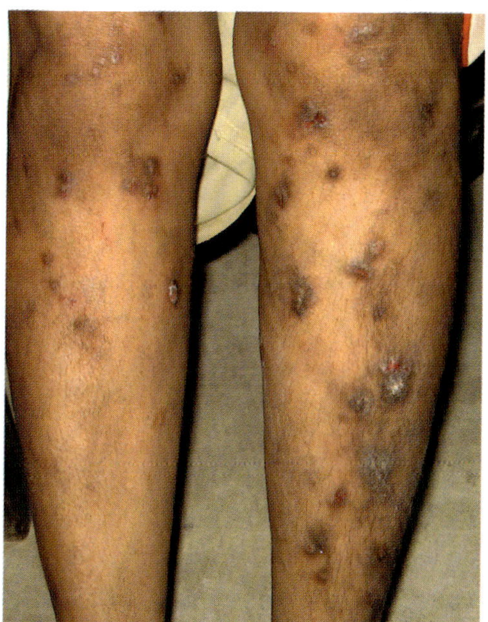

Fig. 38: Crusted and excoriated nodules at lower limbs

- Systemic corticosteroid in recalcitrant cases.
- Doxepin 25-50 mg/day.
- Antibiotic for infection.

Ultraviolet light (UVR) induced changes of the skin

a) Acute/subacute changes: These are due to absorption of UVR by DNA.

* Erythema: UV 300 nm is most erythemogenic
* Pigment darkening
* Delayed tanning
* Epidermal hyperplasia
* Immunologic changes
* Photo-onycholysis
* Pseudoporphyria
* Brachioradial pruritus

b) Chronic changes

* Photoaging
  - Solar elastosis
  - Solar lentigo
  - Poikiloderma of Civatte
  - Ephelid/freckles
  - Favre-Racouchot syndrome
  - Colloid milium
  - Erosive pustular dermatosis
* Photocarcinogenesis
  - Actinic keratosis
  - Basal cell carcinoma: Development cannot be prevented by use of sunscreen.
  - Squamous cell carcinoma: To develop, it requires continuous sun exposure and use of sunscreen may prevent it.
  - Melanoma: Specially lentigo maligna is induced by UVB range.

c) UVA induced erythema

* Deeper red color and more persistent.
* It fades by few to several days.
* Excessive exposure causes edema and blister

formation. If such exposure is widespread, person may develop chills, malaise, pruritus and these may last for 1-2 weeks.

d) UVB induced erythema

* Typical bright red delayed erythema develops by 30 minutes to 8 hours exposure and peak is reached by 12-24 hours and then it is reduced by hours to days.

e) UVC induced erythema

* Erythema is more pink and shorter in duration.
* It starts within hours and is reached to peak by 5-8 hours and fades by hours to days.

f) Pigment darkening

* Immediate grayish tanning lasts for 10-20 minutes in dark person. This is known as Merowosky phenomenon.
* This change is due to photo-oxidation and cellular redistribution of melanin within epidermal melanocyte.
* If pigment persists more than 2 hours, it is known as persistent darkening.
* Gradually color turns into brown and lasts for 24 hours and this is due oxidation of preexisting melanin.
* Delayed tanning persists for weeks to months and it occurs in genetically competent person.

g) Epidermal hyperplasia

* Following hours to days of exposure to UVB/UVC can cause epidermal hyperplasia.
* UVA usually does not cause epidermal hyperplasia.
* UVC increases cellular mitotic activity and increases synthesis of DNA, RNA and protein.

h) Immunologic changes

* UVB, UVC and sometimes UVA alter Langerhans cell function, increase CD8+ cells and modulate cytokines.

i) Vitamin D synthesis

* UVB converts 7-dehydrocholesterol into provitamin D3 within malpighian layer of the skin and finally liver and kidney produce vitamin D.
* Only a low dose of UVB is required to maintain vitamin D synthesis.

j) Pseudoporphyria

* Photosensitization of normal level endogenous substance such as porphyrin causes increased fragility of skin and blister formation.
* There is a loss of elastic fibers in mid-reticular dermis.

k) Brachioradial pruritus

* Pruritus develops at outer arm. It mimics cervical radiculopathy.

l) Solar elastosis

* Thickening and yellow discoloration and marked wrinkling are seen at exposed areas.
* Most commonly it is seen at face and posterior neck.
* Changes at the neck is known as cutis rhomboidalis nuchae.
* Histopathology shows markedly increased elastic tissue.

m) Solar lentigo

* These are evenly colored, light to dark brown, solitary or multiple macules.
* Commonly occurs at sun exposed areas like face, upper trunk, extensors of forearms and dorsa of hands.

n) Ephelide/freckle

* These are light to medium brown macules with size less than 6 mm and few to multiple in number.
* Face, shoulder and anterior arms are the common sites.

o) Poikiloderma of Civatte

* Reticulated red brown patches with telangiectasia.
* Lateral aspect of the neck is the commonest site and spare the perifollicular as well as submental region.

p) Favre-Racouchot syndrome

* Multiple large open comedones at lateral aspect of periorbital area and at nose.

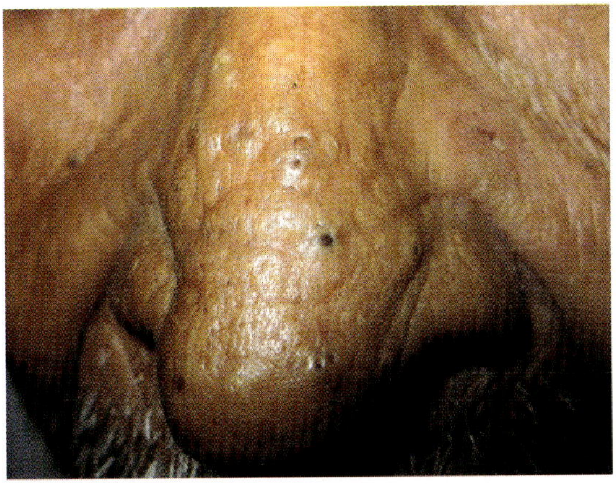

Fig. 39: Multiple open comedones at nose

* Histopathology shows marked elastosis, horn cyst, and dilated pilosebaceous openings.

q) Colloid milium

* These are translucent yellow papules of 1-3 mm size.
* They are numerous in number and closely spaced.
* Common sites are face, neck and dorsa of the hands.

r) Erosive pustular dermatosis of scalp

* Develops at photodamaged bald scalp. Lesions are pustules and erosions with mild inflammation.

s) Photoaging in Indian skin

* Skin becomes darker with dyspigmentation and fine wrinkles.

Polymorphous light eruption (PMLE)

* It is form of allergic contact dermatitis to ultraviolet light.
* Middle aged persons in tropical countries are commonly affected.
* Females are more commonly affected than males due to different cloth habit.
* There is a seasonal variation and usually occurs in summer and rainy seasons. It rarely occurs during winter.
* It manifests with lesions of diverse morphology. But lesions are monomorphic in individual patient. There is a tendency to develop similar type of lesions during recurrence.
* Recurrence is very common. It recurs during a particular season for 3-4 consecutive years. But may be longer than that.
* Actinic prurigo is familial from of PMLE.

Clinical features

- ♦ Primary lesions are confluent groups of tiny papules or papulovesicles, developing at upperback, outer arm and forearms.
- ♦ Common sites in males are back and sides of the neck.
- ♦ Size of this individual group is variable from 0.5 cm to 2.5 cm.
- ♦ Sometimes lesions may be exudative plaques.
- ♦ In some cases lesions are shiny, skin colored or hypopigmented discrete tiny papules, mimicking lichen nitidus. Koebner phenomenon, commonly seen in lichen nitidus which is absent in PMLE.
- ♦ Lesions heal with residual hypopigmentation.

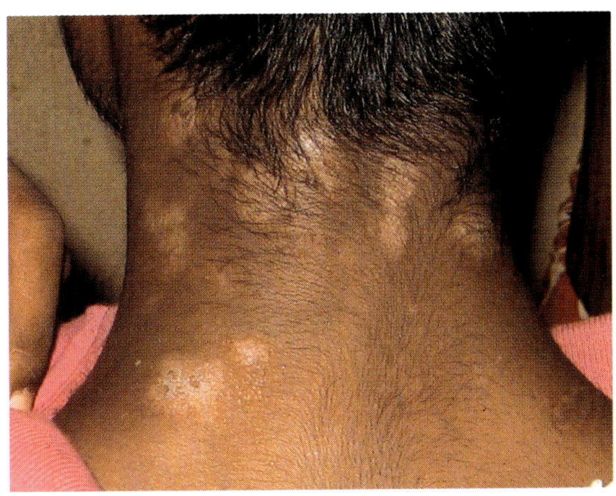

Fig. 40: Plaques studded with tiny papules

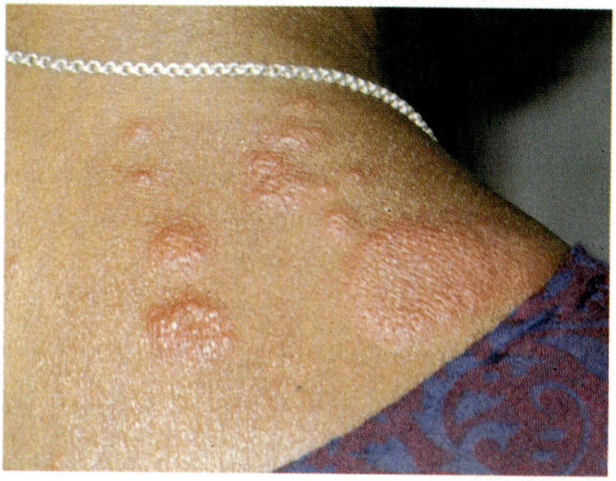

Fig. 41: Erythematous plaques at exposed part of the back

Histopathology

- Mild acanthosis, spongiosis or spongiotic vesicles in the epidermis.
- Mild upper dermal lymphocytic perivascular infiltration.

Treatment

- Potent topical corticosteroid.
- Hydroxychloroquine 200 mg twice daily.
- Systemic corticosteroid, prednisolone, 20-40 mg/day.
- Systemic PUVA to increase tolerance to ultraviolet light.

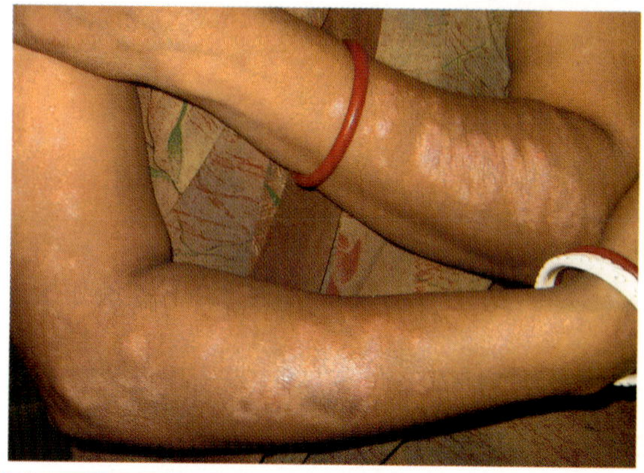

Fig. 42: Irregular plaques, studded with papules at photo-exposed part of the upper limbs

PAPULOSQUAMOUS DISORDERS

CHAPTER C9

Psoriasis

* It is a chronic relapsing papulosquamous disorder, affecting the skin, joints and nails.
* It occurs in 2-3% of general population.
* About 30-45% occur in 10-30 years of age.
* It is a multifactorial disease and it develops due to a complex interaction among genetic, environmental and immunological factors.
* Skin injury and streptococcal infection are well known environmental triggers.
* Disease is also flared by physical and psychological influences.

Genetic influences

* Life time risk:
  - 4%, If no parents are affected
  - 18%, If one parent is affected
  - 65%, If both parents are affected.
* Early onset psoriasis means psoriasis developing < 40 years of age and it is often associated with HLA B27, Cw6 and DR7.
* Guttate psoriasis is associated with HLA Cw6 in 74% cases in comparison to 7.4% in general population.
* PSORS1 gene at chromosome $6p^{21.3}$, was the first gene discovered in relation to psoriasis.

Role of T cell

- Psoriasis is now regarded as a T cell mediated disease where CD8+ T cells predominantly found in epidermis and CD4+ T cells found more in papillary dermis.
- Actually CD8+ T cells play the key role in pathogenesis of psoriasis. An antigen-specific T cell response through TH1 pathway, initiates the psoriatic lesion.
- Activation of T cells may be due to bacterial super antigens like that of beta hemolytic streptococcal superantigens. Here the amino acid sequence of streptococcal M proteins share the sequence of keratin 17 or keratin 6 and may be a target of auto reactive T lymphocytes.
- In this antigen-specific response, activated CD4+ and CD8+ T cells produce a variety of cytokines including IL2, TNFα and IFNγ.
- TNFα stimulates keratinocyte to produce IL8. This cytokine is a potent chemoattractant for T lymphocytes and neutrophils and help to form micro-abscesses.

- IFNγ, profoundly seen in pinpoint psoriatic lesion, acts as an initiator.
- IFNγ expresses ICAM1 in keratinocytes and endothelial cells. This adhesive molecule mediates adhesion and trafficking of lymphocytes into epidermis by binding to its ligand LFA1, present on lymphocytic membrane.
- An inducible protein (IP-10) is also over expressed by keratinocytes and IP-10 has chemotactic and mitogenic properties.
- Majority of T cells in psoriatic plaque are CD45RO+ memory effector cells.

Pathophysiological changes

- There is a complex interaction among altered proliferation, differentiation and immunological dysregulation of keratinocytes.
- Earliest changes observed by electron microscopy in psoriasis:
  - Swelling of keratinocytes and widening of intercellular spaces due to a deficiency in the glycoprotein rich cell surface coating and intercellular adhesions remain limited to the desmosomes.
  - Degranulation of mast cell around the post capillary venules.
  - Activated macrophages, lymphocytes and neutrophils migrate into lower epidermis through altered desmosome-tonofilament complexes.
  - Tonofilaments are decreased in diameter and number and have a reducing tendency to aggregate.
  - Size and number of keratohyaline granules are also decreased and even may be absent.
  - Corneocytes possess thin tonofilaments and they often retain nucleus, known as parakeratotic cells.
  - Corneocytes often fail to form marginal bands and fail to loose their outer plasma membrane.
  - Basal keratinocytes protrude cytoplasmic processes through gaps in the basal lamina and presence of these microherniations correlate with disease activity, such as numerous in active and untreated psoriasis and absent in completely resolved or uninvolved psoriatic skin.
  - There is a correlation between rate of mitosis and parakeratosis.
  - Spongiform pustules located at uppermost portion of spinous and granular layer are collection of neutrophils in intercellular spaces to form multilocular abscesses along with degenerated and flattened keratinocytes, making a sponge like network.
  - Widened lumens of capillary loops at dermal papillae.
  - Bridging of endothelial fenestrations and swelling of endothelial cells and pericytes are present.
  - Thickened vascular basement membrane due to deposition of amorphous substances and collagen fibrils are also seen.
  - Rate of epidermal cell replication is markedly increased in active psoriatic lesion, showing by higher number of mitotic figures in the basal and suprabasal layers.
  - Mitotic activity correlate with degree of parakeratosis such as 5 times increment of mitotic activity when parakeratosis is 91-100% in comparison to 0-20%.
  - Alternating orthokeratosis and parakeratosis correlate with fluctuating epidermal growth activity.
  - Reduction of transit time from normal 53 days to 7 days.
  - Cell cycle time is also reduced from 311 hours to only 36 hours, that means about 8 times faster proliferation than normal. Some studies found cell cycle time is reduced from 200 hours to 100 hours, only doubling of the proliferation rate.
  - Doubling of the recruitment of proliferation population of keratinocytes from 27,000 to 52,000/mm^2 surface area.

- Growth fraction of germinative keratinocytes is increased from 60% in normal skin to 100% in psoriatic skin.
- Source of cycling cells in suprabasal layers is not yet clear. It may be either from basal cells or from the transient amplifying cells which are committed for terminal differentiation.
- Proliferating keratinocytes express keratin 1/keratin 10 and keratin 6/keratin 16, but not keratin 5/keratin 14 which are expressed by basal keratinocytes.
- Keratin 17, normally expressed by deeper cells of outer root sheath (ORS) of hair follicles, but also expressed by interfollicular keratinocytes of psoriatic skin.
- Involucrin appears prematurely at lower suprabasal layers.

Classification of psoriasis

Classical types

- Psoriasis vulgaris
- Pustular psoriasis
- Erythrodermic psoriasis
- Arthritic psoriasis

Morphological variants

- Guttate psoriasis
- Annular, linear and zosteriform psoriasis
- Rupoid, ostraceous and elephantine/lichenified psoriasis
- Follicular and lichenoid psoriasis.

Regional variants

- Sebopsoriasis of scalp
- Flexural psoriasis
- Palmoplantar psoriasis
- Nail psoriasis

Clinical features of psoriasis vulgaris

- Pruritus is the main symptom with variable intensity.
- Primary lesions are well defined, round, erythematous and scaly papules and plaques.
- Lesions start as single or few mild itchy pin point to pinhead sized erythematous papules, usually at elbows, knees, front of the legs and scalp.
- Gradually number and size of the lesions increase and spread widely.
- Amount of scale and erythema are variable from time to time and from site to site in the same patient.
- Early psoriatic lesions shows predominant erythema and minimal scales.
- When lesions are numerous, they are distributed bilaterally and often symmetrically.
- Extensor parts of the limbs, especially elbows and knees, scalp and lower half of the back are commonly affected. But any site may be involved including flexurals like intergluteal fold, umbilicus and groin. But mucosal surfaces are rarely affected.
- Size of the lesions is variable, ranging from pin point or few mm to several cm. Shape is usually round or discoid but may be annular, bizarre, geographic, polycyclic, linear and zosteriform.
- Surface of the lesion contains loosely adherent silvery scales. Scales of the lesions at palms and soles are adherent. Scales are less prominent at lesions of flexural areas.
- Color of the lesions is usually reddish with variable intensity. At dependent areas, red color may become bluish due to sluggish circulation through dilated venules. Skin around a lesion is rather pallor and becomes hypopigmented in a resolving lesion. This hypopigmented area is known as ring of Woronoff.
- Development of psoriatic lesions along a line of trauma, is known as Koebner phenomenon/isomorphic phenomenon. It develops after 7-14 days of trauma and seen in 25% cases. But in some cases psoriatic lesion may disappear following repeated trauma which is known as reverse Koebner phenomenon.

- Nail changes in psoriasis include pitting, discoloration, onycholysis, subungual hyperkeratosis and a tendency to develop bacterial or fungal infection. Nail pits are irregular and minute (< 1 mm) depressions. These represent small intermittent psoriatic lesion developing at proximal nail matrix which produces superficial layer of nail plate. Oil drop sign representing exocytosis, is seen at nail bed.
- Grattage test: It is a clinical test when bleeding points appear following scraping of an early psoriatic lesion and this positive result is known as Auspitz sign. Bleeding occurs due to damage of the basal plasma membrane or Buckley's membrane and papillary dermal blood vessels. It is not specific in psoriasis but also may be positive in actinic keratosis and Darier's disease.

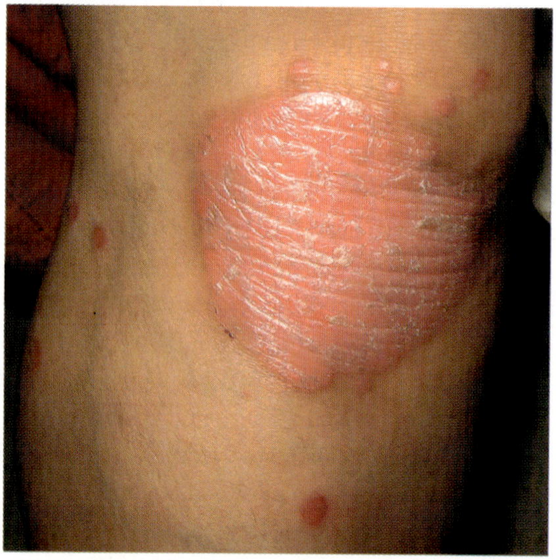

Fig. 1: Well defined plaque with prominent erythema and minimum scale at right knee

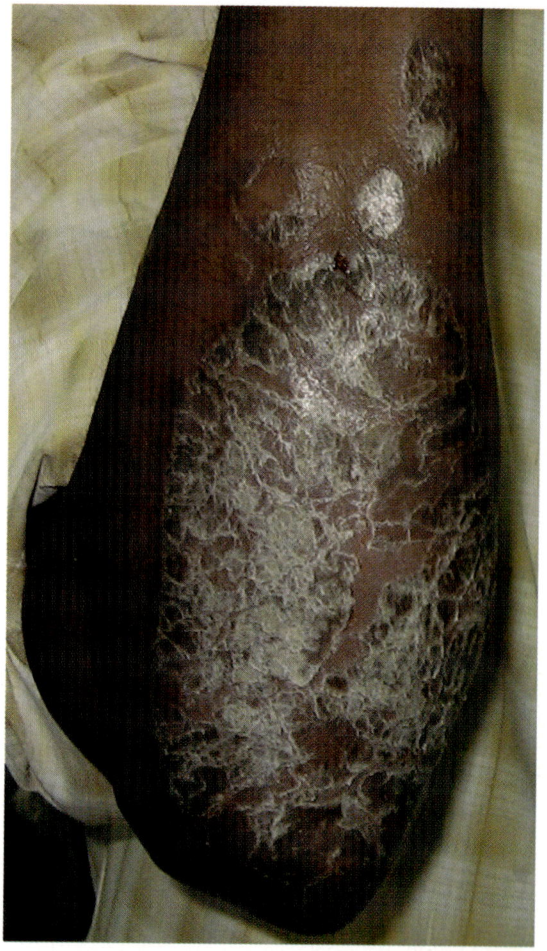

Fig. 2: Well defined plaques with prominent scales and minimum erythema at right elbow

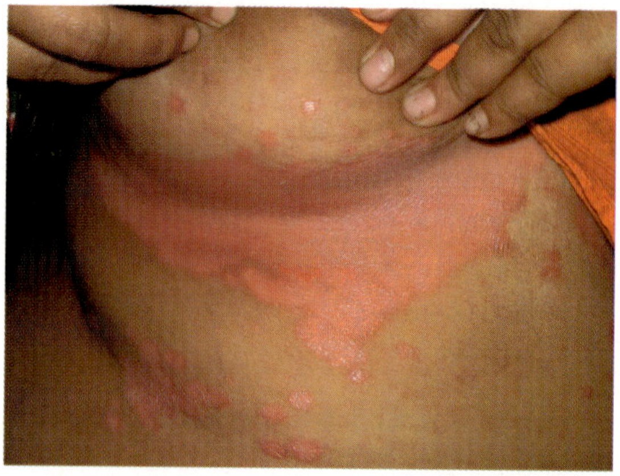

Fig. 3: Flexural psoriasis with minimal scaling at inframammary fold

Differential diagnosis

- BT leprosy with reversal reaction.
- Nummular dermatitis
- Discoid lupus erythematosus
- Bowen's disease.

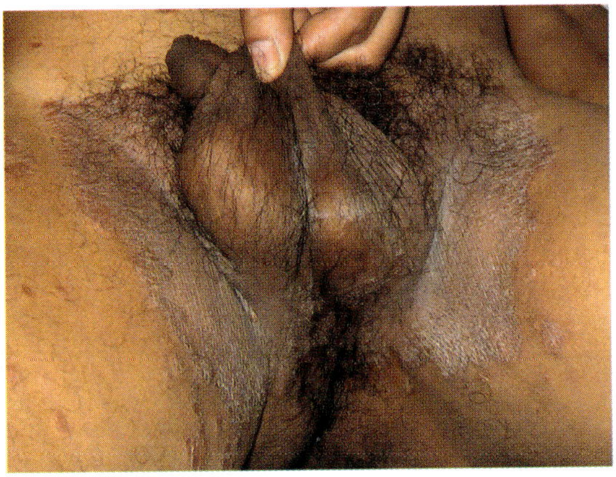

Fig. 4: Well defined scaly plaque at the groin

Differential diagnosis

- Candidiasis
- Erythrasma
- Seborrheic dermatitis

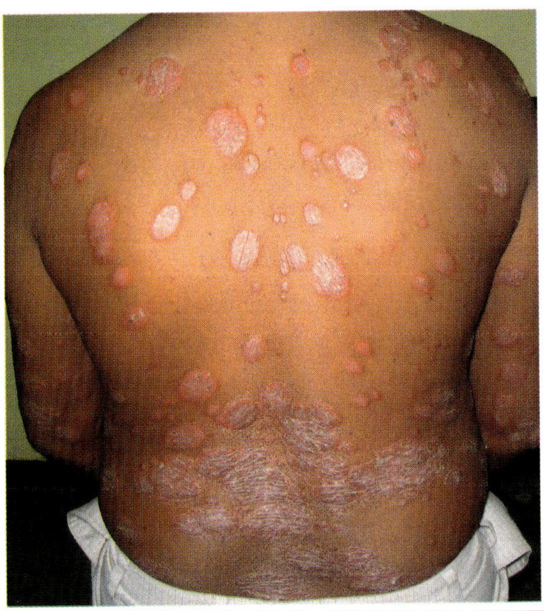

Fig. 5: Numerous discoid scaly plaques and some are coalesced

Differential diagnosis

- Lichen planus
- Discoid lupus erythematosus
- Secondary syphilis
- Sarcoidosis.

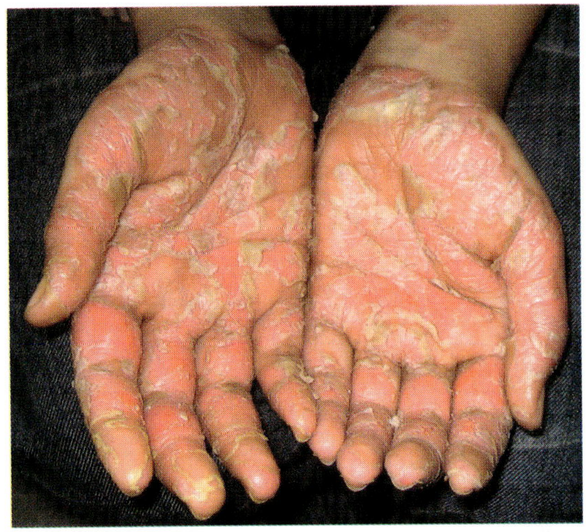

Fig. 6: Palmar psoriasis

Differential diagnosis

- Dyshidrosiform dermatitis
- Tinea manuum.

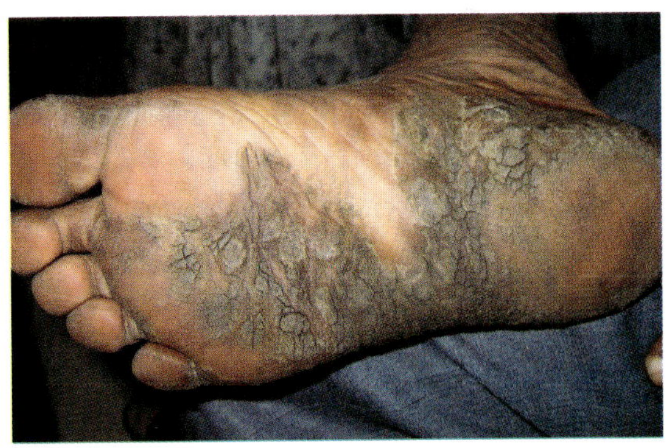

Fig. 7: Well defined scaly plaques with fissurings.

Differential diagnosis

- Tinea pedis
- Dyshidrosiform dermatitis.

Histopathology

- Hyperkeratosis with parakeratosis.
- Collection of neutrophils forming microabscess, known as Munro's microabscess.
- Reduced or absent granular layer.
- Acanthosis with elongated and broadened distal ends of rete ridges, known as elephant foot appearance.

- Suprapapillary thinning.
- Collection of neutrophils as spongiform pustule, known as Kogoj pustule, at tips of the dermal papillae.
- Dilated and tortuous dermal vessels.

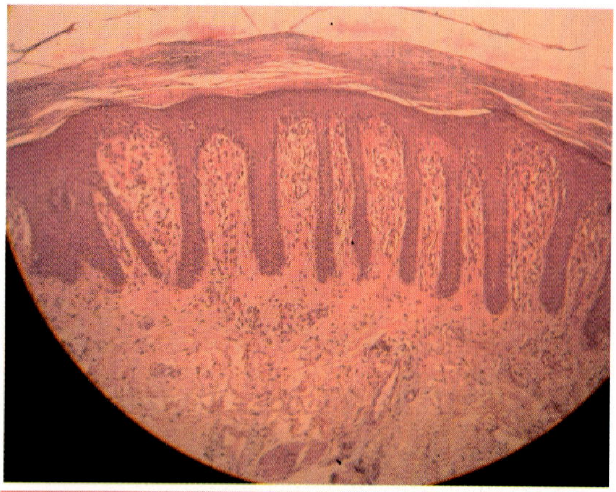

Fig. 8: Shows features of psoriasis

Pretreatment counselling

- It is not contagious.
- Till date, there is no cure of the disease and all treatments are suppressive.
- Spontaneous remission may occur in 50% cases.
- Relapse is the rule.

General plan of treatment

- Topical therapy is indicated for localized lesion when < 30% body surface area is involved.
- Systemic therapy for generalized lesions, when > 30% body surface area is involved, for recalcitrant localized lesion and for lesions at the palms and soles.
- Corticosteroid for both systemic and topical therapy are contraindicated in psoriasis except for lesions at scalp, flexural areas and pustular psoriasis in pregnancy.

Topical therapy for localized lesions

- Calcipotriol and other vitamin D derivatives.
- Coal tar ointment.
- Dithranol ointment.
- Tazarotene.
- Topical PUVA (topical psoralen and ultraviolet A).
- Narrow band UVB therapy.

Treatment outline for localized lesions at specific sites

- Scalp: Coal tar shampoo and topical corticosteroid lotion.
- Face and other flexural areas including umbilicus: Tacrolimus and mild to moderate corticosteroid gel.
- Palms and soles: Topical PUVA, dithranol and tazarotene.

Systemic therapy for generalized lesions

- Systemic PUVA
- Methotrexate
- Acitretin
- Cyclosporine
- Biologicals: Etenercept, alefacept, infliximab, adalimumab and efalizumab.
- Macrolide antibiotic for guttate psoriasis.

Factors to select a particular therapy

- Age of the patient: Dithranol or PUVA is not suitable for a child but only emollient or emollient with systemic methotrexate is favourable.
- Area of involvement: Coaltar, dithranol, calcipotriol, etc. are suitable for localized lesions and for widespread lesions, emollient with systemic therapies like PUVA, methotrexate, cyclosporine, retinoids and biologicals are better options.
- Clinical state of the disease: Coal tar or dithranol is unsuitable for unstable psoriasis.
- Cost effectiveness: One 30 g coaltar ointment costs about Rs 30 and one 15 g calcipotriol costs Rs. 200-1000. Similarly in systemic therapy expense for methotrexate per week is only Rs. 10-40 but for cyclosporine it is about

Rs. 1500 or more than Rs. 10,000 for biologicals. So even for a single lesion in a poor patient, we should not prescribe calcipotriol or cyclosporine and biologicals for extensive lesions.

- Topical therapy is indicated in all forms of psoriasis except pustular psoriasis.

Topical preparations

Coal tar (1-10%)

- It suppresses DNA synthesis and thus inhibits mitotic activity at basal cells. Some of its components also have an anti-inflammatory activity.
- Lotion, cream, ointment and paste forms are available. These are used according to the situation. It is often combined with 2-5% salicylic acid to increase keratolytic effect and for better absorption of coal tar.
- Coal tar is carcinogenic and it may cause allergic reaction and folliculitis. Its color and smell are not well acceptable.
- Goeckerman regimen: Night application of coal tar followed by application of mineral oil on next morning, then sun exposure and tar bath.

Anthralin (0.25-1%)

- Used as short contact therapy such as application of 1% anthralin only for 5 minutes and then removal of it with oil.
- Gradually time will be increased.
- It may cause staining of cloths.
- Ingram regimen: Affected area will be exposed to sun first and then anthralin will be applied.

Calcipotriol/calcipotriene (0.005%): Twice daily application and requires 6-8 weeks to act. It is the topical therapy of choice for localized lesions.

Tazarotene (0.05-0.1%): It is notorious for irritant effect and useful for recalcitrant lesion.

Emollient (liquid paraffin/coconut oil): It is the topical therapy of choice for extensive psoriasis, specially erythrodermic state.

Topical corticosteroid (mild to potent steroid):

- Though it is very popular for shortcut response but use should be restricted for long term adverse effects and tendency to develop pustular psoriasis.
- It is better to use mild to moderate forms only for scalp and intertriginous psoriasis.

Tacrolimus (0.03-0.1%)

- It takes 1-2 months to show response. It is useful for facial and intertriginous psoriasis.

Narrow band UVB (312 nm): It is safe and effective, specially in children.

Topical PUVA

- Topical psoralen is used on the isolated psoriatic lesion and after 30 minutes, the lesion is exposed to sunlight for 15 seconds to 10 minutes with a gradual increment.
- It is particularly useful for palmoplantar psoriasis.

Bath PUVA: 1 ml 8 MOP is mixed with 2 liter of water.

Systemic therapy

* It is indicated in:
  - Extensive lesions where all topical therapies other than emollient are impractical to apply.
  - Single or few lesions but recalcitrant to topical therapies, specially palmoplantar psoriasis.

PUVA:

- 8-Methoxypsoralen is used at a dose of 0.6mg/kg body weight, maximum on every alternate day.
- If it is given daily, drug will accumulate and may produce a severe photosensitivity reaction.

Methotrexate:

- It has antimitotic, antichemotactic and anti-inflammatory roles.

- It is used for severe unresponsive psoriasis, erythrodermic psoriasis, pustular psoriasis and arthritic psoriasis.
- Weekly dose of 5-30 mg is given, either orally or intramuscularly and response is seen after 3-6 weeks.
- Common side effects are nausea, vomiting, headache, anorexia, bone marrow suppression, development of tender and erythematous psoriatic lesions, and mucosal ulceration.
- Subsequent use of daily oral folic acid 1-5 mg, reduces risk of nausea, mucosal ulceration and anemia.

Cyclosporine:

- It inhibits cytokine production by T cells.
- It is used orally at a dose of 5 mg/kg body weight in recalcitrant and pustular psoriasis.
- Common side effects are hypertension, renal and hepatic toxicity, and risks of leukemia, lymphoma, cutaneous carcinoma, etc.

Acitretin:

- It normalizes epidermal differentiation and also has an anti-inflammatory role.
- It is used in erythrodermic and pustular psoriasis at a dose of 0.5-1 mg/kg body weight/ day.
- Common side effects are dryness of skin and mucosae, increased triglyceride level, premature epiphyseal closure, hyperostosis, hepatic toxicity and teratogenicity.

Etanercept:

- It binds with TNFα.
- Dose is 25-50 mg, twice per week as subcutaneous injection.
- It is available in India.
- Major side effects are production of anti-Ds antibody and increased chance of infection.

Alefacept:

- It antagonizes CD2 and thus inhibits T cells.
- Dose is 7.5 mg weekly, given as intramuscular injection.
- There is a chance of antibody formation.

Infliximab:

- It inhibits TNFα while binding to its receptor site.
- Dose is 5 mg/kg of body weight, given as intravenous injection at 0, 2 & 6 weeks.
- Adverse effects are antibody formation and increased risk of infection.

Efalizumab:

- Inhibits CD11a and thus inhibits the function of T cells.
- Dose is 1 mg/kg body weight, given as subcutaneous injection/week. At initial stage of therapy, a flare up of psoriasis is expected and later a rebound phenomenon is seen during withdrawal.

Antibiotic for sore throat: Usually a 7 day course of erythromycin is given, specially in children with guttate psoriasis.

Guttate psoriasis

- Drop like round or oval, 2-3 mm to 1 cm sized lesions are distributed symmetrically over trunk and proximal extremities.
- Children and young adults are commonly affected as a first manifestation of psoriasis.
- It is often aggravated by streptococcal infection at oropharynx or perianal region and in 2/3 cases, a history of upper respiratory infection found 1-3 weeks prior to onset of guttate psoriasis.

Scalp psoriasis

- Frequently it presents as first sign of psoriasis, having classical well defined erythematous plaques.
- However, lesions at eyebrows, retroauricular areas, and external auditory canals have greasy scales like seborrheic dermatitis, and then these lesions are designated as sebopsoriasis.
- Lesions of psoriasis often extend beyond hair line whereas lesions of seborrheic dermatitis remain within the hair line.

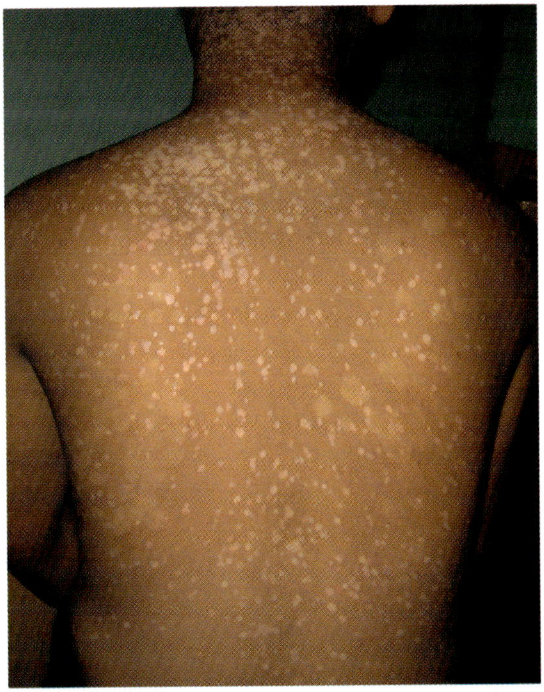

Fig. 9: Widespread rain drops like scaly papules of guttate psoriasis

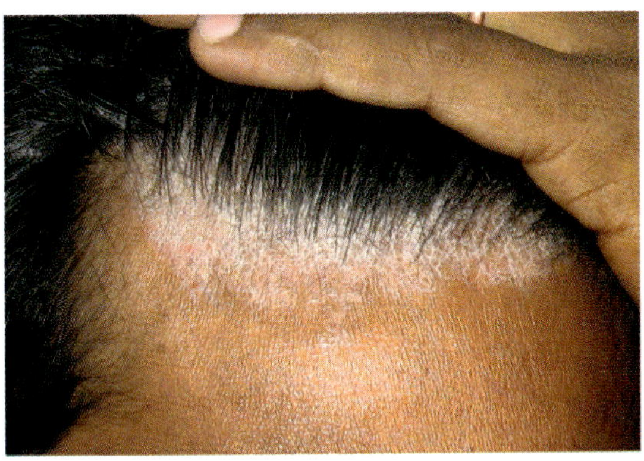

Fig. 10: Scaly plaque at scalp, crossing the hair line in scalp psoriasis

Parapsoriasis

- This is a chronic and uncommon dermatosis, having papulosquamous lesions and mimicks psoriasis.
- It usually occurs at middle age.
- Lesions develop gradually over months to years.
- Pruritus is a rare symptom.

Types

- Small plaque parapsoriasis (SPP).
- Large plaque parapsoriasis (LPP)

- SPP does not progresses to mycosis fungoides (MF) but LPP may transform into MF.

Clinical features of SPP

- Lesions are round to oval erythematous patches with minimal scaling.
- Cigarette paper wrinkling is present on the surface.
- Linear or finger like or digitate lesions are distributed along the line of cleavage. Here lesions are commonly seen at trunk, proximal extremities and buttocks.
- Size of individual lesion is less than 5 cm.

Histopathology of SPP

- Hyperkeratosis and parakeratosis.
- Spongiosis and exocytosis.
- Mild superficial perivascular lymphohistiocytic infiltration.

Clinical features of LPP

- Lesions are well defined dusky-red mild elevated patches or plaques.
- Surface usually have slight scaling; but it may be atrophied and smooth.
- Size of the lesion is more than 5 cm.
- Shape of the lesion is usually round; but may be irregular.
- Lesions are distributed randomly at trunk, female breasts, buttocks and extremities.

Histopathology of LPP

- Epidermal atrophy in later stage.
- Mild exocytosis.
- Vacuolar degeneration of basal layer with band like lymphocytic infiltration.
- Mild capillary dilatation at upper dermis.

Lichen planus

- This is an acute, subacute or chronic papulosquamous disorder of unknown etiology, affecting the skin, mucous membranes, hair follicles and nails.
- It may occur at any age and in any sex. But commonly seen at age between 30-60 years.

Electron microscopical changes

- Degenerations of desmosomes and hemidesmosomes of basal cells.
- Reduction of tonofilaments in early lesions but increases in late lesions.
- Fragmentation of lamina densa due to lymphocytic invasion, followed by duplication and irregular folding.
- Nercotic keratinocytes undergo filamentous degeneration to form colloid bodies.
- Cytolysis of the basal cells produces subepidermal cleft.

Clinical features

- It is a very common disease, presenting with an insidious onset of pruritic, solid and elevated skin lesions.
- Though the lesions are pruritic, it is interesting that the patient does not scratch but rub and in 20% cases lesions may be nonpruritic.
- Primary lesions are firm papules and plaques with varying amount of scales. New lesions may develop along the line of trauma, known as Koebner phenomenon.
- Color of the lesions is variable from purple to violaceous. Surfaces are smooth in early lesions, but scaly in older lesions. Sometimes whitish streaks, known as Wickham's striae, are seen on the surface.
- Number of the lesions varies from few to numerous. These may be discrete or confluent and localized or generalized.
- Size is variable from 1-2 mm to 10 mm. But hypertrophic variety may be of several cm.
- Shape is polygonal or irregular and margin is well defined.
- Lesions commonly develop at and around wrists, ankles and knees. But any site may be affected including oral and genital mucosae, palms, soles and scalp. Flexor surfaces are commonly affected in comparison to psoriasis where extensor surfaces are more affected.
- When the lesions subside, hyperpigmented atrophic patches develop and these may persist for many years.
- Nails are affected in 10% cases and is characterized by roughening, longitudinal ridging, thinning and dystrophy. Pterygium formation may be seen.

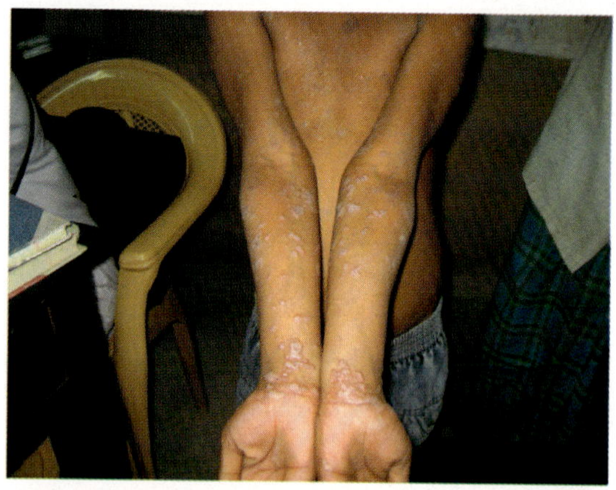

Fig. 11: Lesions at wrist and flexor surface of forearm

Differential diagnosis

- Psoriasis
- Secondary syphilis
- Sarcoidosis

Histopathology

- Orthokeratotic hyperkeratosis, except drug induced lesion where parakeratosis may be present.
- Wedge-shaped hypergranulosis.
- Acanthosis with irregularly elongated and sawtooth rete ridges.

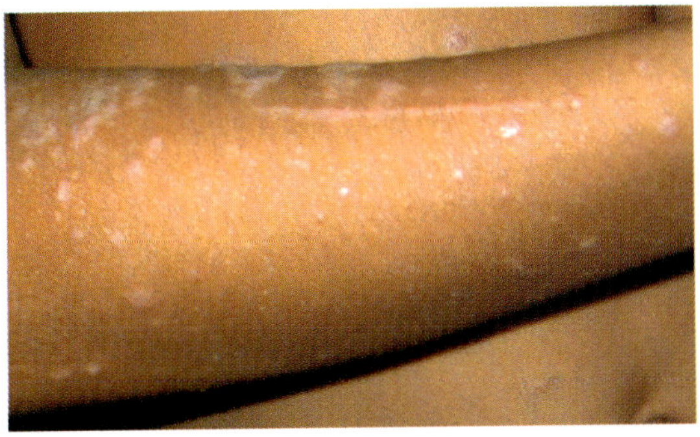

Fig. 12: Koebner phenomenon, showing by a linear lesion at right forearm

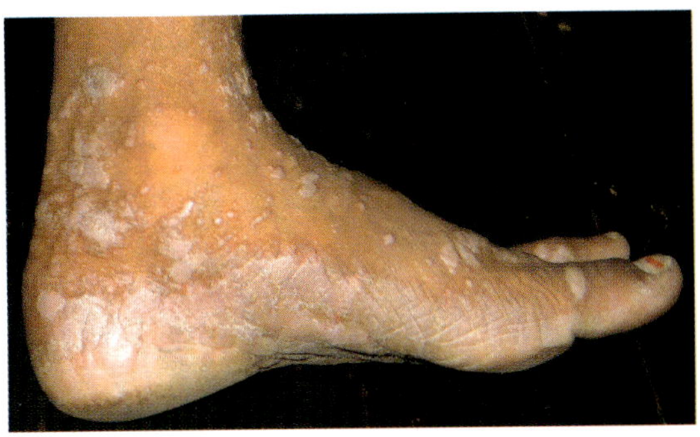

Fig. 13: Lesions around the ankle

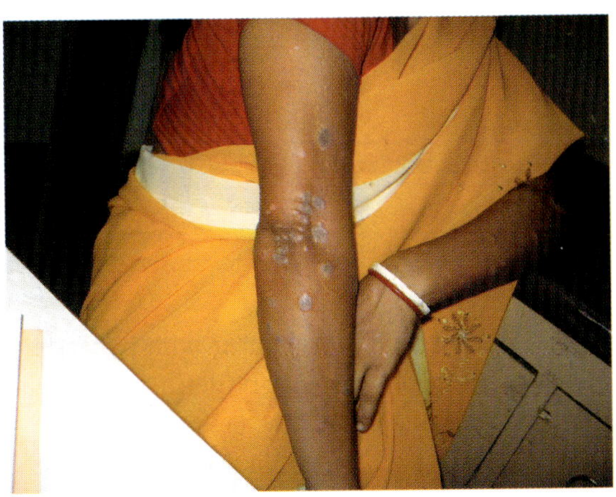

Fig. 14: Violaceous and scaly plaques at right elbow

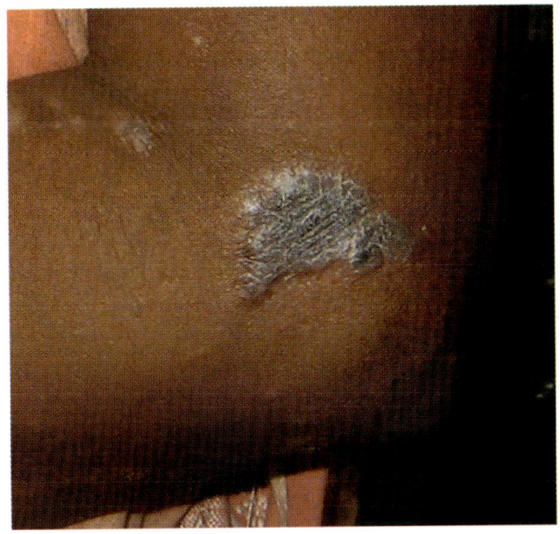

Fig. 15: Violaceous plaques, studded with whitish streaks

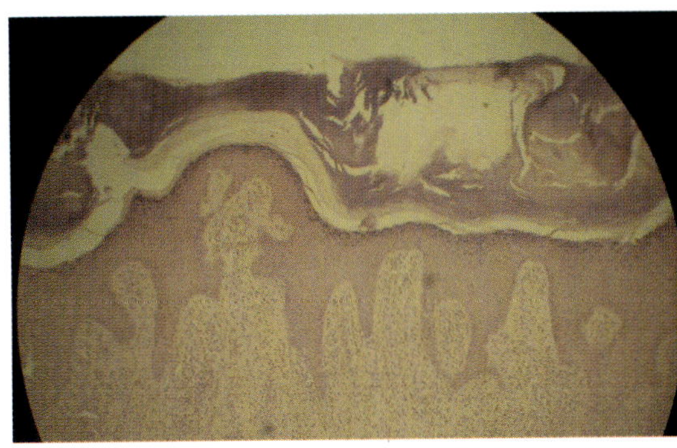

Fig. 16: Orthohyperkeratosis, irregular acanthosis, sawtooth rete ridges and upper dermal infiltration

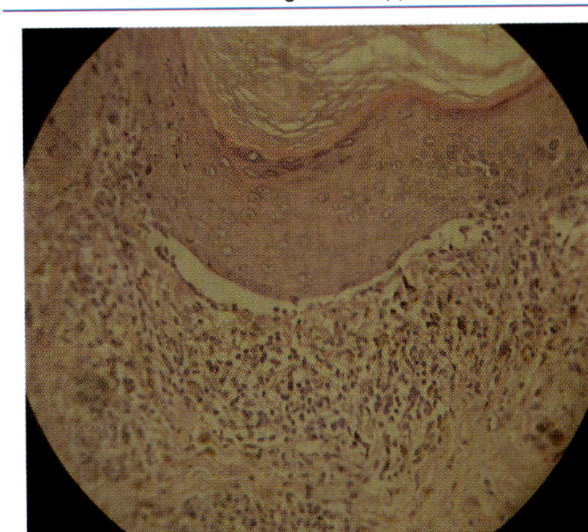

Fig. 17: Orthohyperkeratosis, acanthosis, Max-Joseph canal and band like infiltration

- Basal layer degeneration with pigment incontinence and formation of colloid bodies or Civatte bodies.
- Band like mononuclear cell infiltration along the dermoepidermal junction.
- Artificial cleft formation just below the epidermis, known as Max-Joseph canal.
- In case of bullous lichen planus or lichen planus pemphigoides, the subepidermal cleft is formed as a disease process.

Direct immunofluorescence

- Shaggy deposits of fibrinogen at the dermoepidermal junction.
- Occasionally granular deposition of IgM or linear deposition of C3 or both, at the dermoepidermal junction.
- IgG and C3 depositions along the basement membrane are seen in lichen planus pemphigoides.

Treatment

- For localized lesions, moderate to potent steroid (betamethasone, triamcinolone, mometasone, clobetasol, halobetasol) in cream or ointment form are useful but it takes long time for clearance.
- For hypertrophic lesion, intralesional triamcinolene (10 mg/ml) at 3-4 weeks interval till the lesion subsides.
- For oral mucosal lesion, triamcinolone acetonide in orabase, an adhesive vehicle, is safe and effective as a topical therapy. In resistant cases intralesional triamcinolone (10 mg/ml) may be given at 3-4 weeks interval or systemic steroid as in generalized form.
- For generalized lesions, i.m. injection of triamcinolone acetonide 0.5-1 mg/kg per month for 3-6 months, is the most effective therapy. Prednisolone 1 mg/kg/day for 2-4 weeks, then to be tapered gradually to stop within another 3 weeks.

Variants of lichen planus

- Atrophic, hypertrophic, actinic and follicular
- Eruptive, erosive, bullous and lichen planus pemphigoides
- Linear, zosteriform and annular
- Lichen planus pigmentosus
- Nail and mucosal LP
- Palmo-plantar LP

Eruptive or exanthematous type

- Lesions are intensely pruritic, flat-topped and polygonal papules with purple to violaceous color.
- Lesions are numerous in number and widely distributed.
- Trunk is the commonest site.

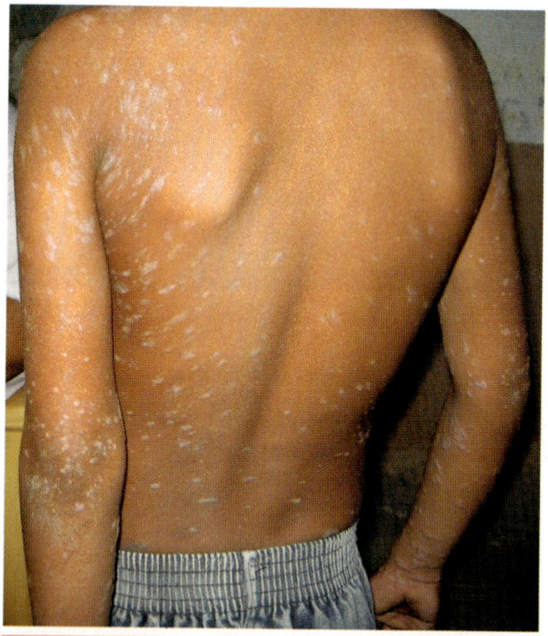

Fig. 18: Numerous lesions involving the trunk and upper limbs

Hypertrophic type

- Lesions are few in number with hyperkeratotic, thickened, sharply defined and long standing plaques. These are having irregular or verrucous surface with variable shape, size, color and itching.
- Shins and ankles are the commonest sites.

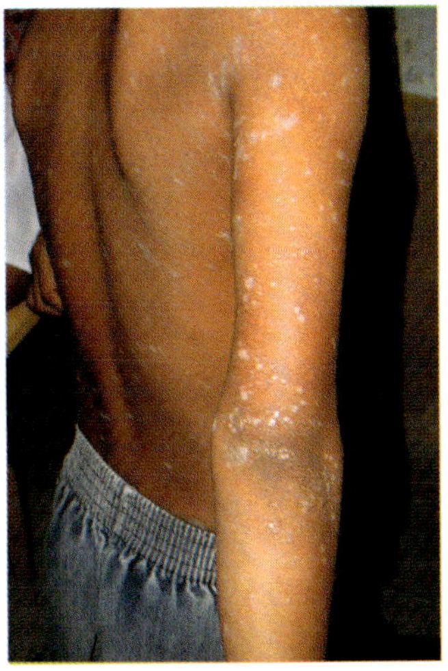

Fig. 19: Lesions around the elbow

Follicular/lichen planopilaris

- Lesions are pigmented and hyperkeratotic follicular papules.
- Scarring alopecia develops when these occur at scalp.

Actinic type

- It commonly affects age group of 20-30 years.
- Presence of pruritus is minimum or absent.
- Lesions are red to brown annular plaques or melasma like hyperpigmented patches at sun-exposed areas.
- Common sites are forehead, face, neck, and dorsal surface of arms and hands.
- A hypopigmented ring may present around the annular lesion and commonly reported from middle east countries.
- Onset is at spring and summer among children and young adults.

Annular type

- Lesion develops when a papule spreads at periphery with central clearing.
- Edge of the lesion is slightly raised and typically purple to violaceous in color.
- Central part may be hyperpigmented or skin colored.
- About 10% of lichen planus may have annular lesions.
- Common sites are axillae, penis, extremities and groin.
- Most are asymptomatic except few may have itching.

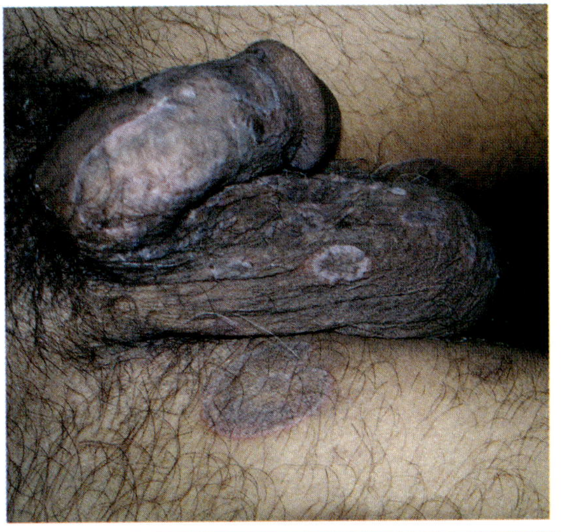

Fig. 20: Multiple annular plaques at genitalia

Linear/zosteriform

- Lesions develop in a linear fashion or become localized within a dermatome.

Bullous type

- Vesicle or bulla develops on pre-existing lichen planus lesion.

Bullous pemphigoid type/lichen planus pemphigoides

- Vesicle or bulla develops on normal skin in association with lichen planus lesion elsewhere.

Mucosal lichen planus

- Oral mucosal involvement occurs alone in 50% cases and remaining 50% occur in association with lesions at other areas.
- Buccal mucosa is the commonest site where the lesion usually starts from the angle of the mouth. Lips, gingival mucosa and tongue are also affected.

- Lesions are asymptomatic, whitish plaques.
- Surface of the lesion is irregular and lacy pattern. Subsequently erosion develops, producing pain and burning sensation. This erosive form may turn into squamous cell carcinoma in 0.8% cases.

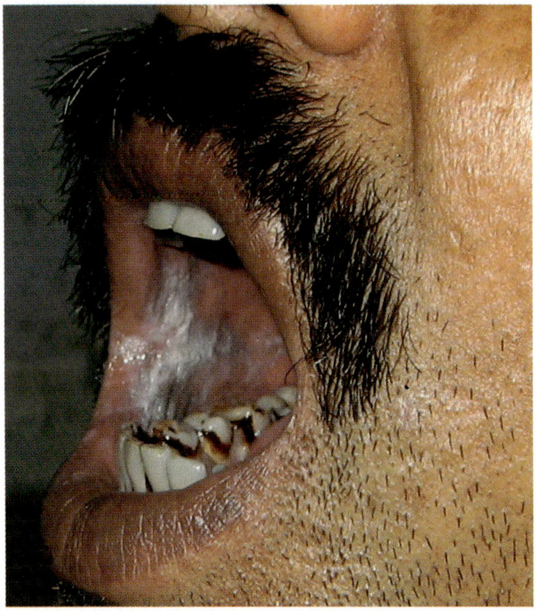

Fig. 21: Whitish plaque at buccal mucosa

- Penile mucosa is also affected, presenting with erosion or annular plaque. Sometimes prepuce may be involved with whitish fissured plaque. This is very often misdiagnosed as candidiasis.
- Vaginal lichen planus is presented with erythematous desquamative vaginitis and increased fragility. Adhesion of vaginal walls or labia minora leads to painful intercourse.
- Vulvovaginal-gingival syndrome is a form of lichen planus, characterized by erosion and desquamation of the vulva, vagina and gingiva. Gingival mucosal lesions are like buccal mucosal lesions, having erythema, erosion and whitish-lacy or-reticulated appearance.

Lichen planus at plams and soles

- Lesions: Waxy papule and plaques with intense itching.
- Classic purple or violaceous color is absent.
- Surface shows a characteristic honeycomb appearance.

Ashy dermatosis

- Asymptomatic, slowly spreading well defined blue gray macules and patches, commonly occur in children and young adults. In acute stage margin may be raised by 1-2 mm.
- Histopathology shows mild hyperkeratosis, acanthosis, hydropic change at basal layer, dermal pigment incontinence, cytoid body, mild perivascular or superficial lichenoid lymphocytic infiltration. No band like lymphocytic infiltration is detected.

Idiopathic eruptive macular pigmentation

- Asymptomatic discrete bluish macules, 0.5-2 cm in size, occur in children and young adult.
- Site: Neck, trunk and proximal extremities.
- Histopathology: Increased pigmentation at basal layer, pigment incontinence, melanophages, perivascular lymphocytic infiltration at papillary dermis.

Lichen planus pigmentosus

- It is commonly found in Indian subcontinent.
- Pruritus may or may not be present.
- Lesions are well defined bluish colored macules and patches with variable shape and size.
- Often lesions become diffuse. In dark skin, sometimes margin may be difficult to find out.
- Common sites are upper limbs, trunk, neck and face.
- Treatment: Clofazimine, DDS, vitamin A (1,00,000 IU/day for 3 weeks in a month for 6-8 months) showed variable result.

Lichen nitidus

* It may or may not be a variant of lichen planus. But both may coexist.

Clinical features

- Pruritus is usually absent.
- Lesions are tiny flesh colored papules, commonly affecting upper limbs, lower abdomen and shaft of the penis. But lesions may be generalized.
- Koebner phenomenon is often present and helps to differentiate from lichenoid polymorphic light eruption and lichen scrofulosorum.

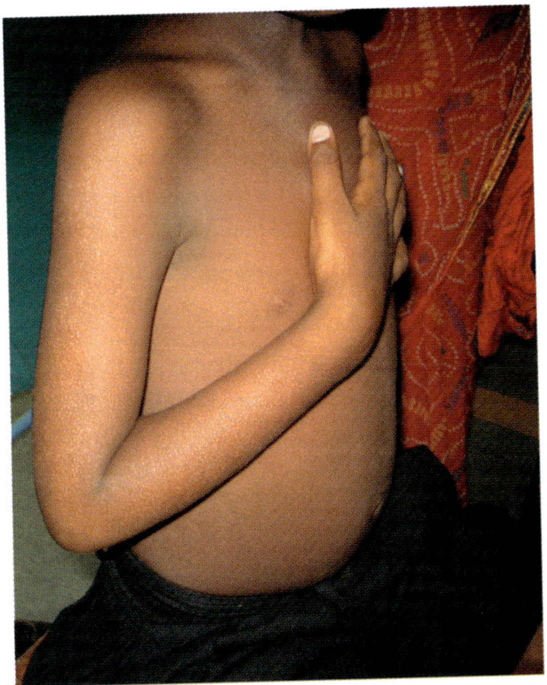

Fig. 22: Numerous tiny well defined papules

Differential diagnosis

- Lichen spinulosa
- Lichenoid polymorphic light eruption.

Histopathology

- Epidermal atrophy at the center and elongated rete ridges at the margin appear in such a way as they are clutching the dermal infiltration as a ball.
- Basal layer degeneration.
- Dermal lymphohistiocytic infiltration and granulomatous infiltration in older lesion.

Treatment

- Intramuscular triamcinolone injection 10-40 mg at 2-3 weeks interval till the lesions subside.

Pityriasis rubra pilaris

* There are two peak age of onset, one is first 5 years of age and second one is 50-55 years.

Clinical features

- Primary lesions are scaly follicular papules which may coalesce to form scaly patches and are often associated with diffuse palmoplantar keratoderma.
- Papules are pinhead in size having a central keratotic plug. Some of the papules may remain discrete and others may be confluent or may coalesce to form reddish-brown and scaly patches.
- Lesions usually starts just as erythema and scaling at scalp and follicular lesions gradually spread with a cephalo-caudal fashion.
- Lesions are distributed bilaterally and more or less symmetrically having a predilection for sides or back of the neck, trunk, extensors of the extremities and dorsa of first and second phalanges.
- Gradually new lesions develop to cover up whole body and the surface of the patches is felt like nutmeg grater.
- In extensive involvement, characteristic small islands of normal skin area may be seen within the affected areas.
- When erythroderma develops, follicular keratotic papules become less prominent.
- Palmoplantar hyperkeratosis shows a tendency of fissuring and may extend upto the sides appearing as sandal.
- Nails become dull, brittle, thickened, rough or striated and sometimes pitted.

- Itching is the only symptom present in early stage in few cases.

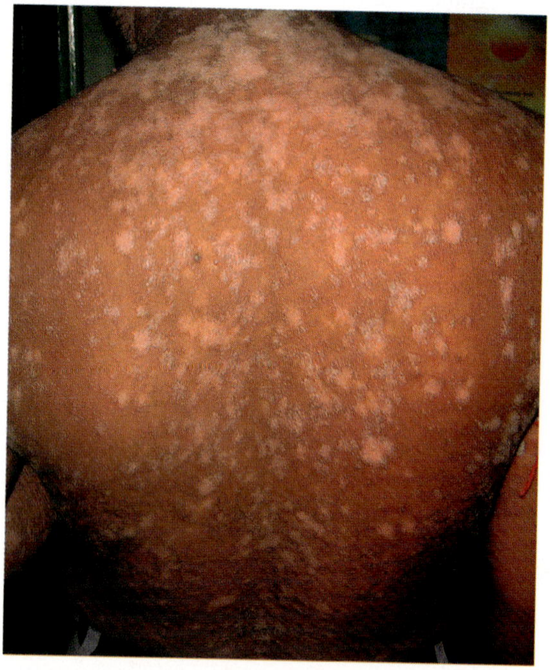

Fig. 23: Numerous erythematous follicular papules

Histopathology

- Orthohyperkeratosis with alternate parakeratosis, oriented both horizontally and vertically, appearing as checkerboard pattern.
- Focal or confluent hypergranulosis.
- Acanthosis with short and thick rete ridges and suprapapillary thickening.
- Corresponding follicular lesion shows orthokeratotic follicular plugging and perifollicular shoulder parakeratosis.
- Erythrodermic lesion shows thinned or even absent corneal layer with presence of plasma and hypogranulosis.
- Slight spongiosis may be present.
- Mild perivascular mononuclear cell infiltrations and moderately dilated vessels in the dermis.

Treatment

- Oral isotretinoin 0.5-1 mg/kg/day for 6-9 months.
- Methotrexate orally or intramuscularly 2.5-30 mg/week till remission.

Variants of PRP

- Type I, the classic adult type and most common type which in 80% cases involutes within 3 years.
- Type II, atypical adult type, has a poor prognosis and associated with ichthyosis.
- Type III, classical juvenile type, has a good prognosis as usually clears within a year.
- Type IV, atypical juvenile type, has circumscribed confluent follicular papules, bearing poor prognosis and palmar sclerosis.
- Type V, associated with HIV infection and may have acne conglobata, hidradenitis suppurativa and lichen spinulosa along with PRP.

Commonest differential diagnosis

- For classical type: Psoriasis,
- For atypical circumscribed type: Phrynoderma, frictional follicular keratosis and follicular dermatitis.

Pityriasis rosea

* It is a mild inflammatory exanthema of unknown etiology with some association with herpes virus –6 or –7.
* It commonly affects age group 15 to 40 years and occurs in spring and autumn.
* Drugs causing pityriasis rosea-like eruptions are captopril, ketotifen, clonidine, metronidazole, barbiturates, ergotamine, etc.

Clinical features

- Pruritus is the commonest symptom with variable intensity.
- Lesions start as discrete and mild erythematous papules which usually involute from their center to form annular patches.

- Size of the lesions is varying from 2 mm to 2 cm, except the herald patch which is larger.
- Larger lesions are oval in shape and have characteristic collarette of scales at the periphery. If the lesion is stretched along its long axis, scales show a tendency to become folded across the lines of stretch, and this is known as Hanging curtain sign.
- In 70% cases, lesion starts as a single lesion, known as herald patch or mother patch, which slowly enlarges and when it begins to involute numerous smaller lesions appear within 1-2 weeks.
- Lesions are characteristically distributed at trunk, neck, face and proximal parts of extremities. Long axis of the lesions are arranged parallel to the line of normal cleavage.
- Rarely palms, soles, eyelids, penis and oral mucosa are affected.
- Some atypical presentations are inverse type involving only extremities, papular type, purpuric type, vesicular type, combination of other types along with classical type, or single herald patch without developing other lesions.
- Lesions may disappear without treatment after 3-8 weeks but rarely recur.

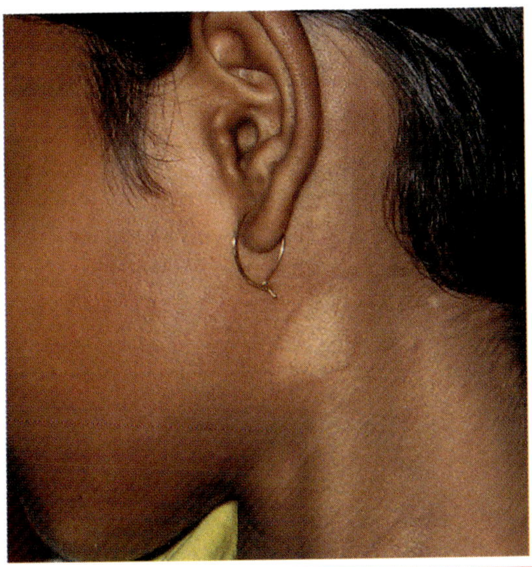

Fig. 24: Multiple oval patches with collarette of scales at the periphery

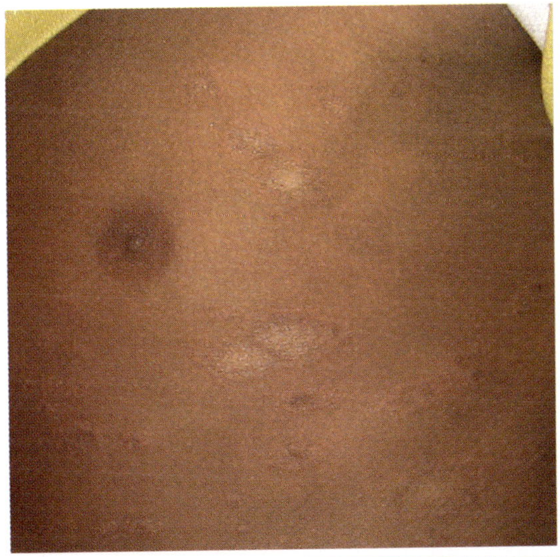

Fig. 25: Multiple oval scaly patches along the ribs

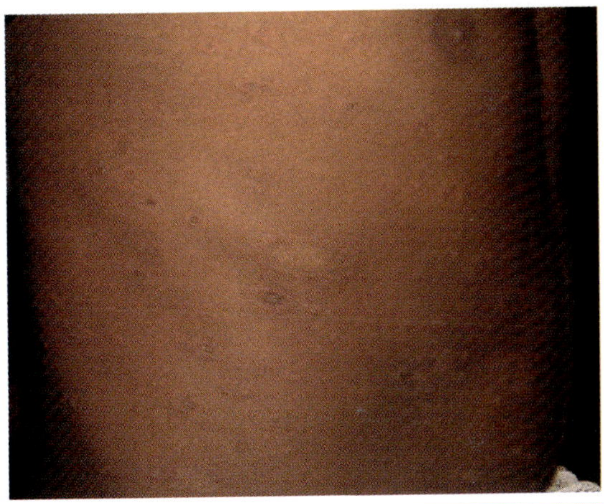

Fig. 26: A large patch (herald patch) surrounded by smaller patches

Differential diagnosis

- Tinea corporis
- Impetigo circinata
- Pityriasiform seborrheic dermatitis
- Papular syphilid
- Pityriasis lichenoides chronica.

Histopathology

- Mild acanthosis, focal parakeratosis, extravasated RBCs into the epidermis, spongiosis and perivascular lymphocytic infiltration.

Treatment

- Emollient and topical corticosteroid
- Systemic corticosteroid
- High doses of acyclovir.

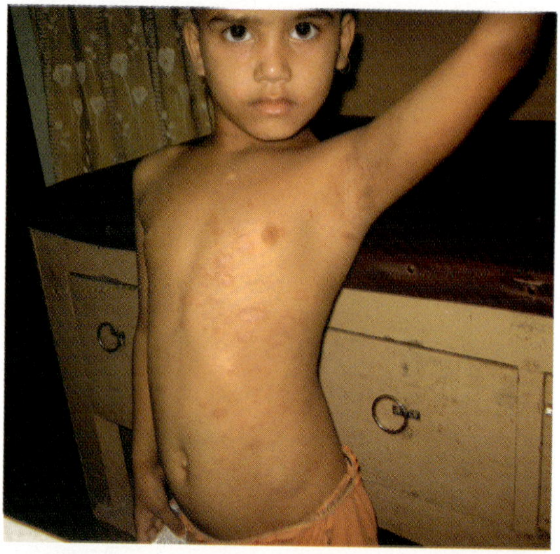

Fig. 27: Oval scaly patches with collarette of scales at the margin

Reiter's disease

- It is an chronic inflammatory disease, having recurrent episodes of arthritis, urethritis, conjunctivitis and mucocutaneous eruptions.
- It usually occurs in a genetically susceptible person, following an infection of the genitourinary tract due to chlamydiae and ureaplasma (postvenereal group) or following an attack of dysentry due to shigella, salmonella, campylobactor and yersinia (post-dysentric group).
- Postvenereal group is mostly seen in USA and Britain, but post-dysentric group is seen in Asia, other parts of Europe and North Africa.
- Male-female ratio in post-venereal group is 99:1 and in post-dysentric group is 9:1.
- It is an episodic disease and each episode lasts about 3 months and it may remit earliest by 2 weeks or may last for a year.
- It recurs in 40% cases.
- Interval between the infection and initiation of the disease is variable from 1-3 months.

Clinical features

- In severe cases general symptoms are fever, malaise, anorexia and weight loss.
- Mucocutaneous lesions are seen in 50% cases and are prone to develop at skin, genital or oral mucosae and nails.
- Skin lesions are seen in 30% cases and classical lesions are known as keratoderma blenorrhagica which commonly affects the palms, soles and toes.
- Lesions start as erythematous macules which turn into vesicles, followed by formation of pustules. When pustules are dried up, papules and plaques, covered with thick crusts are developed.
- At palms and soles, lesions are covered with mollusk-like thick crust.
- Skin lesions appear as relief map or mountain range appearance.
- Balanitis occurs in 25-50% cases. Lesions start as vesicles which rupture and form erosions at glans or corona. These small erosions gradually enlarge as well as coalesce to form a circinate pattern and designated as circinate balanitis.
- In uncircumcised glans, lesions are moist, but in circumcised glans, lesions are covered with thick crust which are similar to keratoderma blenorrhagica of the palms and soles. Lesions may last for days to years.
- Lesions of the oral mucosa is seen in 40% cases. It affects palate, tongue, buccal mucosa, lips, gums and even pharynx and nasal septum.
- Lesions of the mouth start as vesicles which rupture to form erythematous and painless erosions.

- These oral lesions last only for few days.
- Nail involvement is usually seen in those nails which are having adjacent skin lesions. Subungual hyperkeratosis is a common change. Nail plates become thickened, yellow, opaque, rigid and brittle which subsequently shed off.
- Urethritis is a nonspecific feature and may be associated with concurrent gonococcal infection. It may go unnoticed. It is characterized by prolonged abacterial mucoid discharge with dysuria, pyuria and rarely hematuria. It may be associated with cystitis, prostatitis, pyelonephritis, and cervicitis or vaginitis.
- Eye involvement presents as conjunctivitis (red eye) in 50% cases. It is usually transient and may be unnoticed. It may be associated with iritis and keratitis.
- Joint involvement presents as seronegative, asymmetric and polyarticular arthritis. It mostly affects large joints. It may be associated with achilles tendinitis and plantar fasciitis in 20% cases. Unilateral sacroilitis also may be present.
- Neurologic features are acute meningoencephalitis, acute psychotic reaction, cranial nerve palsies, seizures, personality disorders, and cervical or lumbar radiculopathy.
- Cadiovascular system may be affected with conduction defect and aortic insufficiency.
- Secondary amyloidosis may develop.

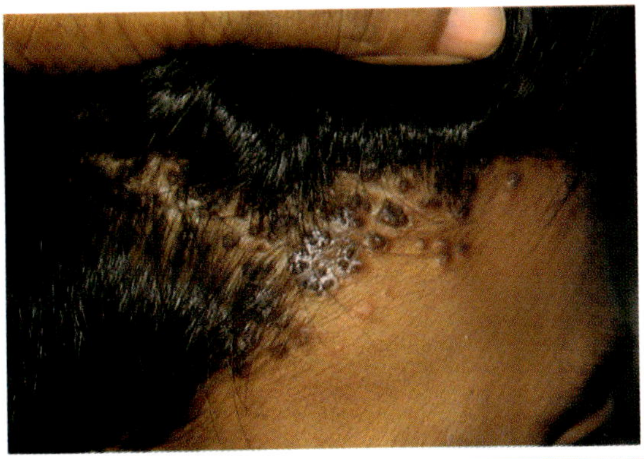

Fig. 28: Cone shaped keratotic papules

Histopathology

- Orthohyperkeratosis with or without parakeratosis in older lesion
- Mound parakeratosis in newly formed lesion.
- Macropustules in the upper epidermis.

Discoid lupus erythematosus

* It is the chronic form of cutaneous lupus erythematosus.
* Lupus erythematosus is not primarily a keratinizing disorder but due to presence of scales, it mimicks many other scaly disorders.

Clinical features

- Erythematous and indurated papules and plaques are presenting with thick adherent scales, follicular plugging, dyspigmentation, atrophy and scarring, and sometimes telangiectasia.
- Cutaneous horn may develop on the lesions.

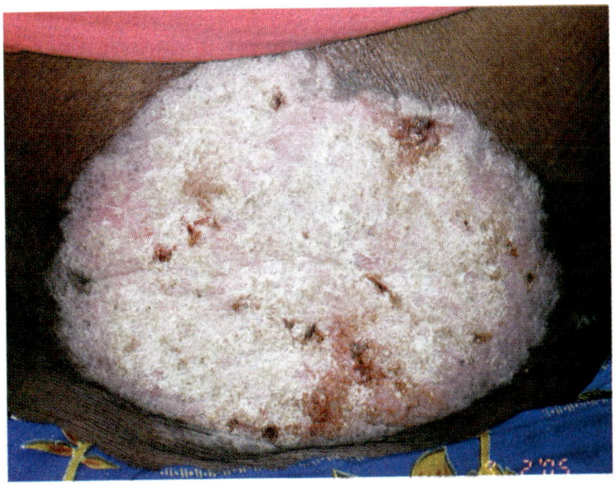

Fig. 29: Well defined erythematous plaque with adherent scales and hemorrhagic crusts at places and hyperpigmented margin

Histopathology

- Hyperkeratosis with or without parakeratosis.
- Follicular plugging.
- Irregular acanthosis with focal atrophy.
- Focal vacuolar degeneration of basal layer and

pigment incontinence and colloid body formation.

- Patchy lymphocytic infiltration in the dermis, specially around the appendages and vessels.

Treatment

- Topical corticosteroid and sunscreen.
- Oral chloroquine or hydroxychloroquine.
- Systemic corticosteroids.

Variants

- Localized type, affecting only head and neck regions.
- Widespread type, affecting other areas along with head and neck regions.
- Hypertrophic type, lesions are very much keratotic and indurated.
- Mucosal type, commonly affecting the lips.

Subacute lupus erythematosus (SCLE)

* This is a widespread photosensitive dermatosis, belonging the group of lupus erythematosus.
* It is having a good prognosis with different immunological pattern and few systemic involvement.
* Women are more commonly affected than men.
* Features of SLE are seen in 60% cases.
* Anti SS-A and anti SS-B are often positive.

Pattern of clinical presentation

- Papulosquamous pattern.
- Annular pattern.

Clinical features

- Erythematous scaly patches and plaques which are distributed symmetrically at sunexposed areas of arms and trunk.
- Lesions have a tendency to coalesce.
- Sometimes lesions become annular with crusted margin. These lesions start as scaly papules and enlarge gradually. During evolution, central scales or crusts shed off with persisting peripheral one and thus take the annular shape.
- Sometimes lesions appear as erythema multiforme like lesions and this is known as Rowell syndrome.
- Arthritis is frequently associated but rarely the renal system is involved.

Histo-and immunopathology

- Interface dermatitis with vacuolar basal cell degeneration and superficial dermal infiltration.
- Deposition of IgG and C3 along the basement membrane of the lesional skin in 50-60% cases.

CHAPTER

C10

ACNEIFORM DERMATOSES

Acne vulgaris

- This is a disease of the pilosebaceous units, developing during puberty.
- Seborrhea and alopecia of the scalp are frequently associated with acne.
- Irregular menstrual period, infertility and hirsutism also may be associated with acne in females.
- Family history of acne is also noted in some cases.
- Sebaceous glands are distributed all over the body except palms, soles, dorsa of the feet and lower lip. But acne develops at the areas where the glands are in high concentration.
- Exacerbation of acne occurs with menstruation and stress.
- It commonly affects areas, rich in sebaceous glands like face, upper back and chest with a varying degree of severity.
- Commonest presenting age group is 16-18 years. But it may develop at later age like 25 years or even 35 years of age.
- Lesions begin as early as 8-10 years of age. In girls these may precede menarche by one year.
- Severe acne occurs frequently in males, but more persistent in females.
- In majority of the cases, lesions start to subside after 22 years of age and rarely persists beyond age of 25 years. But sometimes it crosses the age of 40 years.
- In many cases when facial acne resolves, truncal acne starts to develop.
- Tetracycline, doxycycline and minocycline, the main drugs for acne, are contraindicated in pregnancy and lactation.

Main pathogenic factors

- Hyperkeratinization of pilosebaceous follicle.
- Increased sebum production by hormonal and genetic influences.
- Increased colonization of *Propionibacterium acne* organisms.
- Varying degree of inflammation.

Pathogenesis

- Acne is a disease of the pilosebaceous unit. Sebum, the product of the sebaceous glands, has the primary role in pathogenesis of acne. Sebaceous glands normally harbour an anerobic organism, known as *Propionibacterium acne*.

- In adolescent period, sebum secretion is increased with the influence of sex hormone testosterone as well as *P. acnes* proliferate excessively. These modify the sebum products to make them more comedogenic and altered follicular epithelial lining prevents the easy expulsion of sebum.
- Increased amount of cornified cells remain attached (retention keratosis) along the pilosebaceous canal, just above the opening of the sebaceous duct as a plug. Thus a microcomedone is formed.
- When the duct is closed and the sebum products deposit behind it, a closed comedone or white head is formed.
- If the collection remains behind a small dilated duct, an open comedone or a black head is formed.
- *P. acne* generates various enzymes like lipases, proteases, hyaluronidase, and many chemotactic factors.
- Lipases hydrolyze sebum and produces free fatty acids. These free fatty acids are comedogenic and help to form retention keratosis at the opening of the pilosebaceous duct.
- Chemotactic factors attract neutrophils which liberate hydrolases. Hydrolase enzymes dissolve the wall of the duct and so the contents of it poured into the dermis.
- An inflammatory reaction starts around this sebum contents. If the inflammation is very acute and superficial pustules are developed.
- Subacute inflammation at deeper level gives rise to nodule formation. If further an acute inflammation occurs, cysts are developed.

Evolution

- Earliest lesions are the comedones. These are 1-2 mm sized papules with whitish center, known as white heads or closed comedones and 2-5 mm sized lesions with dark-topped center, known as black heads or closed comedones.
- Comedones may persist or subsequently may turn into erythematous papules, pustules, cysts, abscesses and interconnected sinuses.

Clinical features

- In mild cases it is asymptomatic and considered as a very minor age related problem. Rarely it is associated with itching, specially in postadolescent acne.
- But in severe cases, nodules and pustules often produce pain, followed by anxiety or depression due to fear of disfigurement.
- More than 50% of the patients present with comedones, papules and pustules.
- Comedones may be white head/close comedones and black head/open comedones.
- Other lesions are noncomedogenic papules, pustules, nodules, cystic nodules, cyst and sinuses.
- Erythema and purulent or bloody odorless discharge are often associated with pustular and nodular lesions.
- Also pustular and nodulocystic lesions produce crusts and necrotic ulcers.
- When lesions heal, postinflammatory hyperpigmentation, pock-like pitted scars, hypertrophic scars and keloids may be formed.

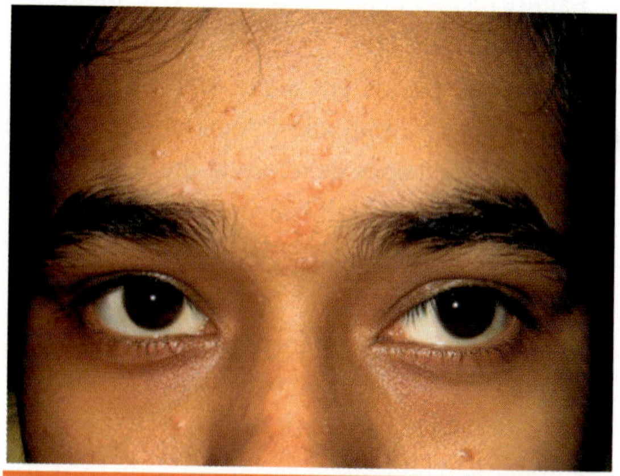

Fig. 1: Few papules and whiteheads in mild form of acne

Differential diagnosis

- Perioral dermatitis
- Acne agminata.

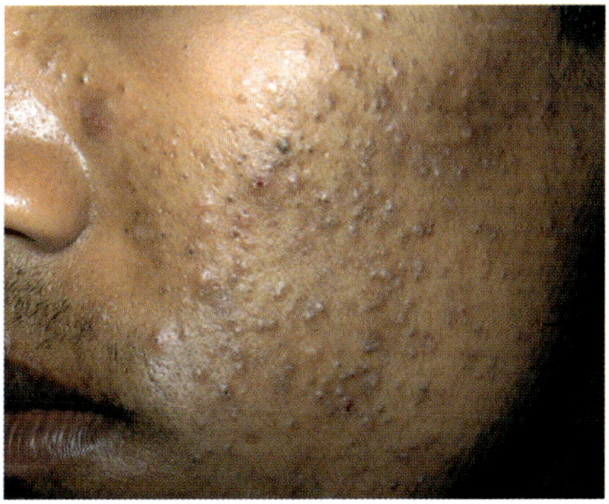

Fig. 2: Multiple papules, blackheads, whiteheads and few pustules in moderate acne

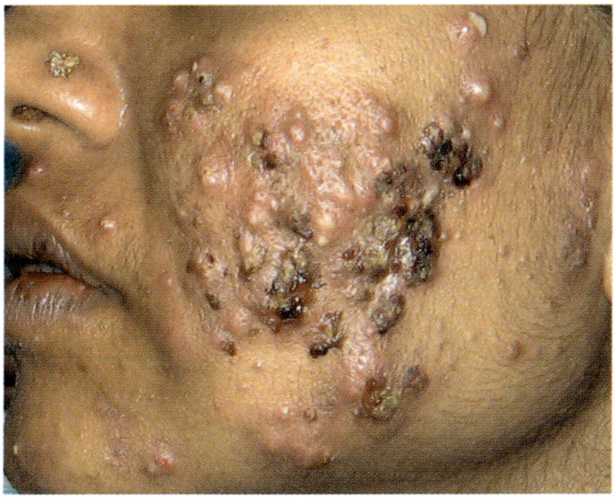

Fig. 3: Multiple nodulopustules with crusting in severe acne

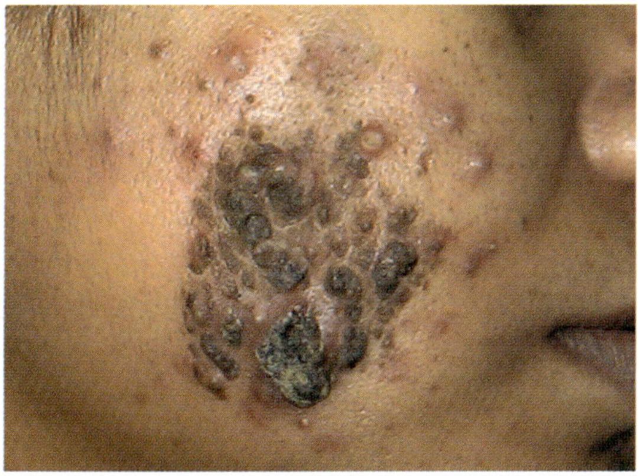

Fig. 4: Monomorphic pustules of pyoderma faciale with crusting in a middle aged women

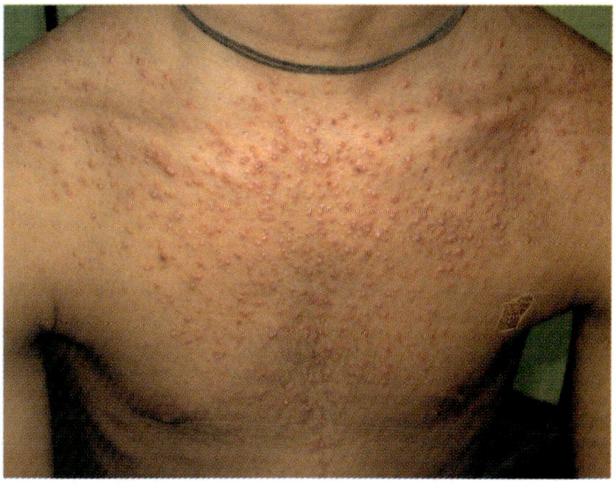

Fig. 5: Monomorphic papulo-pustular lesions of steroid induced acne

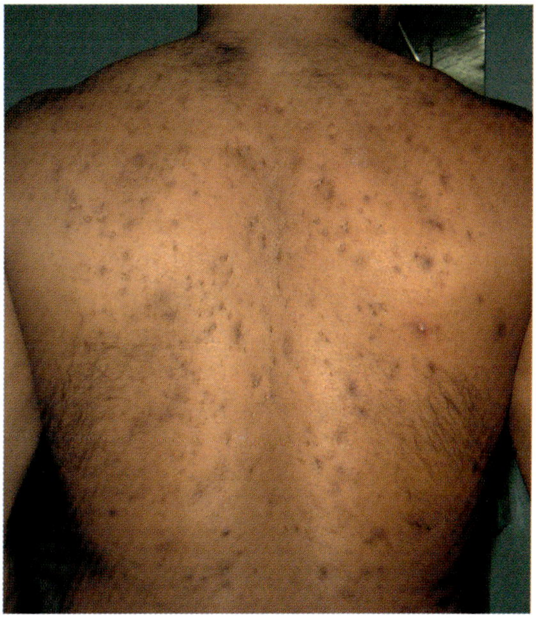

Fig. 6: Multiple acne scars with few active pustules of truncal acne

Differential diagnosis

- Pityrosporum folliculitis.

Grading of acne for treatment

Mild acne

- Comedones.
- Noninflammatory, noncomedogenic dome-shaped yellowish papules or skin colored papules.

Moderate acne

- Pustules less than 20 in number.
- ± Lesions of the mild acne.

Severe acne

- Pustules more than 20 in number.
- Nodulocystic lesions.
- ± Lesions of the mild acne and moderate acne.

Pretreatment counselling regarding misconceptions in acne

- Constipation: Usually the patients or their relatives firmly believe that acnes are due to constipation. So, we should confirm them that it is not at all related.
- Oily food: At the age of puberty, the boys and girls are very much fond of oily/fast foods but the parents does not like it. So, very often the parents request the doctors to tell them that their acne is due to their frequent taking of oily food. So, we should tell their parents that this is not due to oily food.
- Semen or white discharge: Though not very often but sometimes the patients may ask whether it is related or not. Because in the same age the boys recognize that color of the semen and the girls recognize the color of the white discharge and they believe that semen or white discharge are coming out as content of acnes.
- Use of corticosteroid: Some particular brand of corticosteroids are used as fairness cream, specially by females of all ages, commonly in suburban areas. After application of few tubes when the users start to develop adverse effects like excess hair grown, perioral dermatitis and telangiectasia, they come to the dermatologist. Then the dermatologist can feel how tough it is to tackle these complications.

Pretreatment counselling regarding course of the disease during therapy

- Very frankly speaking the result of treatment is to some extent unpredictable. With same regimen in two different patients of similar type of acne will not give same result after a fixed period of treatment.
- In an average minimal result is expected after 8 weeks of treatment and lesions are expected to be clear not before 6 months.
- An average improvement is seen after 4 months.

* Regarding diet:
  - Some studies confirm that there is a relation with hyperglycemic carbohydrate rich food.
  - The theory behind this is that this type of foods produce a hyperinsulinemia state which disturbs the balance of other hormones.
  - Androgenic hormones get a chance to act on sebaceous glands.

Pretreatment counselling regarding forceful excoriation

- This is a very bad habit nurtured by the patient. They are forced to do it when they stand in front of the mirror or get a leisure time.
- It is often an outburst of the psychological impact due to their acne induced disfigurement.
- The result is excessive post acne complications like scars and pigmentation. So, definitely we should discourage this habit.

Pretreatment counselling regarding use of cosmetics

- Use of any form of cosmetics should be avoided.
- But the female patients often request to allow them to use it during on occasion.
- In such a situation only nongreasy and water-based compound may be allowed but only for few hours.

Pretreatment counselling regarding facewash

- It must be clear that acnes are not due to any dirt. Exessive washing must be discouraged.

- It makes the skin more irritable and thus interferes with treatment modalities.
- Face-wash can be done 2-3 times per day but it should be done very gently and any cream-based cleansers to be avoided.

Pretreatment counselling regarding use of oral contraceptive

- Pills containing antiestrogenic progestogens like norgesterol and norethindrone provoke the acne.
- So, it is better to avoid these preparations.

Pretreatment counselling regarding technique of application

- Face should be cleaned gently two to three times a day with mild soap.
- Wait for 20-30 minutes to dry up the face before application of any antiacne preparation.
- Medicine must be applied on entire affected areas of the face, not just on the lesions.
- A pea-sized amount of medicine is enough for whole face.
- For peeling agents like retinoids or benzoyl-peroxide, sensitive areas of the nose, mouth and eyes and chin, are to be avoided.
- Initially these peeling agents are used on alternate day or on every third day. This simple procedure will drastically reduce the irritant effect.

Pretreatment counselling regarding long-term systemic antibiotics

- Very often patients express their concern when they are informed about long term systemic antibiotics.
- But our experience is that it is a safe practice and patients must be reassured.

Therapy to control the abnormal keratinization at pilosebaceous duct

- Topical retinoids
- Systemic isotretinoin

Therapy to control proliferation of *P. acne*

- Benzoyl peroxide
- Topical antibiotics
- Oral antibiotics

Therapy to control acute inflammation

- Isotretinoin which acts indirectly.
- Intralesional corticosteroids
- Oral corticosteroids
- Systemic antibiotics which act indirectly.

Therapy to control sebaceous gland function

- Oral isotretinoin
- Estrogens in oral contraceptive pills
- HPA suppression with low dose prednisone or dexamethasone.
- Anti-androgens like spironolactone or ciproterone acetate.

Therapy for mild acne

- If patient is having only comedones, topical therapy is enough and if it fails, comedones extraction is the definitive treatment.
- Retinoids are the best topical therapy.
- Adapalene is less irritant but costly than tretinoin.
- Alternatives are benzoyl peroxide and azelaic acid preparations.
- Tazarotene is for recalcitrant cases.

Therapy for moderate acne

- Topical clindamycin or clarithromycin or benzoyl peroxide.
- Oral doxycycline (100-200 mg/day) or minocycline (100-200 mg/day) or azithromycin (250 mg/day) for 2-4 months.
- When severity will be reduced, treatment to be followed as mild acne.

Therapy for severe acne

- Oral isotretinoin 40 mg/day for at least 4 months, when lesions are mostly nodular or nodulocystic.

- Minocycline 200 mg per day for at least 8 weeks, when lesions are predominantly pustular.
- Intralesional triamcinolone (2.5 to 5.0 mg/ml) injection may be used for dramatic response.
- When severity will be reduced, treatment to be followed as moderate acne and mild acne.

Retinoids

- These preparations basically increase cell turnover of the follicles and reduce cohesion between keratinized cells. Thus help in fragmentation and expulsion of the pluggings from the pilosebaceous ducts.
- These also convert closed comedones into open comedones and prevent new comedones formation.
- These can cause facial dryness, chapping, peeling and erythema, temporarily making the acne worse.
- Moreover continuous use at this stage leads the skin thin, more susceptible to sunburn and irritating from wind, cold, soap or face-wash.
- Solution or gel is more effective but more irritating than cream form.
- As this group of preparations has direct action on microcomedones, always expected to be a first line therapy in all forms of acne.

Tretinoin

- Available as 0.025% and 0.05% cream/gel/solution.
- Cream is for dry skin and solution/gel is for oily skin.

Tazarotene

- It is available as 0.05% and 0.1% gel and cream forms and is applied once daily.
- It is more effective for papules, open comedones and pustules.
- Initially alternate day therapy or short contact therapy for few minutes and washing it off, is more tolerable.

Adapalene

- It has an additional antiinflammatory role without any photosensitivity reaction. It is available as 0.1% gel.

Azelaic acid

- It has an additional antimicrobial activity without any chance of bacterial resistance.
- It has no photosensitivity reaction and no significant local irritation.
- It is best used for maintenance therapy when systemic therapy is stopped.

Benzoyl peroxide

- It has strong antimicrobial activity without any chance of bacterial resistance.
- It is available as 2.5% and 5% gel. Mild erythema and scaling are expected during the first few days of application.
- So better to start with low concentration and not more than once per day application. Gradually frequency and concentration both may be increased.
- Sometimes peeling and fissuring may become severe but it does not cause any residual wrinkling.
- In 2% cases suddenly diffuse erythema and vesicles may develop. These are due to allergic contact dermatitis to benzoyl peroxide and the medicine should be stopped immediately.

Tetracycline

- Dose is initially 500 mg twice daily for 3 to 6 weeks or more to get a significant improvement, followed by 250 mg twice daily till the new lesions develop. But if no change even after 6 weeks, an alternative drug is to be started.
- The drug is cheaper.
- It should not be taken with foods specially dairy products which prevent intestinal absorption.

- It may produce photosensitivity when given in a higher doses and increases incidence of candidal vulvovaginitis.
- Rarely it penetrates blood brain barrier and impairs intracranial pressure. Thus it develops pseudotumor cerebri syndrome with self-limiting features like severe headache, transient visual disturbances or diplopia and pulsatile tinnitus. The incidence is increased when it is used along with oral isotretinoin.

Doxycycline

- Dose is 100 mg once or twice daily and duration of therapy is like tetracycline.
- It is also cheaper and can be taken with any food.
- Incidence of photosensitivity is still less than tetracycline but increases with higher doses.

Minocycline

- Dose is 50-100 mg twice daily and it is the most effective drug in comparison to tetracycline or doxycycline.
- So patient compliance is very good; but it is costly. If patient can afford, it should be the first drug for pustular acne; otherwise it is kept reserve for tetracycline or doxycycline failure cases.
- Foods inhibit its absorption to some extent.
- Blue-gray pigmentation occurs at skin, nails, oral mucosa, sclera, bones and thyroid gland after taking for a long period and at high doses.
- Skin pigmentation is seen mostly at depressed acne scar and at the sites of any skin inflammation.
- Skin pigmentation may also appear as macules like bruise on the lower legs and as diffuse suntan. Pigmentation of the incisal half of the crown in adult is reported.
- It enters the cerebrospinal fluid easily for its high lipid solubility and causes ataxia, vertigo, nausea and vomiting in some patients.
- When it crosses the blood brain barrier may produce pseudotumor cerebri syndrome as with tetracycline.
- Moreover it is associated with autoimmune hepatitis, serum-sickness-like features and lupus-like reactions.

Clindamycin

- Dose is 75-300 mg twice daily. It is very effective; but costly and notorious for pseudomembranous colitis.

Ampicillin/amoxicillin

- Dose is 500 mg twice daily. These are safe drugs and so useful in pregnancy and lactation with mild to moderate inflammatory acne.
- These are also useful in long-term antibiotic induced Gram-negative pustular and cystic acne.

Cephalosporin

- It is indicated for antibiotic resistant pustular acne.

Trimethoprim (160 mg) and sulfamethoxazole (800 mg)

- Dose of the combined drug is once or twice daily.
- It is indicated for tetracycline resistant acne and for Gram-negative folliculitis.

Macrolide antibiotics

- Dose for erythromycin is 250-500 mg twice daily and due to long half life of azithromycin, dose is 250 mg on alternate day.
- P. acne becomes resistant to erythromycin and for that now it is not considered as a first line drug.

Neonatal acne

- These occur as comedones or pustules at birth or within few days of life. Maternal androgen is responsible for it.
- As gradually, the androgen will be degraded from the body, the lesions are expected to be disappear within 6 months of age and so, no treatment is required.

Childhood acne

- These often appear between 6-16 months of age. Lesions may be mild, moderate or severe forms including comedones, papules, pustules or even nodulocystic acnes.
- Retinoids for comedones and benzoyl peroxide for inflammatory acne are useful.
- For moderate to severe acnes systemic therapy like erythromycin 125 mg or trimethoprim 100 mg twice daily for quite along time, upto 18 months, rarely more than 24 months, is required.
- The time of clearance is varying from 6-18 months.

Post adolescent acne

- This entity is specially for professional women. Lesions are mostly closed comedones, papules and only a few pustules.
- Very often these women pass their adolescent period without any acne and become very astonished by seeing the lesions at this age. Premenstrual flare is also a common history. Chronic stress is another factor which probably increase androgenic activity.
- The mean age of onset is 20 years, mean age for visiting a dermatologist is 37 years and mean duration is 20 years.
- Rarely other features of hyperandrogenism like hirsutism, irregular menses, androgenic alopecia, seborrhea and acne distribution at lower face, mandibular line, or neck.

Senile acne

- Lesions are mostly larger comedones including both open and closed comedones. Excessive sun exposure is a precipitating factor.
- Commonest sites are temples and areas around the eyes. Topical retinoids and comedone extraction are the treatment of choice.
- Retinoids are used to loosening of the firmly compact contents of the comedones.

Variants of acne

* Physiological acne
  - Neonatal acne
  - Childhood acne
  - Senile acne
* Physical acne
  - Acne cosmetica
  - Acne excoriee/mechanical acne
  - Actinic or tropical acne
* Morphological acne
  - Comedones
  - Papules
  - Pustules
  - Nodules
  - Cysts
  - Nodulocysts
  - Acne conglobata
  - Acne fulminans
  - Pyoderma faciale or Gram-negative folliculitis.

Rosacea

* It is an acne like disease, followed by a chronic course with episodes of activity and a variable quiescent period.
* Pathogenesis is unknown. It occurs after the age of 30 years.
* Sun exposure precipitates an acute episode.
* Alcohol aggravates erythema but not the lesions.
* Similarly heat of the hot drinks like coffee, not due to caffeine of coffee is responsible for transient erythema or flushing.
* A significant increase in hair follicle mites, *Demodex folliculorum* is seen. Mites probably cause a mechanical blockage of the follicles or act as a vector for other orgamisms to provoke an inflammatory or allergic reaction.

Clinical features

- Symptoms are mainly due to eye involvement. A feeling of heat or redness of the face and aggravation of the skin lesions are seen on exposure to sunlight or during expression of anger.

- A burning or stinging or foreign body feeling of the eyes, dryness, itching, photosensitivity and blurred vision.
- Primary lesions are clusters of papules and pustules with a background of erythematous and edematous skin.
- Telangiectasia is frequently associated. In full blown cases nose becomes erythematous, edematous and bulbous.
- This irreversible hypertrophy of the nose is known as rhinophyma. But all features may not be found at early stage.

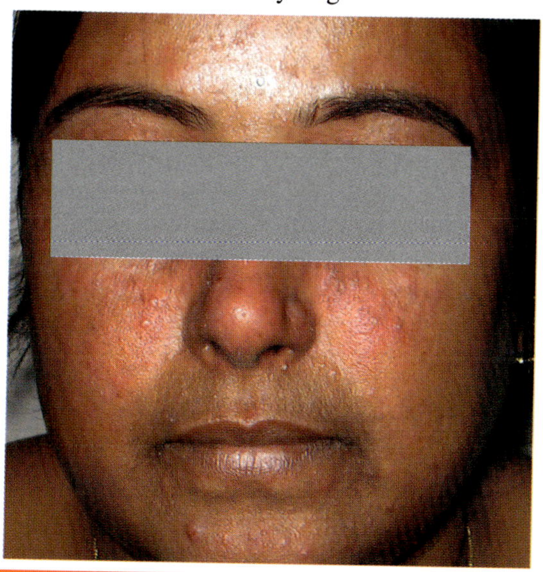

Fig. 7: Multiple pustules on erythematous background at central face.

- Rarely very firm papules and nodules may present which is known as granulomatous rosacea.
- Central parts of the face including forehead, cheeks, nose and chin are affected. Occasionally periorbital areas may be affected.
- The eye changes are interpalpebral conjunctival hyperemia, conjunctivitis, telangiectasia of the conjunctiva, irregularities of the eyelids, blepharitis, chalazion, hordeolum(stye), punctuate keratitis, marginal keratitis and corneal infiltration or ulcer formation.

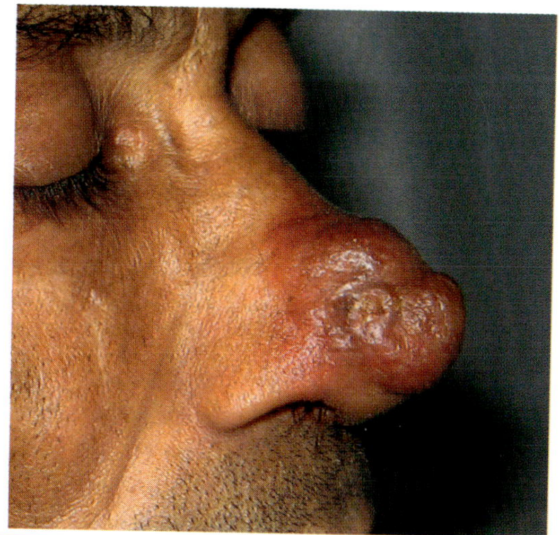

Fig. 8: Erythematous lobulated plaque, studded with pustules.

Histopathology

- Pustules show perifollicular and perivascular neutrophilic infiltrations.
- Long standing papules show granulomatous infiltration containing histiocytes and sometimes giant cells also.

Treatment

- The most effective topical therapy is 0.75-1% metronidazole gel. It is applied once or twice per day.
- 20% Azelaic acid cream is also effective.
- Clindamycin 1% gel is also useful but less effective.
- If response is poor with topical antibiotics, presence of mites of *D. folliculorum* is to be suspected and topical crotamiton (10%) is to be applied.
- Doxycycline 100 mg once or twice daily singly or along with metronidazole 200 mg twice daily is indicated.
- In refractory cases isotretinoin 0.5 mg/kg/day for 20 weeks is indicated.
- Systemic therapy is to be continued till all pustules are cleared. Rate of relapse is unpredictable. So, topical therapy is to be maintained for a long period.
- Even after that if relapse occurs, a low dose

systemic antibiotic or isotretinoin is to be continued.

Perioral dermatitis

Precipitating factors

- Prolonged use of topical steroid, specially fluorinated preparations.
- Cosmetics, specially moisturizing agents with foundation.
- An atopic background and dry skin force to apply excessive moisturizing creams. This hydrates the stratum corneum and alters the stratum corneum and its barrier function, helping proliferation of existing normal flora.

Clinical features

- Symptom is itching.
- Primary lesions are papules and pustules.
- An erythematous or mild scaly background is often associated.
- Number of the lesions is variable from few to numerous. Cheeks, chin and nasolabial folds are the primary sites of involvement sparing a clear zone around the vermilion border.
- Pustules at the cheeks, near the nostril are very characteristic of this entity. In children, pustules are rare. Perioral, perinasal and periorbital areas are affected in them.

Treatment

- Initially stop all topical applications and give only systemic antibiotics like doxycycline 100 mg once or twice daily, tetracycline or erythromycin 500 mg twice daily for 3-4 weeks.
- When relapses occur, an additional course of antibiotic is indicated or sometimes long-term maintenance therapy is required.
- In resistant cases a short course of topical steroid like desonide or hydrocortisone may be given for quick result and definitely for patient's compliance. But this should not be given for more than 2 weeks.
- If relapse is frequent, topical tacrolimus 0.03 or 0.1% ointment may be tried.

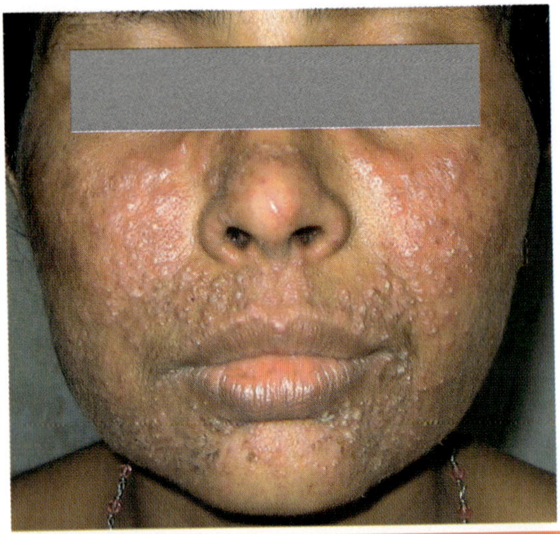

Fig. 9: Numerous papules and pustules.

Acne agminata (Lupus miliaris disseminatus faciei)

- Primary lesions are discrete dull brown acneform papules with yellowish centers.
- Number of the lesions may be few or numerous.
- Eyebrows, cheeks, chin and temples of the face are commonly affected. Rarely arms, axilla, trunk and legs are also affected.
- Initially lesions are soft and translucent. Gradually these become pustular and crusted. Spontaneous healing is expected after a course of 12-24 months but left by scars. During this course, a mixture of scars and active lesions is characteristic.

Histopathology

- Granulomatous infiltration in the dermis.

Treatment

- Dapsone is treatment of choice. But I personally did not get good response in my patients.
- It responded very well to systemic steroid like triamcinolone 12 mg daily for 2 weeks, then 8 mg daily for 2 weeks and then 4 mg daily for another 2 weeks.

CHAPTER C11

NUTRITIONAL DISORDERS

Vitamin A deficiency

- Daily rcquirement: 700-900 μg/day
- Serum level: 30-80 μg/dl.

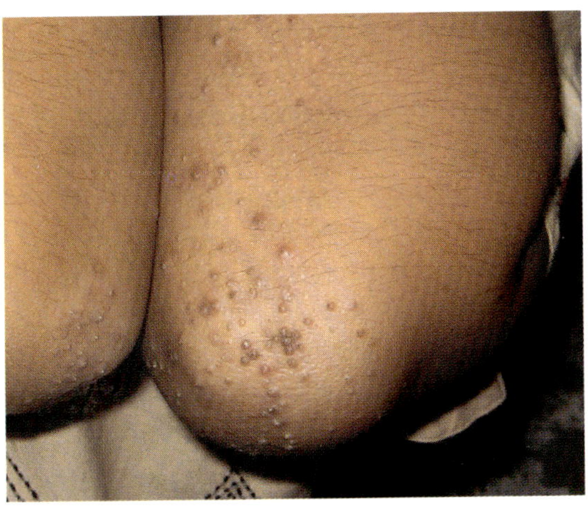

Fig. 1: Keratotic papules at elbows

Clinical features

- Xerosis
- Phrynoderma
- Nyctalopia
- Xerophthalmia
- Keratomalacia
- Bitot's spot
- Impaired bone growth
- Cranial nerve involvement.

Treatment

- 10000-300000 IU/day for weeks to months.

Vitamin B2 deficiency

- Daily requirement: 1-1.3 mg/day
- Serum level: 4-24 μg/dl.

Clinical features

- Angular stomatitis
- Cheilosis
- Magenta glossitis
- Seborrhea-like dermatitis
- Scrotal dermatitis.
- Vulval dermatitis
- Anemia
- Mental retardation
- EEG changes

Treatment

- For infant: 1-3 mg/day.
- For adult: 10-20 mg/day.

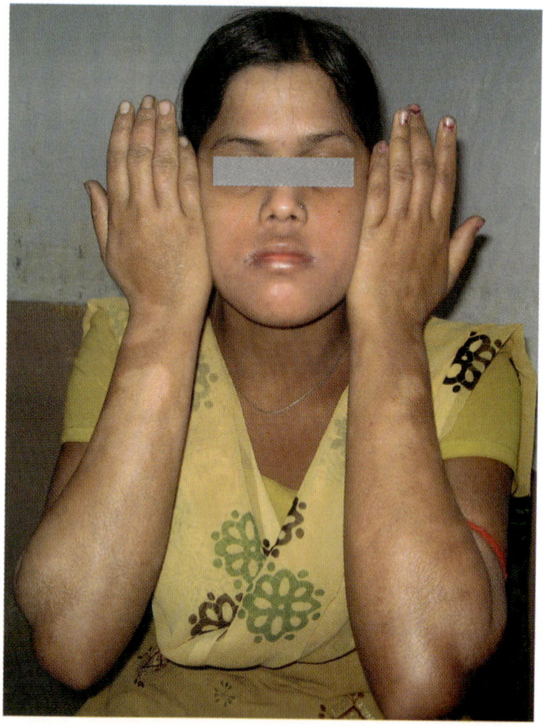

Fig. 2: Seborrheic dermatitis-like lesions at face and extensors of the upper limbs

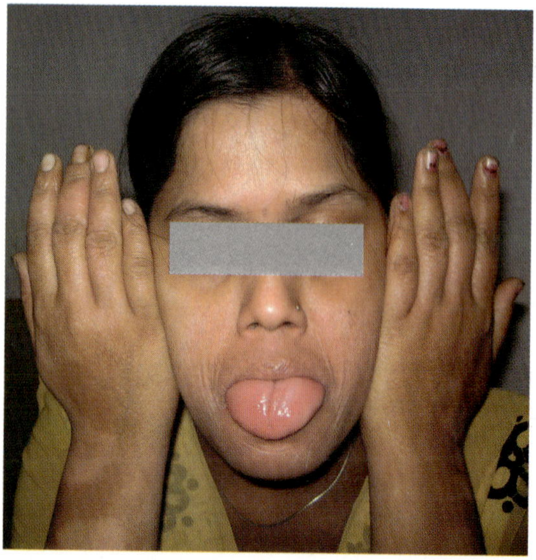

Fig. 3: Reddish tongue with seborrheic dermatitis like lesions at face and dorsa of the forearms and hands

Vitamin B3 (niacin) deficiency (pellagra)

- Daily requirement: 10-20 mg/day.
- It is often associated with other vitamin deficiencies and protein energy malnutrition.
- It occurs in chronic alcoholics and patients with anorexia nervosa, gastrointestinal carcinoma, worm infestation and carcinoid syndrome.
- Drugs causing reduction of endogenous niacin production are isoniazide, pyrazinamide, ethionamide and azathioprine.
- Photosensitivity is due to deficiency of production of urocanic acid which protects the skin from UVB. Kynurenic acid, a metabolic byproduct, accumulated within the skin due to result of nicotinic acid deficiency, sensitises the skin to UVA.

Clinical features

- Three key features are dermatitis, diarrhea and dementia (3 Ds). Actually there is no dementia, the term is used to make 3rd D and stands for neuropsychological changes. But 4th D stands for sudden death due to central pontine myelinolysis.
- Intensely erythematous, symmetrically distributed scaly plaques develop at sunexposed areas like face, V-area of the neck (Casal's neckless appearance), dorsa of the hands (Gaunlet appearance) and forearms and dorsa of the feet (Boot appearance). When these plaques subside, hyperpigmented patches develop.
- Lesions of the perianal and genital areas become eroded and painful, probably due to heat, friction and moisture.
- Increased skin fragility due to altered collagen and elastic tissue synthesis.
- In mild cases seborrheic dermatitis-like lesions develop at face, scalp and neck.
- Vesicles may develop in severe cases, known as wet pellagra.

- Oral changes are angular stomatitis, reddish and cracked lips, and fissured or smooth red tongue.
- Anorexia and weakness.
- Neuropsychiatric changes are anxiety, psychosis, burning sensation, dizziness, and headache.

Histopathology

- Psoriasis form epidermal hyperplasia including hyperkeratosis, parakeratosis, loss of granular layer, presence of scattered necrotic keratinocytes and dyskeratosis. But epidermal atrophy occurs at late stage.
- Vacuolated cells within basal layer and spinous layer.
- Perivascular infiltration in early stage and dilated vessel at late stage.
- Sebaceous hyperplasia with dilated follicle in early stage but atrophy at late stage.
- Swelling of the elastic and collagen fibers and fragmentation of the elastic fibers.

Treatment

- Diet includes egg, meat, milk and vegetables.
- Supplementation of nicotinamide 100 mg thrice daily for several weeks.

Vitamin B6 (pyridoxine) deficiency

* Daily requirement:
  - Physiological: 1-2 mg/day
  - With isoniazide/birth control pills: 30 mg/day
  - With penicillamine: 100 mg/day.
* Plasma level: 5-30 ng/ml.

Clinical features

- Angular stomatitis
- Seborrhea-like dermatitis
- Glossitis
- Oral erosions
- Cheilosis
- Pellagra-like dermatitis
- Anorexia
- Anemia
- Lymphopenia
- Sensory neuritis
- Somnolence
- Confusion

Vitamin B12 deficiency

* Daily requirement: 2.5 μg.
* Serum level: 200-835 pg/ml.

Clinical features

- Generalized hyperpigmentation
- Hyperpigmented macules
- Beefy red tongue
- Poliosis
- Megaloblastic anemia
- Ataxia
- Paresthesia
- Altered reflexes
- Mental status changes

Treatment

- Parenteral vitamin B12 as 1 mg/week for 4 weeks, then 1 mg/month.

Vitamin C deficiency (scurvy)

* Daily requirement: 65-75 mg/day
* Plasma level: 0.5-1.5 mg/ml.

Clinical features

- Corkscrew hairs
- Follicular hyperkeratosis
- Perifollicular hemorrhages
- Swollen and friable gums
- Closed space hemorrhages
- Poor wound healing
- Sjogren-like syndrome
- Hypotension
- Anemia
- Weakness
- Fatigue

Treatment

- Vitamin C 100-300 mg/day for 2-3 weeks.

Vitamin D3 deficiency

* **Serum level:** 25-45 pg/ml

Clinical features

- No skin change
- Rickets
- Osteomalacia
- Muscle weakness

Treatment

- 200-400 IU/day

Vitamin K deficiency

* **Daily requirement:** 0.04 mg/kg/day
* **Serum level:** 80-1160 pg/ml

Clinical features

- Intracutaneous hemorrhage
- Nasal, gastrointestinal, subgleal and intracranial hemorrhage.

Treatment

- Vitamin K 5-10 mg/day.

Biotin deficiency

- Intertriginous and periorificial dermatitis (seborrheic dermatitis-like)
- Xerosis
- Neuropsychiatric changes
- Alopecia

Treatment

- Biotin 150 μg/day

Zinc deficiency

* **Daily requirement:** 15 mg/day
* **Serum level:** 70-150 μg/dl
* Deficiency may be acquired or genetically determined.
* Genetically determined type is known as acrodermatitis enteropathica.

Clinical features

- Acral and periorificial pustulobullous dermatitis
- Pustular paronychia
- Angular stomatitis
- Glossitis
- Hypogeusia
- Anorexia
- Impaired sexual development
- Growth retardation
- Neuropsychiatric changes
- Gastrointestinal changes
- Profound immune defects.

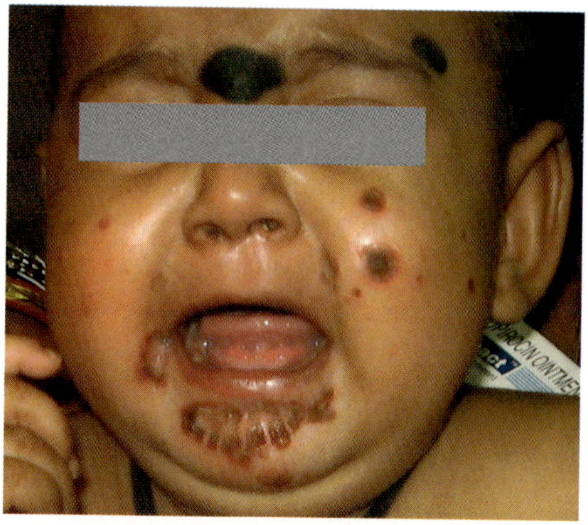

Fig. 4: Well defined crusted and erosive plaque.

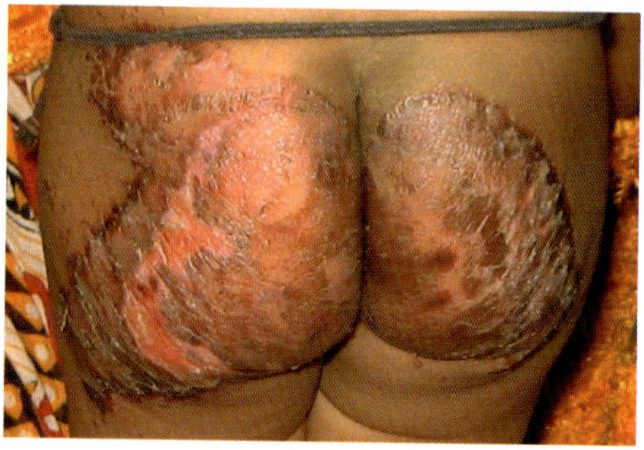

Fig. 5: Well defined crusted erosions at both buttocks.

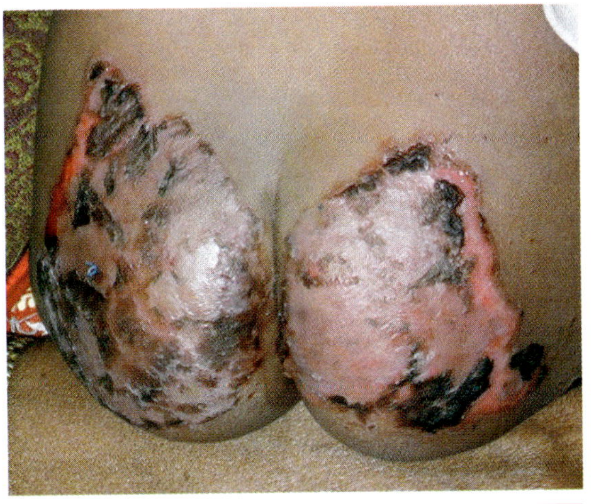

Fig. 6: Well defined crusted erosions at both buttocks

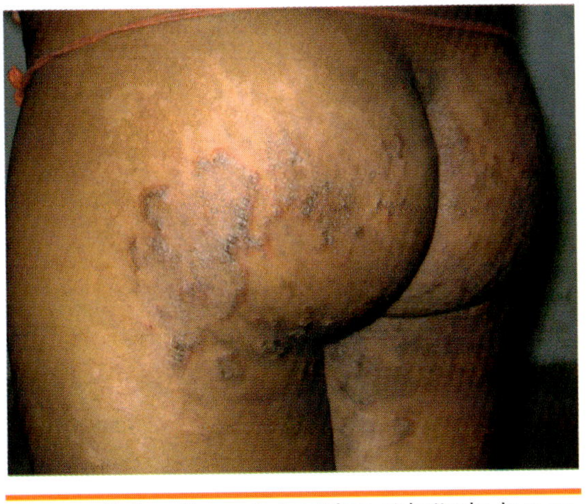

Fig. 7: Polycyclic crusted patches at buttocks in a patient of nephritic syndrome

Treatment

- Supplement with zinc sulfate 1-2 mg/kg/day for several days in acquired deficiency state and 3 mg/kg/day for life long in genetically determined cases.

Copper deficiency

Clinical features

- Menkes characteristic facies
- Pilitorti
- Hypothermia
- Neuropsychiatric changes
- Mental retardation
- Bony changes
- Tortuous arteries

Marasmus

* A form of protein energy malnutrition with profound weight loss.

Clinical features

- Xerotic and wrinkled skin
- Alopecia
- Loss of subcutaneous fat
- Wasting of muscle.

Kwashiorkor

* A form of protein energy malnutrition with excess amount of carbohydrate.
* Weight loss 20-40%.

Clinical features

- Generalized hypopigmentation of the skin, starting at perioral and pretibial areas.
- Hyperpigmented waxy plaques develop at elbows, ankles and intertriginous areas.
- Skin loses its elasticity and becomes xerotic.
- Skin with extensive desquamation, erosions and fissuring, appears as crazy pavement or flaky paint.
- Hair changes include diffuse alopecia, alternating normal and hypopigmented bands at hair shaft, known as flag sign and unusual reddish brown discoloration, known as hypochromotrichia.
- Smooth tongue and angular stomatitis.
- Perianal, nasal and intertriginous erosions are present.
- Hypothermia, cold extremities and peripheral edema.
- Irritability, anorexia and psychological changes.
- Fatty liver change and hypoalbuminemia.

Essential fatty acid deficiency

Clinical features

- Amenorrhea
- Increased transepidermal water loss.
- Hypotension.
- ECG changes.
- Skin changes mimic zinc and biotin deficiencies. But periorificial involvement as well as nail and mucous membrane affection in less prominent.
- Generalised xerosis.
- Widespread reddish skin.
- Intertriginous exudative dermatitis.
- Diffuse alopecia and light coloured hair.
- Poor wound healing and increased chances of secondary infection.

Anorexia nervosa

Clinical features

- Xerosis
- Brittle nails
- Orange yellow skin
- Lanugo hairs
- Alopecia.

Iron deficiency

- Daily requirement: 1.8-2.4 mg/day
- It is very common nutritional deficiency disorder, specially among menstruating women.

Clinical features

- Koilonychia, glossitis and angular stomatitis
- Telogen effluvium
- Pruritus
- Plummer-Vinson syndrome includes anemia dysphagia and glossitis, occurring in middle aged women. Other features are thin lips, smaller mouth, smooth atrophic tongue, koilonychia and alopecia.

CHAPTER C12

PIGMENTARY DISORDERS

Vitiligo

* It is the most common acquired pigmentary disorder, affecting 0.1-2% of world population.
* It is common in India, Mexico and Japan.
* Familial history is found in 30% cases.
* There is less than 10% chance to develop vitiligo in children when parents are affected.
* Really, it should be a disease of little medical significance but on cosmetic ground it gets a lot of importance, specially before making a matrimonial relation in Indian subcontinent.
* It occurs in both sexes equally and at any age.
* Though the disease does not do any harm to the internal organs but produces a lots of psychological distress to the patients and brings them to the dermatologists.
* The term leukoderma is used to denote depigmented lesion secondary to some other dermatoses or to physical and chemical trauma or to intralesional injection of corticosteroids or to application of potent topical steroid with salicylic acid.
* Circumscribed area of white hair analogous to vitiligo is called poliosis.
* Till date, there is no precise etiology and pathogenesis. But it is clear that etiology and pathogenesis are a complex one and interrelated with genetic, immunological, neural and self-destructive mechanisms.
    - Autocytotoxic hypothesis is based on degeneration of melanocyte by accumulated H_2O_2 within the epidermis.
    - Oxidative stress hypothesis is based on alteration in the antioxidant pattern, such as higher levels of superoxide dismutase in skin, erythrocytes, mononuclear cells, and serum of vitiligo patients. Also, there is a reduction of catalase activity in the keratinocytes, melanocytes and mononuclear cells.
* It may be associated with systemic autoimmune diseases or endocrinal disorders like hypothyroidism, Addison's disease and pernicious anemia.

Types

- Focal vitiligo: Localized lesions and single or few in number.

- Lip-tip vitiligo/acrofacialvitiligo: A form of focal vitiligo involving only lips, glans and tips of the digits.
- Segmental vitiligo: Lesion is localized within a dermatome.
- Vitiligo vulgaris: Lesions are scattered and widespread.
- Universal vitiligo: Almost every part of the skin is affected.
- Previtiligo lesion: Earliest lesion with incomplete depigmentation or hypopigmentation.

* Lesions at face and proximal parts of the body respond better than lesions at the mucosal surfaces, digital tips, knuckles, elbows, knees, ankles, palms and soles and female waist.
* Course of the disease and response to therapy are very unpredictable. Usually it progresses slowly but may be stable for long time or spread rapidly or rarely repigment spontaneously.
* Often new lesions continue to develop along with treatment.
* Sometimes few lesions show repigmentation when few lesions deteriorate at the same time.

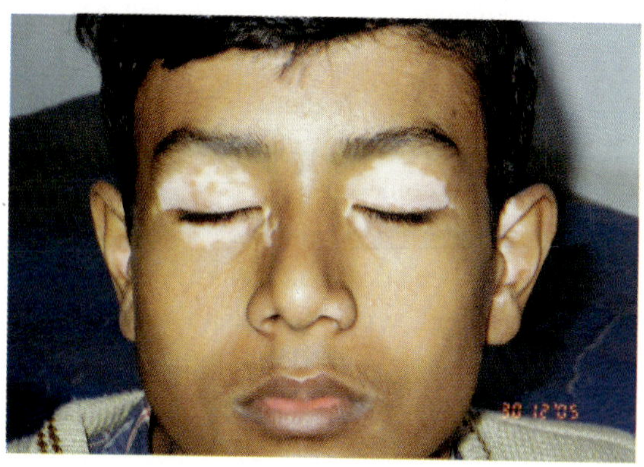

Fig. 1: Depigmented patches at the eyelids

Clinical features

- It is characterized by ivory or chalky white macules or patches, affecting any area of the skin.
- Depigmented hair may be present and bears a bad prognostic sign.
- Some lesions show central depigmentation and peripheral hypopigmentation, surrounded by hyperpigmented nonvitiligo skin. This is usually seen during treatment with psoralen.

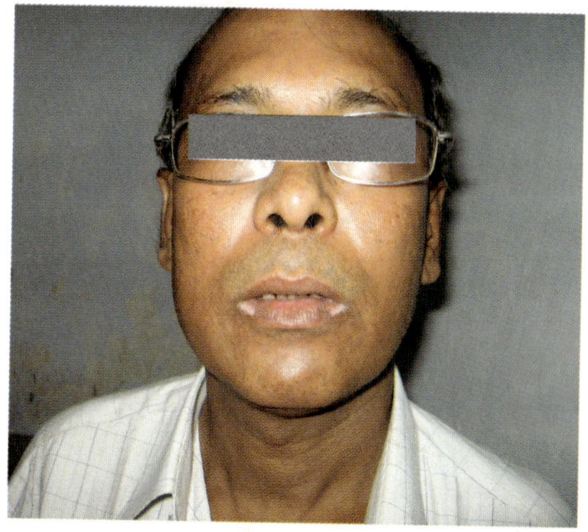

Fig. 2: Angular vitiligo, very commonly seen in Bankura, a district of West Bengal

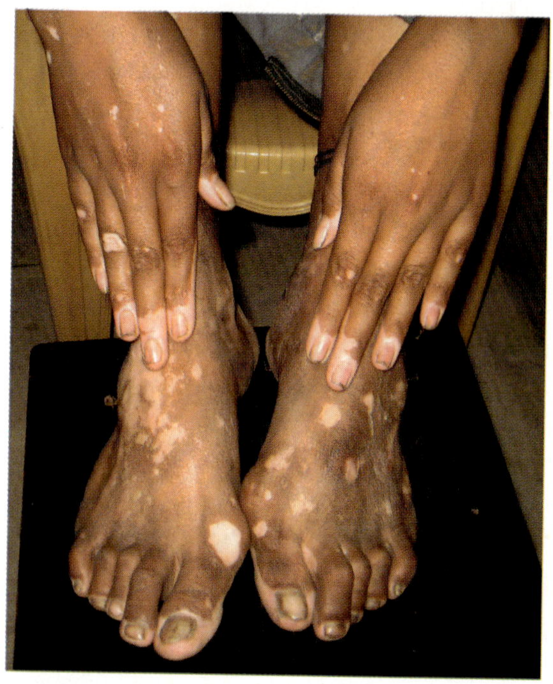

Fig. 3: Acral vitiligo

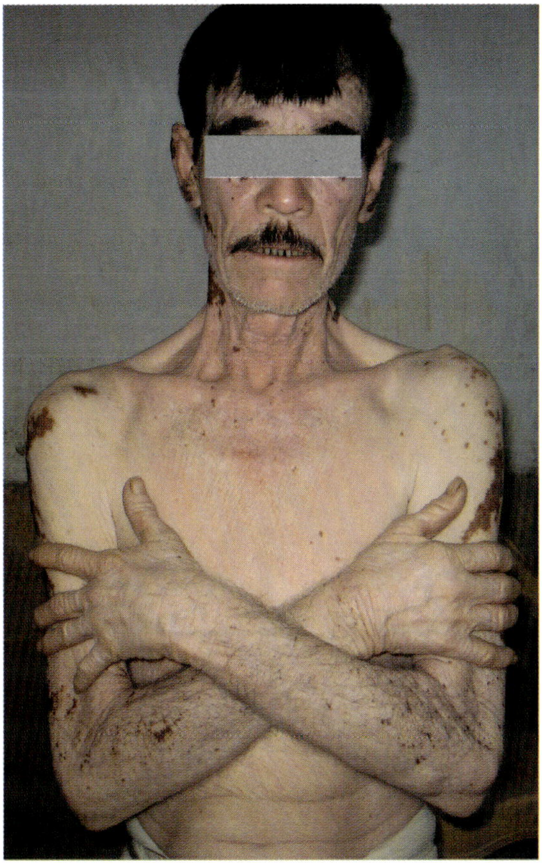

Fig. 4: Generalized vitiligo

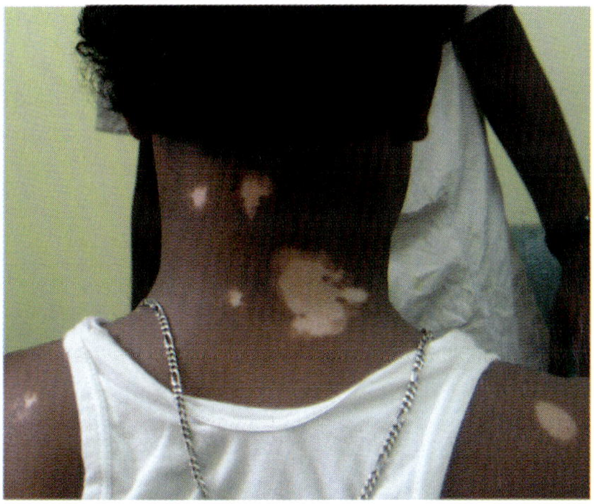

Fig. 5: Trichrome sign, clearly seen in largest lesion

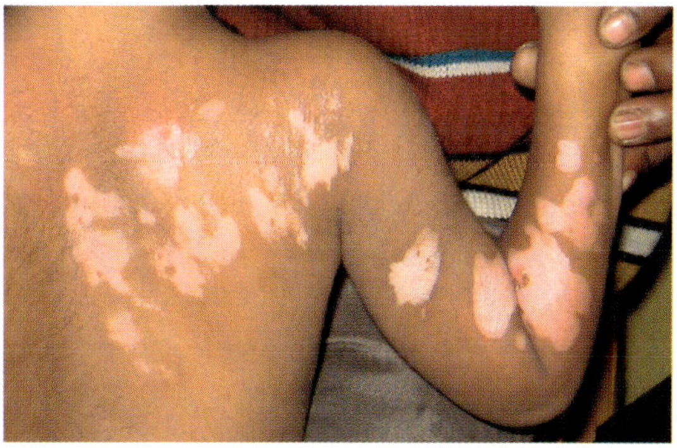

Fig. 6: Post burn leukoderma

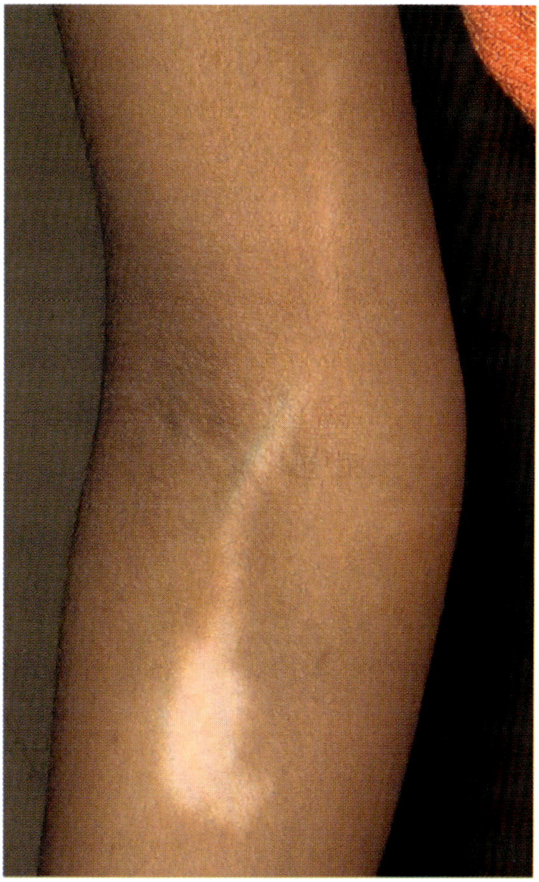

Fig. 7: Post steroidal leukoderma along the course of a vein, following intralesional injection

Differential diagnosis

- Pityriasis alba
- Hypopigmented pityriasis versicolor.

- Hypopigmented LL or BT leprosy
- Hypopigmented lesion of post kala-azar dermal leishmaniasis
- Hypopigmented mycosis fungoides
- Postinflammatory hypopigmented lesions specially in pityriasis rosea, guttate psoriasis and pityriasis lichenoides chronica
- Ash-leaf macule of tuberous sclerosis
- Albinism
- Nevus anemicus
- Hypochromic nevus
- Hypomelanosis of Ito
- Depigmented lesions associated with piebaldism, Vogt-Koyanagi-Harada syndrome, Chediak-Higashi syndrome and Waardenburg syndrome.

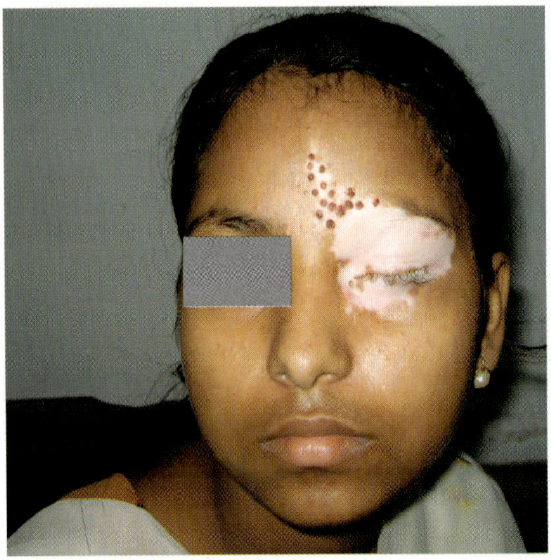

Fig. 8: Punch grafting in a segmental vitiligo (Courtesy: Tanushree Sarkar, PGT)

Wood lamp examination

- Previtiligo lesion in dark skin or vitiligo in lighter skin becomes more obvious.

Histopathology

- Epidermis is normal except the absence of melanocytes.
- Sparse lymphocytic infiltration in dermis.

Electron microscopy

- It confirms the absence of melanocytes and absence of melanosomes in keratinocytes.
- It also recognizes spongiosis, exocytosis, basal layer vacuolation and apoptosis.

Treatment for localized lesions in children and adults

- Tacrolimus ointment (0.03% or 0.1%), twice daily.
- Mometasone, clobetasol or halobetasol ointment, once daily for 2 weeks, followed by 1 week steroid holiday.
- Topical PUVA
- Narrow band UVB.
- Skin grafting.

Treatment for extensive lesions in adults

- Systemic PUVA.
- Corticosteroid pulse therapy.

Treatment for extensive lesions in children

- Corticosteroid pulse therapy.

Treatment for extensive lesions/universal vitiligo in adults

- Some patients have only few normally pigmented areas.
- Sometimes these patients want complete depigmentation of normal pigmented areas to match the remaining major depigmented part.
- Monobenzylether (20%) ointment is used to decolorize the normally pigmented areas. But this depigmentation is irreversible and so proper counselling to be done before doing such procedure.
- Success rate is more than 90%.

Topical PUVA

- Patient is asked to apply 0.75% 8-methoxypsoralen solution on alternate day between 11 am to 1 pm to get maximum amount of UVA.
- To wait for 30 minutes and expose to sunlight initially for 5 seconds only and subsequently exposure time will be increased day by day upto 15 minutes.

- ♦ Instead of diluting the drug, which is a difficult job but preferred by many dermatologists, I like to dilute the time. This is done to avoid severe phototoxic reaction which often causes blister formation.
- ♦ After sun exposure, the area will be washed with soap vigorosly.
- ♦ For rest of the day lesion should be covered with cloth or sunscreen.

Systemic PUVA

- ♦ Patient is asked to take oral psoralen (0.6 mg/kg) on alternate day between 9 am to 11 am and after 2-2.30 hours of intake, lesions will be exposed to sunlight, initially for 5 minutes and exposure time will be increased day by day, maximum upto 30 minutes.
- ♦ Initially 5-methoxypsoralen is used and followed by 8-methoxypsoralen or khelin.
- ♦ Treatment must be continued for at least 6 months.
- ♦ During sun exposure eyes must be protected during and for rest of the day with UV protective glasses like α-plano, SP2, β_2 torid, etc.
- ♦ It is contraindicated in children below 10 years of age.
- ♦ Repigmentation is first noticed as tiny pigmented macules around the follicles.
- ✶ Treatment of choice for segmental vitiligo is skin grafting.
- ✶ Narrow band UVB (311 nm) is treatment of choice in children below 6 years of age.
- ✶ Excimer laser (308 nm) gives best result in facial lesion.
- ✶ Camouflaging: Various color-shades are matched with normal skin and placed on the lesion to produce an immediate cover up. Basically it helps to hide the vitiligo lesion temporarily.

Albinism

- ✶ It is an autosomal recessive disorder with presence of normal number of melanocytes and absence of tyrosinase enzyme activity.
- ✶ It affects skin, hair follicles and eyes.
- ✶ It manifests since birth.

Clinical features

- ♦ Patients can not tolerate bright light and develop sunburn on repeated sun exposure.
- ♦ Skin color is variable from snow white to light tan.
- ♦ Hair may be red to light brown.
- ♦ Eye problems are nystagmus, reduced visual acquity, translucent iris, reduccd retinal pigmentation, foveal hypoplasia and strabismus.
- ♦ Complications include development of dermatoheliosis, actinic keratosis and epithelioma.

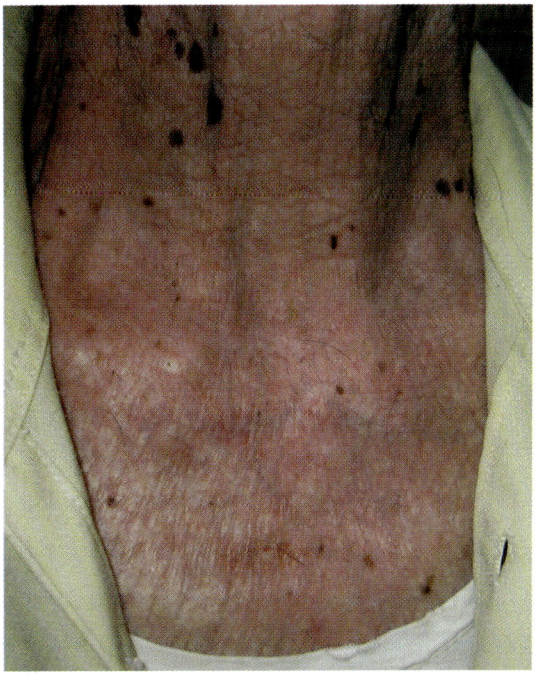

Fig. 9: Generalized depigmentation with dermatheliotic changes

Histopathology

- ♦ Melanocytes are normally present at skin and hair bulb.
- ♦ DOPA reaction is markedly reduced or absent in the melanocytes of the skin and hair bulb.

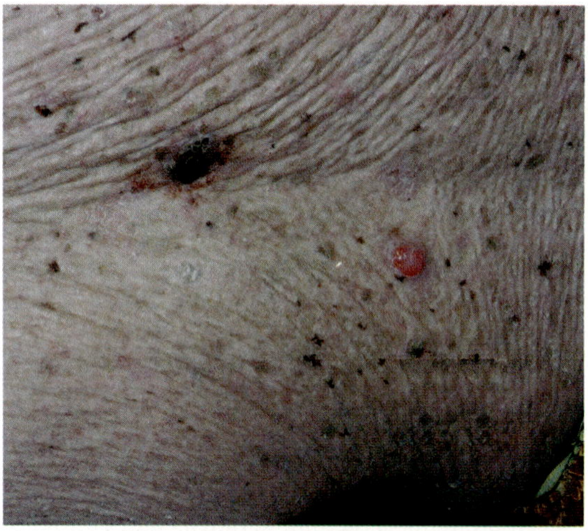

Fig. 10: Generalized depigmented skin with dermatoheliosis, actinic keratosis and early squamous cell carcinoma

Electron microscopy

- It confirms the presence of melanocytes in the skin and hair bulb.
- It detects absence to reduced melanosomes in the keratinocytes.

Molecular testing: It detects the specific genetic defects.

Treatment

- Sun protection with clothing and sunscreens.
- Ophthalmological care.
- Prophylactic use of topical tretinoin for dermatoheliosis and solar keratosis which often turns into squamous cell carcinoma.

Idiopathic guttate hypomelanosis

- This is a common hypopigmented disorder of unknown etiology.
- It commonly occurs after the age of 50 years; but may start even just after age of 30 years.
- Lesions are asymptomatic except creation of a panic following misdiagnosis as vitiligo.

Clinical features

- Lesions are sharply circumscribed white macules predominantly on sun exposed extensor surfaces of the extremities. But lesions also develop at trunk.
- Number of the lesion is variable from few to numerous.
- Size of the lesion is variable from 2-6 mm in diameter.

Histopathology

- Fontana-Masson stain shows markedly reduced melanin content in DOPA positive melanocytes.
- Melanin granules are irregularly distributed.
- Immunoperoxidase confirms an absolute decrease in the number of melanocytes.

Piebaldism

- It is an autosomal dominant disorder, occurring due to mutation of genes, responsible for melanocyte migration into hair follicles and epidermis.

Clinical features

- Depigmented patches of irregular shapes present at center of the face, front of the chest and abdomen, i.e., ventral surface of the body.
- White forelock arising from a depigmented patch is seen in 85% cases.
- Small islands of hyperpigmented patches of 1-5 cm in diameter are often seen within the depigmented areas.

Histopathology, immunohistochemistry and electron microscopy

- Confirm the absence of melanocyte in depigmented patches.

Chediak-Higashi syndrome

- It is an autosomal recessive disorder with irregularly shaped giant melanosomes within melanocytes.
- Giant lysosomal azurophilic granules are also seen within neutrophils, melanocytes and Langerhans cells.

* Due to lysosomal defect, there is a high susceptibility of infection and it causes an accelerated lymphohistiocytic phase, often responsible for death.
* Prenatal diagnosis can be done by fetal blood sampling or study of amniotic fluid or chorionic villous cells.

Clinical features

- Presence of lighter colored skin with silvery sheen hair.
- Presence of intensely pigmented patches or speckled pigmentation at acral and sun exposed areas like ears and nose.
- Ulceration of oral and gingival mucosae.
- Accelerated phase is characterized by fever, hepatosplenomegaly, gingival hyperplasia, and pseudomembranous sloughing of the buccalmucosa.
- Decreased iris pigmentation, causes red reflex and photophobia.

Histopathology and Fontana-Masson's stain

- Sparse melanin granules in keratinocytes, some of which are larger than normal, some are discrete and some are grouped.
- Melanophages in the upper dermis also show irregularly shaped large melanin granules.

Idiopathic guttate hypomelanosis

* This is a very common age-related asymptomatic and hypopigmented disorder, affecting 80% of patient above 70 years of age. Lesions start to develop after age of 40.
* It occurs in both sexes and all races, irrespective of skin types. But the lesions are more prominent in dark skin.

Clinical features

- Primary lesions are hypopigmented macules.
- Size of individual lesions is varying from 2-6 mm.
- Usual number is 10-30 but may be numerous.
- Though limbs are commonly affected, other areas may be involved including trunk and sparing face, palm & soles.
- Shape of the lesion is usually round but may be irregular.
- Margin of thc lesion is sharply defined.

Histopathology

- Orthohyperkeratosis.
- Flattened dermo-epidermal junction.
- Focal absence or reduced melanin content at basal and suprabasal keratinocytes.
- Moderate reduction of DOPA-positive melanocytes.
- Many melanocytes contain reduced amount of melanosomes and many keratinocyte show variable amount of melanin.

Freckles and lentigines

* These are pinpoint macular pigmentary disorders of unknown etiology.
* In freckles, number of melanocytes remains same but production of melanin increases.
* Freckles closely mimic lentigines in which number of melanocytes as well as production of melanin both are increased.
* Lips are commonly affected with lentigines in Peutz-Jegher's syndrome.

Clinical features

- These are pinpoint to pinhead sized brown macules, developing at sunexposed areas, specially at face.
- Color of the freckles may vary from season to season as increase in summer and fade in winter.
- Lentigines usually appear in childhood as brown to dark brown, pinpoint macules. Lesions gradually increase in number during second and third decades and then may remain or may disappear spontaneously.

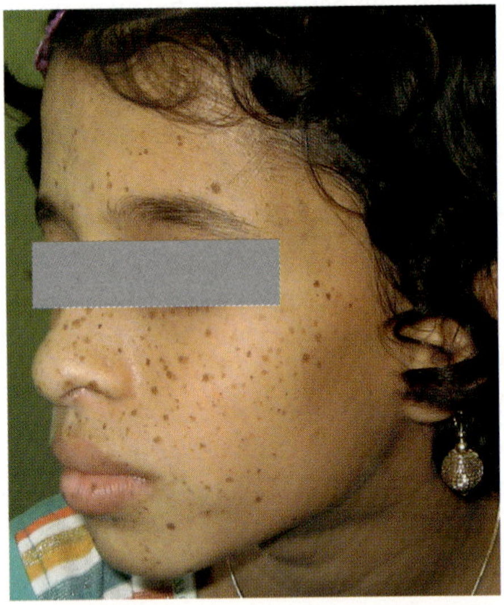

Fig. 11: Brownish macules of freckles

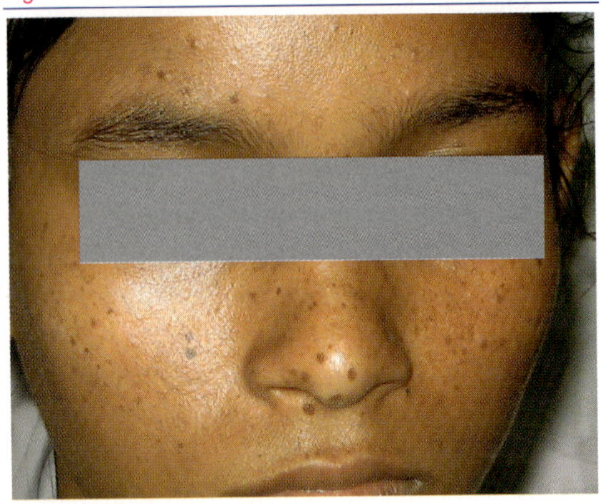

Fig. 12: Dark brown macules of lentigines

Treatment

- Spot chemical peeling with 88% phenol for freckles.
- Laser surgery for lentigines.

Melasma

- This is a common acquired hyperpigmented disorder.
- Though it is asymptomatic, bears a tremendous cosmetic importance.
- It often complicates the patient with an inferiority complex.
- It occurs in adults, specially in the age group of 25-45 years.
- Females are more affected than males.
- Lesions may disappear spontaneously, specially when precipitated by pregnancy.

Precipitating factors

- Sunlight.
- Oral contraceptive pills or estrogen and progesterone therapy.
- Pregnancy.

Types

- Epidermal: Respond to therapy very well.
- Dermal: Responds to therapy poorly.
- Mixed: Responds to therapy partially.

Clinical features

- Well defined hyperpigmented macules or patches.
- Intensity of color is variable from light or dark brown to black.
- Margin may be serrated or irregular.
- Shape is usually geographic.
- Common sites are central parts of the face including cheeks, nose, forehead and supraorbital regions.
- It may also affect chin, upper lip and dorsa of the forearms.

Wood's lamp examination: It helps to recognize the type as epidermal type becomes more prominent and dermal type becomes less prominent.

Histopathology

- Melanin is significantly increased in all epidermal layers.
- DOPA stain shows an increase in the number and activity of melanocytes.

Treatment

- Initiation phase:
  - Application of sunscreen at day time.
  - Application of a combination of hydroquinone (4%), tretinoin (0.025-0.05%) and corti-

costeroid (mometasone, hydrocotisone) for 2 months.
- ♦ Laser may be done in fair patient.

* Maintenance phase:
  - ♦ Application of sunscreen at day time is to be continued.
  - ♦ Application of kojic acid, azelaic acid or glycolic acid at night.

Riehl's melanosis/melanodermatitis toxica

* It occurs due to contact sensitivity or photocontact sensitivity to various chemicals, specially to fragrance in cosmetics.

Clinical features

- ♦ There is a reticular or confluent, brown to black or bluish pigmentation of the face and neck.

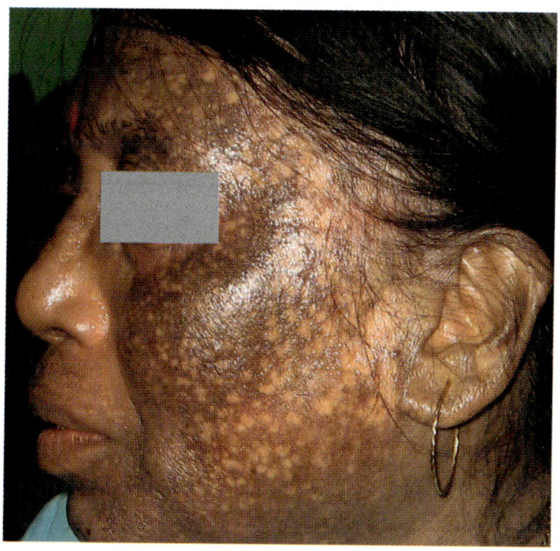

Fig. 13: Reticular pigmentation due to use of photosensitive cosmetics

Berloque dermatitis

* It is a form of localized hyperpigmentation which occurs at the site of contact with perfume containing bergamot oil.
* Bergamot oil contains bergapten or 5-methoxy psoralen, causing photoinduced pigmentation.
* Other plants such as lime, parsnip, fig and carrot containing furocoumarin produce a postinflammatory hyperpigmentation.
* In celery induced dermatitis, furocoumarin is produced by fungus infecting celery.

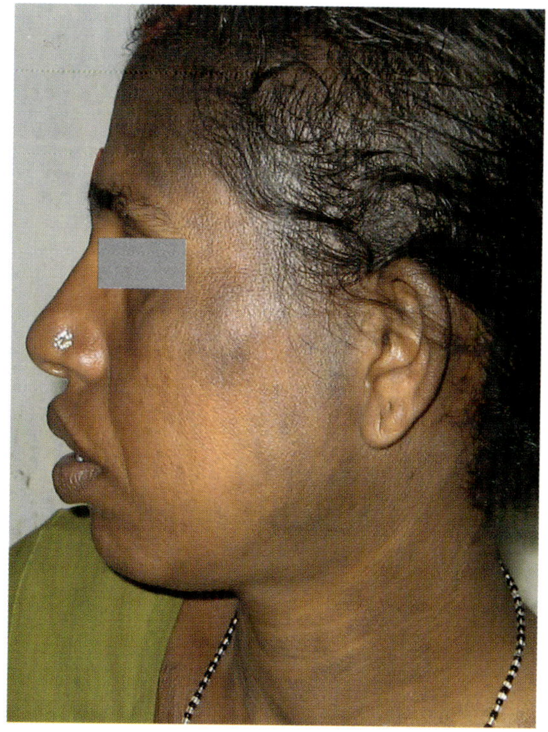

Fig. 14: Hyperpigmentation spreading from face to neck

Clinical features

- ♦ It is characterized by pigmented drop like or streaky patches, resembling pendants.
- ♦ Usually sides of the neck and retroauricular areas are affected.

Post-inflammatory hyperpigmentation

* It is a frequent problem in dark skin people.
* It often occurs following healing of lichen planus, bullous disorders, drug reactions including fixed drug reaction and toxic epidermal necrolysis.
* Pigmentation is characteristically localized within the area of pre-existing lesions.

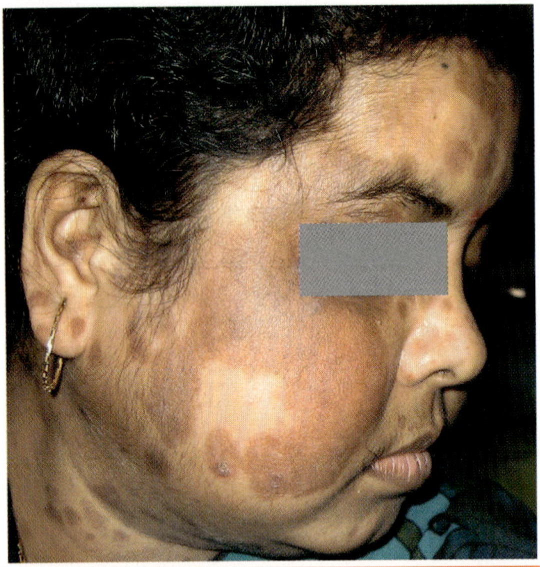

Fig. 15: Irregular hyperpigmented patches after healing of vesicular bullous pemphigoid

Acanthosis nigricans

* It is a common dermatosis, presented with pigmented lesions.
* Hyperpigmentation is due to hyperkeratosis, not due to melanin.
* Types:
  - Benign type
  - Malignant type.
* Malignant type is associated with malignancy, specially with gastric carcinoma.
* Malignant type differs from benign type by the followings:
  - Onset usually after age of 40 years.
  - Extensive, aggressive and persisting lesions,
  - Presence of itching.
  - Involvement of mucosae.

Frequent associated abnormalities

- Obesity
- Insulin resistance and type II diabetes mellitus
- Malignancy: Carcinoma of the stomach, lungs and breast.
- Drugs: Corticosteroid, oral contraceptive pill, nicotinic acid and niacinamide.
- Dermatoses like systemic lupus erythematosus, dermatomyositis and scleroderma
- Syndromes like HAIR-AN syndrome, Bloom syndrome, Crouzon syndrome, Lawrence-Seip syndrome and polycystic ovary syndrome.

Clinical features

- It is characterized by accentuated skin markings with hyperpigmentation and thickening, resulting in a velvety appearance.
- Common sites are lateral sides of the neck, axillae, groins, folds of elbows, ankles and knuckles.
- Occasionally it affects oral mucosa, eyelids, conjunctiva, tongue and lips.
- Rarely it becomes generalized.
- Children with acanthosis nigricans have greater body mass, body fat mass, and greater basal and stimulated insulin levels during glucose tolerance test.

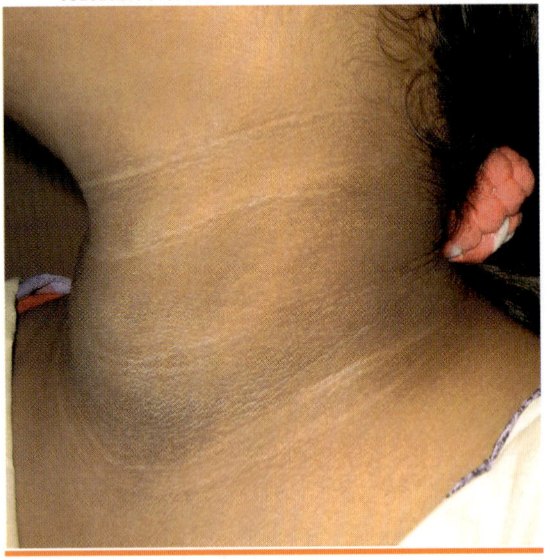

Fig. 16: Velvety hyperpigmentation

Histopathology

- Hyperkeratosis, papillomatosis, and irregular acanthosis.
- Valleys between upwardly projected papillae are filled up with keratotic material.
- Epidermis at the tips and sides of the papillae becomes thin.
- Pseudohorn cyst may be formed.

Treatment

- ♦ Removal of the underlying cause, reduction of body weight, topical retinoids, lactic acid, emollient containing keratolytics like salicylic acid and urea.
- ♦ Oral retinoids for generalized involvement.
- ♦ Results of any of the treatment is not satisfactory.

Pigmented purpuric dermatoses (PPD)

- ⋆ This is a group of dermatoses, presented with mostly asymptomatic pigmented lesions.
- ⋆ This is impotant for cosmetic concern and often misdiagnosed as a feature of vasculitis or thrombocytopenia.
- ⋆ Etiology is not yet clear. Basically a mild form of capillaritis causes extravasation of erythrocytes and degradation of RBCs produces pigmentation due to deposition of hemosiderin.
- ⋆ Onset is insidious and evolves slowly, except drug induced one.
- ⋆ Drug induced PPD develops quickly and becomes generalized.
- ⋆ All types are asymptomatic except lichenoid type.

Proposed etiological factors

- ♦ Local trauma and chronic pressure.
- ♦ Prolonged standing.
- ♦ Drugs like acetaminophen, ampicillin, diuretics, meprobamate, nonsteroidal antiinflammatory drugs, etc.

Types

- ♦ Schamberg disease or progressive pigmented purpuric dermatosis.
- ♦ Majocchi disease or purpura annularis telangiectodes: Lesions take an annular or archiform pattern.
- ♦ Gougarot-Blum disease or pigmented purpuric lichenoid dermatitis: Lesions are macules with lichenoid papules and plaques.
- ♦ Lichen aureus: Lesions are reddish or golden colored solitary or few plaques, involving trunk and limbs.

Clinical features of Schamberg's disease

- ♦ Lesions are asymptomatic or mild pruritic, discrete cluster of reddish to brown pinhead sized macules or irregular confluent patches.
- ♦ Initial lesions are red and appear as cayenne pepper color. Gradually color changes to brown.
- ♦ Diascopy proves pinpoint hemorrhage.
- ♦ Commonest sites are areas of lower third of the legs.

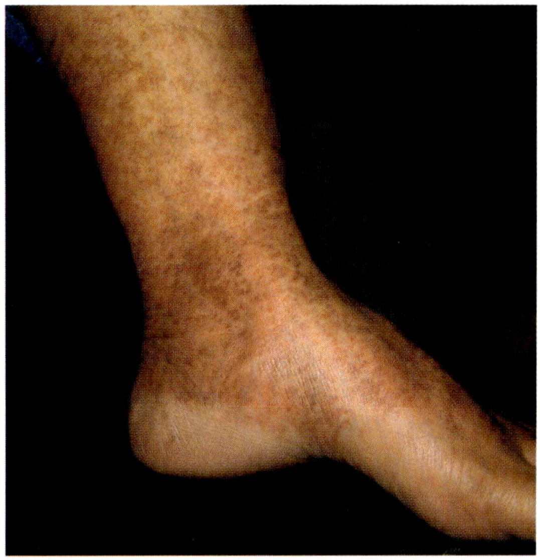

Fig. 17: Cayenne pepper like pigmentation

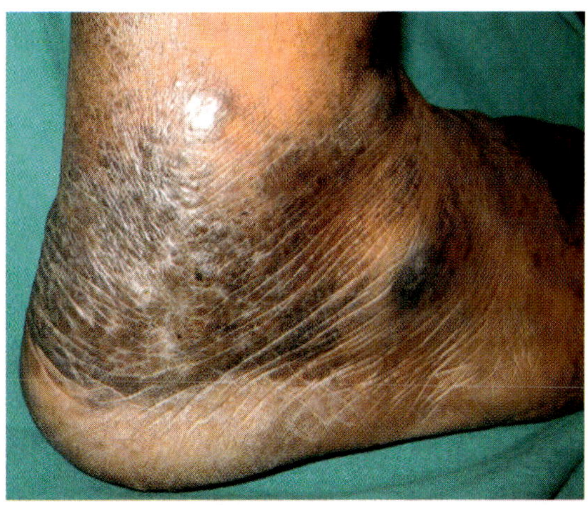

Fig. 18: Pigmented lichenoid papules, coalescing to form an irregular plaque

Histopathology

- Inflammation of the capillaries with perivascular and interstitial lymphohistiocytic infiltration.
- Extravasation of erythrocytes.
- Hemosiderin-laden macrophages are also seen, specially in lichen aureus.

Treatment

- Reassurance.

Reticulate pigmentary anomalies

* There are many cutaneous disorders, characterized by patterned hyperpigmentation.
* Pigmentation may appear as reticular or retiform or fishnet-like.
* Pigmentation is due to melanin in the epidermis.

Histopathology

- Hyperpigmentation of basal keratinocytes with either a normal or slightly increased number of melanocytes.
- Interface vacuolization of basal cells and dermal melanophages are seen in dyskeratosis congenita.
- Digitate elongations of hyperpigmented reteridges in acropigmentation of Kitamura and Dowling-Dego's disease and also have a tendency to spare the suprapapillary epidermis.
- Infundibula of hair follicles are affected in Dowling-Dego's disease.
- Clumps of melanin-laden melanophages are seen in papillary dermis in a patchy pattern without overlying epidermal pigmentation in dermatopathia pigmentosa reticularis.
- Patchy distribution of melanin within the amyloid globules in macular amyloidosis.

Macular amyloidosis

- Reticular pigmentation is seen at interscapular area, outer aspects of upper and lower limbs.

Acropigmentation of Dohi

- Hyper- and hypopigmented macules appear on the face and acral areas.

Acropigmentation of Kitamura

- Slightly depressed hyperpigmented macules present on the dorsal hands and feet. Face, neck and trunk are also affected.
- Gradually lesions are evolved into reticular pattern.
- Palmoplantar pits may be present.

Dowling-Dego's disease

- Heavily pigmented reticular macules with a tendency to coalesce.
- Lesions present at flexurals like axillae, lateral sides of the neck, inframammary and inguinal folds, anticubital and popliteal fossae and intergluteal fold.
- Other sites like genitalia, inner thighs, chest, face and abdomen are also affected.

Dyskeratosis congenita

- Reticular brownish hyperpigmentation appears at first decade of life.
- Common sites are neck, upper chest and arms.
- Other features are nail dystrophy and leukoplakia.
- Associated features are bone marrow suppression and development of malignancy.
- Commonest cause of death is aplastic anemia.

Naegeli-Franceschetii-Jadassohn syndrome

- It is an autosomal dominant disorder and presents with reticular pigmentation.
- Common sites are neck, perioral, periocular areas and other flexurals.
- Other associated features are hypohidrosis, keratoderma, hypoplasia of dermatoglyphics of the fingers and abnormalities of nails and teeth.

Dermatopathia pigmentosa reticularis

- It presents with reticular pigmentation.
- Common sites are limbs and trunk.

Progressive cribriform and zosteriform hyperpigmentation

- Reticular pigmentation starts at second decade of life.
- It affects the lower half of the trunk and thighs and lesions are distributed in a dermatomal fashion.

Reticular erythematous mucinosis

- It is a form of cutaneous mucinosis, presented with reticular pigmentation.
- It may be a presenting sign of systemic lupus erythematosus.

Clinical features

- Lesions are well defined, irregular, reticulated and erythematous patches.
- In some cases papules may be studded within the patches.
- Common sites are center of the chest and center of the upper back. But areas like arms and face may be affected.

Histopathology

- Small amount of dermal mucin deposition on seen.
- Mild to moderate mononuclear cells infiltration is seen around the vessels and hair follicles.
- Mucin deposition is seen as blue and mucicarmine stain. It stains metachromatically with toluidine blue and Giemsa stain.
- Increased number of factor XIIIa bearing dendritic cells.

Treatment

- Chloroquine or hydroxychloroquine orally.

Lichen planus pigmentosus

- This is a macular variety of lichen planus, commonly found in India.
- Middle aged, between 20-40 years males and females are commonly affected.

Clinical features

- Lesions start as slate gray to blue-black macules. Gradually size and number of the lesions increase. Lesions may be slightly elevated plaque.
- Lesions are usually well to ill defined or ill defined.
- Most of the lesion are confluent; but they may coalsece to involve an extensive area. Sometimes lesion take a reticular pattern.
- Initial shape may be oval but larger lesions are irregular.
- Common sites are face, sides of the neck, flexor surfaces of the upper limbs and abdomen. But other areas may be affected except palms, soles, scalp and mucosae. Rarely lesions may be distributed unilaterally.
- Lesions are asymptomatic or mildly pruritic.

Histopathology

- Normal or mild acanthotic epidermis.
- Basal layer vacuolation.
- Pigment incontinence.
- Sparse lichenoid lymphocytic infiltration in the papillary dermis.

Erythema dyschromicum perstans/ashy dermatosis

- It is an acquired chronic, progressive pigmentary dermatosis of unknown etiology.
- It occurs in children and adults and both males and females.
- It is more common in dark skinned people.
- Lesions may be cleared within few years.

Clinical features

- Lesions usually start as asymptomatic slate gray macules with occasional presence of transient elevated border.

- Common sites are trunk and upper limbs. But any area may be affected except scalp, palms, soles and mucous membrane.
- Size is variable from few mm to several cm, covering an extensive area.

Histopathology

- Hydropic degeneration of basal layer.
- Pigment incontinence and lichenoid lymphocytic infiltration in the upper dermis.

Mongolian spot

* It is a type of dermal melanocytosis, commonly seen in Mongoloid and Negroid infants and sometimes in Caucasoid infants.
* Extensive and persistent lesions are seen in association with bilateral nevus of Ota.
* Lesion is present at birth and disappears spontaneously within 3-4 years.

Clinical features

- Asymptomatic bruise-like uniformly pigmented blue patches are classically present at sacrococcygeal region.
- Rarely lesions may present at middle or upper part of the back.
- Shape is oval or round and margin is ill defined.
- Size is variable from few to several centimeter.
- Number is usually single but may be multiple.

Histopathology

- Elongated, slender and slightly wavy dendritic cells are present at lower dermis.
- These nevus cells are sparse and scattered within collagen bundles.
- They lie parallel to the skin surface like collagen bundles and contain melanin pigment.

Nevus of Ota/Nevus fuscoceruleus ophthalo maxillaris

* It is a type of dermal melanocytosis, occurring unilaterally in 90% cases.
* Lesion may be present at birth or may develop within first year of life or even during adolescent period.
* Nevus of Ito is similar to nevus of Ota except the sites of involvement and these sites are supraclavicular, scapular and deltoid regions.

Clinical features

- Unilateral blue to brown patches or confluent macules are commonly present at face, including periorbital region, temple, forehead malar area and nose.
- Lesions are slowly progressive.
- It is frequently present with blue discoloration of ipsilateral sclera.
- It rarely affects conjunctivae, cornea and retina.
- Color of the lesion may be uniform brown to slate blue or mottled. Rarely some areas of the patches may be slightly raised. Sometimes blue nevi like discrete nodules may present within the patches.

Histopathology

- Elongated dendritic melanocytes scattered among the dermal collagen bundles.
- These cells may be seen even at subcutaneous tissue.
- Melanophages are rarely seen.

Becker's nevus

* It is common dermal melanocytosis, appearing in adolescent period.
* Males are affected more than females.
* It commonly appears at second decade of life.

* Excessive hair growth is seen only after hyperpigmentation and no hypertrichosis is seen in many cases.

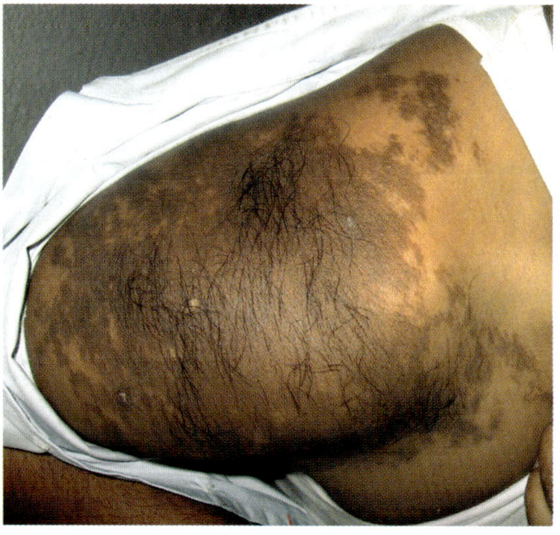

Fig. 19: Unilateral irregular pigmented patch with isolated nodules and excessive hair growth

Clinical features

- It presents as a large unilateral hyperpigmented patch with hypertrichosis.
- Usually the patch is sharply defined but often irregular due to formation by coalescing of multiple lesions.
- Common sites are shoulder, back and chest; but other areas also may be affected.
- Number is usually single and may be multiple or even bilateral.
- Some lesions show cerebriform growth and dermatomal distribution.

Histopathology

- Slight acanthosis and elongated rete ridges.
- Hyperpigmentation of basal layer and melanophages are seen in the upper dermis.
- Increased number of melanocytes and hair follicles may be normal or increased in number.
- Smooth muscle fibers may be increased.

CHAPTER C13

PRURITUS AND URTICARIA

Pruritus

Definition

* It an unpleasant, nonadaptive and poorly localized sensation which compels to scratch. Pruritus and itch, both the words are used synonymously.

Pathophysiology

* Mediators of pruritus:
    - Histamine
    - Proteinases: Tryptase, chymase.
    - Prostaglandin (PGE1)
    - Substance P
    - Opoid peptides: Morphine, nociceptin
    - Neurotrophins: Nerve growth factor (NGF), neurotrophin 4
    - Cytokines: Interleukin 1 (IL1), interleukin 6 (IL6), interleukin 31 (IL31), TNFα
    - Other peripheral mediators: TRPV1 (transient receptor potential vanilloid receptor), TRPM8 (thermosensor for coolness induced by menthol), GRPR (gastrin related peptide receptor), acetylcholine, angiotensin converting enzyme (ACE), neural endopeptidases, serotonin, kinin, bradykinin, nitric oxide, etc.

Conducting nerve of pruritus

- A subset of cutaneous nonmyelinated C fibers comprising of less than 5% of total C fibers.
- Its velocity of conduction is very slow i.e., < 2m/s.

Interaction between nerve and mediators of pruritus

- Direct activation of C fibers.
- Secondary activation.
- Augmentation
- Desensitization.

Variants of pruritus

- Pruritus in aged skin
- Pruritus scalp
- Pruritus vulvae
- Pruritus scroti
- Pruritus ani
- Pruritus scar
- Postburn pruritus.

Different character of pruritus

- Burning
- Pricking
- Feelings of insect crawling
- Tickling
- Allokinesis: The term is used when some stimuli like touch or gentle warming which normally do not cause pruritus, induces pruritus.

Cutaneous causes of pruritus

- Infection/infestations
  - Tinea infection
  - Chronic folliculitis
  - Scabies
  - Pediculosis
  - Insect bite reaction
  - Cutaneous reaction to worm infestation
- Inflammatory dermatoses
  - Atopic dermatitis
  - Seborrhoeic dermatitis
  - Pompholyx
  - Nummular dermatitis
  - Asteatotic dermatitis
  - Allergic contact dermatitis
  - Miliarial dermatitis
  - Lichen planus
  - Psoriasis
  - Urticaria
  - Mastocytosis
  - Dermatitis herpetiformis
  - Urticarial bullous pemphigoid
- Neoplastic dermatoses
  - Cutaneous T cell lymphoma.
- Genetic/nevoid dermatoses
  - Inflammatory linear verrucous epidermal nevus
  - Darier's disease
- Miscellaneous
  - Eosinophilic pustular folliculitis
  - Dermatomyositis
  - Scleroderma.

Systemic causes of prutitus

- Renal
- Hepatic
- Hematologic
- Malignancy
- Endocrine
- Pregnancy
- HIV/AIDS
- Psychogenic.

Pruritus due to drugs

- Drugs causing cholestasis
  - Chlorpromazine
  - Erythromycin estolate, sulfonamide
  - Oral contraceptive pill.
- Drugs causing hepatotoxicity
  - Acitaminophen
  - Isoniazide, minocycline, amoxicillin-clavulanic acid, phenytoin, sulfonamide
  - Testosterone.
- Drugs causing sebostasis/xerosis
  - B-blockers
  - Retinoids
  - Tamoxifen.
  - Busulfan
  - Clofibrate.
- Drugs causing phototoxicity
  - 8-Methoxypsoralen (8 MOP).
- Neurologic drugs
  - Hydroxyethyl starch.
- Idiopathic mechanism
  - Chloroquine
  - Clonidine
  - Lithium.

Features of renal pruritus

- Localized or generalized paroxysmal pruritus, associated with chronic renal failure, not with acute renal failure.
- Pruritus is more when patient is on hemodialysis and it reaches at the peak after two days of without dialysis.

- Pruritus does not correlate with severity of the disease.
- Pruritus may be due to increased number of mast cells/parathyroid activity/plasma histamine level, or accumulation of opoids, or immunological alteration with increased pro-inflammatory cytokines like IL1, IL6, IL31.

Features of hepatic pruritus

- Nearly all hepatic diseases are associated with pruritus specially biliary cirrhosis, obstructive choledocolithiasis and chronic hepatitis C infection.
- Localized or generalized migratory pruritus which is not relieved by scratching, and becomes worst at hand, feet and body areas having tight clothing.
- Pruritus is aggravated at night.
- It may precede several years before manifestation of any liver disease.
- Probable mechanisms of pruritus are increased bile acids, central neuromodulation and unknown pruritogens in the plasma.

Features of hematologic pruritus

- Iron deficiency pruritus may be localized or generalized. If localized it often affects perianal or vulvar regions.
- Polycythemia vera causes aquagenic pruritus which may precede several years before diagnosis of it. Only 30-50% cases are associated with pruritus.
- Pruritus is probably due to release of serotonin from aggregated platelets.

Features of malignancy associated pruritus

- Any malignancy can cause pruritus, specially Hodgkin's lymphoma, non-Hodgkin's lymphoma and chronic lymphocytic leukemia.
- Only in Hodgkin's lymphoma, pruritus correlate with severity of the disease.
- Persistent, unexplained pruritus which does not respond to conventional antihistamines.
- Localized pruritus at tip of the nose may be associated with brain tumor.
- Probable mechanism of pruritus are toxic products from necrotic tumor cells, production of chemical mediators by the tumor, allergic reaction to tumor specific antigens, increased proteolytic activities and release of histamine.
- Reed-Sternberg cells in Hodgkin's lymphoma can produce IL5 which is responsible for peripheral eosinophilia leading to pruritus.

Features of endocrinal pruritus

- Hyperthyroidism causes severe generalized pruritus, probably due to direct effect of thyroid hormones on skin.
- Hypothyroidism causes localized or generalized pruritus probably due to dryness of the skin.
- Diabetes mellitus causes generalized pruritus or localized pruritus specially at genital or perianal area. Localized pruritus in diabetes mellitus is related to poor glycemic condition and candidiasis. Diabetic neuropathy is associated with pain, burning, pricking and pruritus.

Features of pruritus in HIV/AIDS

- Pruritus may be an initial presenting symptom in HIV or AIDS and it may be severe with poor response to conventional therapy.
- In 50% cases mechanism of pruritus is beyond explanation. Other probable mechanisms are acquired ichthyosis, pruritic papular eruption, eosinophilic folliculitis, severe seborrheic dermatitis, psoriasis, scabies, drug eruption and increased sensitivity to insect bite reaction.
- Increased IgE level/eosinophils or altered Th1/Th2 cytokines are also responsible for pruritus.
- Increased IgE level inversely relates with CD4 cell count.
- Intractable pruritus correlate with viral load.

Features of psychogenic pruritus

- To designate psychologic pruritus is possible only after exclusion of all other causes.

- Intensity of pruritus correlates with depth of emotional state.
- Sleep pattern remains unaltered.
- Secondary skin changes are excoriation, lichenification and development of some specific disease like prurigo simplex/nodularis or lichen simplex chronicus.

Laboratory evaluation

- It is required to correlate with the suspected systemic cause, to exclude some other disorders and to make choice of therapy.

Treatment

- Topical preparations:
  - 5% Doxepin cream acts as potent antihistamine.
  - Capsaicin cream acts on vanilloid receptors.
  - Menthol acts on TPR M8.
  - Pramoxine and salicylate act as anesthetic.
  - Pimecrolimus and tacrolimus act as immunomodulators.
  - Cannabinoids act on opoid receptors.
  - Barrier cream
  - Future topical therapy includes neurotrophin inhibitors.
- Systemic therapy:
  - Antihistamines act as most common antipruritic drugs.
  - Opoid antagonists/agonist/agonist-antagonist: Naltrexone, naloxone and nalfurafine.
  - Mirtazapine reduces central itch perception.
  - Thalidomide/gabapentin blocks neuropathic afferent pathway.
- Surgery for tumor
- For renal pruritus:
  - Erythropoietin, ondansetron, lidocaine, cholestyramine, etc.
- For hepatic pruritus
  - Ursodeoxycholic acid, cholestyramine, phototherapy, ondansetron, sertraline, naltrexone, naloxone, thalidomide and stanozolol.
- For hematological pruritus
  - Phototherapy, aspirin for polycythemia vera to reduce platelet aggregation and IFNα.
- For malignancy
  - Paroxetine, mirtazapine and thalidomide.
- Non-pharmacological treatment like cutaneous field stimulation and behavioural therapy.

URTICARIA

- It is an acute and chronic relapsing dermatosis which may continue for hours, days, weeks or even for years, causing a considerable distress.
- It has a compex pathophysiology. Mast cells are the main effector cells which when degranulate by various stimuli release histamine and some other mediators like leukotrienes, causing dilatation of dermal blood vessels and leakage of serum to produce a wheal.
- Most common stimuli are viral infection, drug, food and autoantibody and in a major portion of urticaria, no definite stimuli is elicitable.
- Urticaria may be acute, when the total episodes of the disease, not individual lesion, persists less than 6 weeks and it may be chronic when total episodes of the disease, not individual lesion persists more than 6 weeks.
- Patients of acute urticaria often attend either general physician or at emergency but patients of chronic urticaria often attend dermatologist to get permanent relief.
- Children suffer from acute urticaria more commonly whereas adults suffer from chronic urticaria more commonly.
- Histopathology shows papillary dermal edema, dilatation of dermal vessels and sparse perivascular lymphocytic infiltration, containing macrophages, lymphocytes, eosinophils and neutrophils.
- When neutrophils are predominant in histopathology, urticaria may not respond to antihistamines, but requires colchicines, dapsone or systemic steroid.

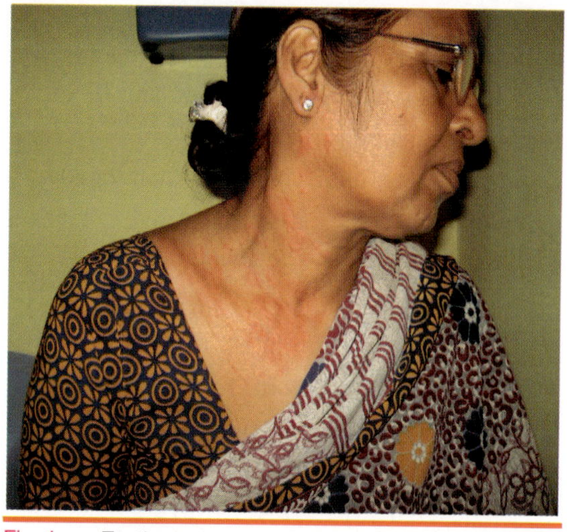

Fig. 1: Erythematous and edematous papules and plaques

- All forms of urticaria are having more or less similar clinical feature as follows:
  - Most common symptom is intense pruritus, but rarely burning sensation.
  - Primary lesion is a wheal, having well circumscribed, pink or pale and edematous plaque with elastic consistency.
  - Lesion is surrounded by varying degree of erythema.
  - Size is variable from few mm to several cm and shape is also variable from round, arcuate, annular, bizarre and linear to any form.
  - Number of the lesion is variable from few, multiple, numerous or diffuse involving entire body.
  - Lesions are distributed not only randomly but also asymmetrically.
  - Individual lesions usually resolve within 24 hours and rarely persist till 36 hours.

Acute urticaria

- It is common in both children and adults with a life-time prevalence of about 15-20% among general population.
- In 50% cases of acute urticaria, the etiology is still unknown.
- Other causes of acute urticaria
  - Upper respiratory tract infection in 40% cases.
  - Drugs like penicillin, nonsteroidal anti-inflammatory drugs and opioids in 9% cases,
  - Food, specially sea food and fruits only in 1% cases. But it is blamed more frequently.
  - Insect bite.
- Infection and food are the most common causes in children whereas drugs are the most common cause in adults.
- A complete resolution is expected within a period of 6 weeks and in 90% cases it occurs within a period of 3 weeks.

Chronic urticaria

- Causes of chronic urticaria:
  - Physical cause in 35% cases
  - Idiopathic in 25% cases
  - Autoimmune in 25%
  - Pseudoallergy in 5% cases
  - Infection in 5% cases
  - Drugs in 5% cases.
- Individual lesions are same as acute urticaria but episodes of urticaria persist more than 6 weeks.

Angioedema

- It is variant of urticaria where edema occurs at reticular dermis and subcutaneous tissue in comparison to acute or chronic urticaria where edema occurs in papillary dermis.
- In about 40% patients, urticaria is associated with angioedema.
- It is associated with pain, instead of pruritus as in urticaria.
- It appears as focal cutaneous or mucous membrane swelling with indistinct border.
- Individual lesion usually persists longer than urticaria as long as 72 hours.
- Common sites are lips, eyelids, extremities and genitalia.

Dermatographism

* It is often associated with chronic urticaria.
* It may be acute or delayed type.
* Acute type develops immediately following a certain pressure.
* Delayed type develops immediately following release of a continuous pressure over 4-8 hours.

Anaphylaxis

* It is the most dangerous condition, must be differentiated from acute urticaria for proper management.
* It has not only the features of urticaria like severe pruritus, wheal or diffuse erythema, also has cardiovascular, respiratory or gastrointestinal tract complications.
* Onset is very sudden.
* Common causes are hymenoptera venom, food and drugs.
* Increased serum tryptase level may confirm the diagnosis.

Urticarial lesions in other dermatoses

* Following other dermatoses may present with urticarial lesions:
  - Urticarial dermatitis
  - Arthropod bite reaction
  - Urticaria pigmentosa
  - Bullous pemphigoid
  - Pruritic urticarial papules and plaques of pregnancy (PUPPP)/polymorphous eruption of pregnancy.
  - Urticarial vasculitis
  - Interstitial granulomatous dermatitis
  - Eosinophilic cellulitis (Wells syndrome)
  - Neutrophilic eccrine hidradenitis
  - Urticaria like follicular mucinosis.
* Urticarial lesions of above conditions differ from ordinary urticaria on following points:
  - Lesions are more infiltrated or indurated rather than edematous lesions in ordinary urticaria.
  - More persistent as > 24-36 hours whereas < 24-36 hours in ordinary urticaria.
  - Lesions are distributed symmetrically, not randomly as in ordinary urticaria.
  - Lesions resolve with signs like hypo/hyperpigmentation/scarring whereas no residual sign in ordinary urticaria.
  - Usually not associated with angioedema as 40% cases of angioedema are associated with ordinary urticaria.
  - Papules, vesicles, scaling and crusts may be associated with it but not with ordinary urticaria.

Urticaria pigmentosa

* Most common form of cutaneous mastocytosis occurs frequently in children.
* Increased local concentration of soluble mast cell growth factor stimulates proliferation of mast cells and melanocytes leading to urticaria and pigmentation.
* Adulthood cases progress to systemic disease and rarely develop hematologic disease.
* Anemia, thrombocytopenia, and associated hematologic disorders are poor prognostic indicators.

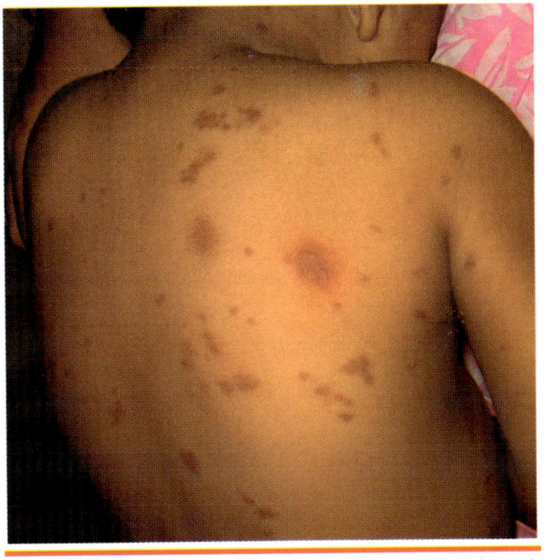

Fig. 2: Urticarial papules and plaques at back with positive Darier sign

Clinical features

- Pruritic, oval to round macules, papules and plaques are present.
- Lesions may turn into vesicles in infancy.
- Number of the lesions is variable from few to numerous.
- When lesions are stroked, they become more erythematous, edematous and pruritic. This is known as Darier sign.
- 50% Children with isolated urticaria pigmentosa is resolve by adulthood.

Histopathology

- Mast cell infiltration in the dermis.
- Cytoplasm of mast cell contains metachromatic granules.

Treatment

- Antihistaminics.
- Systemic glucocorticosteroids.

VESICULO-BULLOUS DISORDERS

CHAPTER C14

Pemphigus

* It is an autoimmune blistering disorder, affecting the skin and mucous membrane.
* Desmoglein is a desmosomal and transmembrane protein of the keratinocytes. It plays a key role to maintain the cell-cell adhesion.
* Desmoglein is of 4 types, such as Dsg 1, Dsg 2, Dsg 3 and Dsg 4.
* Dsg 1 and Dsg 3 are related with pemphigus.
* Actually an aminoterminal residue segment of the desmoglein 3 at the extracellular domain is responsible for cell-cell adhesion.
* In pemphigus, autoantibody is formed against this desmoglein. An antigen-antibody complex is likely to induce proteinases and causes separation of keratinocytes from one to another, known as acantholysis. This results in blister formation.

Types of pemphigus

- Pemphigus vulgaris
- Pemphigus foliaceus
- IgA pemphigus
- Pemphigus herpetiformis
- Paraneoplastic pemphigus
- Drug-induced pemphigus
- Benign familial pemphigus

Variant of pemphigus vulgaris

- Pemphigus vegetans

Variants of pemphigus foliaceus

- Pemphigus erythematosus
- Endemic pemphigus

* IgG is the main antibody, directed against desmoglein.
* In pemhigus vulgaris, major antigen is desmoglein 3 (Dsg 3) and in pemphigus foliaceus, major antigen is desmoglein 1 (Dsg 1).
* In paraneoplastic pemphigus, antigens are not only desmoglein but also plakin molecules of the desmosomes.
* Not only epidermis of the skin, but oral mucosa also contains Dsg 3 and so, it is very often affected in pemphigus vulgaris.

* In IgA pemphigus, major antigen is desmocollin 1 and definitely the antibody is IgA, as the name of the disease is implied.
* Histopathology shows intraepidermal cleft. In pemphigus vulgaris, it is suprabasal and in pemphigus foliaceus, it is subcorneal.
* Direct immunofluorescence (DIF): IgG deposition is seen in 100% cases of pemphigus vulgaris, pemphigus foliaceus and paraneoplastic pemphigus.
* Probable causes implicated in pemphigus are trauma, ionizing radiation, viral infection, drugs and PUVA.
* Rare associations with pemphigus vulgaris:
    - Internal malignancy
    - Castleman's disease
    - Thymoma, myasthenia gravis
    - Graves' disease
    - Localized scleroderma
    - Systemic lupus erythematosus

Pemphigus vulgaris

* Pemphigus commonly occurs in the age group of 40-60 years, but any age may be affected.
* In 10% cases, earliest manifestation is painful oral ersions.
* Oral mucosa is affected in more than 80% cases.

Clinical features

- When oral mucosa is affected, patient feels difficulty in chewing and pain during swallowing (odynophagia) or presents with hoarseness of voice.
- When there is only oral lesions without any skin lesion, very often patient's first visit to ENT department and also it is misdiagnosed as oral candidiasis.
- Primary lesions are vesicles which gradually increase in number to affect all over the body. They rupture easily or enlarge to some extent to form bullae but ultimately rupture to form erosions.
- These erosions continue to spread at the periphery without any tendency of healing spontaneously and often bleed with minor trauma.
- Erosions are being covered with dirty reddish or brownish crusts, depending on presence of bleeding or infection or both.
- Intact vesicles are rarely seen in oral mucosa due to repeated trauma within the oral cavity during chewing of the foods.
- Lesions are initially tense but within few hours they turn into flaccid due to thin covering of the vesicles, through which evaporation occurs quickly.
- Common sites other than oral mucosa, are axillae, groin, genitalia and trunk.
- **Bullae spreading sign** becomes positive and **Nikolsky's test** shows positive result.

Bulla spreading sign/Asboe-Hansen sign

- If a slow and steady pressure is given on the top of an intact vesicle or bulla with the pulp of the index finger, it will spread at the periphery.

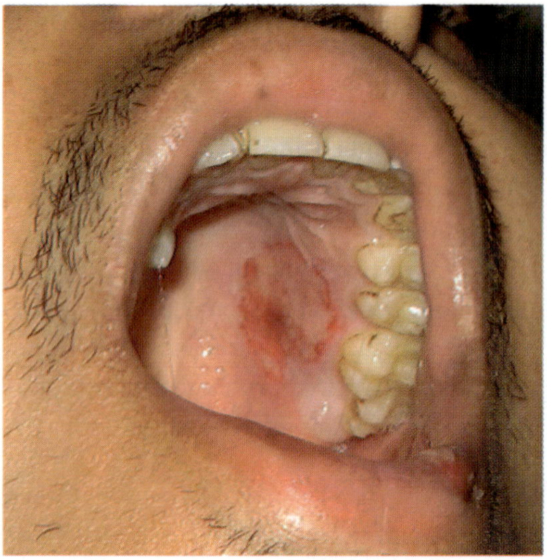

Fig. 1: Palatal erosion without any skin lesion in pemphigus as an earliest feature

Nikolsky's test

- When a tangential or shearing pressure is given by thumb on normal appearing skin over a bony prominence and near a vesicle/bulla, superficial skin may be peeled off.

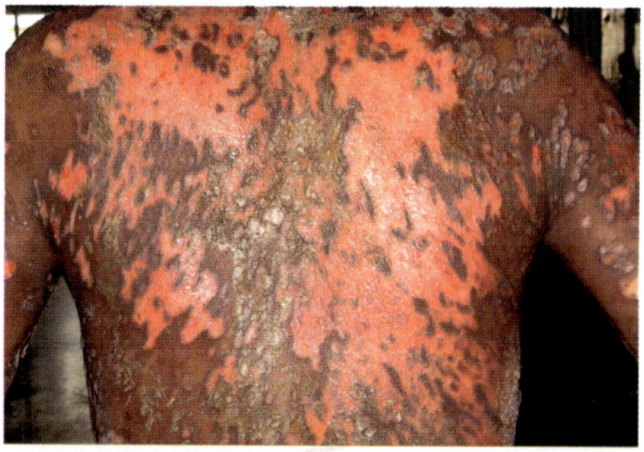

Fig. 2: Extending erosions at the back

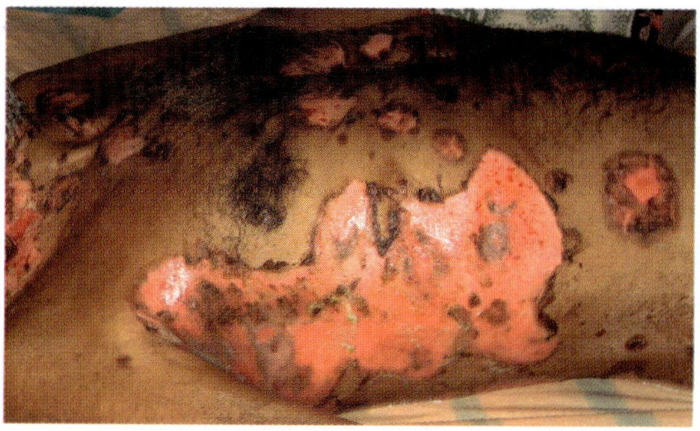

Fig. 3: Huge erosions with crusting at places

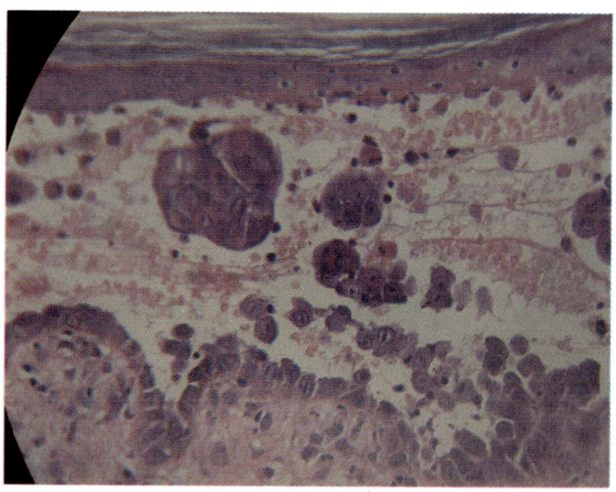

Fig. 4: Suprabasal cleft containing single as well as cluster of acantholytic cells and tombstone appearance of basal layer

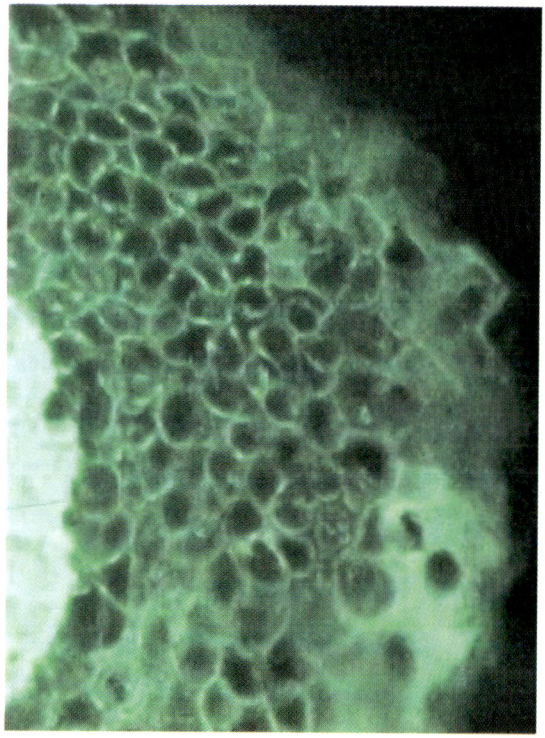

Fig. 5: Fishnet appearance due to immunofluorescence along the margin of the keratinocytes. (Courtesy: Abhishek De, Assistant Professor, IPGMER, Kolkata)

Histo- and immunopathology

- Suprabasal cleft with single row basal cells, known as tombstone appearance, at the floor of the cleft.
- Acantholytic cells present within the cavity.
- Direct immunofluorescence (DIF) test shows fishnet pattern of intercellular immunofluorescence.
- Indirect immunofluorescence (DIF) test (IIF) often becomes positive.
- Tzanck smear shows presence of acantholytic cells.

Treatment

- Systemic corticosteroid, predinsolone, 60-120 mg/day (1-2 mg/kg body weight).

- ♦ Cyclophosphamide, 50-200 mg/day (1-3 mg/kg/day) and DC pulse therapy.
- ♦ Rituximab, an antiCD20, 375 mg/m^2 once weekly for 4 weeks.
- ♦ Azathioprine (2-5 mg/kg/day) and mycophenolate mofetil (2 g/d).
- ♦ IVIG 400 mg/kg/day for 3-5 days per month.
- ♦ Etanercept, a TNFα antagosist.
- ♦ Daphentin, an antimalarial
- ♦ Allogenic hematopoietic stem cell transplantation.
- ♦ Dsg 3 peptide.
- ♦ Pyridostigmine bromide, a cholinergic agonist.

Pemphigus foliaceus

- ✶ It is a variant of pemphigus vulgaris where the target antigen is desmoglein 1 (dsg 1), another component of desmosomal proteins. Upper layers of the epidermis is rich in dsg 1 and so, cleft develops through the granular layer. Oral mucosa is usually spared as dsg 1 is rarely present there.

Clinical features

- ♦ Lesions start as very superficial vesicles which rupture to form erosions. Erosions go on spreading at the periphery as well as coalesce to form a polycyclic margin. As the erosions are becoming older, scales and crusts cover them.
- ♦ Foul smell and burning sensation are often associated.
- ♦ Common sites are face, scalp, upper trunk, but any site may be affected.
- ♦ As vesicles or bullae are very superficial, they rupture quickly to form larger areas of erosions.
- ♦ Nikolsky's test and bulla spreading sign, both are positive.

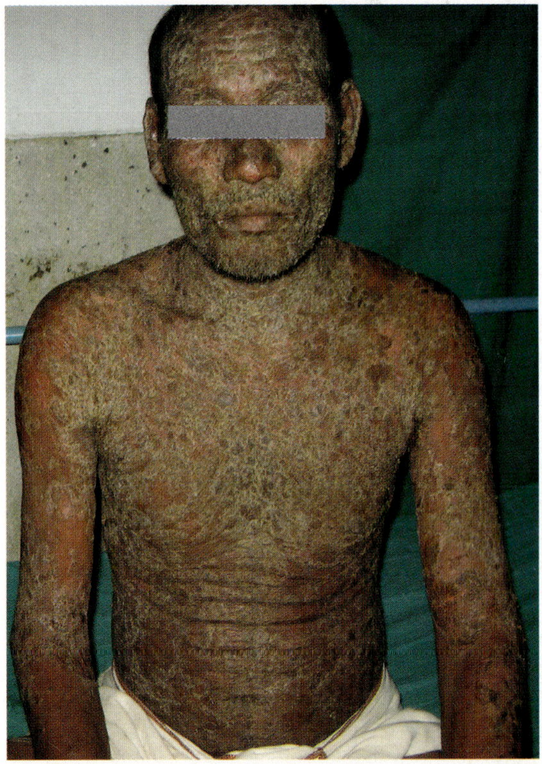

Fig. 6: Generalized crusted erosions

Differential diagnosis

- ✶ Subcorneal pustular dermatosis
  - ♦ Primary lesions are pustules
  - ♦ Multiple polycyclic and crusted erosions are developed.
- ✶ Seborrheic dermatitis
  - ♦ Moist scales affecting seborrheic areas.
  - ♦ No history of vesicle formation.
- ✶ Toxic epidermal necrolysis (TEN)/Stevens-Johnson syndrome (SJS).
  - ♦ Presence of history of drug intake.
  - ♦ Sudden onset.
  - ♦ Burning sensation.
  - ♦ Tender erythematous macules or patches which turn into deep brown to black due to necrosis and skin easily sloughs out to form extensive erosions in TEN or develops erythe-

ma multiforme like lesions, turning into blisters and erosions in SJS.

- Mucosal involvement is a must.

* Erythroderma
  - Generalized erythema, edema and scaling.
  - No history of vesiculo-bullous lesions.
  - History of papulosquamous lesions are often present.

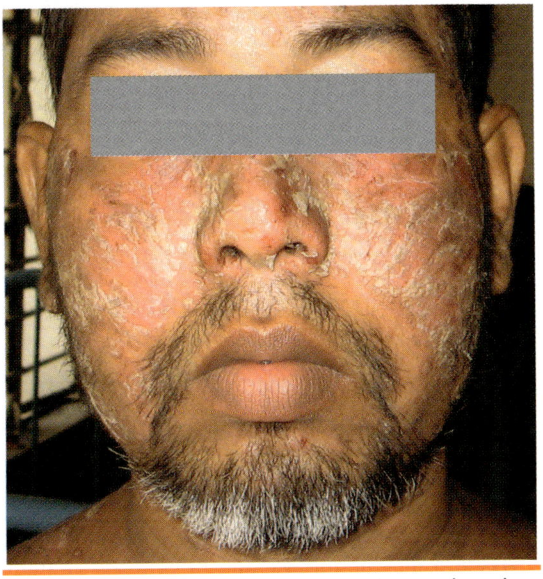

Fig. 7: Well defined erythematous and crusted erosions at malar areas of the face

Differential diagnosis

- Seborrheic dermatitis
- Malar rash
- Upgrade type 1 lepra reaction in BT Hansen.

Bullous pemphigoid

* It is a common immunobullous disorder, occurring mostly in older age.
* Antigens are BPAg1 and BPAg2.
* Antibodies are of IgG group.
* Antigen-antibody combination activates plasminogen and causes subepidermal blister.
* Blisters are tense for initial period due to thicker covering which prevents quick evaporation. But when a bulla persists for longer time, it will become flaccid.
* Inflammatory cells and complement C_3 also play a role in pathogenesis.
* In 50% cases elevated IgE and sometimes eosinophilia are present correlating with pruritus.

Types of pemphigoid

- Generalized
- Localized

Variants of generalized pemphigoid

- Urticarial
- Erythrodermic
- Cicatricial
- Vesicular
- Childhood
- Herpes gestationis
- Lichen planus pemphigoides

Variants of localized pemphigoid

- Dyshidrosiform
- Vulvar
- Nodular
- Vegetating

Clinical features

- Symptom is mild to moderate itching and signs are initial nonbullous forms and various bullous forms.
- Any age may be affected. But commonly occurs in older age group.
- Primary lesions originate from the normal or erythematous skin. Lesions of classical bullous pemphigoid are vesicles and bullae with variable number and size. Number may be numerous and size may be upto 10 cm.
- After few days when the primary lesions rupture following friction or spontaneously, secondary lesions arise as crusted ulcers with a tendency of healing without scarring. But post-inflammatory hyperpigmented macules or patches and milia are formed.
- Mucosal lesions are less common as only in 10-35% cases.

- Commonly affected sites are lower abdomen, inner thighs and flexor of forearms.
- Initially the blisters are tense due to subepidermal position but after few days these become flaccid due to evaporation.
- Primary lesions contain clear or hemorrhagic fluid.
- Nikolsky's test is negative.
- Bulla spreading test is usually negative but may be positive in some cases.

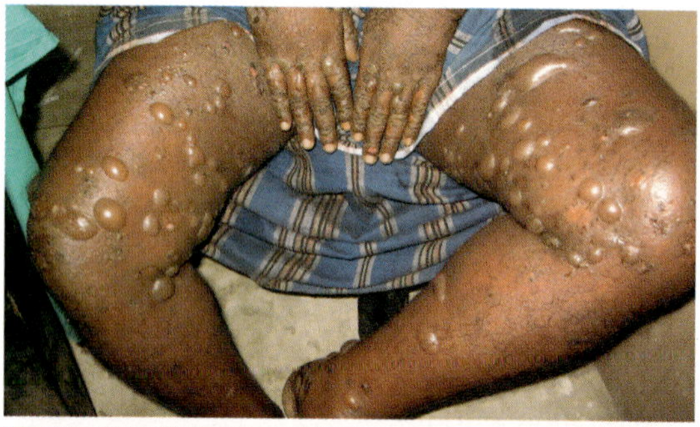

Fig. 8: Tense vesicles and bullae at upper and lower limbs

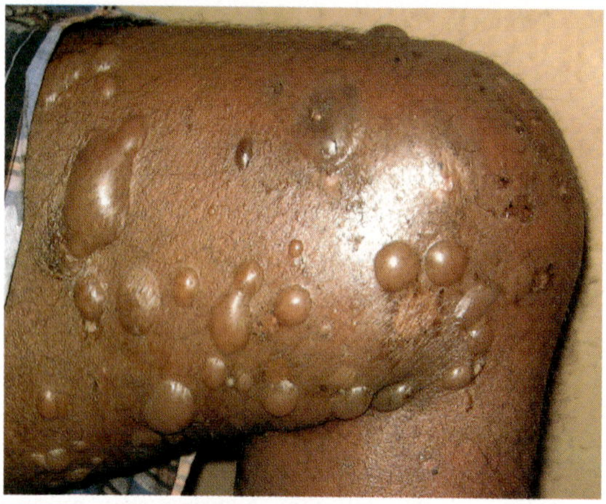

Fig. 9: Tense vesicles and bullae

Histo- and immunopathology

- Subepidermal blister containing sparse neutrophils and eosinophils.
- DIF shows linear pattern of C3 and IgG at BMZ.
- Indirect IF is positive in 70-80% cases and shows circulating IgG. Titer does not correlate with disease activity or severity.

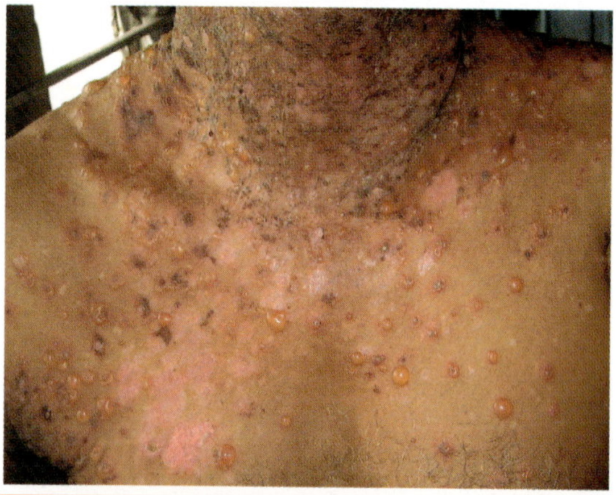

Fig. 10: Numerous monomorphic tense vesicular eruptions with crusted erosions of vesicular bullae pemphigoid

Dermatitis herpetiformis (DH)

- DH is basically cutaneous manifestation of celiac disease and biopsy of the small intestine shows, it is associated with gluten hypersensitive enteropathy in more than 90% cases.
- HLA-DQ2 genotype is strongly associated in both the cases.
- IgA antiendomysial antibodies are formed against tissue transglutaminase and in skin the antigen is epidermal transglutaminase.
- Gluten is a protein, present in wheat, rye, barley or in their hybrids like kamut, spelt, triticale, etc., but not present in oat.
- Gliadin is the alcohol soluble extract of gluten which is probably the real culprit for the disease.
- Instead of its strong association with enteropathy, symptomatic malabsorption is seen only in 20% cases of DH.
- Deposition of IgA antiepidermal transglutaminase antibodies, causes infiltration of activated neutrophils from the circulation into the dermal papillae and proteases released from degranulated neutrophils disrupt lamina lucida to produce a subepidermal cleft.

* DH responds to dapsone dramatically while worsens with inorganic iodine ingestion.
* Common age group involved is 30-40 years but it may develop at any age from 20-90 years.

Clinical features

- Primary lesions are intensely pruritic papules, papulovesicles and sometimes urticarial plaques and these develop with an erythematous background.
- Sometimes no primary lesions are seen except excoriated and crusted lesions due to vigorous scratching. Ultimately this results in burning sensation instead of pruritus and formation of hemorrhagic crusts.
- Lesions are arranged in groups or in herpetiform pattern. They are distributed usually bilaterally and symmetrically.
- Common sites are scalp, elbows-knees, extensors of forearms, buttocks and lower back.

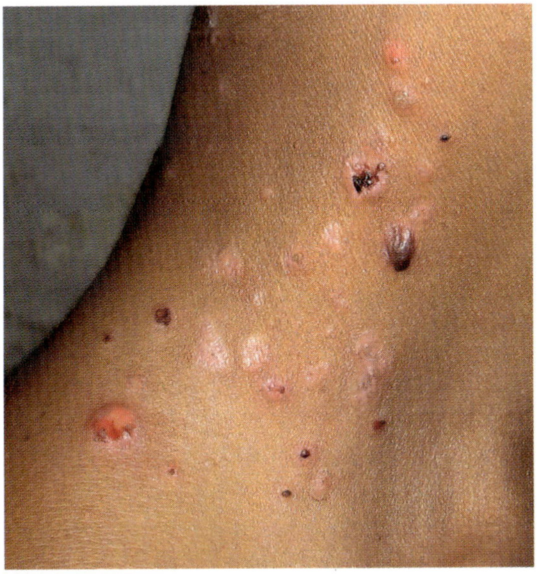

Fig. 11: Grouped vesicles with hemorrhagic crusts at the neck

Histo- and immunopathology

- Papillary dermal edema, collection of neutrophils at papillary dermis.
- Subepidermal cleft containing predominantly neutrophils and perivascular lymphocytic infiltration.
- Granular IgA deposition in the papillary dermis.

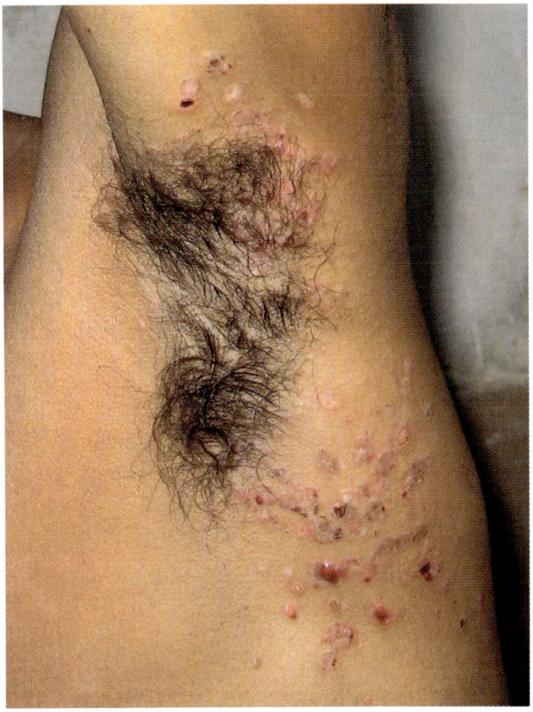

Fig. 12: Grouped vesicles with hemorrhagic crusts

Treatment

- Dapsone is given orally, initially at a dose of 50-300 mg/day in adult and 0.5 mg/kg/day in children. Maximum maintenance dose is 100 mg/day.
- Systemic steroid is required in recalcitrant cases.

Herpes gestationis

* This is a form of bullous pemphigoid, occurring in 2nd to 3rd trimester of pregnancy.
* Associated increased risks of fetal morbidity and mortality have been reported.
* This may recur in subsequent pregnancy, during menstrual periods or due to oral contraceptive pills.

Clinical features

- ♦ Intensely pruritic urticarial lesions develop which gradually turn into tense vesicles and bullae.
- ♦ Infant may be born with transient vesiculobullous eruption.

Linear IgA dermatosis (LAD)

- ✶ This is a group of immunobullous disorder, mediated by IgA antibody, directed against basement membrane zone antigens.

Histo- and immunopathology

- ♦ Subepidermal blister with uniform neutrophilic infiltration along the dermoepidermal junction.
- ♦ DIF reveals linear pattern IgA deposition along the basement membrane zone.

Subtypes

- ♦ Adult type
- ♦ Childhood type or chronic bullous dermatosis of childhood (CBDC).
- ♦ Cicatricial pemphigoid-like
- ♦ Drug induced: Drugs are Vancomycin, lithium, diclofenac, captopril, cefamandole, somatostatin, etc.

Chronic bullous dermatosis of childhood (CBDC)

- ✶ It occurs in childhood and rarely in infancy.
- ✶ It usually remits within age of 10 years. But about 10% cases may persist till later life.

Clinical features

- ♦ Primary lesions are tense vesicles and bullae with or without an erythematous base.
- ♦ New lesions often develop around the scar of the healed lesions or subsiding lesions. This arrangement takes an annular or polycyclic shape and appears as string of pearls.
- ♦ Common sites are buttocks, lower abdomen, inner thighs and genitalia.

Adult type

- ✶ It usually occurs above the age of 40 years.
- ✶ Females are slightly more affected than males.
- ✶ Cutaneous lesions are heterogeneous and may mimic other bullous disorders.

Clinical features

- ♦ Primary lesions are mild pruritic tense vesicles and bullae.
- ♦ Common sites are scalp, scapula, buttocks, elbows and knees. But palms, soles, oral mucosa and conjunctiva may be affected.

Bullous systemic lupus erythematosus

- ✶ It commonly occurs in black women.
- ✶ Majority of the patients have past history of lupus erythematosus.
- ✶ Lesions do not correlate with disease activity.

Clinical features

- ♦ Primary lesions are non-pruritic tense vesicles and bullae.
- ♦ Lesions are discrete and they are asymmetrically and widely distributed.
- ♦ Sun exposed areas are commonly affected.
- ♦ Rarely associated other cutaneous features of chronic or subacute lupus erythematous or systemic lupus erythematosus.

Epidermolysis bullosa acquisita

- ✶ This is a non-inherited bullous disorder and clinical manifestation occurs due to acquired skin fragility.
- ✶ It may be associated with lymphoma, amyloidosis or colitis.

Clinical features

- ♦ Primary lesions are tense vesicles and bullae with a non-erythematous background.
- ♦ Lesions usually develop at acral areas.
- ♦ Following healing, scarring and milia formation are very common.
- ♦ Nail dystrophy and alopecia are other features.

- Some patient show a tendency to involve oral and conjunctival mucosa like cicatricial pemphigoid.

Histo- and immunopathology

- Subepidermal blister.
- Dermis may or may not be inflammatory.
- If inflammation is present, infiltrate contains lymphocytes, neutrophils and eosinophils around the vessels as well as at interstitial areas.
- DIF reveals linear deposition of complement at basement membrane zone and IIF reveals anti-basement membrane zone antibodies in 50% cases.

Porphyria cutanea tarda

* It is the commonest form of porphyria, occurring due to decreased catalytic activity of uroporphyrinogen decarboxylase.
* Uroporphyrin and coproporphyrin can be detected in urine.
* Isocoproporphyrin can be detected in feces. Presence of porphyrin in urine can be detected by help of Wood's lamp examination or by sunlight.
* History of photosensitivity and skin fragility must be present.
* It is precipitated by alcohol, estrogen, polychlorinated hydrocarbons, hemodialysis in renal failure patients, hepatitis C and HIV infections.

Variants

- Type I or acquired sporadic type: Enzymatic deficiency exclusively expressed in the liver.
- Type II or autosomal dominant hereditary type: Enzymatic deficiency expressed in all tissues.

* Ratio of type I and type II is 3-4:1.

Clinical features

- Primary lesions are blisters developing at sun-exposed areas.
- Blisters rupture and turn into crusted erosions, and subsequently heal by postinflammatory hyperpigmentation, milia and scar formation.
- Associated features are hypertrichosis, scarring alopecia, morphea form or sclerodermoid changes.

Histo- and immunopathology

- Subepidermal cell poor blister with a characteristic festooning of the dermal papillae.
- Deposition of PAS positive glycoproteins around the upper dermal vessels.
- DIF reveals deposition of immunoglobulins (mainly IgG and less commonly IgM), complement and fibrinogen along the dermoepidermal junction and around the papillary dermal vessels.
- Fibrosis present in the sclerodermoid lesions.

Epidermolysis bullosa

* This is a group of genetically determined mechanobullous disorders.
* There are more than 20 types.
* Every type differs in genetic defect, clinical presentation, associated features and prognosis.
* They are divided into three main types, depending on the level of blister.

Types

- Epidermolysis bullosa simplex (EBS): The level of blister is intraepidermal or through the basal layer.
- Epidermolysis bullosa junctional type (JEB): The level of blister is through the dermoepidermal junction.
- Epidermolysis bullosa dystrophica (DEB): The level of blister is subepidermal or intradermal.

Variants of EBS

- Generalized EBS (Koebner)
- Localized EBS (Weber-Cockayne)

- EB herpetiformis (Dowling-Meara)
- EBS Ogna and EBS superficialis
- EBS with muscular dystrophy.

Variants of JEB

- JEB Herlitz
- JEB with pyloric atresia
- Generalized JEB
- Cicatricial JEB

Variants of DEB

- Hyperplastic DEB (dominant)
- Albopapuloid DEB (dominant)
- Localized DEB (recessive)
- Inverse DEB (recessive)
- Generalized DEB (recessive)

* Ratio of incidence among the types is 11:2:5 (EBS:JEB:DEB).

Genetic defects

- Keratin 5 & 14 in EBS.
- BPAg2 and laminin 5 in JEB.
- Anchoring fibril, type VII collagen in DEB.

* Clinical manifestations may or may not be present at birth. But trauma is the most prominent precipitating factor.

Salient features of generalized EBS

- Tense or flaccid blisters develop at trauma prone sites of the body. Lesions rupture and form erosions. They heal quickly without any scarring and milia formation. But repeated blistering at the same site may produce scar and milia.
- Feet, hands, elbows and knees are the common sites.
- Palmoplantar keratosis may be associated.
- Nails, teeth and oral mucosa are spared.

Salient features of localized EBS

- Lesions appear in childhood or adulthood.
- It is often precipitated by vigorous exercise and ambient temperature.
- Hyperhidrosis of palms and soles is often associated.

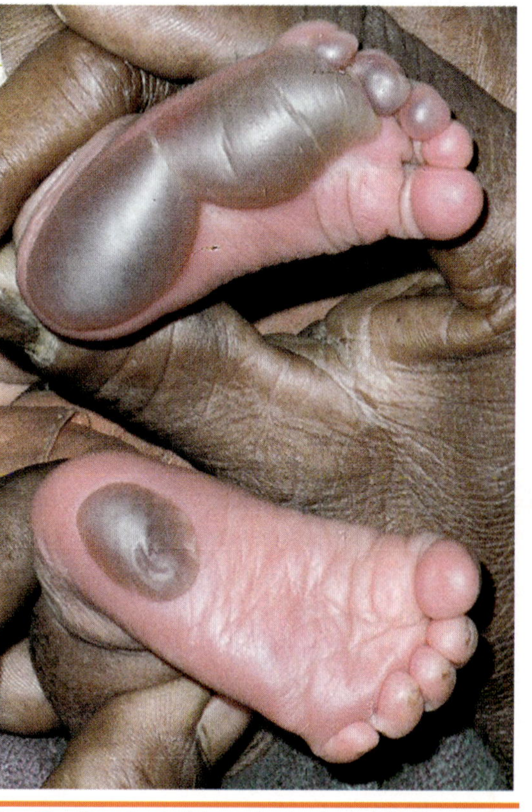

Fig. 13: Localized blisters at soles in an infant

Salient features of JEB gravis

- The mortality rate is more than 40% during first year of life.
- Generalized blisters develop at birth with periorificial granulation tissue and loss of nails.
- Most of the mucosae are involved.
- When the blisters rupture, whole skin becomes eroded and active oozing starts.
- These eroded areas are very painful.
- Blistering affects respiratory, gastrointestinal, genitourinary systems and develops complication.

Salient features of dominant DEB

- Lesions appear in infancy or in childhood.
- Blisters develop at acral areas and they heal by scars and milia formation.
- Scars may be hypertrophic or hyperplastic.
- Nails dystrophy present.
- Mucosa is rarely affected.
- Teeth are normal.

Salient features of recessive DEB

- Blisters appear at birth. They are less severe and localized.
- Acral areas are commonly affected with little or no mucosal involvement.
- Lesions heal with atrophic scars.
- Generalized severe variant is mutilating. Syndactyly with mitten-like deformities are seen at hands and feet. They also develop flexion contracture. Caries and periodontitis are associated. Stricture and scarring develop at oral mucosa, esophagus, urethra, anus and conjunctiva. Other associated features are malnutrition, growth retardation, anemia, development of squamous cell carcinoma.

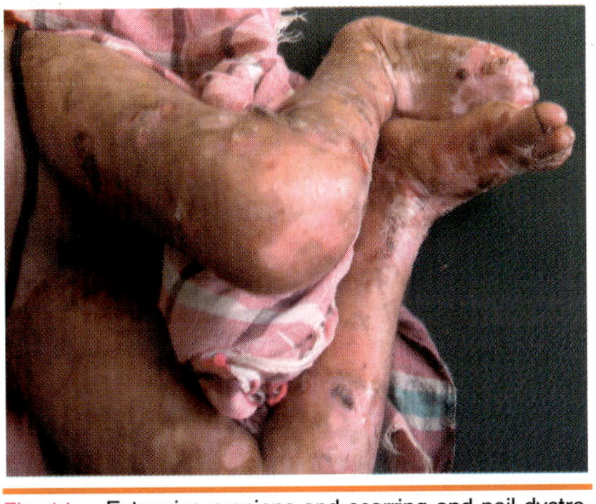

Fig. 14: Extensive erosions and scarring and nail dystrophy

Treatment

- Symptomatic treatment as no curable treatment is available.

Stevens-Johnson syndrome (SJS) and toxic epidermal necrolysis (TEN)

* These are two closely mimicking dermatoses affecting skin, mucosal surfaces and other organs.
* Any age may be affected; but commonly occurs in age > 40 years.
* In almost 90-100% cases are drug induced. But they may be idiopathic.
* Both are life threatening; but TEN is more dangerous due to lack of definite role of corticosteroid or any other medicine.
* SJS responds to systemic corticosteroid.
* SJS is considered as extreme form of erythema multiforme and TEN is considered as a variant of SJS.
* Probably drugs or their metabolites act as hapten and bind with keratinocytes to make antigens and so keratinocytes convert into targets for cytotoxic T cells, leading to cell death or apoptosis.
* Drugs are detoxified in the liver and mostly excreted through the kidneys; so if they are incapable to do their job properly, various drug-metabolites get deposited in the body, resulting in drug reactions.
* Cytokines released by activated lymphocytes and dying keratinocytes cause fever, malaise and death.
* Activation of granzyme-perforin and Fas-fas ligand pathways is one of the proposed route for keratinocyte necrosis in TEN.
* Common drugs are sulfur group, antitubercular drugs, non-steroidal anti-inflammatory drugs, phenytoin, carbamazepine, allopurinol, nevirapine, etc.
* HIV infection increases frequency of drug reactions probably due to altered immune response.
* Time required from first dose of the drug to development of reaction is variable from 1-3 weeks.
* Reaction occurs more rapidly following rechallenge.

* Average mortality rate in elderly due to SJS is 5%; but 30% in TEN.
* Commonest causes of death are sepsis, electrolyte and fluid imbalance, and gastrointestinal bleeding.
* Both SJS and TEN may start as erythema multiforme like lesions; but in 50% cases of TEN do not. They usually start as diffuse erythema, leading to skin necrosis and detachment.

Clinical features

- Prodromal features appear 1-3 days prior to the reaction and these are fever, malaise, headache, etc.
- Symptoms are skin pain, burning sensation or paresthesia, conjunctival burning or itching and painful oral or genital mucosa.
- Early lesions may be morbilliform rash or erythema multiforme-like or diffuse erythema.
- Whatever the presenting lesions, they coalesce rapidly and become crinkled. Then widespread flaccid blisters develop and a sheet of skin start to detach. Slight shearing pressure on the erythematous skin causes separation of the skin, known as Nikolsky's phenomenon.
- With slight trauma necrosed skin detaches and leaves denuded areas with active oozing. This stage mimics second degree burn.
- Lesions usually start at face and extremities, then spread to trunk and mucosae.
- Scalp, palms and soles are rarely affected.
- Mucosal involvement is seen in more than 90% cases. These include oral, genital, conjunctival, upper respiratory tract, proximal gastrointestinal tract, etc.
- Eyes are very commonly affected. Common features are hyperemia, pseudomembranous discharge, adhesion between bulbar conjunctiva and eyelids, keratitis and corneal erosion.
- Nails are commonly involved in TEN with loss of nail plates.
- Dreaded complications are blindness, acute renal failure due to tubular necrosis, gastrointestinal bleeding, cutaneous infection resulting in septicemia.
- Recovery starts within days and almost completes by 3 weeks.
- Irregular postinflammatory hyperpigmentation is commonly seen following recovery.
- Urethral stricture, vaginal synechia, conjunctival synechia and corneal scar are the complications during or after recovery.

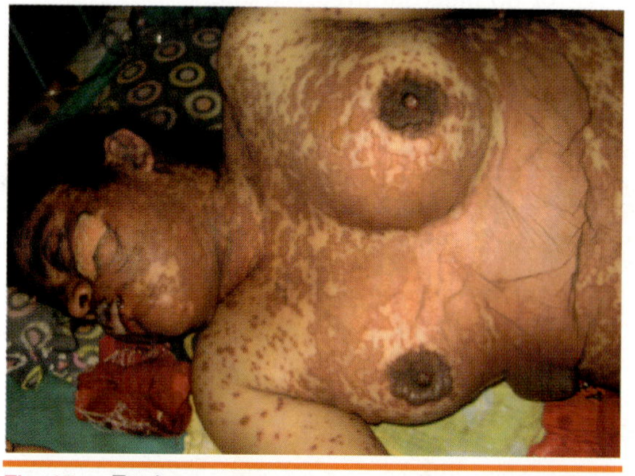

Fig. 15: Erythematous macules and patches with coalesced crinkled skin at the abdomen and denuded facial skin

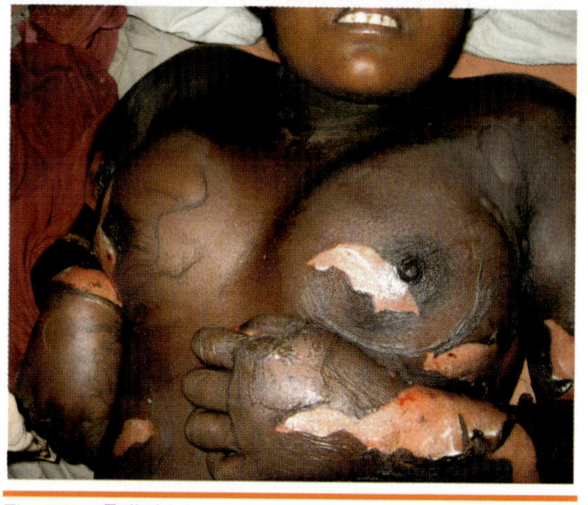

Fig. 16: Full thickness necrosis with denuded areas of the skin

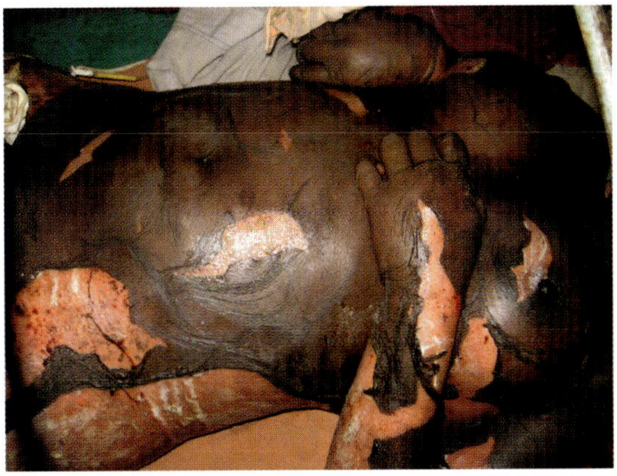

Fig. 17: Generalized necrotic skin with denudation at places

Treatment

- Fluid and electrolytes correction.
- Control of sepsis.
- Guard for organic complications.
- Intravenous immunoglobulin 400 mg/kg/day for 3-5 days, for TEN.
- Short course of systemic corticosteroid, about 60-80 mg prednisolone per day.
- Gentian violet paint may be used to prevent cutaneous infection.
- Oral cyclosporine, 3-5 mg/kg/day.

Staphylococcal scalded skin syndrome

- It is caused by staphylococcal exotoxin.
- Often it is difficult to find out the original site of infection. It may be associated with otitis externa or media, sore throat and pyoderma.
- Infant and children are commonly affected.
- Subcorneal blisters are sterile.

Clinical features

- Sudden development of erythematous and tender skin with fever and irritability. Skin may be denuded following shearing pressure with the thumb and demonstrates positive Nikolsky's phenomenon.
- Flaccid and diffuse blisters develop.
- Large eroded areas appear when blisters are ruptured by minor trauma.

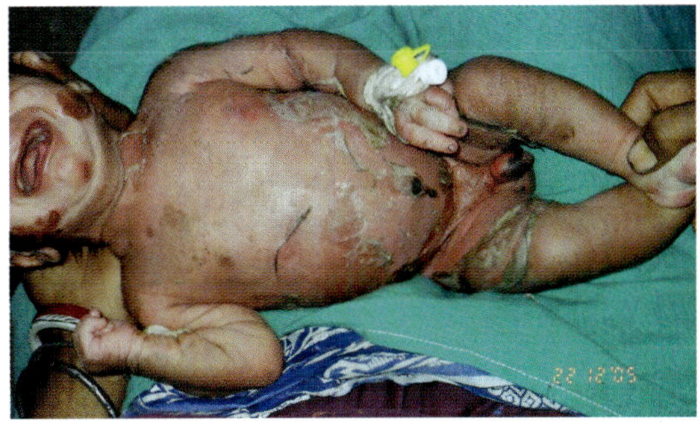

Fig. 18: Scalded skin at trunk and proximal part of the limbs

Treatment

- Antibiotic to control staphylococcal infection.

Hydroa vacciniforme

- It is an eczematous form of herpetic infection and commonly associated with atopic dermatitis.
- Clinically it mimics varicella infection.
- Few other viral infection like Coxsackie and Epstein-Barr virus, also may cause similar manifestation.

Characteristic features

- Erythematous macules and papules which quickly evolve into vesicles and bullae. Gradually center of the lesions collapse and become umbilicated. Formation of hemorrhagic crusts is a characteristic finding.
- Lesions are distributed symmetrically and sun-exposed sites are commonly involved.

Differential diagnosis

- Chicken pox
- Disseminated herpes simplex

Treatment

- Topical calamine lotion
- Systemic acyclovir or valcyclovir.

CONGENITAL AND HEREDITARY DISORDERS

CHAPTER C15

Tuberous sclerosis

* It is an autosomal dominant disorder, associated with development of hamartomas of the skin, brain, eyes, heart, kidneys, lungs and bones.
* Mutations of two different genes are responsible for the disease.
    - Gene TSC_1, encoding hamartin
    - Gene TSC_2, encoding tuberin
* Tuberin and hamartin act as tumor suppressors through GTPase-Rap1 pathway.
* TSC_1 mutation causes milder manifestations than TSC_2 mutation.
* It is characterized by three basic features (Epi-loi-a):
    - Epilepsy
    - Low intelligency
    - Adenoma sebaceum
* Angofibroma or adenoma sebaceum has no relation with sebaceous glands. Lesions are composed of vascular and fibrous tissues. Though angiofibroma is considered to be pathognomonic in tuberous sclerosis, but it is also seen in 43-48% adults of multiple endocrine neoplasia type 1 (MEN1).
* Collagenoma and confetti-like hypopigmented macules are hallmarks of tuberous sclerosis; but these are also seen in MEN1 as 72% and 6% cases respectively. Periungual or subungual fibromas are also considered as pathognomonic.
* Systemic features may produce severe symptoms and signs and may lead to death.
* Pulmonary cysts appear as honey-comb appearance in X-ray.
* EEG shows multifocal high voltage spikes and slow chaotic weaves.
* Brain shows tubers as pale sclerotic patches, causing elevation or broadening of cerebral gyri.
* Fundoscopy shows two types of lesions
    - Multiple mulberry-like raised lesions at or near the optic nerve head.
    - Flat disc-like lesions are seen at the periphery of the retina.

Clinical features

* Hypopigmented macules:
    - These appear in 90% of patients at their birth or shortly after birth. There after, these le-

sions show a tendency to remain stable in shape and size.
- Wood lamp examination makes the lesion more obvious in fair skin.
- Commonest site is trunk.
- Size is variable from few mm to several cm and number ranges from few to more than 75.
- Shape may be oval or thumb print-like or confetti-like, specially at pretibial areas and may be round or linear. But the commonest shape is lance-ovate or ash leaf-like spots.
- Poliosis at scalp or eyebrow may be associated.
- A single early lesion is very difficult to differentiate from nevus depigmentosus (nevus achromicus).

* Cutaneous angiofibroma/adenoma sebaceum:
  - These lesions appear between 2-6 years of age in 65-90% cases. But they may present at birth or may appear even after age of 20 years.
  - Lesions are dome-shaped papules and pink to red in color with smooth surface.
  - Size is variable from 1-4 mm.
  - Common sites are nasolabial folds, cheeks and chin. Often upper lip is spared except area just below the nose.
  - Distribution is usually symmetrical but may be asymmetrical also.
* Collagenoma:
  - Large fibrotic slightly raised plaques or nodules appear at birth in 25% cases. Surface shows depressed follicular openings, appearing as pig skin, elephant skin, orange peel or goose flesh.
  - Common sites are forehead, cheeks and scalp.
  - But in 15-40% cases lesions develop at trunk, specially at lumbosacral area during childhood period. These are also called shagreen patch or peau d' chagrin lesions.
  - Number may be single or multiple and size is variable from 1 cm to palm size.
* Fibroma:
  - These are often periungual or subungual firm papules and known as Koenen's tumor. Lesions may affect gingiva also.
  - They appear after puberty in 50% cases.
* Systemic symptoms:
  - Seizure is seen in 80-90% cases.
  - Mild to severe mental retardation seen in 60% cases.
  - Obstructive hydrocephalus is caused by nonmalignant subependymal nodules.
  - Renal angiomyolipomas are seen in 15% cases. Renal cysts may develop bilaterally.
  - Cardiac rhabdomyomas are most commonly seen in infants and they often regress spontaneously.
  - Retinal glioma, known as phakomas, are described in 50% cases.
  - Bone cysts and periosteal thickening, specially off the hands and feet are seen in 85% cases.
  - Pulmonary cysts, may rupture and form pneumothorax.
  - Round or oval, 1-2 mm sized, punctate tooth pits are seen, specially at permanent teeth.

Neurofibromatosis

* It is an autosomal dominant disorder, presenting with nerve sheath tumors.
* Café-au-lait macules are the hallmarks of neurofibromatosis.

Types

  - Neurofibromatosis type 1 (NF1), commonest type and seen in 90% cases.
  - Neurofibromatosis type 2 (NF2)
* Genetic mutations
  - Gene is localized to chromosome 17q and encodes neurofibromin in NF1.
  - Gene is localized at chromosome 22q and encodes merlin in NF2.
* Neurofibromin negatively acts through GTPase-Ras activation pathway.

* Merlin negatively acts through serine-threonine kinase PAK1-Ras transformation pathway.
* Neurofibromas are composed of Schwann cells, mast cells and fibroblasts.
* Neurofibroma may be itchy due to presence of mast cells.
* In 5% cases of neurofibromas may undergo malignant change.
* Congenital bowing due to tibial dysplasia is pathognomonic of NF1. It is due to thinning of the cortex and sclerosis of the medulla.

Clinical features of NF1

* Café-au-lait macules:
  * These are well defined asymptomatic coffee colored macules and patches, usually appear during first few months of life; but may appear at birth.
  * Gradually number and size of the lesions increase.
  * Lesions may present at any part of the skin.
* Freckles:
  * Presence of axillary lesions is known as Crowe's sign.
  * Lesions may be seen at inguinal regions or may be generalized.
  * Size is 1-4 mm and lesions start to appear between 3-4 years of age.
* Neurofibroma:
  * Dermal or subcutaneous nodules appear during late childhood or adolescent period.
  * Lesions are soft to firm in consistency and size is variable from few mm to several cm.
  * Overlying skin may be violaceous, pink, blue or skin colored.
  * Lesions may be sessile or pedunculated.
  * Number may be few to hundreds with a tendency to increase in size and number.
  * There is no site of predilection and so any area of the skin may be affected.
  * Dermal lesion may invaginate following pressure with a finger and this is known as Buttonholing sign.
  * Replacement of dermal collagen by neural tissue presents as pseudoatrophic macules.
  * Replacement of superficial thick-walled dermal vessels by overlying neurofibroma, appears as red-blue macules.
* Plexiform neurofibromas:
  * These are firm, barely palpable masses.
  * Lesions may be superficial or deep and often they are oriented along the nerve and involve several fascicles.
  * Lesions may be huge with a bag of worm consistency.
  * Rarely they present at birth and have a tendency to affect extremities.
  * Lesions may be studded with hypertrichosis and may be confused with Becker's nevus.
  * Underlying soft tissue and bone may be hypertrophied or bone may be eroded.
* Systemic features:
  * Lisch nodules are asymptomatic, yellow-brown melanocytic hamartomas of the iris, causing vision difficulty. Lesions are seen in adults and best observed by slit lamp examination.
  * Optic gliomas are seen in 15% of childhood patients and presented with decreased visual acuity and visual field defects. Gradually vision may be lost and gross disfigurement may be developed.
  * Brain stem gliomas and meningioma are also seen.
  * Presence of learning disabilities may be seen.
  * Skeletal manifestations are bone dysplasia, pectus deformity and scoliosis.
  * Other features are short stature, macrocephaly and hypertension.

Diagnostic criteria for NF1

* At least two of the following:
  * At least six café-au-lait macules, measuring ≥ 0.5 cm before puberty and ≥ 1.5 cm after puberty.

- ♦ Axillary or inguinal freckles.
- ♦ A plexiform neurofibroma or two or more dermal neurofibromas.
- ♦ At least two Lisch nodules.
- ♦ Optic nerve glioma.
- ♦ Pathognomonic skeletal dysplasia, specially tibial or sphenoid wing dysplasia.
- ♦ An affected first degree relative.

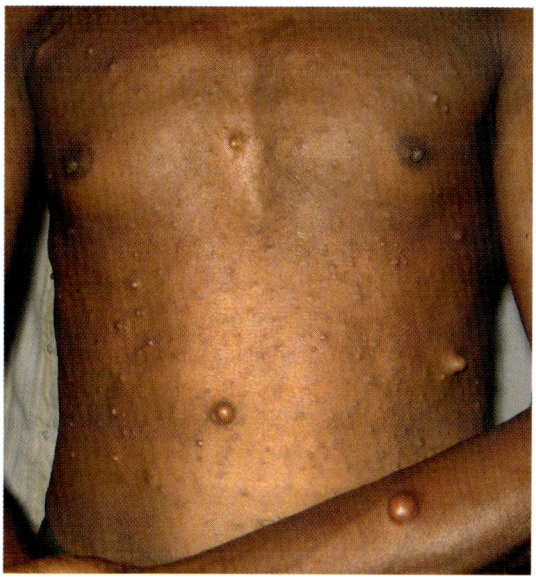

Fig. 1: Numerous papules and nodules of neurofibromatosis

Diagnostic criteria for NF2

- ✶ Any one of the following:
  - ♦ Bilateral vestibular schwannomas, detected by MR1 scan.
  - ♦ First degree relative, suffering from NF2 and unilateral vestibular schwannoma.
  - ♦ At least two of the meningioma, glioma, schwannoma and juvenile posterior subcapsular cataract.

Hemangioma

- ✶ This is a group of benign tumors originating from capillaries, arteries or veins.
- ✶ Lesions may present at birth or often within few days of life.
- ✶ Most of the lesions resolve by 4-7 years of age.
- ✶ About 40% cases appear at birth and 60% appear within 8 weeks of birth.
- ✶ Rapid growth phase is between 4-8 weeks and continues till 6-9 months.
- ✶ Regression starts between 18-24 months and 50% involute within 5 years and 90% within 9 years.

Types

- ♦ Superficial: Lesion starts as a red papule and gradually enlarges to form plaque.
- ♦ Deep: Lesions presents as a nodule with blue-gray color.
- ♦ Mixed: Noduloplaque type of compound lesion with reddish-blue color.

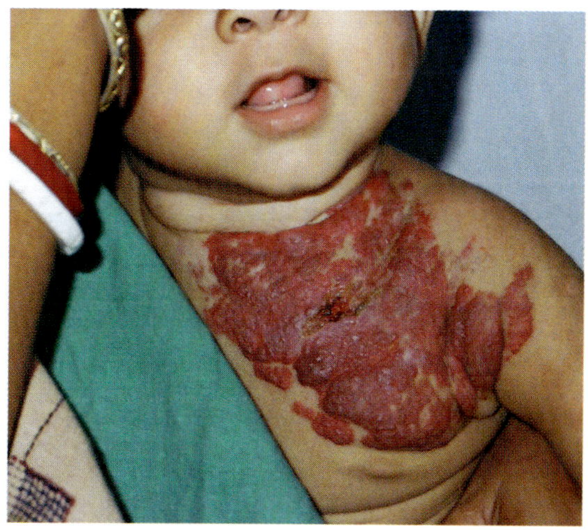

Fig. 2: Huge bright red plaque at upper chest of an infant

Clinical features

- ♦ Earliest lesion is a punctate telangiectatic lesion.
- ♦ Gradually a cluster of small, closely set angiomas appear which enlarge and coalesce to form a plaque.
- ♦ Head and neck region involve in 60% cases.
- ♦ Plaques may be verrucous and deeper lesions are felt like a bag of worms.
- ♦ Ulceration, hemorrhage and infection are common complications.

- Residual lesion may present as hypopigmented or telangiectatic scar or redundant scar.

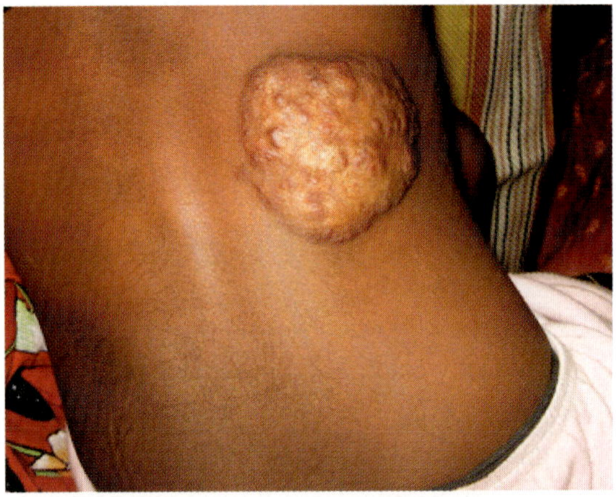

Fig. 3: Involuting lesion at right of the back in a child

Treatment

- Waiting for spontaneous resolution.
- Systemic steroid, sclerotherapy and laser surgery.

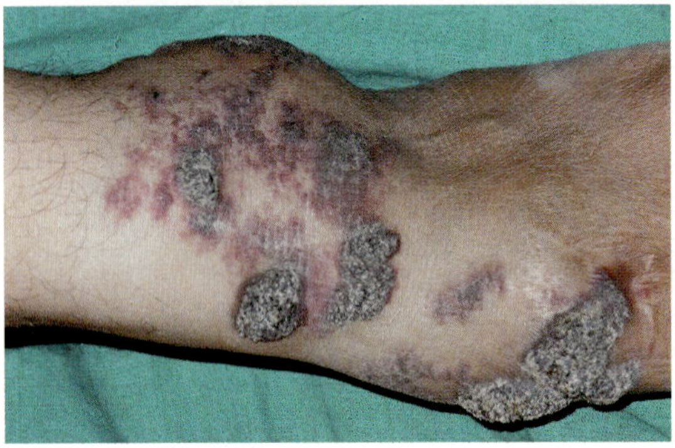

Fig. 4: An irregular verrucous plaque with crusting at dorsum of foot and ankle

Congenital melanocytic nevus

- It usually appears at birth but in some cases may appear by 1 year of age.
- Incidence of small type is 1% newborn, large type is 1:20,000, and giant type is 1:5,00,000.
- Various names are implied such as coat sleeve when trunk is involved and stocking when lower limbs are affected.

Types

- Small: Diameter is less than 1.5 cm.
- Medium: Diameter is varying from 1.5 cm to 19.9 cm.
- Large: Diameter is 20 cm or more.

Clinical features

- Small and medium size
  - Lesions are flat, light to dark brown, well circumscribed patches or plaques.
  - With time surface of the lesions may have coarse dark brown hair, more elevation and more variability in color.
- Large size
  - Lesions are dark brown to black plaques present at birth with verrucous or cobblestone surface.
  - Hypertrichosis may or may not be present and color may be variable.
  - Posterior trunk is the commonest site for large lesions and may have a dermatomal distribution.
  - Under development of the limb may occur, if lesion present on it.
- Very large or giant nevus
  - Lesion appears at birth and continues to grow during infancy.
  - It presents as large brown to black plaques with varying degree of nodularity, color variation, hypertrichosis, erosions, ulcerations.
  - Frequently it has satellite lesions and they may be disseminated over entire skin surface.
  - They produce a lot of cosmetic disfigurement and have a risk of transformation into malignant melanoma.
  - Suspicion of malignancy arises when pigmentation becomes very deep or irregular and grows rapidly. Risk of malignancy is also associated with axial lesions more than lesions of the extremities and risk of malignancy is less when associated with satellite lesions.
  - Life time risk of malignancy is variable from 0-35% and on an average is 4.5-10%.

Mucocutaneous melanosis

- It develops in first 3 years of age in association with large congenital nevus, particularly when head, neck and back are involved or having satellite lesions.
- Due to proliferation of nevus cells in central nervous system (CNS) as leptomeningeal melanocytosis, there is a risk of intracranial pressure or spinal cord compression.
- So, clinical features may be headache, lethargy, irritability, recurrent vomiting, seizure, photophobia, increased head circumference, bulging of anterior fontanelle, papilledema, neck stiffness, occasionally cranial nerve palsies, specially 6th and 7th nerves, etc.
- MRI shows focal areas of high signal as T1-weighted images in one or multiple areas of the brain.
- It bears a poor prognosis with mortality rate >90% before age of 10 years.

Histopathology

- Extension of nevus cells into the deeper dermis and subcutaneous tissue between collagen bundles as single cells.
- They are also distributed around appendages, nerves and vessels.

Treatment

- Surgical intervention according to site, size, type, and risks of disfigurement, malignancy and anesthesia.

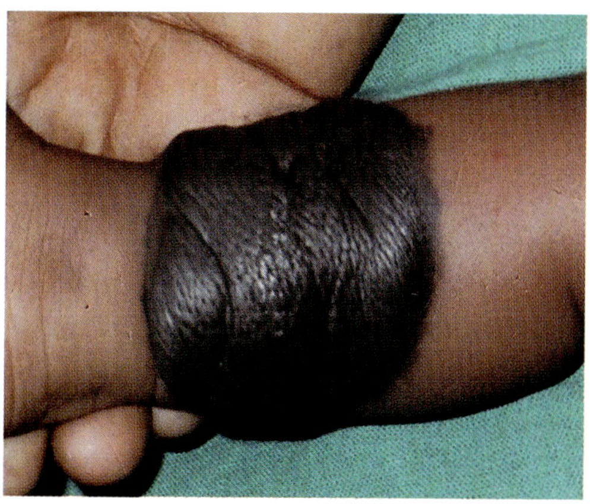

Fig. 5: Well defined jet black mild lobulated plaque

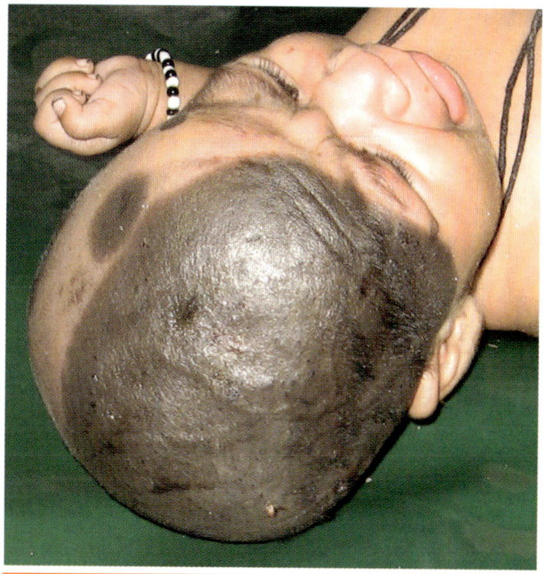

Fig. 6: Scalp lesions in a case of congenital melanocytic nevus

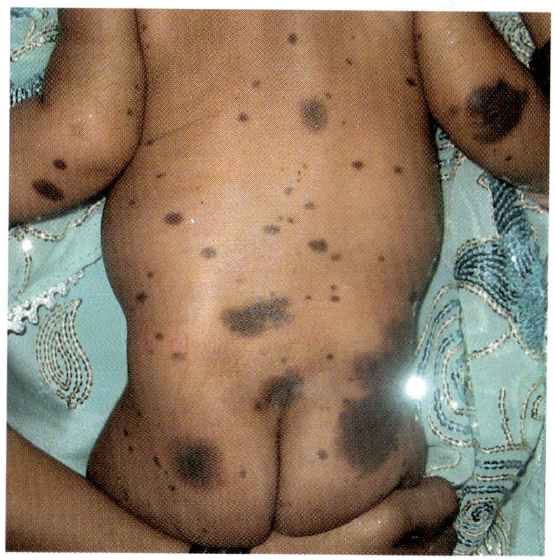

Fig. 7: Numerous lesion of congenital melanocytic nevus

Nevus flammeus

- The term includes two different entities: Salmon patch and portwine stain.
- Both the conditions are congenital and are vascular malformation.
- Salmon patch is present in upto 50% of new-

borns and port-wine stain appears in 0.3% of newborns.

Clinical features

- Salmon patch is characterized by pale pink to red, ill defined macule and commonly affects the nape of the neck, glabella, eyelids, etc.
- Port-wine stain appears as bright red to pink patch or plaque and it is usually unilateral with a predilection for face and limbs.
- Salmon patch has a tendency to involute within first-year of life; but port-wine stain has a tendency to persist and to become thicker and darker.
- Port-wine stain is often associated with other malformation.

Congenital generalized phlebectasia/cutis marmorata telangiectatica congenita

- It is characterized by localized or generalized reticulate erythema which do not disappear with rewarming.
- Lesions are present at birth or shortly after birth.

Clinical features

- Lesions are red to violaceous, reticulated, marbled or mottled patches.
- Localized lesions show a segmental distribution with sharp demarcation at midline.
- Color of the lesions is variable from light pink to dark purple and it is influenced by reduction of ambient temperature.
- Other associated features are limb hypoplasia/hyperplasia, portwine stain, infantile hemangioma, Sturge-Weber syndrome, glaucoma, retinal pigmentation/detachment, macrocephaly, seizure, hydrocephalus, psychomotor retardation, etc.

Congenital erosive and vesicular dermatosis

- It is a rare disease which often occurs in premature infant and presents at birth.
- Etiology is not yet clear may be due to some infection, or amniotic adhesion, or unusual healing defect of immature skin.

Clinical features

- Generalized vesicles, crusts, erosions and scars, involve trunk, extremities, scalp and tongue. But face, palms and soles are spared.
- Scars are reticulated with alternate skin colored or hyperpigmented elevations and hypopigmented depressions.
- Scars at scalp and trunk show a cobble-stone appearance.
- Sweating is absent at scarred areas and compensatory hyperhidrosis is seen at normal areas.
- Patient often feels hyperthermia during warm weather or following exercise.
- Other features are chronic conjunctivitis, corneal scarring, mental/motor retardation, cerebral palsy and seizure.

Aplasia cutis congenita

- It is a congenital defect of the skin, presented with localized absence of epidermis, dermis and subcutaneous tissue.
- At birth presenting feature may be an ulcer with granulating base or superficial erosion or a well formed scar.
- Most cases are sporadic; but it may be associated with teratogens, limb abnormalities, epidermal nevi and epidermolysis bullosa.
- It also may be associated with cleft lip and palate, spinal dysraphism, mental retardation, spastic paralysis, seizures, etc.

Clinical features

- Solitary or multiple sharply defined skin defects with a weeping or granulating base.
- Shape may be oval, round or stellate.
- Size is variable from 1-3 cm.
- Commonest site is the scalp; but other areas like face, trunk and extremites may be involved.

- In 70% cases number is single, in 20% cases double and 10% cases three or more.
- A scalp lesion may have a whorl of hair around the lesion. This is known as hair collar sign.
- Lesions heal spontaneously with scar formation.

Treatment

- Reassurance.
- Antibiotic and antiseptic dressing for secondary infection if at all present.

Nevus sebaceous

- This is a common congenital developmental defect.
- Lesion is usually present at birth, but may appear in early childhood or even in adulthood.
- Yellow color of the lesion is due to sebaceous secretion and this color is reduced after infantile period.
- Lesion increases in size according to the growth of the body; but suddenly enlarges at puberty. This is a classical history of growth pattern.
- Multiple sebaceous nevi may occur in association with cerebral, ocular, skeletal anomalies as a part of the epidermal nevus syndrome and this association is termed as Schimmelpenning syndrome.

Clinical features

- A well circumscribed, hairless, yellow to tan plaque develops at scalp or face.
- Surface is verrucous or velvety.
- Shape may be oval or to some extent linear or irregular.
- Size is variable from few mm to several cm.
- At puberty, lesion becomes more verrucous and thicker and larger size. Lesions become more greasy due to excess sebaceous secretion on hormonal influence during puberty.
- In adulthood, various types of appendageal tumor develop and commonest one is syringocystadenoma papilliferum. It is seen in 10-20% cases.
- Other appendageal tumors are trichoblastoma, trichilemmoma, proliferating trichilemmal cyst, nodular hidradenoma, syringoma, chondroid syringoma and sebaceous epithelioma.

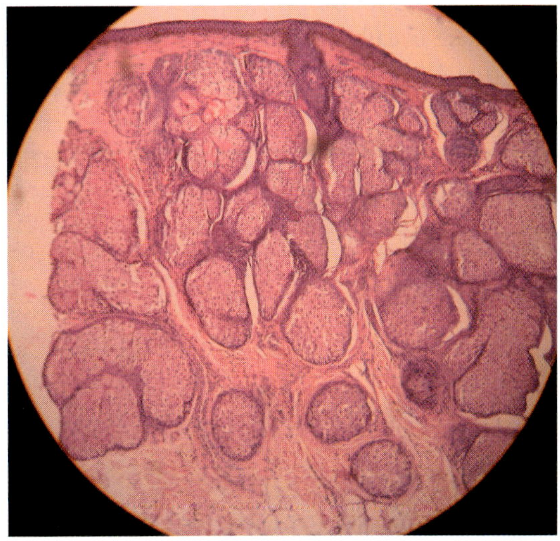

Fig. 8: Dermis is filled up with numerous sebaceous glands

Histopathology

- Sebaceous glands are well developed during infancy.
- Number and size of sebocytes is greatly reduced in childhood; but presence of incompletely differentiated hair structures and some dilated keratin-filled infundibula, help to diagnose at this stage.
- At puberty, epidermis become papillomatous with large number of mature or near to mature sebaceous glands. Hair structures are small with occasional dilated infundibula. Ectopic apocrine glands are seen in 2/3rd cases.
- Basaloid epithelial proliferation, mimicking basal cell carcinoma, is evident in 5-7% cases. True malignant transformation is very rare.

Treatment

- ♦ Surgical excision is the treatment of choice.

Epidermal nevi

- ✶ These are benign congenital lesions, occurring due to hyperplasia of different epidermal structures and affecting both sexes equally.
- ✶ They are usually apparent at birth; but may appear in early childhood.

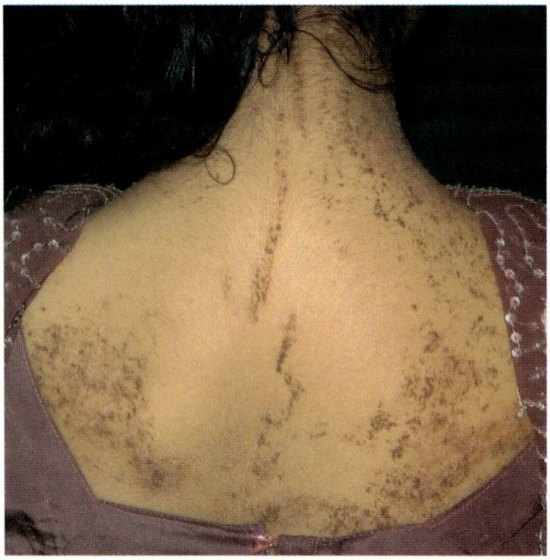

Fig. 9: Bilateral epidermal nevi

Verrucous epidermal nevi

- These are firm well defined plaques with rough verrucous surface.
- Shape is usually linear or zosteriform.
- Color is variable from tan to dark brown.
- Number is usually single; but may be multiple.

Nevus unius lateralis

- The term describes extensive unilateral lesions.
- It usually presents as spiral linear verrucous lesions with a continuous or interrupted pattern, affecting multiple sites.

Systematized epidermal nevi

- The term describes bilaterally distributed extensive lesions with predominant truncal involvement.

Ichthyosis hystrix

- The term describes porcupine quill like hyperkeratosis, associated with epidermolytic hyperkeratosis and epidermal nevus.

Epidermal nevus syndrome

- The term describes a sporadic association of epidermal nevi with abnormalities of other organs.

Nevus comedonicus

- ✶ It originates from hair follicle, seen at birth or within 1st decade of life.
- ✶ Lesion tends to increase in size along with the growth of the body.

Clinical features

- ♦ Primary lesion is a linear plaque, studded with hyperkeratotic umbilicated papules.
- ♦ These papules appear as comedone when they contain horny plugs at their center.
- ♦ Lesions may have varying degree of erythema.
- ♦ Common sites are face, neck, trunk and upper extremities.
- ♦ Comedones sometimes become inflammed and turn into nodules, cysts and abscesses.
- ♦ Scar may develop following healing of the lesion.

Nevus spilus

- ✶ This is a subtype of melanocytic nevi.
- ✶ Lesion is present at birth; but may be noticed in infancy, childhood and or even later.
- ✶ Initial lesion appears as a café-au-lait macule.

* There is no relation with sun exposure. But the darker macules have a potency to develop malignant melanoma.

Clinical features

- This is a solitary non-hairy flat brown patch, sprinkled with darker dot-like macules.
- Size is variable from 1-20 cm.
- Common sites are face, trunk and extremities.

Nevus depigmentosus

* It usually presents at birth or may appear in infancy.
* It has a tendency to persist for life-long.

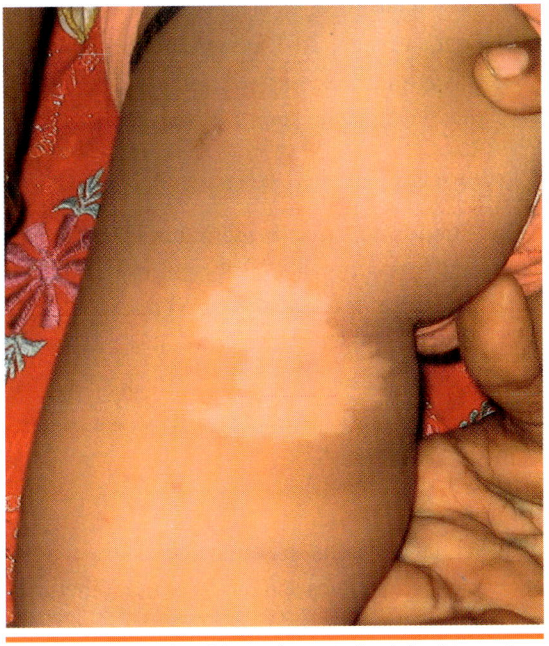

Fig. 10: Well defined hypopigmented patch of hypochromic nevi. Margin is remarkably serrated

Clinical features

- Well defined hypopigmented patch with irregular and serrated margin.

Congenital insensitivity to pain

* An autosomal recessive disorder due to defective genes encoding receptor tyrosine kinase for nerve growth factor (NTRK1).

Clinical features

- It is characterized by absence of reaction to noxious stimuli, self-mutilating behavior and mental retardation.
- Oral self mutilation is very common. These are biting injuries and scarring of soft tissue of mouth and oral mucosa.
- Trophic ulcer may develop at toes mimicking a leprosy complication.

Congenital adrenal hyperplasia/adrenogenital syndrome

* Impaired steroid metabolism in adrenal cortex causes the disease and most common one is 21-hydroxylase deficiency. There are also other defects like 11β hydroxylase and 3β hydroxysteroid dehydrogenase deficiencies.
* Due to any of the above defects cortisol synthesis in adrenal cortex is stimulated by over-production of cortisol precursors and some of these precursors are diverted to produce excess amount of sex hormones.
* Androgen is most important sex hormone, responsible for clinical features of this hyperandrogenism syndrome and side by side aldosterone deficiency causes salt wasting, failure to thrive, hypovolemia and sometimes even shock.
* Prepuberty features due to hyperandrogenism:
  - Precocious sexual development like ambiguous genitalia, large clitoris, rugated and partially fused labia majora, common urogenital sinus instead of separate urethra and vagina in a female child, and subtle hyperpigmentation and enlargement of genitalia in a male child.
  - Development of acne, axillary/pubic hair growth, and hirsutism.
  - Rapid linear growth and acceleration of bone age.
* Postpubertal features if no treatment/inadequate treatment where females are mostly affected:
  - Development of acne, androgenetic alopecia, and hirsutism.

- ♦ Amenorrhea/irregular menses, infertility, deep voice, increased muscle mass and development of male habitus.
- ♦ Early cardiovascular disease and after initial rapid linear growth, due to early epiphyseal closure and ultimate development of short height.

Treatment

- ♦ It must be started between 2-6 months of age with glucocorticosteroid and mineralocorticoid as replacement therapy.

Congenital eythropoietic porphyria (CEP)

- ✶ It is an autosomal recessive disorder.
- ✶ Due to deficiency of uroporphyrinogen III synthase, a marked over production of uroporphyrin I occurs.
- ✶ These porphyrins accumulate in circulating erythrocytes, bone marrow cells, plasma, urine and feces.
- ✶ Passing of red color urine in infancy is a classical complaint.
- ✶ Fluorescence of teeth is due to binding of porphyrin to dental calcium phosphate.
- ✶ Under Wood's lamp urine becomes reddish orange.

Clinical features

- ♦ Photosensitivity starts after age of 1 year and becomes severe in first 2-3 years.
- ♦ In neonates, phototherapy for hyperbilirubinemia may give rise to severe photosensitivity, leading to generalized blistering.
- ♦ Recurrent vesicles and bullae develop at sun exposed areas of the skin, containing fluorescent pink fluid.
- ♦ This results in mutilating ulceration, scarring, loss of acral tissues like ears, tip of nose, eyelids, distal phalanges and nails.
- ♦ Hyperpigmentation and hypertrichosis are other features.
- ♦ At middle age, a presentation with fluorescent teeth, and deformed ears, nose, eyelids give a clue for diagnosis of CEP without active vesicles/bullae.
- ♦ Eye complications are corneal ulceration, keratoconjunctivitis, photophobia, scarring, cataract and blindness.
- ♦ Splenomegaly and hemolytic anemia are also present.
- ♦ Bone fragility is due to expansion of marrow as well as due to toxicity of porphyrin itself.

Treatment

- ♦ Avoidance of ultraviolet light (< 510 nm).
- ♦ Protection of sunlight by clothing or opaque sunscreen.
- ♦ Oral carotene, 30-150 mg/day for children.
- ♦ Blood transfusion, splenectomy and bone marrow or allogenic stem cell transplantation.

Congenital candidiasis

- ✶ Infection is acquired in utero during premature labour, specially when history of use of intrauterine device or cervical suture present.
- ✶ An additional history of maternal vulvovaginitis is often present.
- ✶ It is benign in full term baby, but serious in premature one.

Clinical features

- ♦ Primary lesions are multiple erythematous macules, papules and pustules and sometimes bullae.
- ♦ Lesions are localized in full term baby but widespread in premature one.
- ♦ Common sites are back, extensors of extremities and skin folds, but relative sparing of diaper area.
- ♦ Pustules at palms and soles are also common, a useful diagnostic point.
- ♦ Oral thrush is uncommon and nails show yellow discoloration, thickening and paronychia.

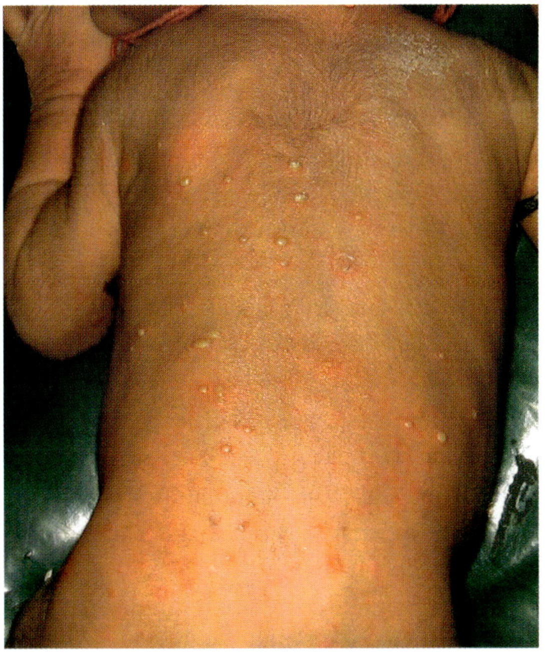

Fig. 11: Multiple pustules in a case of congenital candidiasis

Differential diagnosis

- Erythema toxicum neonatorum
- Bacterial folliculitis/impetigo
- Congenital herpes/varicella
- Congenital syphilis

KOH preparation

- Spores and pseudohyphae are found.

Fungal culture

- It confirms the diagnosis.

Congenital rubella syndrome

* It occurs following maternal rubella infection during first 16 weeks of pregnancy and rarely on later.
* It is manifested with a triad of congenital cataract, deafness and cardiac defect (patent ductus arteriosus).

Clinical features

- The main cutaneous feature is a diffuse eruption of blue red infiltrative papules and nodules, 2-8 mm in size, known as blue berry muffin lesions.
- These lesions are usually present at birth or appear within first 24 hours.
- Other cutaneous features are generalized nonspecific maculopapular eruption, reticulated erythema of the face, hyperpigmentation, recurrent skin infection, and vasomotor instability producing a poor circulation, generalized mottling and acral cyanosis.
- Systemic features are mental retardation, microcephaly, meningo-encephalitis, hepatosplenomegaly, radiolucent bony lesions, pigmentary retinopathy and thrombocytopenia.

Congenital syphilis

* Fetus becomes infected with *Treponema pallidum*, usually after 16 weeks of pregnancy.
* Fetal risk is 70-100% to get infection when mother is suffering from early syphilis.
* Clinical features depend on stage of maternal syphilis, stage of pregnancy at the time of infection, rapidity of maternal diagnosis and treatment and fetal immunological reaction.
* About 40% of congenital syphilis is still born and 2/3 infected new borns are symptom free at birth.
* When manifestations develop before 2 years of age, designated as early syphilis and after 2 years of age, designated as late syphilis.

Clinical features of early syphilis

- Lesions are like that of the secondary syphilis as they spread widely, are more severe and have longer duration.
- Lesions may not manifest at birth but definitely within first month of age.
- Most common cutaneous feature of early syphilis is rhinitis or snuffles, commonly appear-

ing as first sign between 2nd to 6th week of age.

- Diffuse bright pink to reddish papulosquamous lesions affect palms and soles also. If it remains untreated, skin lesions fade to coppery brown over 1-3 months.
- Vesiculo-bullous lesions appear rarely but when palms and soles are affected, it is diagnostic. Otherwise palms and soles become erythematous and fissured.
- Condyloma lata are moist and warty lesions appear at anogenital region, around the nares and angle of the mouth.
- Fissures at angle of the mouth with a tendency of oozing, extend out radially over surrounding skin from mucous membrane. When these fissures become deep, form radial scars after healing, known as rhagades.
- Sometimes intractable diaper dermatitis may present as a feature.
- Nasal mucosal lesions may produce ulceration, leading to destruction of the nasal cartilage to form saddle nose.
- Also in long bones, there may be widening of epiphyseal lines and increased density of shaft and spotty translucent areas, known as moth eaten areas.
- Pseudoparalysis of Parrot, is an extremely painful condition due to subepiphyseal fracture.
- Dactylitis occurs due to osteochondritis of small joints.
- Anemia, fever, wasting, hepatosplenomegaly and lymphadenopathy are also present.
- Sometime syphilitic meningitis develops with bulging of fontanelle and ophisthotonus convulsion may culminate into physical and mental retardation.

* Clinical features of late congenital syphilis:
  - These are mainly the signs of stigmata.
  - Most pathognomonic change of late congenital syphilis is dental changes including tendency of the deciduous teeth to be caries.
  - Hutchinson's tooth shows central notching and tapering of lateral sides towards biting edge, and appears as a screwdriver. Permanent upper central incisors are affected.
  - Malformation in the form of poorly developed cusps crowded together on the crown of the lower 1st molar tooth is known as mulberry molar.
  - Hutchinson's triad includes interstitial keratitis, Hutchinson's incisors and 8th cranial nerve deafness.
  - Higomenaki's sign is unilateral thickening of inner 1/3rd of the clavicle.
  - Bones and joints deformities are Clutton's joint, saber shin, short maxilla and frontal or parietal bossing.
  - Paroxysmal cold hemoglobinuria shows chilled and dark urine within 8 hours of cold exposure.
  - Placental changes like villous enlargement, acute villitis and necrotizing funisitis.

Diagnostic tests

- Demonstration of *Treponema pallidum* by dark ground illumination test (DG1).
- Serological tests are FTA-ABS, VDRL and TPHA. Here interpretation is important. If titer of a serological test is higher in baby than the mother, it is diagnostic. But if titer is less than that of the mother, then it is due to passive transfer and that reverts to normal within 4-6 months of delivery.
- In case of meningitis, cerebrospinal fluid (CSF) examination shows increased protein, mononuclear cell pleocytosis and positive VDRL test.

Treatment

- Aqueous crystalline penicillin 1.5 lac units/kg body weight, in two divided doses, iv for 7 days, followed by three divided doses for another 3 days.

- For meningitis, aqueous crystalline penicillin 2-3 lac units/kg body weight/day in divided doses as 4-6 hours interval for 10-14 days.

Follow up

- Clinical examination to be done at 1st, 2nd, 3rd, 6th and 12th month.
- Serum VDRL test to be done at 3rd, 6th and 12th month.

Congenital varicella syndrome

- It develops when mother is infected within first 20 weeks of gestation with varicella virus and the highest risk lies between 13-20 weeks.

Clinical features

- Intact vesicles or scarring are seen with a dermatomal distribution.
- Low birth weight, mental retardation, seizure, cortical atrophy, encephalomyelitis, contracture, gastrointestinal and genitourinary defects, cataract, microphthalmia and chorioretinitis, etc. are other features.

Ichthyosis

A. Hereditary/congenital primary ichthyosis

- Ichthyosis vulgaris
- Recessive X-linked ichthyosis
- Bullous congenital ichthyosiform erythroderma (epidermolytic hyperkeratosis)
- Non-bullous ichthyosiform erythroderma
- Lamellar ichthyosis
- Collodion baby.

B. Ichthyosiform disorders

- Harlequin ichthyosis
- Erythrokeratodermia variabilis
- Progressive symmetric erythrokeratodermia
- Neutral lipid storage disease with ichthyosis
- Refsum disease
- Peeling skin syndrome
- Netherton syndrome
- Neu-Laxova syndrome
- KID syndrome
- CHILD syndrome
- Conradi syndrome
- CHIME syndrome
- Sjogren-Larsson syndrome
- Gaucher syndrome

C. Acquired

- Old age
- AIDS, sarcoidosis and lymphoma
- Scleroderma, SLE and dermatomyositis
- Sarcoidosis, graft vs host disease and Kava dermopathy
- Clofazimine, lipid lowering drugs and antipsychotic drugs.

Ichthyosis vulgaris

- It is the mildest and most common form of ichthyosis with an autosomal dominant inheritance.
- It is not present at birth. But it starts to develop usually after 3 months of age and becomes prominent during childhood.
- Winter season aggravates dryness and scaling.

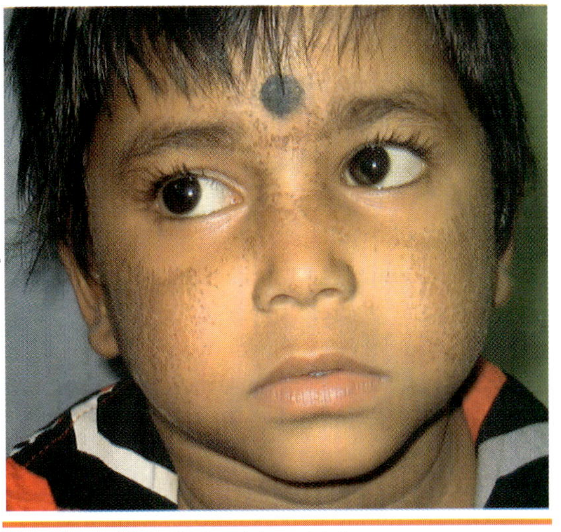

Fig. 12: Ichthyosis involving cheeks

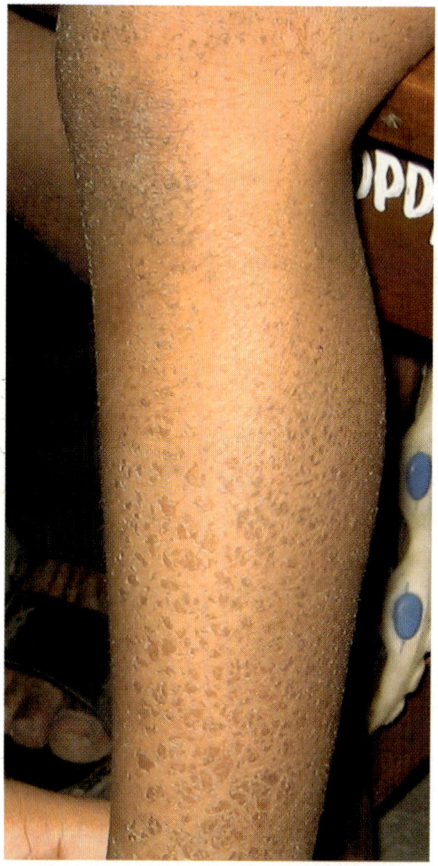

Fig. 13: Ichthyosis involving extensor of the leg

Clinical features

- Extensors of extremities are predominantly affected and flexor surfaces are usually spared.
- Scales at pretibial and lateral aspect of lower legs are large, plate like, resembling fish scales.
- Scales at forehead and cheeks are prominent during childhood and clear by later age.
- Other features are mild palmo-plantar keratoderma, discrete hyperkeratosis at elbows, knees and ankles, tendency to develop atopic dermatitis and keratosis pilaris-like lesion at upper arms, buttocks and thighs.

Histopathology

- Orthokeratotic hyperkeratosis with absent or reduced granular layer.

Treatment

- Application of emollient, keratolytic and humectants.
- Systemic retinoids.

Recessive X-linked ichthyosis

* It starts in early infancy, usually within 3 months of age and rarely after age of 1 year. Even scales may present at birth as collodion membrane.

Clinical features

- Scales are small to large and brown to dark brown in color.
- They may shed or molt episodically during spring and rainy season.
- Entire body is affected including flexor surfaces with accentuation at neck, abdomen, back, front of legs and feet. But it spares palms, soles, central face and flexurals.
- Other features are hypogonadism, cryptorchidism, testicular cancer, corneal opacity, increased blood cholesterol sulfate and increased mobility of B lipoproteins.

Congenital bullous ichthyosiform erythroderma/Epidermolytic hyperkeratosis

* It is an autosomal dominant disorder, having verruciform and thick macerated scales with a disagreeable odor.

Types

* Non-severe palms-soles involvement (NPS type):
  - NPS-1: Generalized involvement with hystrix or porcupine like hyperkeratosis.
  - NPS-2: Generalized with relative sparing of skin between joints and mild form of hyperkeratosis.
  - NPS-3: Presented with exfoliative dermatitis.
* With severe palms-soles involvement (PS type):
  - PS-1: Smooth palmoplantar hyperkeratosis with sharp border and red halo.

- PS-2: Presented with erythroderma with contracure of the digits and ainhum like constricting digital bands.
- PS-3: Generalized involvement with pebbly hyperkeratosis of palms and soles and array in a cerebriform pattern.

Clinical features

- Skin is red and tender at birth.
- Superficial blisters develop within hours to weeks of delivery, resembling epidermolysis bullosa.
- Blisters develop in crops and vary from 0.5 cm to several cm. Erosions develop following rupture of the blisters.
- Hyperkeratosis starts to develop from 3rd month, specially at elbows and knees, followed by grayish brown scales covering most skin surface and verruciform scales at flexors creases and intertriginous areas.
- Nit-like encasement of scalp hair may present.
- Face is involved but without any ectropion.
- Palmoplantar keratoderma is present.
- Hair, eyes, teeth and nails are normal.

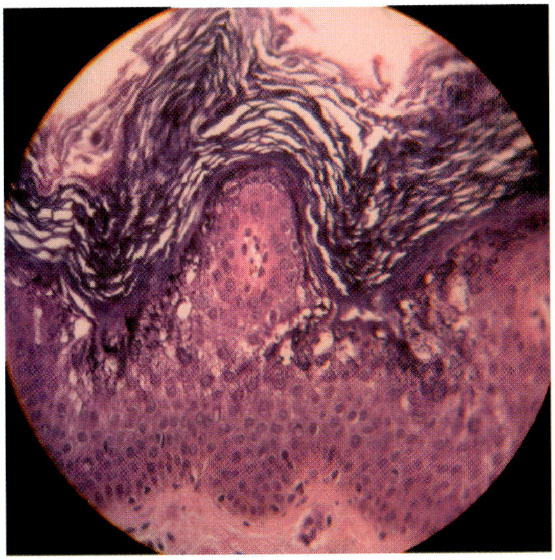

Fig. 14: Hyperkeratosis with acantholytic epidermis

Histopathology

- Gross orthokeratotic hyperkeratosis and acanthosis.
- Vacuolar degeneration of upper epidermis.
- Dense irregular clumped tonofilament masses are seen within granular keratinocytes. These resemble keratohyaline granules.

Congenital non-bullous ichthyosiform erythroderma

- It is a severe unremitting disorder, persisting for whole life and caused by mutation of TGM1 gene encoding keratinocyte transglutaminase 1.
- These lipoxygenases cause inflammation and proliferation of skin.
- Due to obstruction of sweat ducts by hyperkeratosis, patients often feel hyperpyrexia, heat intolerance, difficulty in perspiration and heat exhaustion during hot and humid weather and vigorous physical exercise.

Clinical features

- Prominent erythrodermic component becomes apparent when collodion membrane is shed off after few weeks of birth.
- Presence of plate-like scales at limbs and fine white scales at face, trunk and scalp.
- Mild to variable ectropion and mild palmoplantar keratoderma are present.
- Other features are intrauterine growth retardation, failure to thrive and neurologic abnormalities.

Lamellar ichthyosis

- It is usually inherited as autosomal recessive trait.

Clinical features

- Scales are large, thick, quadrangular and yellow to brown black in color.
- They are attached at the center with raised edges, resembling armor plates.

- Scales are most prominent at face, trunk and extremities with a predilection for flexor areas.
- Cheeks are often red, shiny and taut with minimal scaling.
- Scales are more at forehead than at lower part of the face.
- Scalp also shows scales with partial hair loss.
- Ectropion is seen in severely affected person.
- Palms and soles are affected with exaggerated palmar markings, keratoderma and fissuring of variable degree of severity.

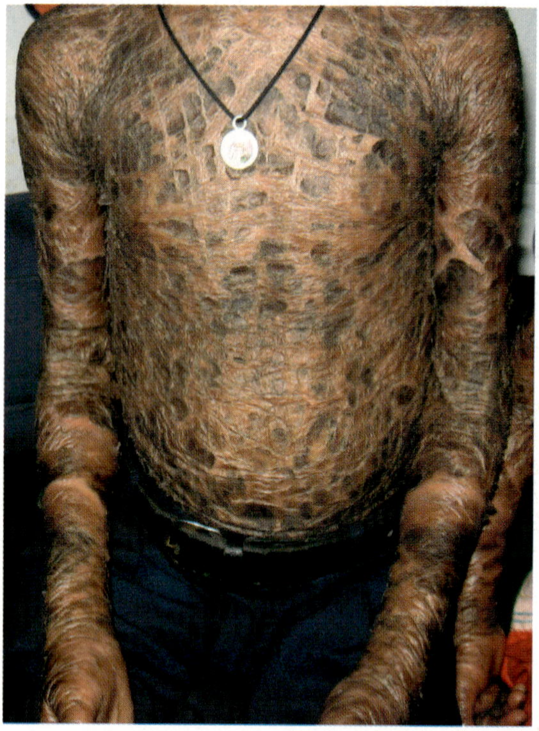

Fig. 15: Dark colored large scales in a case of lamellar ichthyosis. Third isolated hand is of another sibling

Collodion baby

* In this disorder, the baby is born with a membrane like covering, resembling collodion.
* It is not a disease; but just a phenotype of several other diseases.
* These babies are often prematurely born.
* In 60% cases it is associated with development of non-bullous ichthyosiform erythroderma and lamellar ichthyosis. But less commonly Conradi syndrome, trichothiodystrophy and recessive X-linked ichthyosis may develop following shedding of the membrane.
* In 5% cases, normal skin may appear following shedding of the membrane, known as self-healing collodion baby.
* The collodion membrane is made up of thick stratum corneum with poor barrier function.

Clinical features

- At birth, the baby is completely covered with cellophane or oiled-parchment-like membrane.
- The membrane is so taut, that causes distortion of extremities as well as facial expression.
- It also causes flattened ears, everted eyelids, lips and even vulva, and edema of the limbs.
- The baby is unable to suck properly and feels difficulty to expand the chest.
- Other features are cutaneous infection, systemic infection, aspiration pneumonia, excess transcutaneous fluid and electrolyte loss, hypernatremic dehydration, increased metabolic requirement and temperature instability.

Treatment

- Maintenance of nutrition and fluid and electrolyte balance.
- Application of emollient and humectants.
- Antibiotic for infection.
- Oral retinoids.

Harlequin ichthyosis

* This is an autosomal recessive ichthyosis having severe and dramatic form of congenital thickening of skin.
* It is associated with increased epidermal triglyceride, abnormal keratin expression, altered cal-

cium mediated signaling and altered cutaneous phosphatase activity.

Clinical features

- Skin becomes profoundly thickened, armor like gray or yellow colored, dry and hard like tree bark.
- Skin is divided into multiple polygonal or triangular plaques, resembling costume of a harlequin by deep and reddish to brown fissures.
- Rigidity of skin results in marked ectropion and everted lips with a gaping fish mouth appearance. It also causes distorted and flattened ears and nose.

Treatment

- Application of emollient.
- Maintenance of nutrition, fluid and electrolytes balance.

CUTANEOUS FEATURES OF INTERNAL DISEASES

CHAPTER C16

Cutaneous manifestations of diabetes mellitus

* Bacterial infections, presented with
  - Pyoderma, specially boils, carbuncles and cellulitis
  - Malignant otitis externa
  - Necrotizing fasciitis
* Candidial infection, presented with
  - Paronychia
  - Onychomycosis
  - Balanoposthitis
* Noninfective dermatoses
  - Diabetic dermopathy
  - Necrobiotic lipoidica diabeticorum
  - Scleredema diabeticorum
  - Sclerodermatous changes at hands with limited joint mobility. Patient is unable to appose the palms and this is known as Prayer sign.
  - Diabetic bulla
  - Diabetic rubiopathy
  - Peripheral neuropathy
  - Trophic ulcer
  - Reactive perforating collagenosis
  - Acanthosis nigricans
  - Xanthoma
  - Granuloma annulare

Necrobiosis lipoidica diabeticorum

- Red brown papules or nodules which coalesce to form yellow brown plaques, with violaceous, raised and indurated borders.
- Gradually center becomes atrophic and telangiectatic to form a glazed porcelain sheen appearance. Sometimes they become ulcerated.
- Shins are the commonest sites. But other areas like feet, ankles, calves, thighs, upper limbs and trunk may be affected.
- Lesions may be pruritic or painful. Sometimes anesthesia may develop on the lesion.
- Spontaneous remission occurs in 20% cases. But rarely squamous cell carcinoma may develop.

Diabetic dermopathy

- In 72% cases are seen in diabetes, 20% in non-diabetic but may have other endocrinopathy and also seen in 1.5% of healthy persons.

- Lesions are asymptomatic, atrophic, pink to brown scar like macules and size < 1 cm.
- Lesions clear within 1-2 years spontaneously but development of new lesions is going on.

Cutaneous manifestations of hyperthyroidism

- Pruritus
- Intolerance to heat
- Diffuse and nonscarring alopecia of the scalp
- Facial flushing
- Soft and moist infantile skin
- Hyperpigmentation
- Hyperhidrosis, specially at palms and soles.
- Thyroid dermopathy
- Thyroid acropachy
- Palmar erythema
- Plummer nails.

Cutaneous manifestations of hypothyroidism

- Intolerance to cold
- Diffuse and nonscarring alopecia of the scalp.
- Dry and brittle hair.
- Loss of hair at lateral 3rd of eyebrows.
- Retarded growth of hair
- Swelling of face with puffy eyelids.
- Broadened nose
- Thickened lips and macroglossia
- Cold, dry, doughy and wrinkled skin
- Myxedema
- Swelling of fingers with retarded growth of nails.
- Carpal tunnel syndrome
- Hoarseness of voice.

Cutaneous manifestations of Cushing syndrome

- Increased central adiposity, causing moon facies and buffalo hump.
- Thinning of the extremities
- Increased facial redness and telangiectasia
- Acanthosis nigricans
- Acne
- Hypertrichosis
- Thinning of the skin and easy bruisability
- Violaceous striae, > 1 cm breadth
- Rarely hyperpigmentation
- Increased dermatophytic and candidial infection of skin and nail.

Cutaneous manifestations of Addison's diseases

- Hyperpigmentation of skin and mucous membrane
- Longitudinal pigmented bands at nails.
- Reduced axillary and pubic hairs in females
- Calcification of auricular cartilage
- Vitiligo

Cutaneous manifestations of paraneoplastic syndromes

- 100% Association
  - Hypertrichosis lanuginosa acquisita associated with lungs, breasts and gastrointestinal malignancies.
  - Acrokeratosis paraneoplastica of Bazex, associated with oropharyngeal, esophageal and laryngeal squamous cell carcinoma.
  - Necrolytic migratory erythema, associated with glucagonoma-$\propto$ cell pancreatic carcinoma.
  - Paraneoplastic pemphigus, associated with non-Hodgkin lymphoma, chronic lymphocytic leukemia, Castleman disease and thymoma.
- 90% Association
  - Tripe palm, associated with gastric and lung carcinomas.
- 80% Association
  - Scleromyxedema, associated with multiple myeloma.
  - Erythema gyratum repens, associated with lung carcinoma.
  - Necrobiotic xanthogranuloma, associated with multiple myeloma.

* 50% Association
    * Trousseau's syndrome, associated with lung and pancreatic carcinomas.
* 13-30% Association
    * Multicentric reticulohistiocytosis, associated with melanoma, hematologic and breast malignancies.
    * Sweet syndrome, associated with acute myeloid leukemia.
    * Primary systemic amyloidosis, associated with multiple myeloma.
    * Dermatomyositis, associated with ovary, lung and pancreatic carcinomas.
* 3-7% Association
    * Pyoderma gangrenosum, associated with lung cancer.
    * Dermatitis herpetiformis, associated with T-cell, B-cell and non-Hodgkin lymphoma.
    * Scleroderma, associated with lung cancer.
* % Unknown
    * Leser Trelat sign, associated with gastrointestinal adenocarcinoma.
    * Acanthosis nigricans, associated with gastrointestinal adenocarcinoma.
    * Acquired ichthyosis, associated with lymphoma.

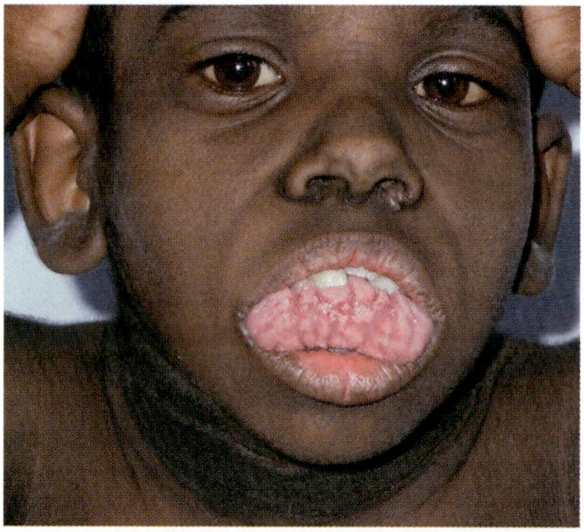

Fig. 1: All flexurals have a velvety appearance including lips and tongue, in case of severe acanthosis nigricans

CHAPTER C17

CUTANEOUS MALIGNANCY

Basal cell carcinoma (BCC)

* It is a locally proliferating carcinoma of the skin without any apparent cause.
* Predisposing factors:
  * Prolonged sun exposure
  * Prolonged intake of inorganic arsenic
* It usually affects adults and rarely seen in children. Syndromes associated BCCs develop at an early age.
* It does not metastasize with a few exceptions. When metastasis occurs, it affects lymph nodes, lungs and bones.
* It usually occurs at face, but any area may be affected. Mucous membrane, palms and soles are often spared.

Clinical types

* Noduloulcerative type, including rodent ulcer, is the commonest type.
* Pigmented type
* Superficial type
* Fibrosing type or morphea-like
* Fibroepitheliomatous type

* Syndromes associated with BCC
  * Unilateral linear nevoid basal cell nevus
  * Nevoid basal cell carcinoma syndrome
  * Bazex syndrome
* Differentiation may be towards any of the appendages like hair, apocrine, eccrine or sebaceous glands.

Clinical features

* Noduloulcerative type:
  * It commonly affects the face.
  * Early lesion appears as a small, round and translucent nodule with visible telangiectasia.
  * It may also present as erythematous or lichenoid papule, keratotic or indurated papule and plaque, or pedunculated papule.
  * Lesion usually progresses slowly with a thread or indurated margin and depressed, ulcerated or crusted center. Ulcerated center with rolled border is known as rodent ulcer.
  * Facial lesion with local invasion may destroy eye, nose and skull bones.

* Superficial type:
    - This type commonly affects the trunk.
    - It is characterized by mild elevated erythematous and scaly plaque.
    - Lesion slowly increases in size by peripheral extension.
    - At least some of the part contains thread like pearly border.
    - Small superficial and crusted ulcer may develop within the lesion.
    - Center of the lesion may be smooth or atrophic.
* Pigmented type:
    - It commonly affects the face.
    - It differs from noduloulcerative type by presence of profuse pigmentation only.
* Morphea form type:
    - It commonly affects the face.
    - It is characterized by solitary, flat or mild depressed, indurated yellowish plaque.
    - Surface of the lesion is smooth and shiny.
    - It ulcerates after a long period.
    - Histopathology shows deep infiltration.
* Fibroepitheliomatous type:
    - It commonly affects the back.
    - Lesions are elevated, slight pedunculated and firm nodules.
    - Surface is usually reddish and smooth.
    - Lesion mimics fibroma.
* Nevoid basal cell carcinoma syndrome:
    - It commonly affects age group 15-35 years.
    - Lesions start as benign small nodules and number of the lesions may be from hundred to thousand.
    - Lesions are distributed haphazardly at face and trunk.
    - Along with age lesions become ulcerated and enter into a neoplastic stage.
    - Some of the facial lesions become invasive and affect eye and brain and metastasize into lungs.
    - In 50% patients also develop palmar pits at second decade of life and these represent the herbinger of basal cell carcinoma.
* Unilateral linear basal cell nevus:
    - Lesions are closely set nodules of BCC and present since birth.
    - Comedones and striae like lesions often intersperse between the lesions.
    - Interestingly lesions do not increase in size along with age.
* Bazex syndrome:
    - Follicular atrophoderma is the main feature.
    - Multiple BCCs develop during adolescent period and sometimes in early childhood.
    - Presence of localized anhidrosis or generalized hypohidrosis.
    - Congenital hypotrichosis at the scalp and other areas.

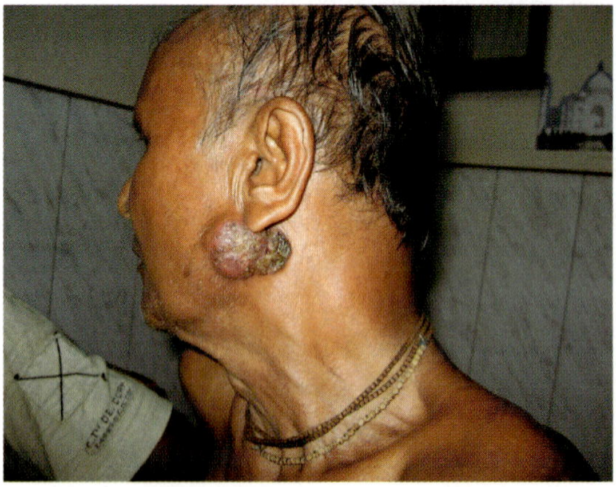

Fig. 1: Noduloulcerative plaque with crusts

Differential diagnosis

- Squamous cell carcinoma
- Malignant melanoma
- Lupus vulgaris.

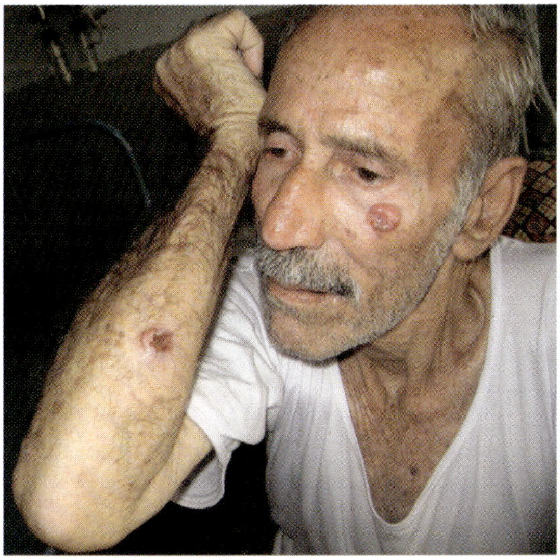

Fig. 2: Noduloucerative Basal cell carcinoma with telangiectasia at left cheek

Differential diagnosis

- Pseudolymphoma
- Keratoacanthoma
- Solitary trichoepithelioma.

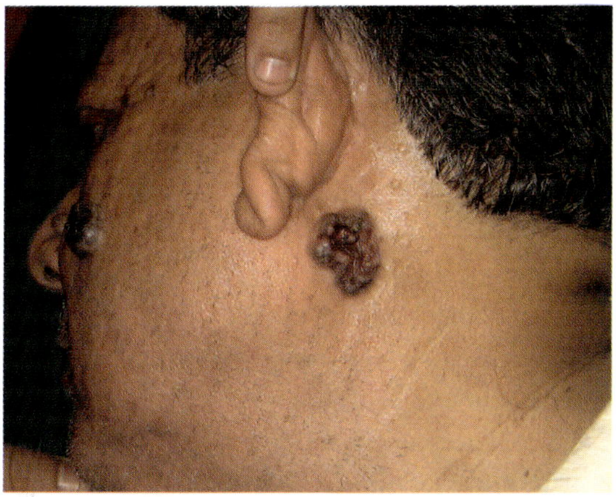

Fig. 3: Pigmented rodent ulcers

Histopathology

- Downward growth of epithelial cells, predominantly of basal cell type.
- Nuclei of peripheral cells of the mass are arranged in a palisading pattern.
- Cells show a variable degree of cytologic atypia and mitotic activity.

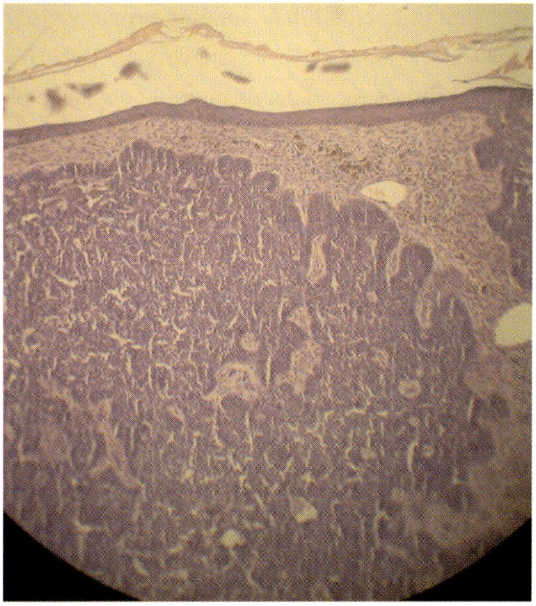

Fig. 4: A mass of basaloid cells in the dermis

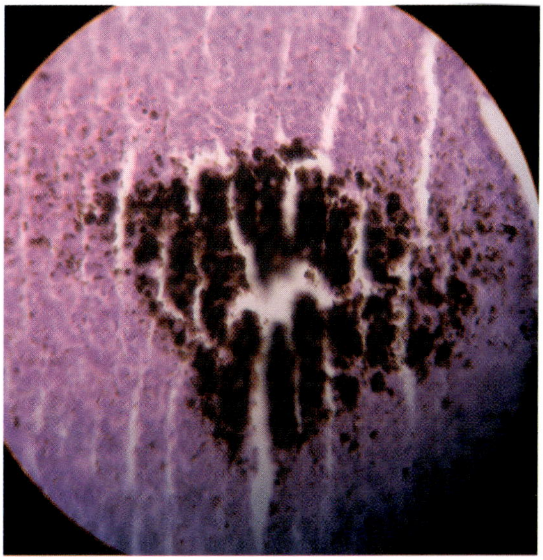

Fig. 5: Profuse pigmentation within the mass of BCC

- Cells are having large, oval or elongated nuclei and less cytoplasm.
- Cytoplasm of the cell is poorly defined and so the cellular mass appears as symplasmatic mass of nuclei.

- Nuclei appear uniform and nonanaplastic.
- Nuclei usually don't show prominent variation in size and their staining property.
- Rarely some cells may have very large hyperchromatic nuclei or multiple nuclei or bizarre starburst mitoses.
- This cell differs from basal cell by higher ratio of nucleus to cytoplasm and by lack of intercellular bridges.
- Cystic spaces may be seen due to cell necrosis or due to loss of intercellular adhesion, specially at the center of the tumor mass.
- Presence of a specialized stroma, proliferating stroma, arranged as parallel bundles around the tumor mass resembling they have a mutual relation to grow.
- Stroma is having numerous young fibroblast and may appear mucinous.
- Presence of artifactual cleft between the epithelium and stroma due to retraction helps to differentiate basal cell carcinoma from squamous cell carcinoma.
- Inflammatory infiltrate may be profuse in ulcerated BCC but scanty in non-ulcerated lesion.
- In infiltrating or aggressive type, cells are arranged as elongated strands of few cell layers with little or no palisading of the peripheral cells.
- Keratotic type shows parakeratotic cells and horn cyst. Horn cysts are formed with interposition of granular cells.
- Adenoid type consists of gland-like tubular structures. Cells are arranged in a interwining fashion around the islands of connective tissue. Ultimately the tumor mass resembles a lace-like pattern.
- Adamantinoid type shows that cells contain elongated nuclei and stellate cytoplasm and they are arranging as thin interconnected bridges through empty spaces as seen in adamantinoma.
- Granular type shows that cells are having numerous cytoplasmic eosinophillic granules.
- Clear cell type shows that cells are vacuoles of different size due to deposition of glycogen.
- BCC with matricial differentiation shows presence of shadow cells as in pilomatricoma.
- In morpheic or fibrosing type, thin strands of tumor cells are embedded in a dense fibrous stroma.
- Superficial BCC shows irregular buds of tumor mass, attached along the undersurface of the atrophic epidermis and presence of fair number of fibroblasts around the tumor masses.
- Noduloulcerative type may be solid, keratotic or adenoid patterns.
- Fibroepitheliomatous type shows long, thin, anastomosing strands, embedded in a fibrous stroma.
- Basosquamous type shows presence of basaloid cells at the periphery and focal keratin pearls and squamous cells at the center. These cells are larger, ligher and better defined than basal cells.

* Histologically BCC is divided into differentiating type and undifferentiating type.
* Differentiating type shows a slight degree of differentiation towards any of the appendages like hair, sebaceous glands, apocrine glands and eccrine glands. Sometimes differentiation may be toward more than single structure.
* Keratotic type differentiates toward hair follicle.
* Adenoid type differentiates toward tubular structures.
* Undifferentiated types are also called solid BCC, which may be circumscribed or infiltrating.

* Basal cell carcinoma with low risk of local recurrence:
  - Nodular
  - Nodulocystic
  - Fibroepithelioma of Pinkus
* Basal cell carcinoma with higher risk of local recurrence:
  - Superficial type
  - Infiltrative type
  - Morpheic type
  - Metatypical type
  - Micronodular type.
* Uncommon variants of BCC
  - Adamantinoid type
  - Granular type
  - Clear cell type
  - BCC with matricial differentiation.

Treatment

- Surgical excision
- Electrosurgical excision followed by application of imiquimod.

Bowen's disease

* It may occur at exposed or unexposed skin.
* It occurs on exposed skin due to sun light and on unexposed skin due to chronic arsenicosis.
* It occurs in association with epidermodysplasia verruciformis, caused by HPV-5.

Clinical features

- Initially a small, reddish, slight elevated and mild scaly papule develops. Gradually it enlarges in an irregular fashion and becomes covered with the moderately adherent scales.
- When scales are removed, a moist, erythematous or granulomatous surface is noticed. But there is no tendency of bleeding.
- Lesion may become hyperkeratotic, ulcerated and crusted. Ulcer indicates invasive carcinoma.
- Trunk is commonly affected. But fingers, nail folds, nail bed, even glans are affected.
- Penile lesion is designated as erythroplasia of Queyrat.

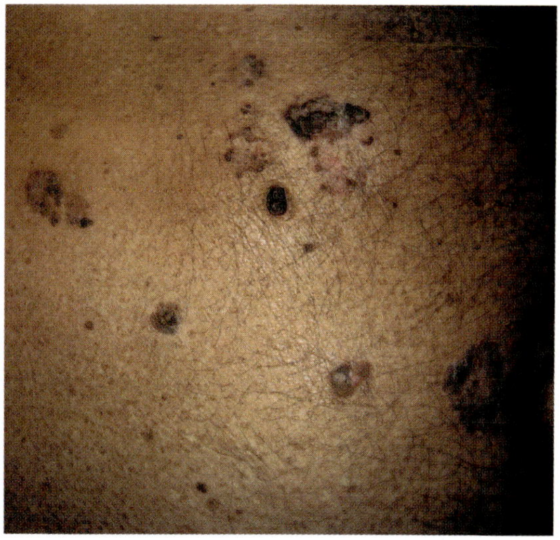

Fig. 6: Irregular but well defined erythematous plaques with adherent scales

Differential diagnosis

- Seborrheic keratosis
- Actinic keratosis
- DLE (Discoid lupus erythematosus)

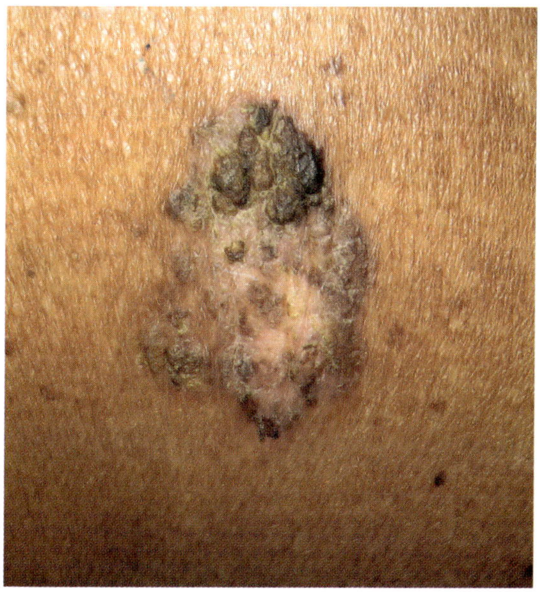

Fig. 7: Irregular erythematous and crusted plaque

Histopathology

- Hyperkeratosis with or without parakeratosis.
- Acanthosis with obliteration of dermal papilla.
- Loss of polarity of the keratinocytes with wind blown appearance.
- Presence of keratinocytes with atypical, pleomorphic, large, irregular, hyperchromatic nuclei.
- Premature keratinization may present in mid epidermis.
- In some cases proliferating cells may be encircled by normal cells, known as Borst-Jadassohn phenomenon.

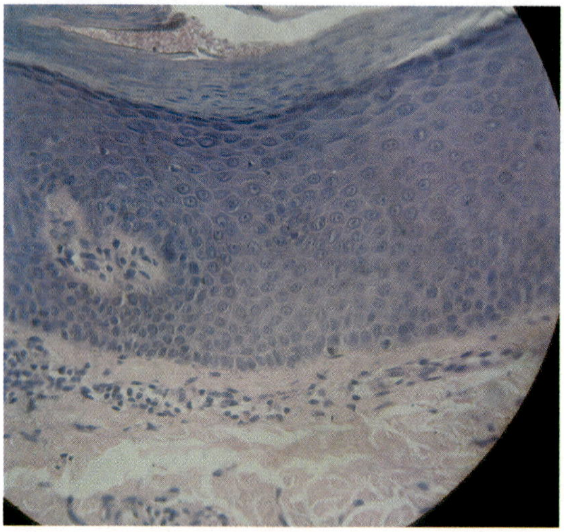

Fig. 8: Homogeneous thickening of the epidermis and obliteration of dermal papillae and loss of polarity of the keratinocytes

Treatment

- Application of imiquimod or 5-fluorouracil (5%) cream,
- Laser-/cryo-/electrosurgery.

Squamous cell carcinoma

* It occurs at any site of the skin including mucosae.
* It usually does not occur at normal appearing skin.
* Its incidence is significantly increased in presence of immunosuppression.
* Predisposing factors:
  - Sun-damaged skin
  - Actinic keratosis
  - Arsenical keratosis
  - Burn scar
  - Marjolin's ulcer
  - Osteomyelitic sinus
  - Radiation

Types

- Adenoid type
- Mucin producing type
- Verrucous type

Clinical features

- Most commonly it arises as a shallow ulcer with wide, elevated and indurated border.
- A red granular base is often concealed by crusts.
- Sometimes raised, hyperkeratotic and verrucous plaque is developed without any ulceration.

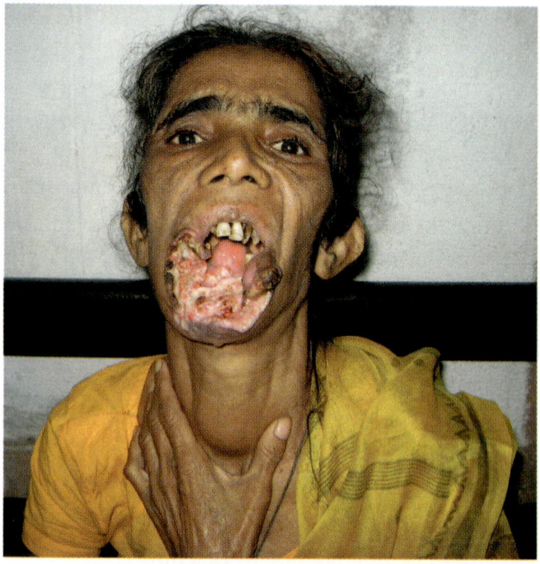

Fig. 9: Fungating ulcerated growth at mouth

Differential diagnosis

- Ulcerated lupus vulgaris
- Pyoderma gangrenosum

Histopathology

- Irregular masses of epidermal cells which proliferate downward into the dermis.
- The masses contain both normal and atypical neoplastic cells in a variable proportion.
- Higher number of atypical cells are seen in poorly differentiating SCC.
- Atypical cells are variable in shape and size. Their nuclei are hyperchromatic and hyperplastic.

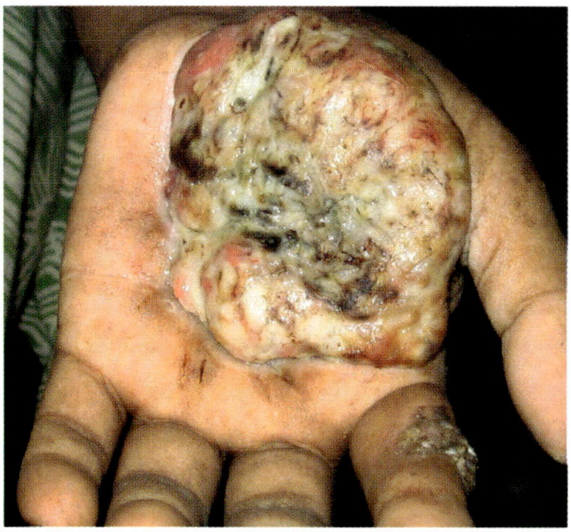

Fig. 10: Cauliflower like ulcerated plaque

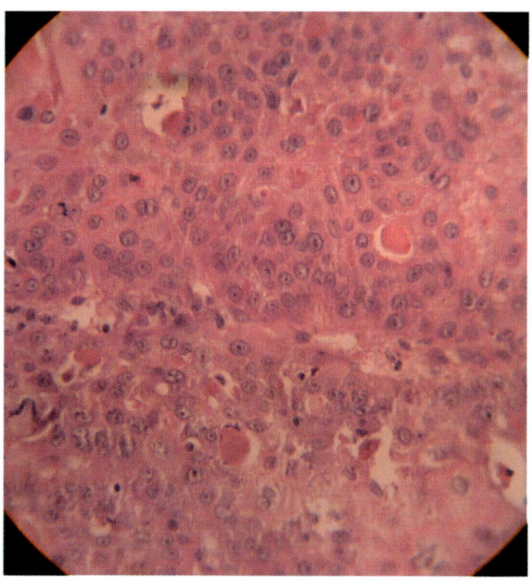

Fig. 11: Anisocytosis of epithelial cell with moderate degree of differentiation and individual cell keratinization

- Individual cell shows keratinization and mitosis. Intercellular bridges are also lost and secondary acantholysis develops.
- There is tendency of keratinization when squamous cells undergo differentiation. Keratinization occurs in the form of horn pearls. The horn pearl is composed of concentric layers of squamous cells which show gradual keratinization with maximum at the center. This central part of the keratinization may be complete or incomplete. Keratohyaline granules are sparse or absent.

Treatment

- Surgical intervention.
- Radiotherapy
- Chemotherapy.

Paget's disease

- It is a form of epithelial adenocarcinoma involving mammary and extramammary tissues.
- It occurs at older age around 50 years, ranging from 32-80 years.
- Paget's disease of the nipple occurs exclusively in females.
- Cutaneous lesion is often associated with carcinoma of the breast.
- Breast lump is palpable in more than 50% cases.
- Mammary Paget's disease (MPD) comprises of only 0.5-4% of breast cancers.
- Very often MPD is misdiagnosed as nipple dermatitis which commonly affects bilaterally and younger age group and lesions are less defined and extremely pruritic.

Clinical features of mammary Paget's disease

- Lesion develops at nipple or areola as well demarcated erythematous flat plaque with scales and crusts. Sometimes oozing present like a subacute dermatitis.
- Lesion always arises unilaterally.
- It gradually extends around the site of origin.

- It may be associated with itching, followed by development of pain or burning sensation and ulceration.

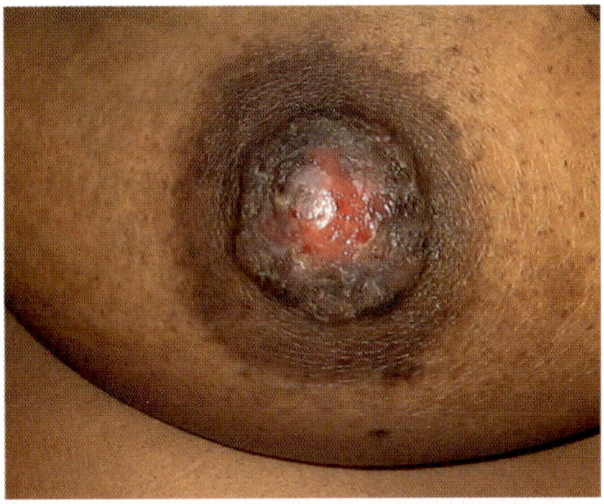

Fig. 12: Well defined unilateral ulcerated plaque with destruction of the nipple

Differential diagnosis

- Nummular dermatitis
- Bowen's disease
- Erosive adenomatosis of the nipple
- Nevoid hyperkeratosis of the nipple

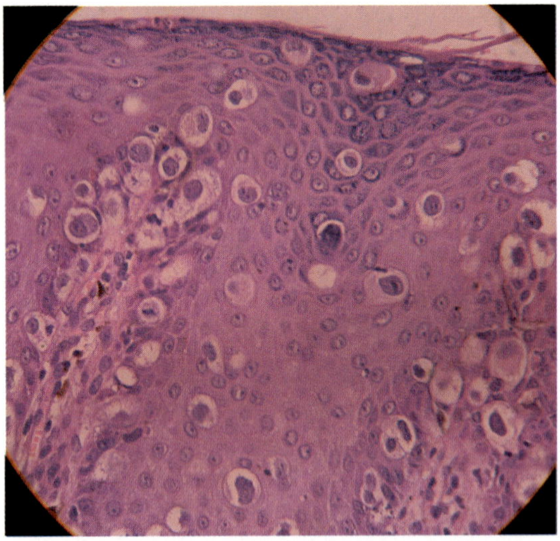

Fig. 13: Owl-eyed keratinocytes or Paget's cells

Histopathology

- Infiltration of epidermis by large and round or oval malignant cells without intercellular bridges, having large hyperchromatic or vesicular nuclei.
- Cytoplasm of the cells contains granules of mucopolysaccharides.

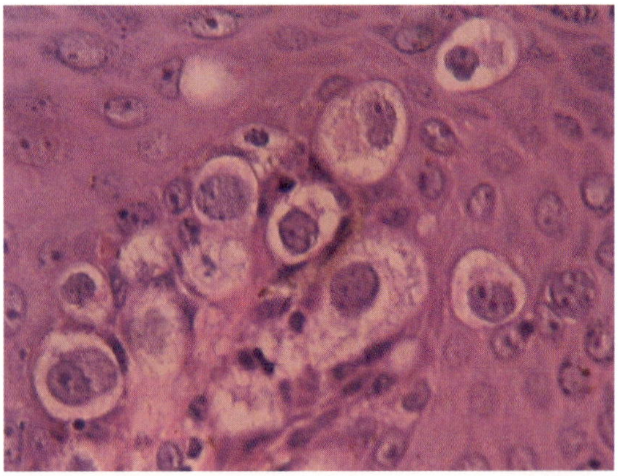

Fig. 14: Close up view of Paget's cell

Treatment

- Surgical excision
- Radiotherapy
- Chemotherapy.

Malignant melanoma

* Most of the melanomas originate from the epidermis and may remain localized within it, known as in situ melanoma.
* When it extends into the dermis, known as invasive melanoma.
* Occasionally invasive melanoma is seen solely within the dermis.
* Invasive melanoma when grows vertically known as tumerogenic and when grows radially, known as nontumerogenic.
* Type of in situ melanoma and nontumerogenic melanoma:
  - Lentigo melanoma (LMM)
  - Superficial spreading (SMM)
  - Acral lentiginous (ALM)
  - Mucosal lentiginous
* Tumerogenic melanoma may develop from any of the above types or may develop as de novo.

- De novo tumerogenic melanoma is known as nodular melanoma.
- Other variants of tumerogenic melanoma:
  - Desmoplastic melanoma
  - Neurotrophic melanoma.
- Spreading pattern of nontumerogenic melanoma:
  - Lentiginous pattern: Contiguous focal proliferation of nevus cells.
  - Pagetoid pattern: Buckshot scatter melanocytes within the epidermis.
- Nodular melanoma has poor prognosis in comparison to superficial spreading melanoma.

Clinical features of nodular melanoma

- It occurs in slightly older persons and more frequently in men.
- It starts as a papule with variable pigmentation.
- Rapidly the papule turns into nodule and often ulcerates.
- Lesion may be pigmented, oligomelanotic or even amelanotic.

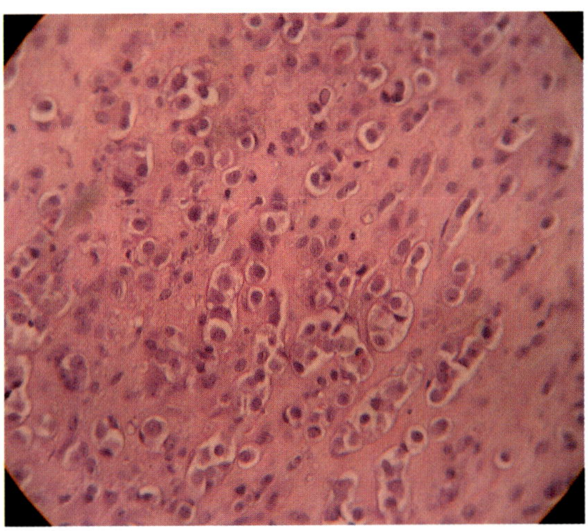

Fig. 15: Clear cells in the dermis

Histopathology of nodular melanoma

- Epidermis may be stretched, attenuated and ulcerated or may be hyperplastic and pseudoepitheliomatous.
- Continuous proliferation of neoplastic melanocytes form a dermal mass.
- This mass is larger than the largest nest in the overlying epidermis.
- Variations are seen in cell size and shape, amount of pigmentation and cell-distribution.
- Tumor mass contains uniformly atypical cells. They grow in nests or in sheets.
- By continuous proliferation, the malignant cells first fill up the papillary dermis and then spaces between the coarse collagen fibers of reticular dermis.
- Tumor cells in the epidermis appear as pagetoid pattern but it is limited within the area confined by the dermal mass. Lateral spread is commonly seen in other forms of primary melanoma like superficial spreading type (SMM), lentigo malignant melanoma (LMM), acral lentiginous melanoma (ALM).
- Due to lack of peripheral extension, it is difficult to differentiate metastatic melanoma of the skin from the primary nodular melanoma and also amelanotic form of other epithelial malignancies.
- Band like inflammatory infiltrate, mixed with melanophages, is often seen at the base of the tumor.
- Lymphocytes infiltrating the mass is a favourable sign of prognosis, as it indicates apoptosis of tumor cells.
- Malignant melanoma cells are of two types: epitheloid type and spindle shaped type.
- Epithelioid type cells are seen in LMM and ALM and they lie in alveolar or nested form.
- Spindle shaped cells are seen in SMM and nodular melanoma and they lie in branching form.
- Spindle cells of nodular melanoma differs from sarcoma or other spindle cell tumors by presence of junctional melanocytic activity.
- Atypical nucleus of melanoma cell is larger than melanocyte or nevus cell and contains

irregular nuclear membrane and hyperchromatic chromatin.

- Mitotic figures are seen at dermal component in 85% cases of nodular melanoma, in comparison to in 1/3rd cases of non-nodular melanomas at their epidermal parts. Mitoses are also seen in adjacent hyperplastic keratinocytes. Nuclei of these keratinocytes are large with prominent nucleoli but they are not irregular or hyperchromatic.

Mycosis fungoides (MF)

* It is form of cutaneous T-cell lymphoma and commonest among the all cutaneous lymphoma.
* Clinical features appear due to intraepidermal and superficial dermal infiltration with small to medium sized malignant T cells.
* Malignant T cells characteristically contain cerebriform nuclear contour.
* It predominantly affects the adult male with 2:1 male: female ratio. Children are occasionally affected.

Clinical features

- Initial lesions are erythematous scaly patches and plaques, unresponsive to conventional anti-inflammatory therapy.
- Lesions are often larger in size with arcuate or polycyclic configurations.
- This disease is slowly progressive. Transformation from patch or plaque to nodule, takes time. Lesions may ulcerate at times.
- Most of the lesions are scaly like psoriasis and often are misdiagnosed as psoriasiform dermatitis. This variant is known as psoriasiform MF.
- Alopecia may occur due to degeneration of hair follicle by the infiltration and mucin deposition. This variant is known as alopecia mucinosa.
- Epidermal atrophy, telangiectasia and hypo- or hyperpigmentation may present within the lesions. This variant is known as poikiloderma vasculare atrophicans.
- Rarely lesion may be solitary and involves acral skin. This variant is known as pagetoid reticulosis.
- Sometimes dermis contains granulomatous infiltration with disintegrated elastic fibers. This variant is known as granulomatous slack skin.
- Rarely nodule may develop at onset and this variant is known as d'emblee MF.
- Diffuse erythroderma may develop as a consequence of patch stage or from blood on outset. The later variant is known as Sezary syndrome.
- Extra-cutaneous organs like lymphoreticular system and lungs may be affected, specially in Sezary syndrome.

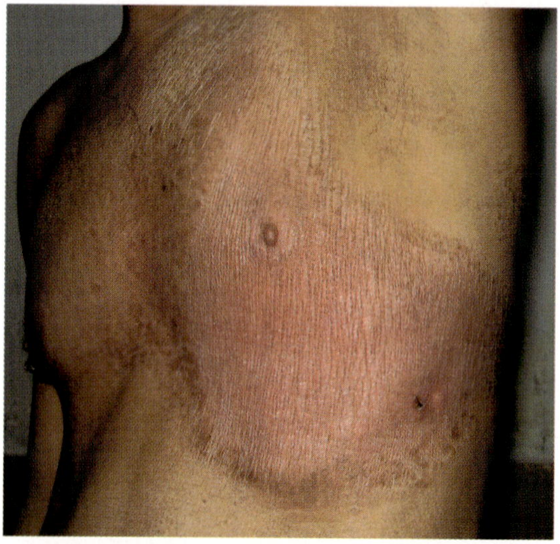

Fig. 16: Erythematous mild scaly patch with wrinkled surface

Differential diagnosis

- Large plaque parapsoriasis
- Pityriasis rotunda.

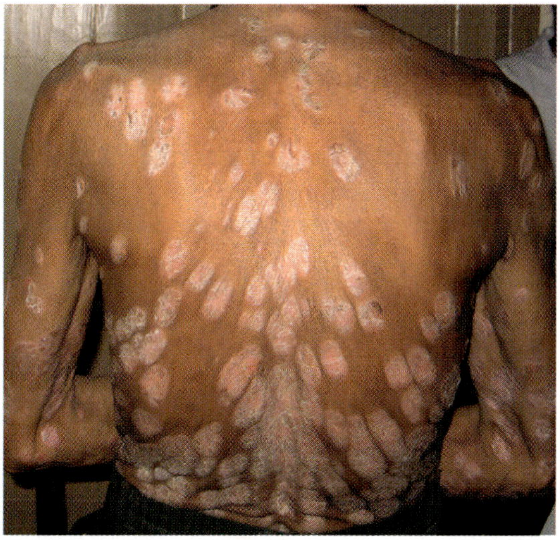

Fig. 17: Multiple well defined scaly plaques

Differential diagnosis

- Psoriasis
- Nummular dermatitis
- Sarcoidosis
- Secondary syphilis

Histopathology

* Early lesion (patch/plaque):
  - Diffuse lymphocytic infiltrate with coarse fibrosis in the papillary dermis.
  - Infiltration is of a mixed type. Other than lymphocytes, it contains eosinophil, plasma cells and monocytes. But it is difficult to find out the cytology of mycosis fungoides cells. Malignant T cell clone may be seen in the epidermis as a result of epidermotropism where epidermis plays a passive role and T cells play an active role.
  - Similarly hair follicle may be invaded by T cells as a result of folliculotropism.
  - T cells may be arranged in a linear pattern along the basement membrane or in a pagetoid pattern with a single cell or a cluster. This cluster is designated as Pautrier microabscess.
  - Malignant T cells are small to medium sized lymphocytes. They are having indented nuclear contour or cerebriform with dense heterochromatin.
  - It is very difficult to find out these malignant T cells among the dermal infiltrate but the epidermotrophic cells are almost exclusively are of this type.
* Late lesion (nodule):
  - Epidermotropism is lost.
  - Dermis contains more number of malignant T cells.
  - Hair follicle involvement produces follicular mucinosis.
  - Eccrine apparatus involvement causes syringometaplasia but no mucinosis.

Clinical staging

- Stage I: Disease confined to the skin
- Stage Ia: Localized lesions
- Stage Ib: Disseminated lesions.
- Stage II: Lymph node enlargement without histological evidence of lymphoma.
- Stage III: Lymph node enlargement with histological evidence of lymphoma.
- Stage IV: Evidence of visceral lymphoma.

Treatment

- 5-FU (5% cream)
- Tazarotene
- Radiotherapy
- Topical corticosteroid
- Systemic PUVA
- Surgery
- Chemotherapy.

Dermatofibrosarcoma protuberans

* It is a locally invasive tumor.

Clinical features

- It is characterized by one or few painless, firm, reddish, dermal nodules.
- Lesions grow slowly and may coalesce to form an irregular protuberant swelling with indurated base.
- Gradually lesion may ulcerate and may be complicated by secondary infection.

Histopathology

- Replacement of dermis by masses of fibroblastic spindle shaped cells which may be arranged in cartwheel or storiform pattern.
- It may invade the subcutaneous fat also.
- CD31 is the marker.

Treatment

- Wide excision.

Histiocytosis X/Langerhans cell histiocytosis (LCH)

* It occurs due to proliferation of Langerhans cells.
* It is a broad spectrum disease with predominant involvement of the skin.

Types

- Acute disseminated LCH is also known as Letterer-Siwe disease and usually occurs in infants. But children or adult are also affected.
- Chronic multifocal LCH, associated with diabetes insipidus, exophthalmos and multiple bony defects. It is also known as Hand-Schuller-Christian disease.
- Chronic focal LCH or eosinophilic granuloma, commonly affects the bones.
- Congenital self-healing reticulohistiocytosis or Hashimoto-Pritzker disease, develops at or just after birth.

Clinical features of acute disseminated LCH

- It is characterized by seborrheic dermatitis like lesions with greasy scales at scalp and mild scaly, discrete, brown or purpuric papules at trunk.
- Lesions may be eroded and crusted at flexural regions. Sometimes nodules develop.
- Rarely vesicular, urticarial or xanthomatous lesions develop.
- Nail beds may be involved.
- Osteolytic lesions of the bones are uncommon except mastoid bone involvement and presents as otitis media.
- Noncutaneous features are pancytopenia, hepatosplenomegaly, persisting aural discharge with deafness, pneumothorax and ascites.
- Associated general features are fever, malaise and failure to thrive.

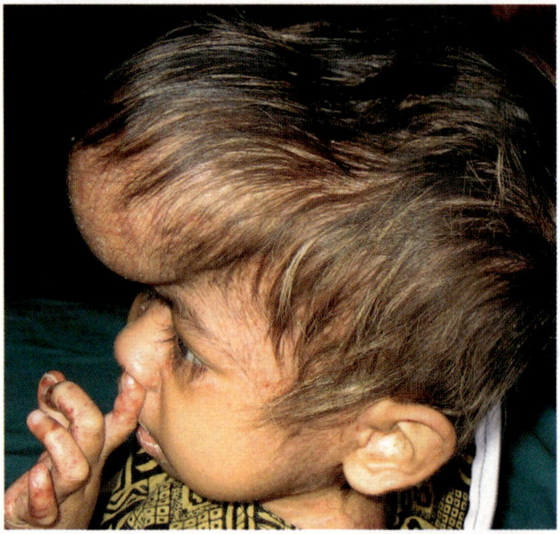

Fig. 18: Frontal bossing and purpuric lesions at fingers

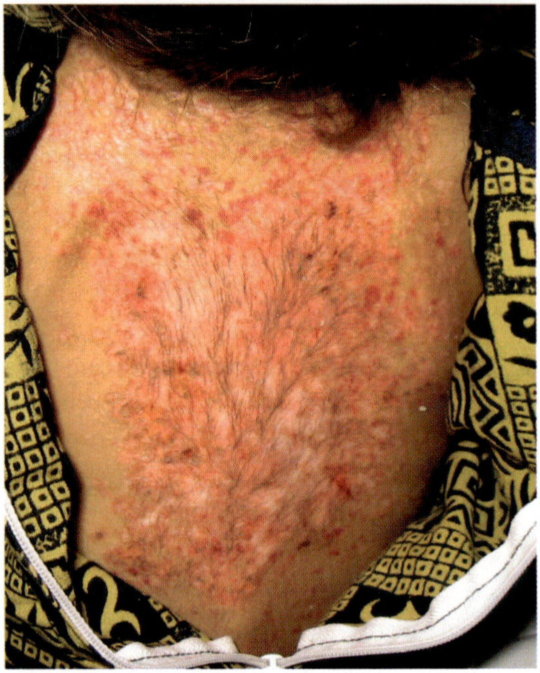

Fig. 19: Crusted and purpuric papules with mild scaling at the back

Differential diagnosis

- Seborrheic dermatitis
- Purpuric allergic contact dermatitis

Histopathology

- Accumulation of large histiocytic cells at upper dermis.
- Cells are having lobulated, bean-shaped or boat-shaped nuclei and pink homogenous cytoplasm.
- Cells are S100 and CD1a positive.

Treatment

- Topical nitrogen mustard.
- PUVA
- Prednisolone (2 mg/kg/day) with chemotherapy containing vinblastin, methotrexate and 6-mercaptopurine.

B-cell lymphomatoid hyperplasia

- The unfortunate term is pseudolymphoma as it is often confused with true lymphomatous infiltrates.
- Dermal infiltration may be of nodular or diffuse pattern.
- It affects superficial dermis, both superficial and deep dermis or predominantly deep dermis including subcutaneous tissue.
- Infiltrate does not destroy the vessels and adnexae. But in some cases hair follicle may be distorted and hyperplastic.
- The hallmark of this entity is formation of true lymphoid follicle.
- Follicle contains lymphocytes with various stages of maturation.
- Lymphocytes may have small and large, cleaved and uncleaved nuclear contours.
- Moreover there may be presence of immunoblasts and macrophages containing basophilic debris at their center, known as tingible body macrophages.

Primary B cell lymphoma

- Follicular centric and marginal follicular type are more indolent.
- Diffuse large cell types are more aggressive and lesion may ulcerate.

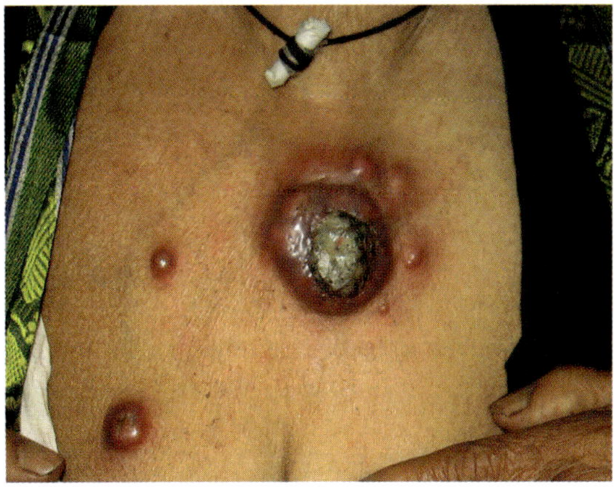

Fig. 20: Erythematous and indurated dome-shaped plaque with central necrotic crater and satellite papules

Differential diagnosis

- Keratoacanthoma
- Metastasis
- Sarcoidosis

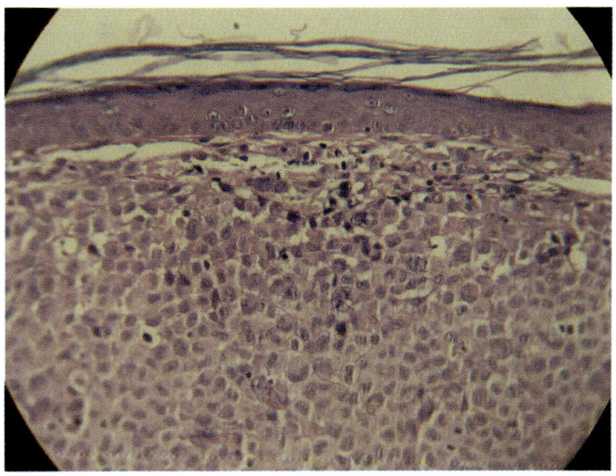

Fig. 21: Diffuse large atypical lymphoid cells in the dermis with presence of grenz zone

Secondary B cell lymphoma

- General symptoms are common including B symptoms, like fever, weight loss and night sweat.

- Other systemic involvement like purpura, hepatosplenomegaly and bone pain.
- Number of the lesions are more.

Follicle centric B cell lymphoma

- Commonest type with indolent course.
- Asymptomatic, red to plum colored single or grouped, papules, plaques and nodules, surrounded by erythema. Lesions rarely ulcerate.
- Site: Scalp, face and neck.

Marginal follicular B cell lymphoma

- Recurrent in nature.
- Asymptomatic, reddish colored, single or cluster, papules, plaques and nodules. Lesions rarely ulcerate.
- Site: Extremities and trunk, mostly upper limb.

Diffuse large B cell lymphoma

- Mostly in female aged more than 60 years are affected.
- Primary lesions are painful plum colored papules, nodules or infiltrated plaques. Lesions may ulcerate.
- Large lesion may be surrounded by satellite lesions.

Kaposi's sarcoma

- It may be sporadic type, endemic type and a type associated with immune deficiency including AIDS.
- Early lesion is presented as a dark-blue or reddish macule and it gradually becomes brownish papule, plaque or nodule.
- Size of the lesion is variable from 5 mm to 3 cm.
- Histopathology
    - Proliferation of capillary spindle cells, replacing dermal collagen tissue and formation of large vascular spaces.
    - Promontory sign may be present.

PART D

MISCELLANEOUS DERMATOSES

DERMATOSES WITH UNIQUE MORPHOLOGY

CHAPTER

D1

Generalized pustular psoriasis

* It may originate on previously quiescent psoriatic plaques or on normal skin.

Clinical features

- There is a dramatic onset of superficial pinpoint to 2-3 mm size pustules. Sheets of such pustules spread to surrounding normal appearing skin with a predisposition at flexurals, webs of the fingers and periungual regions.
- Pustules may be dried up to turn into erythrodermic psoriasis.
- Nails become thickened and separated by subungual lake of pus.
- Mucous membrane sometimes may be affected.
- There is a cyclic remission and relapse for decades.

Differential diagnosis

- Acute generalized exanthematous pustulosis
- IgA pemphigus
- Subcorneal pustular dermatosis

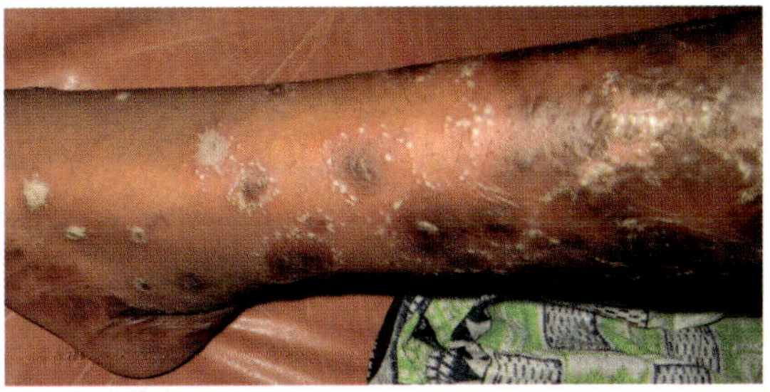

Fig. 1: Pustular lesions at the leg

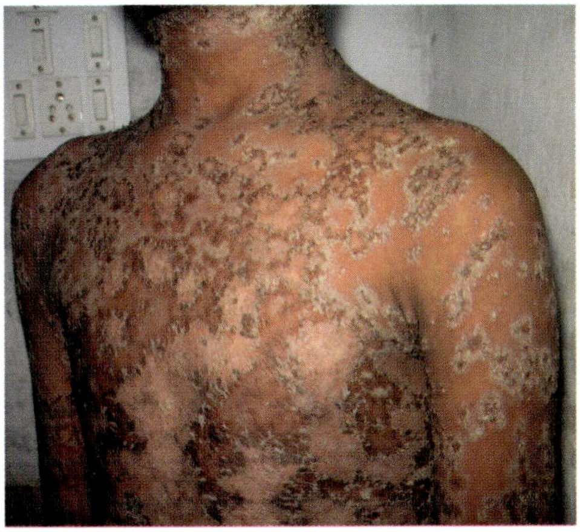

Fig. 2: Generalized pustular lesions

Subcorneal pustular dermatosis (Sneddon-Wilkinson disease)

- It is a form of neutrophilic dermatosis and its exact etiology is not yet clear.
- Pustules are formed due to collection of neutrophils in the epidermis either due to deposition of IgA antibody at intercellular spaces or due to influence of TNFα. In some cases elevated level of TNFα is seen in serum and pustules. Pustules are sterile.
- Sometimes it is associated with monoclonal gammopathy.
- Middle aged females are commonly affected.

Clinical features

- Primary lesions are pustules developing mostly at flexural areas sparing the face and mucosa.
- Intact pustules often show sedimentation at the bottom and clear fluid at the top.
- They evolve into annular or serpiginous crusted erosions.

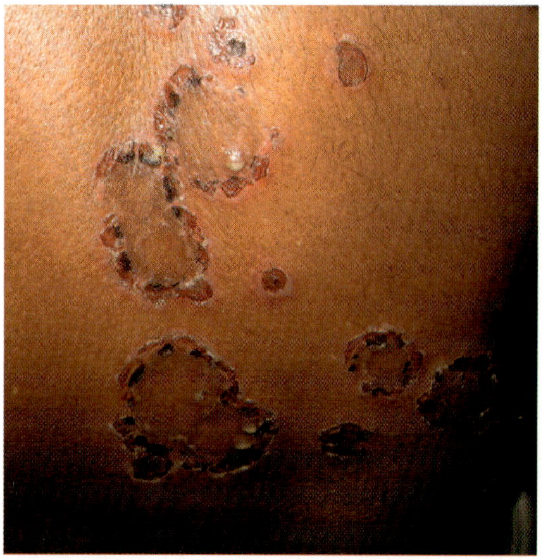

Fig. 3: Pustules spreading in a polycyclic fashion

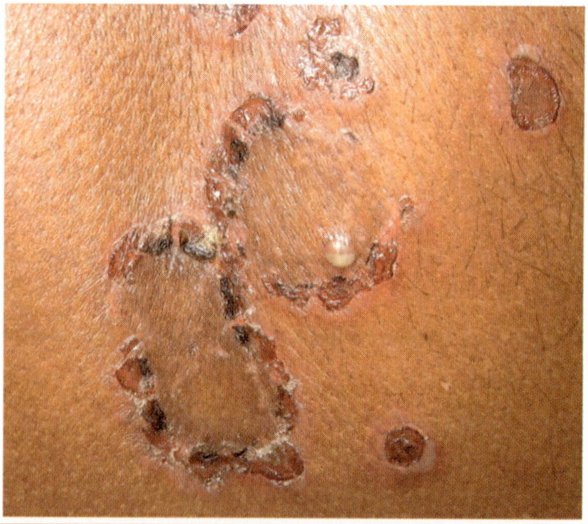

Fig. 4: Typical pustule with a fluid level

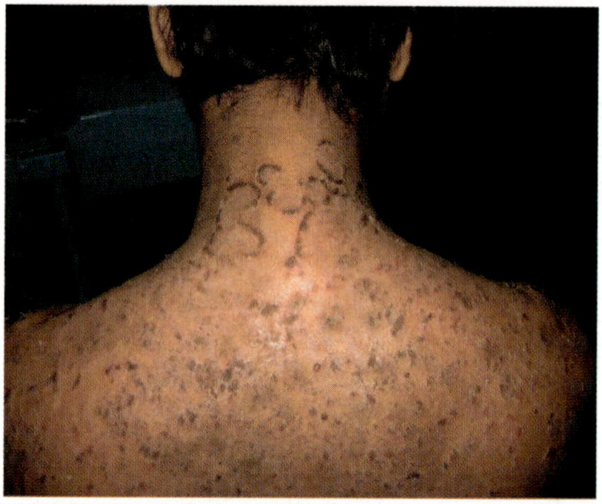

Fig. 5: Generalized crusted erosions with a polycyclic pattern, mimicking tinea corporis

Histopathology

- Subcorneal collection of neutrophils.
- Spongiosis, neutrophilic exocytosis, dilated capillaries at dermal papillae with perivascular mixed inflammatory cells infiltration.
- Sometimes secondary acantholytic cells at the floor of the pustule.

Immunofluorescence

- It is usually negative and in some cases intercellular IgA deposition is seen.

Treatment

- Topical corticosteroid for localized lesion.

- ♦ Dapsone 50-200 mg/day for generalized lesions.
- ♦ Systemic corticosteroid for generalized and resistant cases.

IgA pemphigus

- ✶ This is a pustular form of immunobullous disorder.
- ✶ Clinicopathologically it is of two forms:
  - ♦ Subcorneal pustular dermatosis (SPD) type.
  - ♦ Intraepidermal neutrophilic (IEM) type (Huff syndrome).
- ✶ Sometimes overlapping is seen between the two types.
- ✶ Desmocollin 1 is the main antigen in SPD type and antigen in IEN type is yet to be determined.
- ✶ It affects middle to older aged individuals.

Clinical features

- ✶ SPD type
  - ♦ Primary lesions are pruritic flaccid pustules, developing at erythematous background and affecting the trunk and flexurals.
  - ♦ Usual presenting lesions are crusted annular-erythematous erosions with peripheral flaccid pustules.
  - ♦ When multiple lesions coalesce, a serpiginous or polycyclic pattern is formed. Some of the lesions may be archiform due partial healing from one side.
- ✶ IEN type
  - ♦ Primary lesions are moderately tense pustules with sunflower like arrangement i.e., multiple lesions are arranged like a flower.
  - ♦ Limbs are commonly affected.

Differential diagnosis

- ♦ Bullous impetigo
- ♦ Subcorneal pustular dermatosis

Histopathology

- ✶ SPD type
  - ♦ Collection of neutrophils at subcorneal level.
  - ♦ Minimal acantholysis.
- ✶ IEN type
  - ♦ Intraepidermal collection of neutrophils.

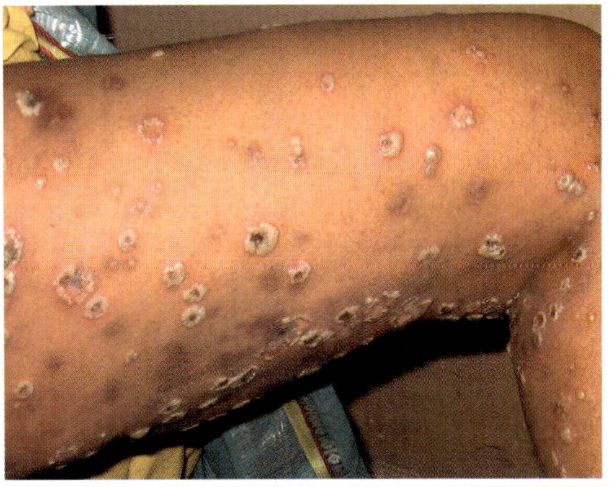

Fig. 6: Multiple pustules with central collapse and peripheral rim of pus

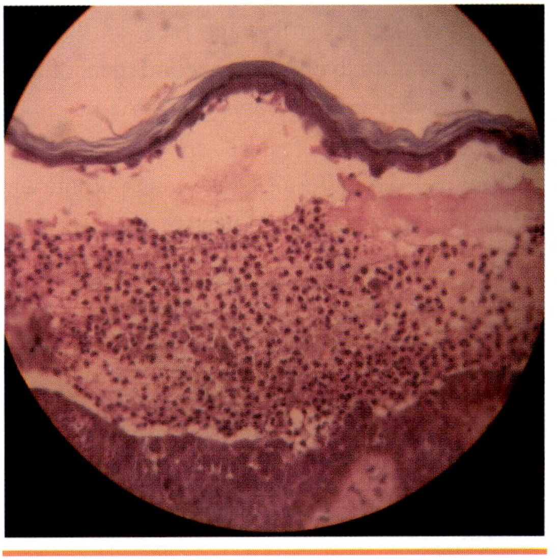

Fig. 7: Subcorneal cleft with neutrophilic infiltration

Immunofluorescence (IF)

- ✶ Direct IF
  - ♦ Deposition of IgA antibody at intercellular spaces throughout the epidermis.
  - ♦ Complement and other antibodies are usually absent.
- ✶ Indirect IF
  - ♦ Positive in 50% cases.

Acute generalized exanthematous pustulosis (AGEP)

- Sudden onset of ill defined erythematous and edematous patches, studded with numerous tiny pustules.
- Drugs is the commonest cause, seen in 90% cases, followed by enterovirus infection.
- High grade fever is often associated with the eruptions but sometimes before or after the onset.

Clinical features

- Symptoms are pruritus and burning sensations.
- Lesions develop within 48 hours of drug ingestion and present as nonfollicular pustules with size less than 5 mm in diameter.
- These initially affect the face, axillae and groins. Gradually they become generalized and may even affect mucosal surfaces.
- Other cutaneous features are vesicles/bullae, erythema multiforme like lesions, purpura and edema of the face and hands.

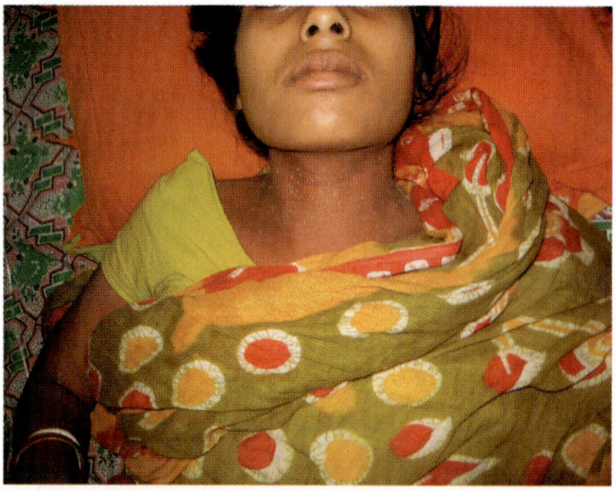

Fig. 8: Nonfollicular pustular eruptions

- Positive patch test with the offending drug is seen in 80% cases.
- Lesions subside within 1-2 weeks following withdrawal of the offending drug.

Histopathology

- Subcorneal spongiform pustules, containing neutrophils and eosinophils.
- Sometimes necrosis of keratinocytes is present.
- Profound papillary dermal edema and vasculopathy are seen. Sometimes true vasculitis may be present.

Treatment

- Topical steroid, emollient and rarely systemic steroid are required.

DRESS syndrome

- The term stands for drug reaction with eosinophilia and systemic symptoms.

Clinical features

- Edema of the face is the hall mark.
- Morbilliform eruptions appear with an edematous background and are associated with follicular accentuation.
- Vesicles and bullae may develop.
- Gradually lesions turn into pustules.
- Pustules may be both follicular and nonfollicular.
- Few purpuric lesions may also be seen.
- Sometimes erythroderma develops.
- Common sites are face, upper trunk and extremities.

Erythema toxicum neonatorum

- It represents probably a transient graft-versus-host reaction, occurring in full-term baby within few days of life.

Clinical features

- Initially it develops as multiple blotchy erythematous macules which gradually become studded with numerous tiny papules or pustules. It involves face, trunk and limbs, sparing the palms and soles.

- Spontaneous recovery is expected within 3 days, followed by exfoliation. But sometimes may persist upto 6 weeks and even may recur.

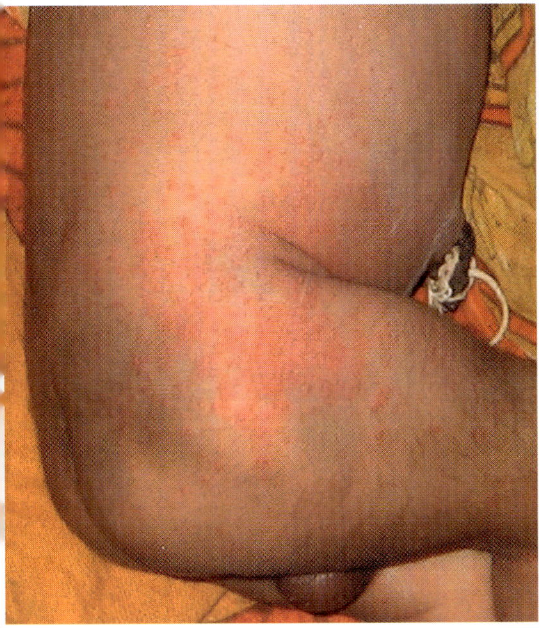

Fig. 9: Micropapulopustular eruptions with an erythematous back ground in a neonate

Miliaria

* This is very common dermatosis of eccrine sweat apparatus.
* It is related to hot and humid climate when excessive sweating occurs. This history is often revealed by the patients.
* Patients are habituated to do self-treatment, such as application of cold water, ice, antiseptic lotions and deodorant powder.
* Application of antiseptic solution often produces irritant contact dermatitis.
* Blockage of the sweat duct is the sole pathology; but how this blockage occurs that is not yet clear.
* Depending on the level of the blockage, clinical features develop.

Types

- Miliaria crystalina/sudamina: Due to blockage of the duct at the corneal layer.
- Miliria rubra/prickly heat: Due to blockage of the duct at spinous layer.
- Miliaria profunda: Due to subbasal or deeper blockage of the duct.

Variants of miliaria rubra

- Miliaria pustulosa: It occurs when polymorphs appear excessively.
- Miliarial dermatitis: It occurs when mononuclear cells appear excessively.

Clinical features

* Miliaria crystalina
  - Lesions are asymptomatic crystal colored tiny vesicles.
  - It occurs mostly at upper trunk, specially at occluded area in a bed-ridden person.
  - It also occurs following a very high fever.
  - Lesions resolve spontaneously after few days with scaling and dryness.
  - Usually patients do not seek any consultation from dermatologist.
* Miliaria rubra
  - Lesions are erythematous tiny papules or papulovesicles with or without few papulopustules.
  - Lesions are intensely pruritic and patients are often compelled to consult dermatologist.
  - Forehead, outer arms and upper back are commonly affected; but any area may be involved.
* Miliaria profunda
  - Lesions are asymptomatic firm papules.
  - They resolve within few hours to days by exfoliation.
* Miliaria pustulosa
  - Monomorphic impetigo like pustules develop with an erythematous halo.
  - Patients often feel mild burning sensation.

- Commonest sites are infra-axillary areas of the trunk, inner side of the thighs and infra-mammary regions.
- Lesions closely mimic candidiasis and impetigo.

★ Miliarial dermatitis

- It commonly occurs in patient having an atopic background.
- Erythematous tiny papules and papulovesicles often become confluent and they coalesce.
- Mild oozing may be present and definitely patient feel severe pruritus and seek consultation from dermatologist.

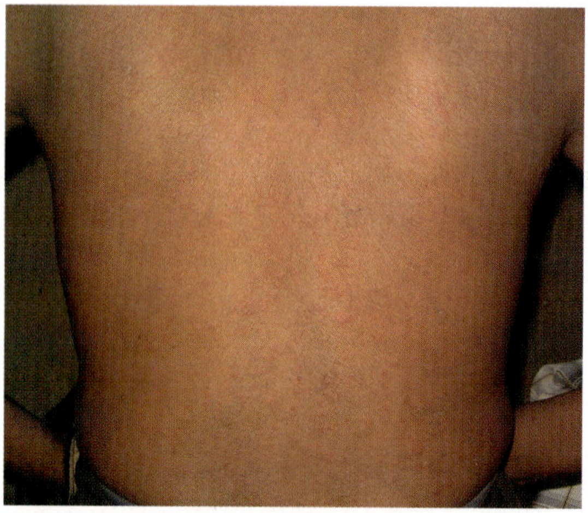

Fig. 10: Tiny erythematous papules and papulovesicles at the back

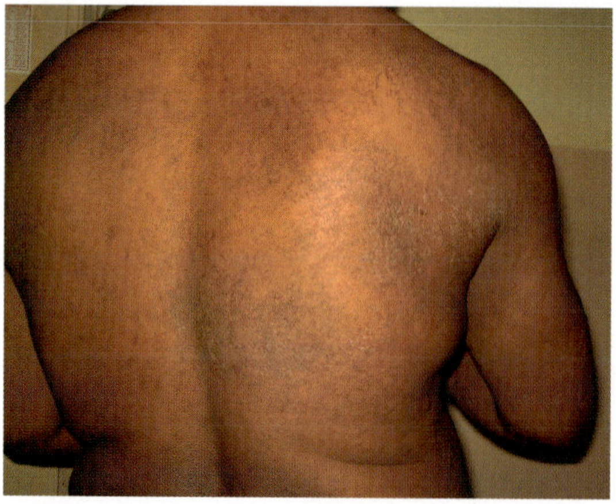

Fig. 11: Post-miliarial exfoliation

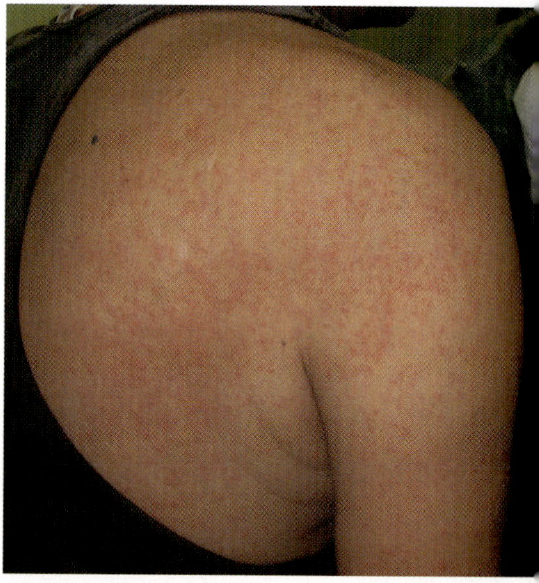

Fig. 12: Erythematous tiny papules of miliaria rubra

Differential diagnosis

- Measles
- Drug eruption
- Viral exanthem.

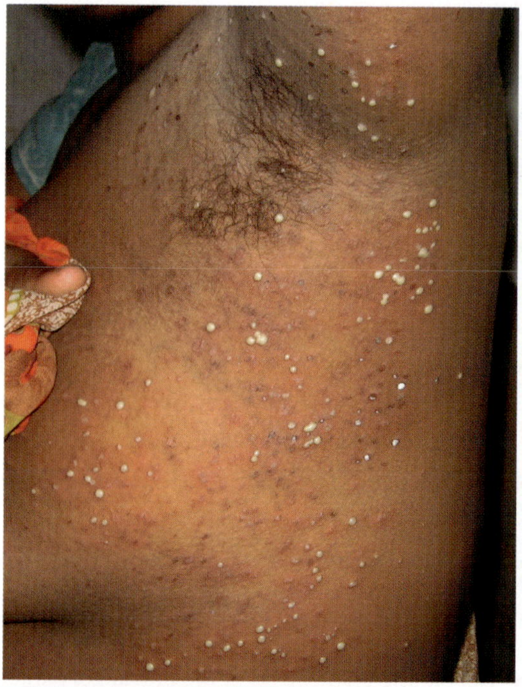

Fig. 13: Pustular miliaria

Differential diagnosis

- Cutaneous candidiasis
- Bullous impetigo
- Acute generalized exanthematous eruptions (AGEP)
- Pustular psoriasis.

Treatment for symptomatic miliaria

- Cold sponging
- Residing in an air-conditioned environment with low humidity.
- Systemic corticosteroid for miliarial dermatitis.

Roseola infantum/Exanthem subitum/ sixth disease

- It is caused by herpes virus-6 (HHV-6); but HHV-7 also may cause the disease. Both the viruses are lymphotropic and replicate within CD4+ T cells.
- Viral shedding from respiratory secretion and inhalation by close contacts, causes the disease.
- It primarily affects infants and toddlers.
- Neurological involvement may be present.
- Viruses enter into a latency phase within salivary glands and peripheral mononuclear cells.
- Viral reactivation occurs following immunosuppression.

Clinical features

- Development of diffuse exanthema during defervescence of preceding high fever (104-105ºF).
- Fever lasts for 3-5 days and it may be accompanied by seizure in 10% cases.
- Exanthem consists of rose pink macules and papules, distributed at trunk, neck, proximal extremities and occasionally at face.
- An enanthem develops with red papules at soft palate and uvula, known as Nagayama's spots.
- Other features are edematous eyelids, injection and edematous eyelids, injection of the tympanic membranes, cervical or occipital lymphadenopathy and bulging of anterior fontanella.
- Neurological features are seizure, encephalitis and aseptic meningitis.

Treatment

- Symptomatic.

Erythroderma

- It is a disease state, characterized by varying amount of erythema, edema and scaling, involving more than 90% of the body surface area.

Causes

- Dermatitis: Seen in 40% cases.
- Psoriasis: Seen in 25% cases.
- Drugs: Seen in 10-15% cases.
- Lymphoma: Seen in 5-10% cases.
- Idiopathic/other causes include pityriasis rubra pilaris, congenital ichthyosiform erythroderma, lichen planus, Norwegian scabies, pemphigus foliaceous, bullous pemphigoid and HIV.

Precipitating factors in psoriatic erythroderma

- Systemic corticosteroids
- Excessive use of potent topical corticosteroids.
- Irritant topical therapy like dithranol.
- Photo- and photochemotherapy.
- Any systemic infection or even emotional stress.

Characteristic features

- Presence of variable degree of itching with feeling of heat and tightness of the skin.
- When it is due to psoriasis, some areas, specially distal parts of the extremities, upper intergluteal fold or scalp may reveal psoriatic plaques. But it may develop without any pre-existing psoriatic lesion.
- Erythema is due to dilated cutaneous blood vessels. Intensity of erythema is variable from patient to patient as well as over a few hours to days in same patient. It is more obvious in

fare skin than dark skin. It is more prominent in drug induced and in psoriatic erythroderma.

- Amount of scale is more prominent in psoriatic erythroderma and eythroderma due to pemphigus foliaceous. Size of the scale may vary from potato chips to <1 mm and its color may be yellowish to white.
- Most cases skin is dry but may be moist and exudative, depending on the intensity of edema of the skin. Edema of the skin is more prominent in dermatitic erythroderma. Due to exudates, scales are converted into crusts. Edema is due to increased cutaneous vasopermeability and due to hypoalbuminemia.
- Postinflammatory hypopigmentation and hyperpigmentation are seen at affected sites in dark skinned patients.
- Alopecia and nail dystrophy or onycholysis may occur due to involvement of hair follicles and nail matrices respectively.
- Lymphadenopathy occurs in 60% cases without any underlying malignancy and hepatomegaly in 20-35% cases. But if splenomegaly is seen, lymphoma must be excluded.
- Dehydration is a major complication due to continuous transepidermal water loss as the cutaneous barrier integrity is lost and so skin looks dry. Normally 400 ml water is lost through the skin per day but remarkably increases in erythroderma.
- Hypoalbuminemia is due to transepidermal leakage of proteins with loss of scales. This leakage of proteins on the surface maintains a healthy environment for the growth of microorganisms.
- Hypoalbuminemia leads to a negative nitrogen balance resulting in muscle wasting.
- Normally 0.5-1 g exfoliated material is lost per day by an adult person from the skin and the body catabolizes 50-60 g protein per day. But in psoriatic erythroderma or in any exfoliative dermatitis an extra 20-30 g of protein is lost through scales.
- Negative nitrogen and potassium balance star when the rate of scaling reached 17 g/sq m day.
- Negative nitrogen balance is also contribute by increased basal metabolic rate. But thyroid function remains normal.
- Imbalanced temperature is manifested a raised skin temperature above 38°C withou evidence of any underlying infection or malignancy. This is due to increased blood flow through dilated blood vessels.
- Total body temperature is lost through radiation and convection. It is clinically manifested as chilling and uncontrollable shivering.
- Hypothermia may occur in extreme cases.
- Tachycardia at rest is due to decreased peripheral resistance of the cardiovascular system as cutaneous vessels are dilated. If it is left untreated patient may undergo cardiac failure.
- Decreased peripheral resistance causes increased renal water conservation resulting in hypervolemia.

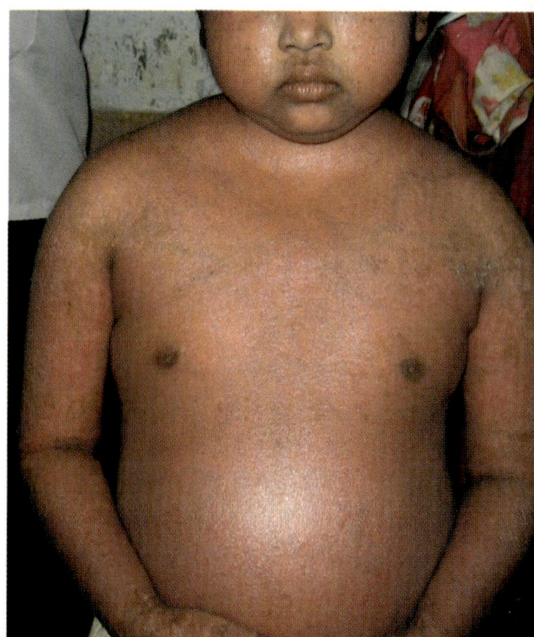

Fig. 14: Generalized erythema and scaling due to drug

Histopathology

- Usually it shows a nonspecific features even in confirmed cases of psoriatic erythroderma.
- In drug induced erythroderma it shows pronounced eosinophils in dermal infiltrates.
- In erythroderma due to mycosis fungoides/ Sezary syndrome, it shows Pautrier's microabscess in the epidermis, epidermotropism without spongiosis and a monotonus band like infiltrate mostly composed of cerebriform-mononuclear cells, specially around the vessels and along the dermoepidermal junction.
- In erythroderma due to dermatitis it shows pronounced spongiosis.

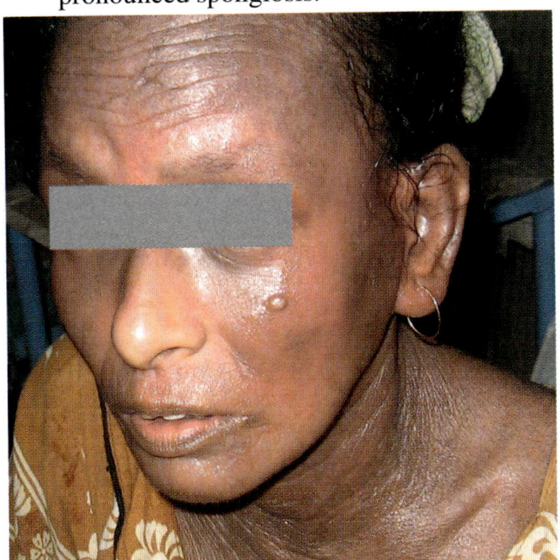

Fig. 15: Generalized erythema and edema but less scaling due to atopic dermatitis

Treatment

- Avoidance of precipitating factors, bed rest, high protein diet and maintenance of fluid, electrolytes and temperature.
- Application of emollient frequently following soaking bath in tepid water to maintain proper hydration and thus to reduce transepidermal losses.
- Use Burrow's solution (12.5% aluminium subacetate)/Condy's compress (potassium permanganate 1:8000 dilution) if oozing is present.
- Antihistaminics for pruritus.
- If response is poor with topical therapies, methotrexate, cyclosporine, acitretin or even PUVA may be used in a case of psoriasis and systemic steroids in other cases if there is no contraindication.
- Antibiotic for any infection.
- Cyclosporine and infliximab are the most rapidly acting agents for the treatment of erythrodermic psoriasis.
- Acitretin and methotrexate are the other first line therapies for erythrodermic psoriasis but work slowly.
- PUVA is also helpful in mycosis fungoides.

Scleroderma

- It is a common connective tissue disorder with increased amount of dermal collagen, including collagen I, III and IV, fibronectin and proteoglycans.
- Female to male ratio is 3-5:1 and commonly affected age group is 30-50 years.

Clinical stages

- Edematous stage: Pitting edema of the fingers is frequently seen.
- Indurated/sclerotic stage: Hard, taut and shiny skin becomes obvious.
- Atrophic stage: Gradual softening of the skin is noted.

Clinical features

- Skin is felt dry and tight, associated with pruritus.
- Microstomia and facial disfigurement with retraction of lips, perioral furrow and beaked nose, are often present.
- Diffuse hyperpigmentation, predominantly present at belt and bra area.
- Focal dyspigmentation contains depigmented macules, sparing perifollicular areas and skin over the superficial veins, appearing as salt

and pepper spots. Dyspigmentation commonly affects upper back, neck and central face, involving both sclerotic and nonsclerotic skin.

- Telangiectasia commonly is seen at lips and palms and appears as matted or squared off macules.
- Hair growth is reduced. But hypertrichosis occurs during resolution.
- Digital ulcers develop due to trauma, ischemia and fibrosis.
- Calcinosis occurs at extremities at near and distal to the joints.
- Digital ulcers are painful, limiting the daily work and leading to osteomyelitis and autoamputation.
- Due to crippled deformities patient may develop depression.
- Pulmonary hypertension and alveolitis lead to pulmonary fibrosis. These changes are diagnosed by bronchoalveolar lavage, pulmonary function test and high resolution CT scan.

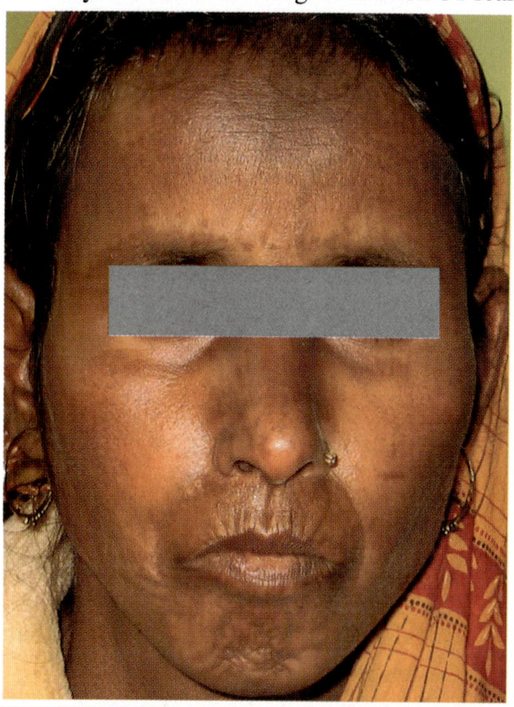

Fig. 16: Presence of radial furrow around the mouth with pinched nose and diffuse hyperpigmentation at face

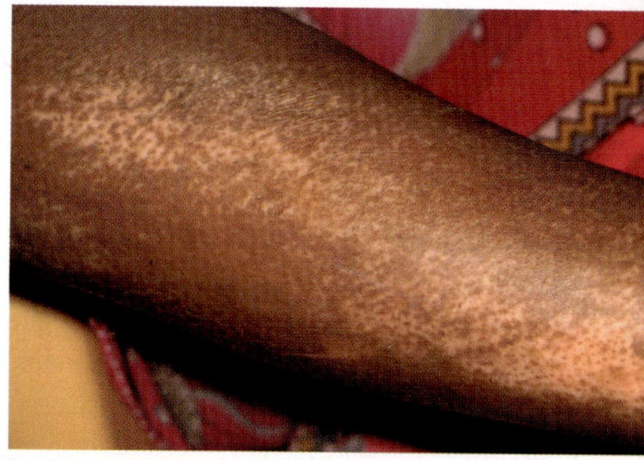

Fig. 17: Hypopigmented macules on indurated skin of the forearm

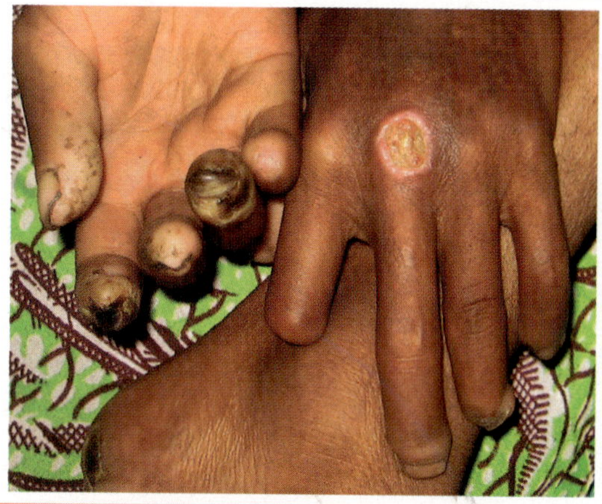

Fig. 18: Deformity of the hands with ulceration

Histopathology

- Increased dermal collagen
- Compact and hyalinized collagen
- Atrophic eccrine and pilosebaceous glands.
- Eccrine glands are trapped by collagen.
- Loss of subcutaneous fat as it is replaced by collagen.
- Sparse lymphocytic infiltration at dermis and subcutaneous tissue.

Antinuclear antibodies

- Nucleolar and speckled patterns.
- Positive anticentromere antibody mostly associated with limited form.
- Antibody to RNA polymerase I and III are associated with diffuse form.

- Positive Scl-70, indicates presence of interstitial lung disease.
- Antifibrillar antibodies become positive in < 10% cases of diffuse form.

Treatment

- D-Penicillamine, an inhibitor of collagen cross-links, is one of the commonly used drugs.
- Azathioprine, methotrexate, chlorambucil, PUVA, etc are used with variable result.
- Ketotifen, a mast cell stabilizer, may be used.
- Relaxin: Increases collagenase activity.
- Epoprostenol/prostacycline: Useful in pulmonary arterial hypertension.
- Bosentan: Endothelin receptor antagonist.
- Sildenafil: Regularises vascular abnormality.
- Sitaxsentan: Endothelin receptor antagonist.
- Anti TGF-B1 monoclonal antibody.
- Anti CTGF (C for collagen).
- Hematopoietic stem cell transplantation.

Diagnostic criteria for diffuse form: Diagnosis required either one major or two minor criteria.

- Major criteria:
  - Symmetric cutaneous sclerosis proximal to metacarpo or metatarsophalangeal joints.
- Minor criteria:
  - Sclerodactyly.
  - Digital pitting or loss of subcutaneous fat from finger pads.
  - Bibasilar pulmonary fibrosis.

Types of scleroderma

- Type 1: Acral scleroderma, involving forearms and arms.
- Type 2: Acral scleroderma, involving arms and trunk.
- Type 3: Involving trunk and face.
- CREST syndrome.
- Limited form: Distal extremities and face are involved.
- Diffuse: Trunk is involved along with limited form.

Relative frequency of various features of diffuse scleroderma

- Arthralgia: 98% cases.
- Sclerodactyly: 95% cases.
- Raynaud's phenomenon: 90% cases.
- Positive ANA: 90% cases.
- Proximal limb weakness: 80% cases.
- Esophageal dysmotility: 80% cases.
- Tendon friction rub: 70% cases.
- Interstitial lung disease: 70% cases.
- Anticentromere antibody: 5-30% cases.
- Anti Scl-70 antibody: 20-60% cases.
- Renal crisis: 20% cases.
- Sicca syndrome: 15% cases.
- Cardiomyopathy: 15% cases.

Relative frequency of various features of limited scleroderma

- Raynaud's phenomenon: 99% cases.
- Sclerodactyly: 90% cases.
- Mat telangiectasia: 90% cases.
- Arthralgia: 90% cases.
- Esophageal dysmotility: 90% cases.
- ANA: 90% cases.
- Anticentromere antibody: 50-90% cases.
- Small bowel involvement: 60% cases.
- Proximal limb weakess: 60% cases.
- Anti Scl-70: 10-15% cases.

Worse prognostic feature

- Male patients
- Black patients
- Late onset
- Trunk involvement
- Internal organ involvement
- High ESR.

Survival rate in diffuse scleroderma

- 5 years: 70% cases.
- 10 years: 50% cases.

Survival rate in limited scleroderma

- 5 years: 90% cases.
- 10 years: 70% cases.

Systemic sclerosis sine scleroderma: Presence of only Raynaud's phenomenon and interstitial lung disease without any skin involvement.

Rat bite ulcer: Painful fingertip ulcer.

Heuck-Gottron sign: Loss of nail cuticle and presence of telangiectasia.

Thibierg-Weissen syndrome: Main feature is calcinosis in extremities.

Sclerodermoid disorders

* Metabolic
    - Porphyria cutanea tarda
    - Diabetes
    - Phenylketonuria
* Reactive
    - Scleredema
    - Scleromyxedema
    - Nephrogenic fibrosing dermopathy
    - Chronic graft vs host disease
    - Toxic oil syndrome
    - Drugs
* Syndromes
    - Stiff skin syndrome
    - Carcinoid syndrome
    - Werner's syndrome
    - POEMS syndrome (polyneuropathy, organomegaly, endocrinopathy, monoclonal gammopathy and skin changes including diffuse pigmentation and hemangioma).

Scleredema

* It is characterized by diffuse induration of the skin due to increased amount of dermal collagen and deposition of mucin.
* Though etiology is unknown, it is often associated with diabetes. Collagen probably becomes irreversibly glycosylated and becomes resistant to degradation by collagenase and thus the amount of collagen increases.
* Other probable causes are excess insulin stimulation, microvascular damage, hypoxia, streptococcal hypersensitivity and paraproteinemia.
* There are three forms depending on presence or absence of preceeding illness or diabetes.

Clinical features

* First type
    - It primarily affects women and sometimes the children.
    - It is preceded by upper and lower respiratory infection with fever and malaise.
    - Suddenly the skin of the face and neck becomes indurated which gradually extends to trunk and proximal parts of the limbs.
    - Face becomes expressionless with difficulty in opening the mouth.
    - Swallowing may be difficult when tongue and pharynx are involved.
    - It usually resolves by few months, ranging from 6 months to 2 years.
* Second type
    - It is not preceded by any illness.
    - It is very subtle in onset but it persists for years.
    - It is often associated with paraproteinemia.
* Third type
    - It commonly affects obese middle aged men.
    - It is associated with insulin dependent diabetes and so, this type is termed as scleredema-diabeticorum.
    - Skin of the posterior neck and upper back is commonly affected.
    - Onset is insidious but persists for long period.
    - Skin becomes erythematous and indurated with peau d' orange appearance.

Histopathology

- Thickened collagen bundles in reticular dermis.

- Separation of collagen bundles due to deposition of mucin, leading to fenestrated appearance of the dermis.
- No increment in the number of fibroblast.
- Reduced elastic fibers.
- Sparse perivascular lymphocytic infiltration.

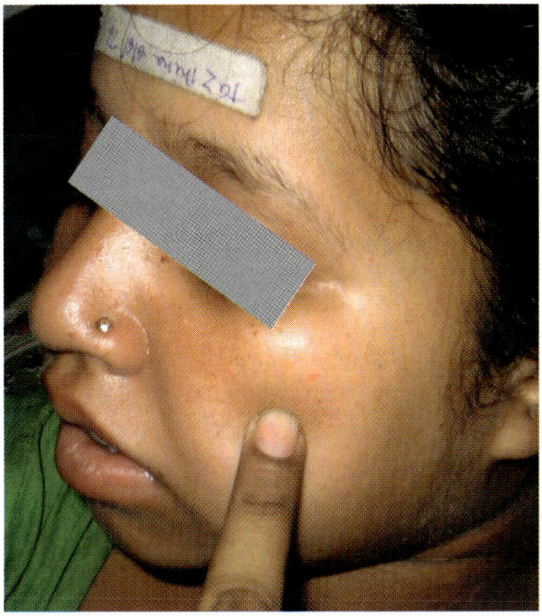

Fig. 19: Smoothly indurated skin with expressionless facies

Treatment

- PUVA
- Dexamethasone-cyclophosphamide pulse therapy
- Cyclosporine

Scleromyxedema

* It is a form of fairly uncommon chronic idiopathic dermatosis characterized by indurated skin due to dermal deposition of mucin and increased amount of dermal collagen.
* Though the exact etiology is not yet clear, an association with monoclonal gammopathy is almost always seen.
* It commonly affects middle aged people, irrespective of sex.

Clinical features

- Lesions start as closely spaced waxy papules of 2-3 mm in size.
- These are strikingly arranged in a linear array.
- Gradually surrounding skin becomes indurated or sclerodermoid with deep longitudinal furrowing.
- Lesions are distributed widely and symmetrically. But mucous membrane and scalp are spared.
- Commonly affected sites are distal parts of the upper limbs, head, neck, trunk and thighs.
- Sometimes skin becomes erythematous and edematous with a brownish pigmentation.
- When the disease progresses skin becomes stiff with development of sclerodactyly and limited joint movement.
- Pruritus may be present.
- General features are dysphagia, peripheral neuropathy, muscle weakness, arthropathy and carpal tunnel syndrome.

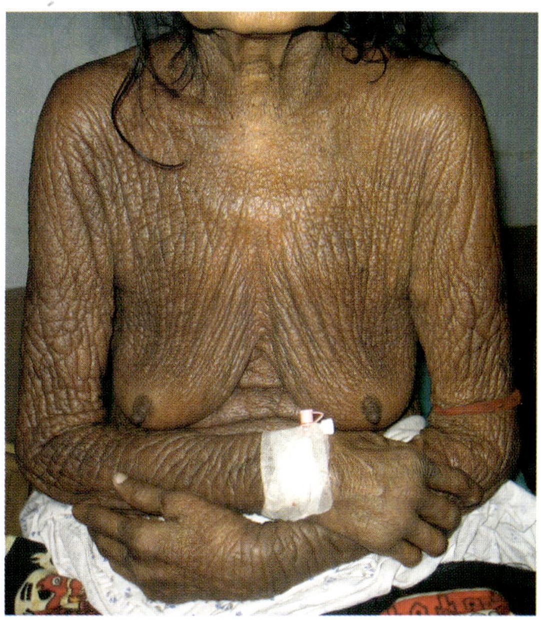

Fig. 20: Generalized thickened skin with closely set papules and deep furrows

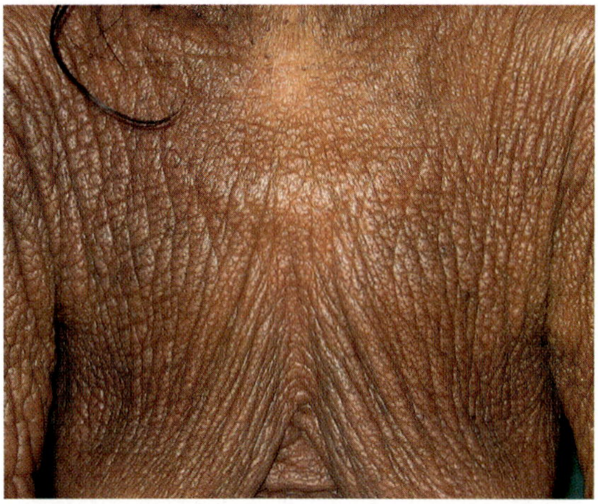

Fig. 21: Closely-set papules in linear array with deep furrows

Differential diagnosis

- Scleroderma
- Scleredema
- Nephrogenic systemic fibrosis.

Histopathology

- Normal or thinned epidermis.
- Diffuse deposition of mucin in the upper and mid reticular dermis.
- Increased amount of collagen.
- Irregularly arranged fibroblasts with marked proliferation.
- Follicular atrophy.
- Mild lymphoplasmacytic perivascular infiltration.

Treatment

- Cyclophosphamide, melphalan and methotrexate.
- Linalidomide and thalidomide
- Bortezomib.
- Dexamethasone.

Nephrogenic fibrosing dermopathy/ Nephrogenic systemic fibrosis

- In 90% cases it is related with dialysis in chronic renal failure but 10% cases never have such treatment.
- It may be due to deposition of gadolinium ions of contrast media or aberrant targeting the tissue by the circulating fibrocytes.

Clinical features

- Ill defined indurated plaque with irregular advancing border as ameboid appearance, distributed symmetrically at limbs and trunk.
- Color of the lesions may be erythematous to brown.
- It may be associated with joint contracture and calciphylaxis.
- Scleral plaque may be seen with sclerosis of the internal organs.

Chronic graft vs host disease

- It develops in more than 50% cases of allogenic transplant recipients who survive more than 100 days.
- It is a frequent complication of allogenic hematopoietic stem cell transplantation.

Clinical features

- Early stage
  - It is characterized by erythematous or violaceous papules and plaques.
  - Commonly affecting sites are dorsa of the hands and feet, forearms, and trunk. But may be generalized also.
  - Individual lesion is less angulated than lichen planus.
  - Lesions often waxe and wane.
  - Oral mucosa may be affected with lacy whitish lesions.
  - Salivary glands are frequently affected and are presented like Sjogren's syndrome.
- Late stage
  - Initially morphoea-like focal sclerotic plaques are formed, followed by generalized sclerotic change as scleroderma.
  - Morphoea-like stage is reversible and it is very essential to diagnose at this level.

- Poikilodermatous changes may be seen at face and trunk.
- Other features are subacute LE-like eruptions, scarring alopecia, multiple hemangiomas and nodular fibromas.
- Occasionally muscle weakness, pain and contracture are present.
- Sometimes fasciitis develops at lateral trunk and extremities.

Histopathology

* Lichenoid lesion
  - Hyperkeratosis, irregular hypergranulosis and mild acanthosis.
  - Vacuolization of the basal layer.
  - Apoptotic keratinocytes with formation of colloid bodies.
* Late stage
  - Dermal band like infiltration.
* Sclerodermoid lesions
  - Epidermal atrophy
  - Dermal fibrosis.

Stiff skin syndrome

* It may be congenital or may develop in early childhood.
* Probably it is caused by disturbance in organization of the dermal collagen and glycosaminoglycans of the dermal extracellular matrix.
* Rock hard indurated skin is seen at thighs and buttocks, sparing the inguinal folds, hands and feet.
* Mild hypertrichosis is seen on affected areas.
* It is slowly progressive.
* Restricted movement of the hip and knee joints may be noticed.
* Histopathology shows giant amianthoid-like collagen fibers.

Morphea

* It is a localized form of dermal sclerosis.

Clinical features

- It is characterized by indurated and hyper-/hypopigmented or brown colored plaque.
- Center in some of the lesion may be slightly or grossly depressed. Grossly depressed lesion is termed as en coup de sabre which commonly affects the forehead.
- Along with hair loss and sweat loss, there may be slight sensory impairment which then closely mimicks borderline tuberculoid leprosy.
- Any site may be affected, such as trunk and limbs.
- Surface is usually smooth and shiny.
- Shape of the lesion is variable such as oval, round, linear or bizarre.

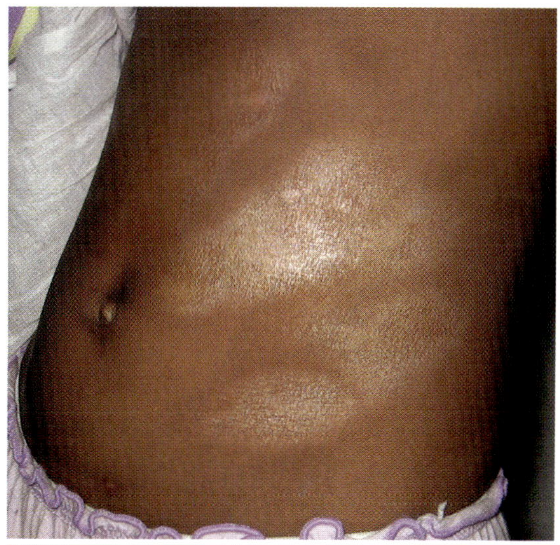

Fig. 22: Indurated plaques with mottled hypopigmentation

Differential diagnosis

- BT leprosy
- Lichen sclerosus et atrophicus
- Pityriasis rotunda.

Histopathology

- Normal or atrophied epidermis.
- Thickening of the dermis with degenerated, homogeneous and eosinophilic collagen fibrils at papillary dermis.
- Coarse and dense collagen at reticular dermis, engulfing the subcutaneous fat.
- Loss of dermal appendages and subcutaneous fat.

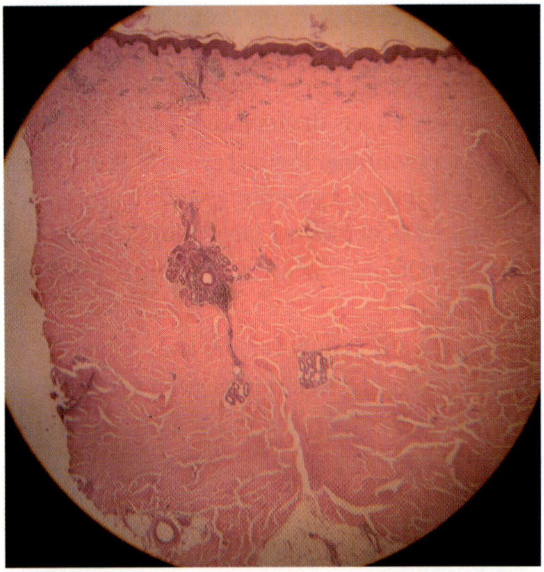

Fig. 23: Thinned out epidermis with grossly thickened dermis

Treatment

- No curable treatment is available.
- Only progression of the lesion may be halted by giving intralesional triamcinolone injection at the border, with concentration of 10 mg/ml and 0.1-0.3 ml/site at every 3-4 weeks interval.

Lichen sclerosus et atrophicus (LSA)

- It is a chronic atrophic disorder affecting both male and female genitalia as well as skin of the other areas.
- Though it commonly occurs in adult but also occurs in children 1-12 years of age.
- Females are commonly affected and the ratio between female and male is about 10:1.
- Nongenital LSA is usually asymptomatic but genital lesions may be symptomatic with pruritus, burning sensation, pain, dysuria, dyspareunia and recurrent balanitis.
- Course of the disease waxes and wanes and spontaneous resolution usually occurs in girls.
- Squamous cell carcinoma may develop in vulval and penile lesions.

Clinical features

- Genital, specially vulval lesion is extremely pruritic and nongenital cutaneous lesion is not pruritic.
- It starts as ivory white or porcelain white sharply defined papules.
- Lesions gradually coalesce to form larger plaque.
- Though the lesions are initially elevated but gradually become flattened as normal skin and even depressed at places.
- Surface of the lesion, usually have dilated pilosebaceous orifices, studded with keratin plugs, known as follicular plugging and dilated sweat duct orifices, studded with keratin plugs, known as dells.
- When these plugging are profuse, lesion becomes verrucous.
- Purpura and telangiectasia may be present and often help in diagnosis.
- Lesions may be eroded and sometimes frank bulla may be formed.
- Vulval lesion often becomes eroded and macerated and in later stage it becomes atrophic and shrunken. When vulval lesion extends towards the perineum, it takes a figure of 8 appearance.
- Clitoris, labia minora and vaginal orifice are notoriously affected. Labia majora and minora may be fused and vaginal introitus is reduced in size.
- In uncircumcised male, prepuce is first affected, becomes sclerotic and it can not be retracted as in phimosis. When glans is affected, it appears as mother of pearl with purpuric lesions and urethral orifice is reduced.

Histopathology

- Initially hypertrophy of the epidermis, followed by atrophy in late stage with follicular plugging or dell.
- Homogeneous and edematous papillary dermis, sometimes cleft formation.

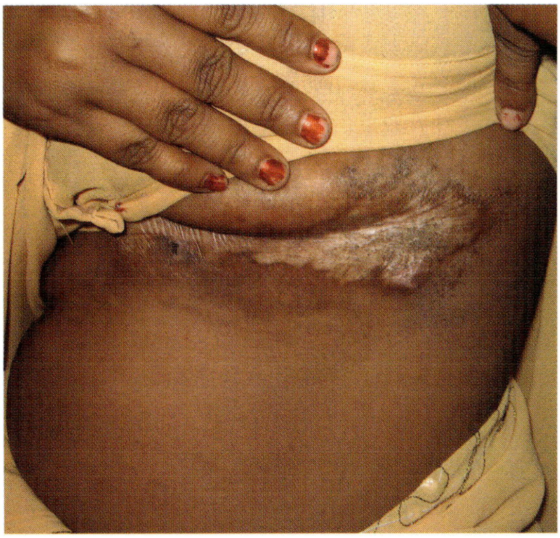

Fig. 24: Whitish indurated plaque with follicular plugs and irregular hyperpigmentation

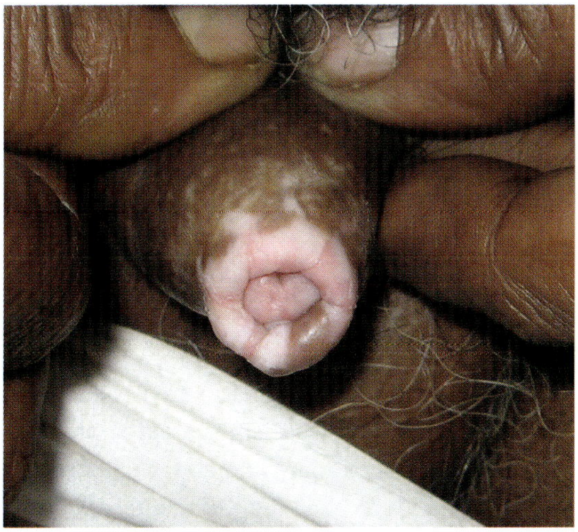

Fig. 25: Thickening and tightening of the prepuce, and whitening of the prepuce and glans

Treatment

- Application of potent topical glucocorticoid preparations like clobetasol propionate or halobetasol for 6-8 weeks only.
- Topical tacrolimus and pimecrolimus.
- Topical androgens.
- Systemic hydroxychloroquine, 200 mg/day for weeks to few months.
- Circumcision for phimosis.

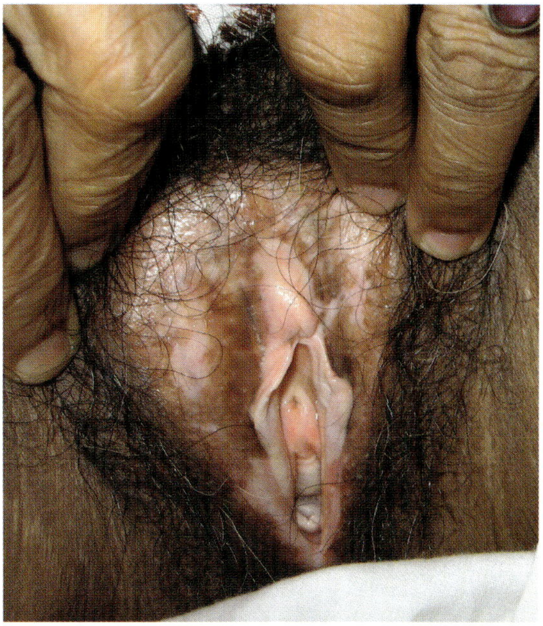

Fig. 26: Depigmented, indurated and atrophic vulval skin

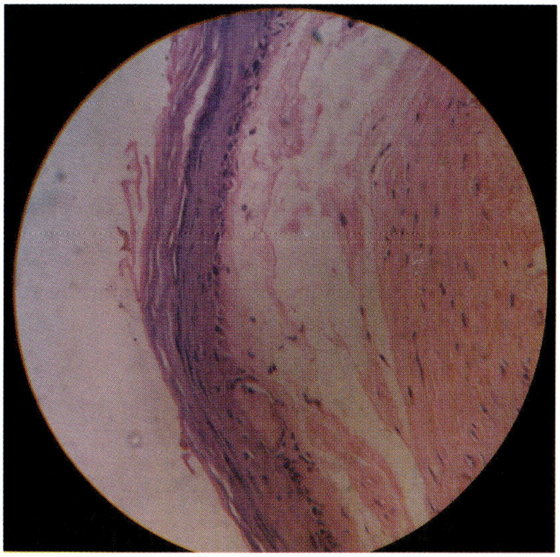

Fig. 27: Hyperkeratosis with homogenization of the reticular dermis

Sclerema neonatorum

- Wax like tight, cold and indurated skin in premature infant.
- Diffuse rapidly spreading non-pitting hardening of subcutaneous fat in first few days of life.

- Baby is cyanotic at birth with difficulty to maintain temperature.
- Histopathology shows lipid crystal as needle-like cleft in routine processing. There is little evidence of fat necrosis in most cases, rather increased thickening of subcutaneous fat, increased size of fat cells and rarely presence of giant cells.

Lipodystrophy

Acquired generalized lipodystrophy

- Onset is childhood or adolescence with male-famale ratio 1:3.
- Fat is lost from face, arms, legs, palms and soles, sparing fat of the eye and bone marrow.
- It is often associated with acanthosis nigricans and voracious appetite.
- It may be associated with juvenile dermatomyositis, diabetes mellitus and hepatic steatosis.

Lipodystrophia centrifugalis abdominalis infantilis

- It occurs in children with onset at age of 3 years and male-female ratio is 1:2.
- Depressed areas due to loss of fat are predominantly seen at groin in 80% cases and axillae in 20% cases.
- Lesion is surrounded by an erythematous ring with mild scaling and is associated with regional lymphadenopathy.
- Individual lesion extends centrifugally for 3-8 years and stops at puberty. When expansion stops, erythematous ring and lymphadenopathy disappear.

Lipoatrophia annularis

- Females are more affected than males and upper limbs are commonly involved.
- Lesion starts as an annular erythematous swollen ring like a bracelet. Gradually whole limb becomes tender and the ring becomes atrophic due to loss of fat. This constriction ring divides the limb into two parts. The depth of the ring may be 2 cm which is often more than breadth. It may persist for 20 years.
- Lesion may be preceded by arthralgia and accompanying pain at the limb.

Localized lipodystrophy

- It occurs after 6 months to 2 years at the site of insulin injection.
- Children and females are more affected than males.
- Lesions are mostly atrophic rarely hypertrophic.
- It improves when nonhuman insulin is replaced by human insulin.

HIV associated lipodystrophy

- It occurs during non-nucleoside antiretroviral therapy.
- These drug also inhibits γDNA polymerase of mitochondria leading to adipocyte apoptosis.
- Accumulation of fat is seen at neck, upper back and abdomen.

Atrophoderma

- This is a disease of unknown etiology, occurring between 2nd to 3rd decade of age.

Clinical features

- Lesions are asymptomatic areas of slightly depressed skin with slight gray color, without any other surface changes. Centers of the old lesions are felt slightly indurated.
- Size of the lesion varies from 1-10 cm.
- Margin of the lesion is sharply demarcated by irregularity and shows a cliff-off pattern mostly due to an optical effect of the slate gray color.
- Lesions are distributed bilaterally and symmetrically at back of the trunk.
- Histopathology of an early lesion shows slight nonspecific lymphocytic infiltration and some thickening of collagen.
- Histopathology of old lesion shows no inflammatory infiltrate and thickened, tightly packed

and hyalinized collagen bundles at deeper layer.

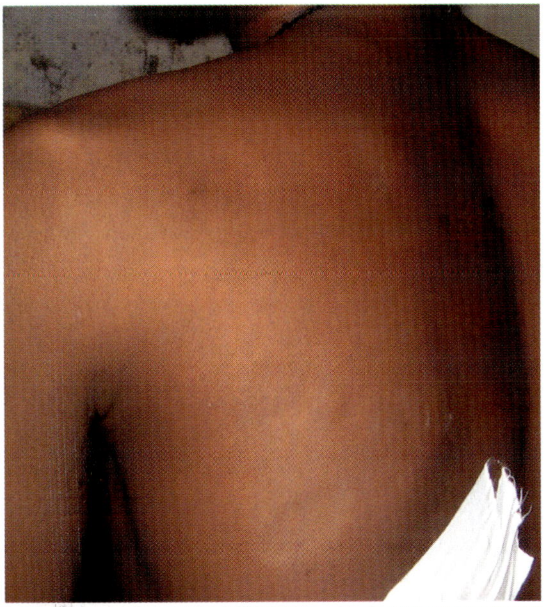

Fig. 28: Multiple depressed plaques at back

Anetoderma

- It is characterized by focal dermal defect of elastic tissue due to an unknown etiology and affects the young adults.
- It may be primary, secondary and familial.

Types of primary anetoderma

- Jadassohn-Pellizzari type, where inflammation preceeds the lesion.
- Schweninger-Buzzi type, where no inflammation precedes the lesion.

Causes of secondary anetoderma

- Secondary syphilis, tuberculosis, leprosy, HIV, varicella and molluscum contagiosum.
- Sarcoidosis, granuloma annulare, lichen planus, prurigo nodularis, urticaria pigmentosa, porphyria, scleroderma, discoid or systemic lupus erythematosus and antiphospholipid syndrome.
- Pilomatricoma, dermatofibroma, involuted infantile hemangioma, juvenile xanthogranuloma and melanocytic nevi.
- B-cell lymphoma, plasmacytoma and cutaneous lymphoid hyperplasia.
- Drugs like penicillamine.

Clinical features

- Primary lesions are circumscribed areas of flaccid and slack skin, which may be elevated as sack like protrusions or macular lesions or depressed lesions.
- Color of the lesions may be skin-color in dark complexion and blue-white in fair complexion. Some lesions may coalesce.
- Surface of the lesion is usually normal but may be wrinkled.
- Buttonhole sign is positive as in neurofibroma. Examining finger sinks into the lesion with feeling of a distinct margin like a hernia ring and bulge of the lesion reappears when finger is withdrawn.
- Number of the lesions varies from few to hundreds and size of the lesions varies from 1-2 cm in diameter.
- Common sites are chest, back, neck and upper extremities.
- Histopathology shows normal elastic tissue in early lesion but reduced or absent in old lesion. Elastophagocytosis may be present.

Darier disease

- It is an autosomal dominant disorder, with a chronic course and without any spontaneous remission.
- Course of the disease is fluctuating which often deteriorates and rarely improves.
- It occurs due to mutation of ATP2A2, encoding SERCA2 (endoplasmic reticulum Ca^{2+} ATPase) and results in dysfunction of intracellular Ca^{2+} mediated signaling.
- This causes impairment of junctional proteins (desmoplakin), leading to acantholysis.
- It starts between the age of 6-20 years in most of the cases with a peak age group 11-15 years.

- It is associated with moderate itching.
- Presence of foul smell leads to social isolation.
- Secondary infection often complicates the papillomatous lesions.
- Aggravating factors
  - Summer season
  - Sweating
  - Heat
  - Occlusion
  - Lithium
  - Infection

Variants

- Acral hemorrhagic type: Irregularly shaped blue-black sharply defined macules present at palms, soles and dorsal aspects of the hands as an additional finding. Color of the lesions is due to hemorrhage in the vesicles.
- Segmental type 1: Lesions are unilateral, along Blaschko's lines.
- Segmental type 2: Lesions are generalized with a streaky pattern.

Clinical features

- Primary lesions are keratotic dirty papules, developing at seborrheic areas.
- Lesions often become confluent and coalesce to form papillomatous plaque.
- Some of the lesions become crusted and macerated, specially at axillae, groin and perineal area.
- Color of the lesion may be reddish or brown.
- Common sites are scalp, trunk, face, lateral sides of the neck, axillae, inframammary regions, groin and perineal area.
- Lesions are usually follicular; but not always.
- Hypomelanotic macules of 2-3 mm in size along with keratotic papules are also present.
- Rarely sterile vesicles or bullae are seen.
- In 50% cases skin colored or brownish flat papules are seen at the dorsa of the hands and feet.
- Keratotic papules and keratin filled depressed papules are present at palms and soles. Palmar print shows subtle lesions by disruption of dermatoglyphic pattern.
- Whitish painless palatal papules are seen and appear as cobble stone. Buccal mucosa, gingiva and tongue are also affected.
- Nails show longitudinal red and white bands, longitudinal ridges and subungual hyperkeratosis.

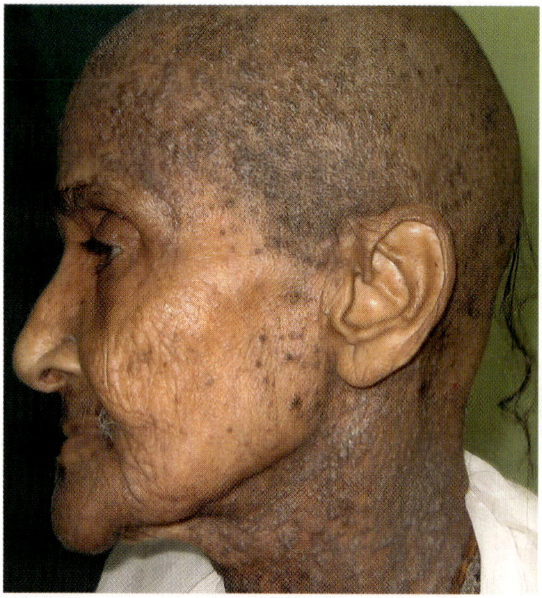

Fig. 29: Keratotic papules at seborrheic areas

Histopathology

- Hyperkeratosis, acanthosis and papillomatosis.
- Formation of dyskeratotic cells, known as corps ronds and grains.
- Suprabasal acantholysis with formation of cleft. It may contain partially keratinized acantholytic cells.
- Formation of villi due to upward protrusion of dermal papillae, lined by single layer of basal cells within the cleft.
- Grains are formed within corneal layer.
- Corps ronds are having central homogeneous basophilic pyknotic nuclei, surrounded by a

clear halo and a basophilic dyskeratotic shell is present at the periphery. In some cases halo may be replaced by homogeneous eosinophilic dyskeratotic material. All these changes make the cells very conspicuous.

- Grains are like larger parakeratotic cells. Nuclei are elongated and grain shaped. Nuclei are surrounded by basophilic or eosinophilic dyskeratotic material.

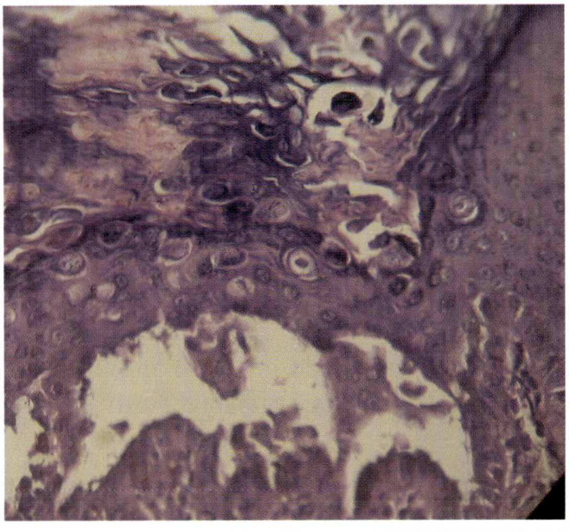

Fig. 30: Superbasal cleft with villi and presence of dyskeratotic cells at upper spinous layer (corp ronds) and at corneal layer (grains)

Treatment

- Topical tretinoin for localized lesions.
- Isotretinoin or acitretin for generalized lesions.

Benign familial pemphigus/Hailey Hailey disease

- It is an autosomal dominant disorder, caused by mutation of ATP2C1, encoding for hSPCA1 protein.
- This hSPCA1 protein is responsible for transport of Ca^{2+} and Mn^{2+} and sequestration of Ca^{2+} in Golgi lumen. Depletion of Ca^{2+} in Golgi, results in impaired processing of cellular junctional proteins and thus acantholysis occurs.
- Initial manifestation is seen in 2nd to 3rd decade; but also seen in 4th to 5th decade.
- Initial lesions rupture easily and very often they are overlooked for a long time.
- Course of the disease is unpredictable.
- Complete remission, followed by exacerbation is a common feature. It is often complicated by secondary bacterial, fungal and viral infection.

Aggravating factors

- Heat and sweating
- Summer seasons
- Staphylococcal, candidal or herpetic infections.

Clinical features

- Primary lesions are flaccid vesicles on normal or erythematous skin.
- Lesions rupture easily, leaving by macerated or crusted erosions.
- Erosions show a tendency to spread at the periphery and produce a crusted circinate border.
- Moist and malodorous vegetative plaques, studded with painful fissures are developed, specially at groin.
- Common sites are intertriginous areas like axillae, groin, perianal region, lateral aspect of neck, lower abdomen and inframammary regions.
- Healing occurs without any scarring but with postinflammatory hyperpigmentation.

Histopathology

- Early lesion shows small suprabasal cleft or lacunae and fully developed lesion shows vesicle or bulla.
- Upward protrusions of dermal papillae, lined by single layer of basal cells within the cleft are known as villi.
- Sometimes, a narrow strand of epidermal cells may protrude downward into the dermis.

- Large portion of viable epidermal cells undergo acantholysis. But cells are not completely detached from each other in comparison to pemphigus vulgaris. This partially detached appearance is known as dilapidated brick wall appearance.

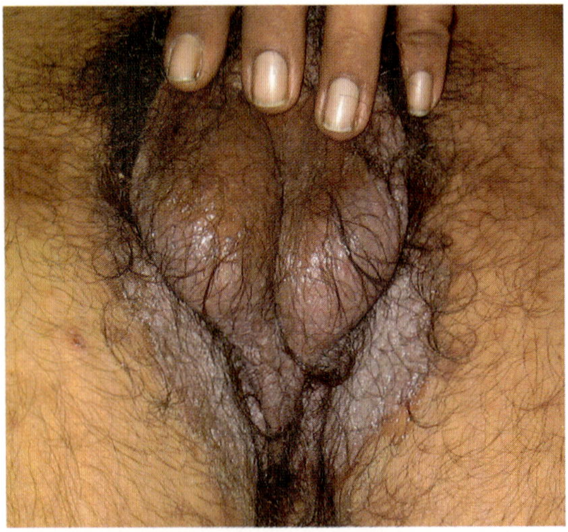

Fig. 31: Vegetative plaques at the groins

Differential diagnosis

- Pemphigus vegetans (Hallopeau type).
- Lymphangioma circumscriptum
- Condyloma lata.

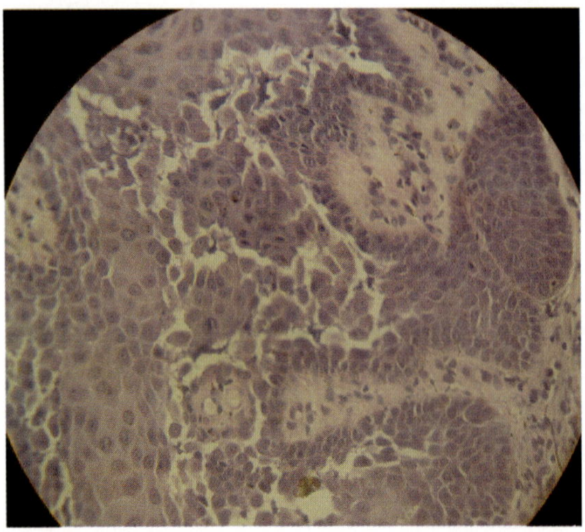

Fig. 32: Suprabasal cleft with irregular, dilapidated masses of keratinocytes

- Some of the partially detached or fully detached epidermal cells undergo premature keratinization to form dyskeratotic cells. They have a homogenized cytoplasm, mimicking corps ronds and grains of Darier's disease.

Treatment

- To control bacterial, fungal and viral infection if present.
- To keep the affected area dry with Condy's compress.
- Systemic therapy shows limited response with prednisolone, cyclosporine, methotrexate and dapsone.

Lichen amyloidosis

* It is a form of cutaneous amyloidosis.

Clinical features

- Lesions are persistent and pruritic, small, hyperpigmented and dirty looking, discrete, keratotic papules, involving mostly shins of the legs.
- Sometimes papules may coalesce to form a plaque.
- Lesions may be generalized.

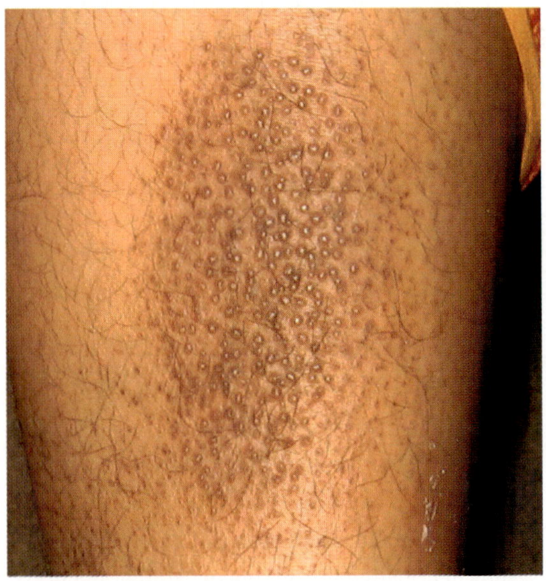

Fig. 33: Brownish papules at the shin

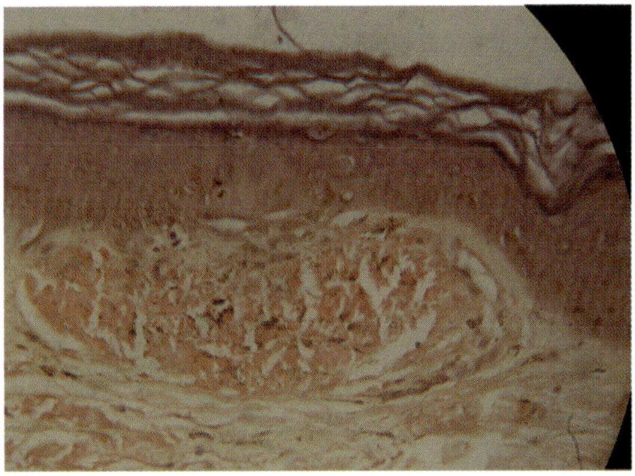

Fig. 34: Deposition of pink material at upper dermis

Histopathology

- Deposition of amyloid at papillary dermis, specially at dermal papillae, with hyperkeratosis and hyperplasia of the epidermis.

Treatment

- Application of topical steroid with salicylic acid preparations and topical retinoids.
- Dermabrasion.

Actinic keratosis

* It commonly occurs in fair skinned people or patient with albinism.

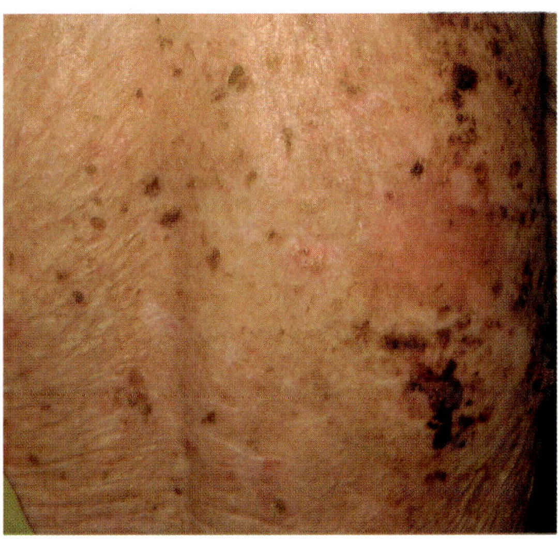

Fig. 35: Hyperkeratotic papules with irregular surface

Clinical fatures

- It initially appears as collection of telangiectatic capillaries of 1-2 mm in size and gradually becomes covered with dry, rough and adherent scales.
- When scales are removed, bleeding points appear, resembling Auspitz sign in psoriasis.
- Common sites are dorsa of the hands, forearms, back, face, upper chest, sides of the neck and ears.

Treatment

- Imiquimod (5%) cream, 5 days in a week for 6 weeks.
- 5-Fluorouracil (5%) twice daily for 3-4 weeks.
- Cryo- or electrosurgery.

Actinic prurigo

* It commonly occurs in young girls and is presented with pruritic, erythematous, excoriated and crusted papules on exposed parts of the body.
* Lesions are aggravated by sunlight.
* Commonly affected sites are face and distal parts of the limbs and relative sparing of proximal parts of the limbs and forehead.

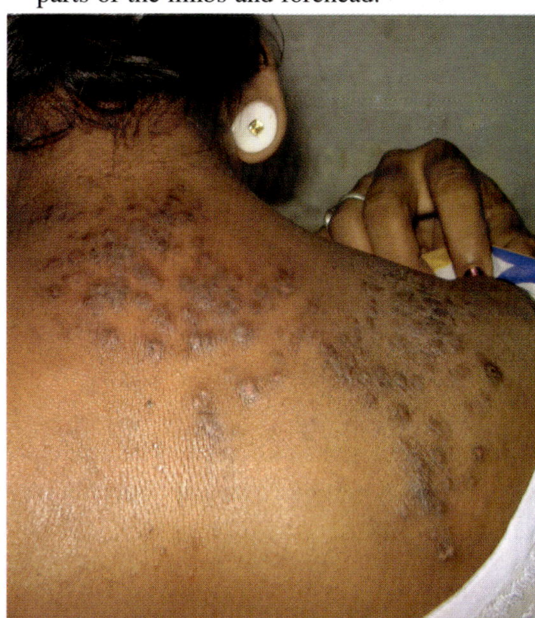

Fig. 36: Excoriated and keratotic papules at upper back

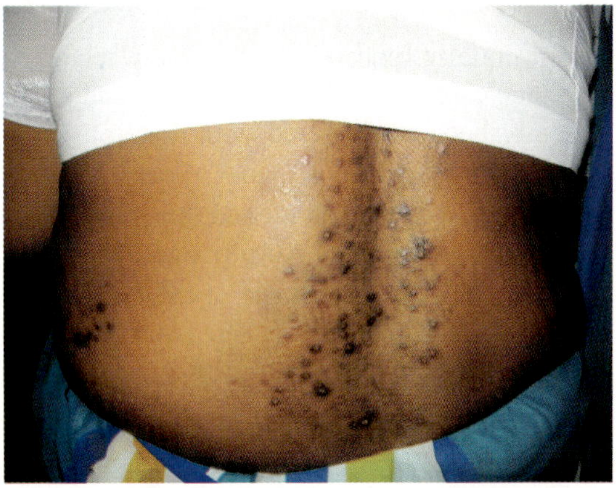

Fig. 37: Excoriated and keratotic papules at lower back

Treatment

- Avoidance of sunlight and application of sunscreen.
- Prophylactic use of UVB or PUVA therapy.
- Topical or intralesional steroid.
- Intermittent thalidomide in a dose of 50-100 mg per day.

Papular urticaria

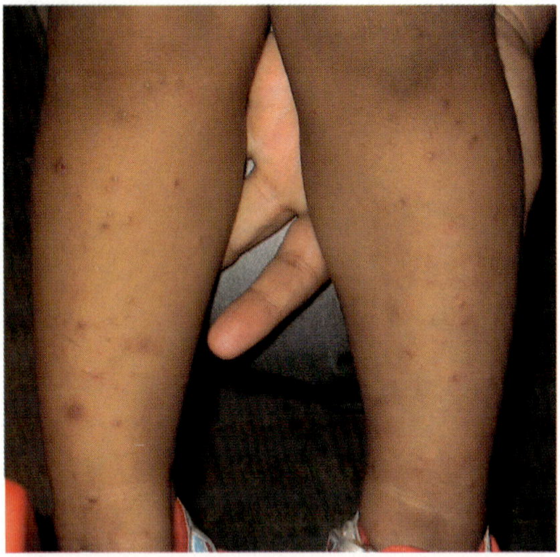

Fig. 38: Papular excoriated lesions at extensor of lower limbs

* This is an extremely pruritic dermatosis exclusively occurring in young children and it is aggravated by insect bite, specially by mosquito.
* Lesions are excoriated papules, involving extensors of both upper and lower limbs, and dorsa of both hands and feet. Trunk and face are relatively spared. Webs of the fingers and toes are also spared.

Pulicosis

- Tiny, red-brown, hard-bodies, wingless insects, are capable of jumping approximately 2 feet.
- Their flattened abdomens allow them to travel through hairs of the hosts.
- They live in floor-mats and bodies of the animals.

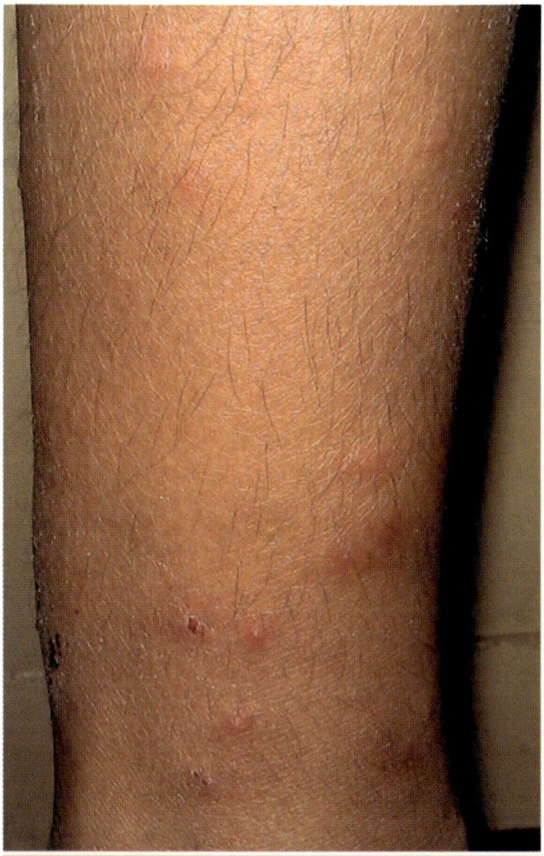

Fig. 39: Erythematous papular eruptions at lateral side of the leg

- They jump on the human body.
- They may spread bubonic plague after feeding from infected rats.
- Erythematous papules with or without cen-

tral punctum of the bite are seen at approachable areas of the fleas like lower legs.

- In a family only one member is usually affected, others are resistant but how still not known.

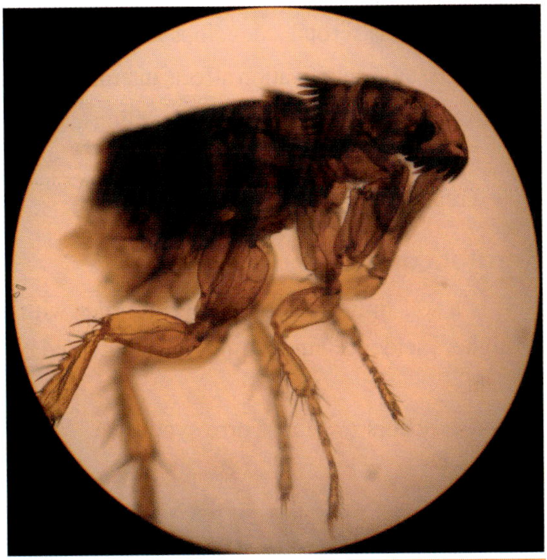

Fig. 40: Picture of the flea

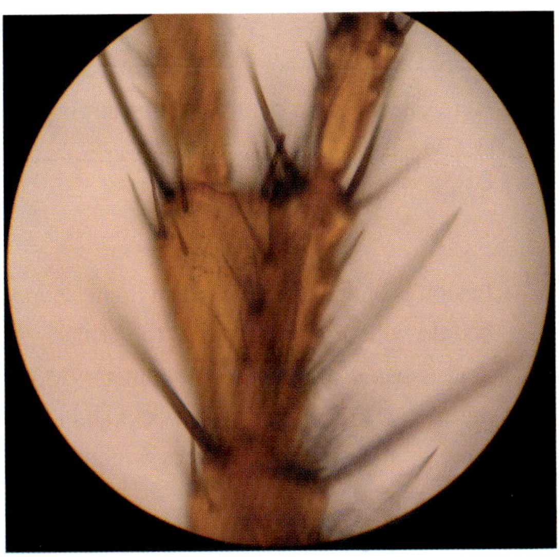

Fig. 41: Cactus-like leg of the flea

Lichen spinulosus

- It is commonly seen along with atopic dermatitis.

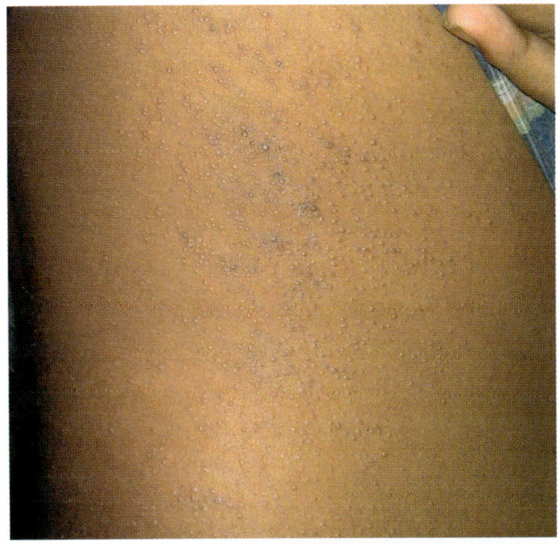

Fig. 42: Discrete spiny tiny papules at trunk

Clinical features

- Numerous asymptomatic round tiny skin-colored or hypopigmented or barely hyperpigmented, dry, spiny papules.
- Lesions are discrete, may be confluent, but never coalesce.
- Trunk and extremities are commonly affected.

Treatment

- Application of emollient.

Papular acrodermatitis of childhood/Gianotti-Crosti syndrome

- It is associated with Hepatitis B infection, but other viruses are also may be responsible. These are cytomegalovirus, Coxsackie viruses, EBV, parvovirus B19 and rotavirus, etc.
- It also may occur following vaccination like MMR, Hemophilus, oral polio, DPT and hepatitis B.
- It occurs predominantly in children between 1-6 years of age.
- Lesions resolve spontaneously by 8-12 weeks with postinflammatory hypopigmentation.

Clinical features

- Prodromal features are fever, cough, rhinorrhea and lymphadenopathy.
- Exanthem consists of erythematous and edematous monomorphous papules. Occasionally lesions may be papulovesicles. Sometimes lesions may coalesce to form larger plaques. Sometimes purpuric lesions are seen.
- Lesions are distributed symmetrically at face and extensors of upper and lower limbs. Buttocks may be involved but trunk is usually spared.

Calcinosis cutis

- It is due to the aberrant deposition of calcium into the soft tissue.

Clinical features

- It presents as firm to hard papules, plaques or nodules due to cutaneous deposition of calcium.
- Lesions may be painful and may ulcerate to discharge chalky materials.

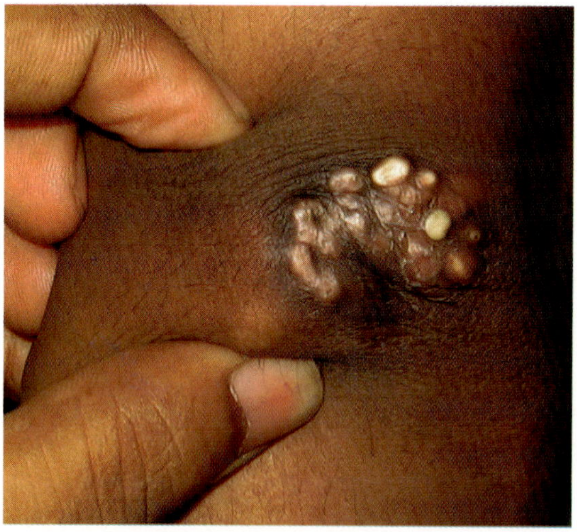

Fig. 43: Combined, circumscribed, ulcerated papules forming an irregular plaque and subcutaneous nodule at left elbow

- Calcinosis universalis is having multiple lesions with symmetrical distribution.
- Calcinosis circumscriptum is a localized lesion.
- Pinnal calcification develops at pinna.
- Calcinosis scrotalis develops at scrotum.
- Metastatic calcification affects internal organs.
- X-ray shows radio-opaque deposition and confirms the diagnosis.
- Treatment is simple excision.

Keratoacanthoma

- It is a self limiting keratinizing disorder with a higher incidence among immunosuppressed patients.
- It also occurs in Muir-Torre syndrome.

Types

- Solitary
- Multiple

Variants of solitary keratoacanthoma

- Giant keratoacanthoma
- Keratoacanthoma centrifugum marginatum (KCM)
- Subungual keratoacanthoma.

Clinical features of solitary keratoacanthoma

- Lesion is characterized by firm dome shaped nodule with a horny crater at the center.
- Size is usually 1-2.5 cm in diameter. Maximum size is reached by 6-8 weeks and rarely more than 2 months and takes 6 months to 1 year to involute.
- In 95% cases it occurs at exposed areas. Palms, soles and mucosae are usually spared.
- KCM is characterized by annular plaque with rolled margin. It is having a tendency of peripheral speading and central healing with scarring.

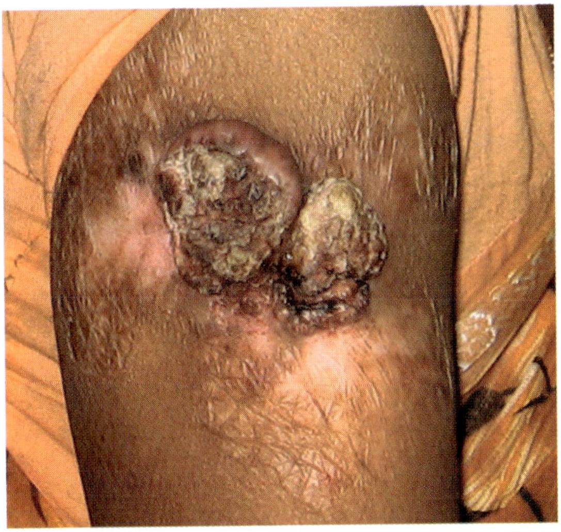

Fig. 44: Dome shaped plaques with central crater

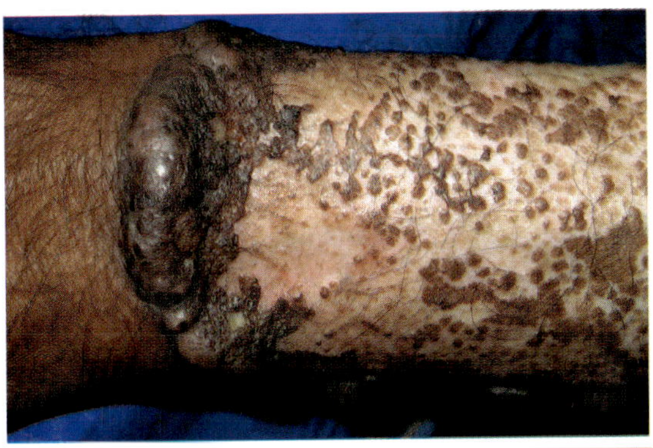

Fig. 45: Annular plaque with rolled border in a case of KCM

Histopathology

- Keratin filled epidermal invagination or crater is seen and the epidermis extends like a lip or buttress over the sides of the crater.
- Epidermis grows upward irregularly from the base of the crater.
- Also, strands of epidermis enter the dermis below the base of the crater.
- Many areas of these strands are poorly differentiated from the stroma.
- Keratinization is extensive and well advanced. But one or two layers of basophilic nonkeratinized cells are present at the periphery of the epidermal growth.
- There are many horn pearls with complete keratinization at their centers.
- Base of the growth is usually does not cross the level of the sweat glands.
- Nuclear atypia and many mitotic figures are seen within these poorly differentiated areas.
- Some areas show fair amount of keratinization and appear glassy and eosinophilic.
- Pronounced dermal infiltration is found.

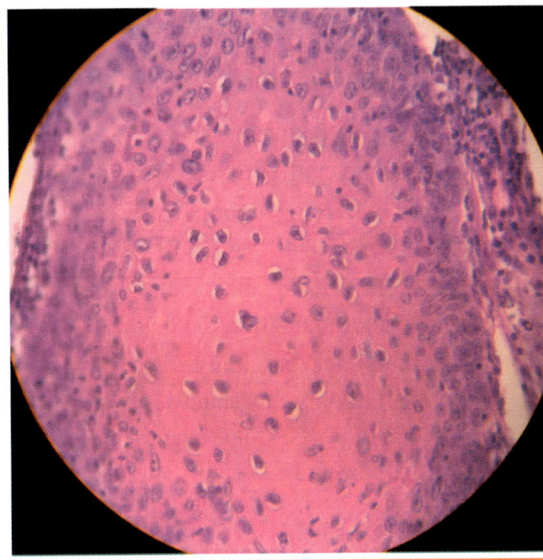

Fig. 46: Extensive keratinization within the epidermal growth with one or two layers of nonkeratinized cells at the periphery

Pilomatricoma

- It is a benign neoplasm or cyst originated from follicular matrix.
- It occurs due to mutation of CTNNB1 gene, encoding β-catenin.
- It commonly affects young adults; but may develop at any age.

Clinical features

- It presents as solitary skin-colored to faint-blue nodule or cyst.
- Lesions are very firm in consistency due to calcification.
- Head and upper trunk are common sites.
- Rarely lesions may be multiple.

Histopathology

* Early evolving lesion
    * It shows a cyst with matrical cornification.
    * Wall of the cyst consists of basaloid matrical cells.
    * Center of the cyst shows presence of anucleated cornified cells, named as ghost cells or shadow cells.
    * Sometimes at transition zone between the nucleated peripheral zone and anucleated central zone, few pink trichohyaline granules are seen.
* Late, fully developed lesion
    * Lost of cystic configuration.
    * Presence of varying amount of basaloid matrical cells and shadow cells.
    * Central cornified area shows fibrosis and granulomatous inflammation.
    * In very late stage, basaloid cells may be totally absent and only few shadow cells are buried within fibrosis. Calcification and ossification may occur.

Dermatofibroma

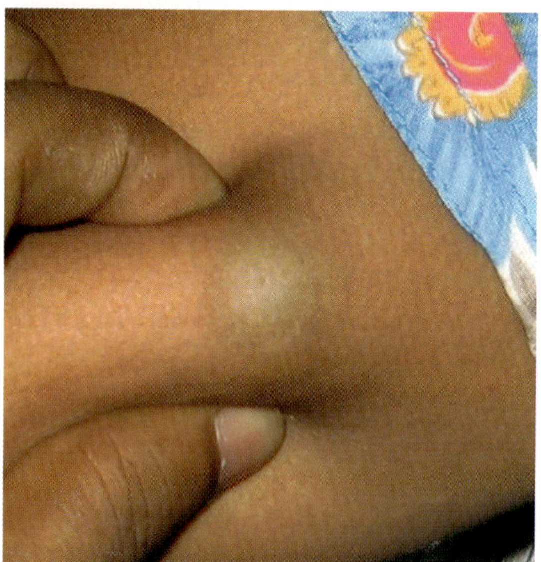

Fig. 47: Firm nodule, better felt on palpation than inspection

* This is a common fibrohistiocytic tumor of the skin.
* It commonly occurs in adults.
* Dermatofibroma is more superficial and factor XIIIa+ in comparison to dermatofibrosarcoma which is deeper and CD34+.

Clinical features

* Firm, nontender, minimally elevated dermal nodule which is attatched with overlying epidermis.
* Color of the lesion is variable from hyperpigmentation to pink, according to the skin color.
* Usual size is 1-2 cm in diameter.
* Lower limbs are the commonest sites; but it may arise from any site.
* Pinching of the lesion leads to downward movement and this is known as Dimple sign/ Fitzpatrick sign.

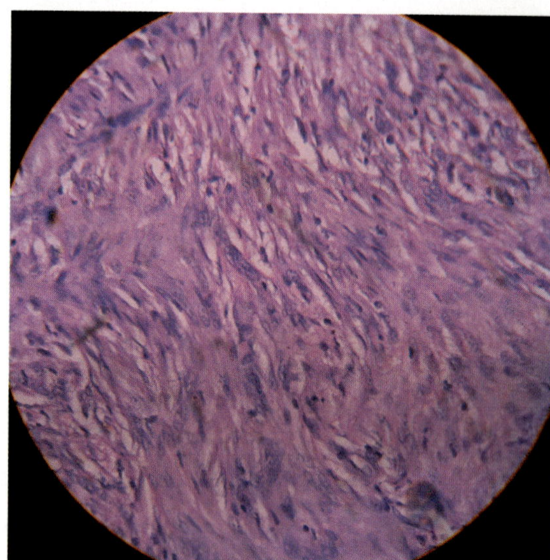

Fig. 48: Storiform pattern of fibrohistiocytic cells

Histopathology

* Pseudoepitheliomatous hyperplasia of the epidermis.
* Collection of fibrohistiocytic cells within collagen bundles in the mid dermis which are arranged in a storiform/cartwheel pattern.

Leiomayoma cutis

- This is a form of benign smooth muscle tumor and the muscle is the arrector pili muscle, attached with the hair follicle.
- Lesions are painful during winter season.
- Pain may be provoked by cooling the lesion with ice. This is known as pseudo-Darier sign.
- Histopathology confirms the dermal mass consisting of smooth muscle fibers.
- Lesions usually start in puberty.

Clinical features

- Lesions appear as pink or coppery color nodules.
- Size may be upto 1.5 cm.
- Number may be single or few or multiple.
- Common sites are extremities.

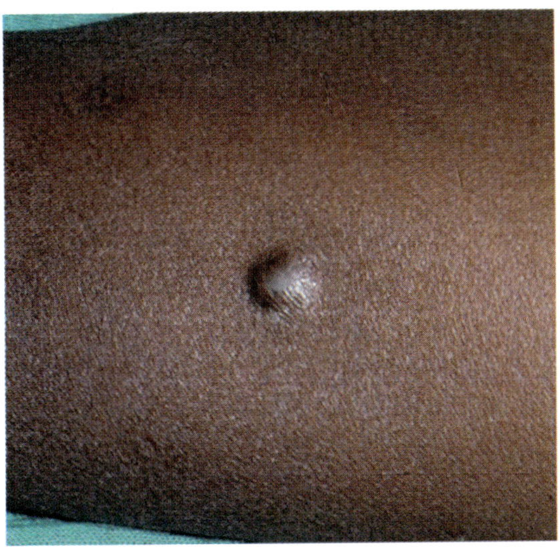

Fig. 49: Coppery color nodule at the arm

Differential diagnosis

- Dermatofibroma
- Spitz nevi
- Keloid
- Neurofibroma.

Treatment

- Simple surgical excision.

Erythema elevatum diutinum

- This is a form of cutaneous small vessel vasculitis.
- Exact etiology is not yet clear.
- Histopathology shows leukocytoclastic vasculitis.

Clinical features

- Primary lesions are reddish-brown papules and nodules. Lesions are distributed with a tendency of symmetry.
- Common sites are dorsa of the hands and fingers, elbows, knees and shins.

Treatment

- Dapsone
- Intralesional corticosteroid.

Xanthoma

- This is a common cutaneous manifestation of lipid metabolism.

Tuberous xanthoma

- These are lobulated yellowish plaques.
- Common sites are elbows, knees, face, knuckles, toes and axillary and inguinal folds.
- Shape and size of the lesions are variable.
- Hypercholesterolemia is often associated.

Tendinous xanthoma

- These are slowly developing subcutaneous nodules and remain attached with tendons or ligaments.
- Common sites are ankles and elbows.
- Hypercholesterolemia is often associated.

Plane xanthoma

- These are yellowish orange macules or slight elevated plaques.
- Common sites are neck, eyelids, flexors and trunk.
- Presence at palmar creases is an pathognomonic sign of type III dysbetalipoproteinemia.
- It may be associated with chronic biliary obstruction.

Xanthoma disseminatum

- Lesions are erythematous yellowish brown papules of varying shape and size and distributed bilaterally and symmetrically.
- Common sites are face, trunk and extremities.
- Histopathology shows collection of spindle shaped mononuclear cells, foamy histiocytes lymphocytes, neutrophils and eosinophils.

Eruptive xanthoma

- Lesions are pinhead to larger yellowish papules with an erythematous background.
- These appear in crops.
- Common sites are buttocks, arms and extensors of the limbs.
- These lesions may resemble with papular lesions of lepromatous leprosy and sarcoidosis.

Keloid

- It is characterized by a firm, reddish or hyperpigmented papule or plaque due to overgrowth of connective tissue and usually develops from the scar of a previous injury. But it often develops spontaneously, specially at suprasternal region.
- Common sites are chest, upper back, shoulders and upper arms.
- It extends beyond the original margin of the previous injury.

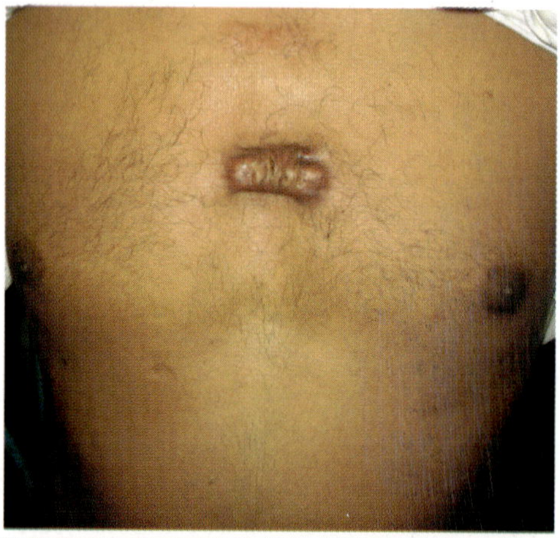

Fig. 50: Firm and hyperpigmented palques with claw-like extensions and irregular surface at chest

- It closely mimics hypertrophic scar which remains localized within the site of injury. Both may be painful or itchy.

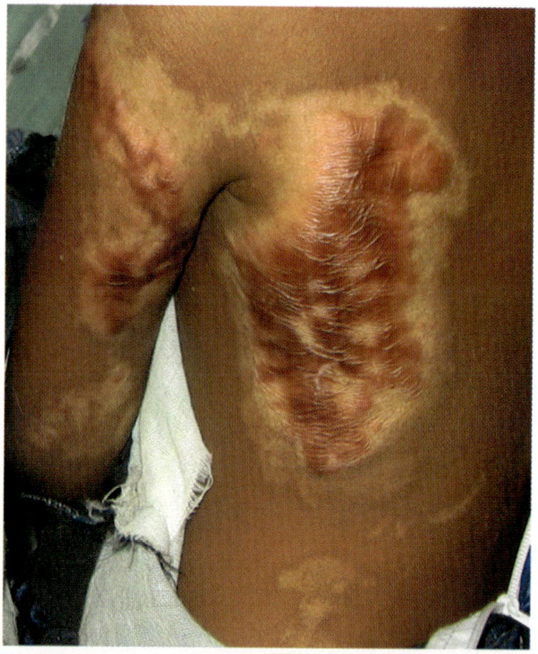

Fig. 51: Hypertrophic scar on burn scar

Differential diagnosis

- Hypertrophic scar
- Lobomycosis

Treatment

- Pressure bandage after applying silicon sheet on the lesion.
- Intralesional injection of triamcinolone (40 mg/ml) at a dose of 0.1-0.3 ml/cm^2 area, initially weekly, followed by 2-3 weeks interval.

Mycetoma

- This is a chronic infective dermatosis, caused by two-sets of organisms and present as two different types.
- It affects the skin and underlying bones.

Types

- Eumycetoma, caused by true fungi and responds to antifungals.

- Actinomycetoma, caused by filamentous bacteria and responds to antibiotics.

Fungi causing eumycetoma

- *Madurella mycetomatis*
- *Madurella grisea*
- *Leptopheria senegalensis*
- *Pyrenochaeta romarei*
- *Acremonium*
- *Aspergillus*

Filamentus bacteria causing actinomycetoma

- *Actinomadura madurae*
- *Actinomadura pelletieri*
- *Nocardia asteroides*
- *Nocardia brasiliensis*
- *Streptomyces somaliensis*

Color granules produced by the organisms

- Black granules by *Madurella mycetomatis* and *Madurella grisea*.
- Red granules by *Actinomadura pelletieri*.
- White granules by *Acremonium* and *Aspergillus*.

Demonstration of the organisms

- Crushed granules dissolving with 20% KOH.
- Histopathological examination can detect the granules.
- Special fungal stain for eumycetoma or ZN stain and Gram stain for actinomycetoma.
- Culture from the sinus tissue.
- X-ray shows bony erosions in eumycetoma.

Clinical features of mycetoma

- It is characterized by a triad of indurated swelling, discharging sinuses and discharge of granules.
- Sprouting of granulation tissue at the openings of the sinuses is commonly seen in actinomycetoma.
- Feet and ankles are the commonest sites in eumycetoma.
- Actinomycetoma commonly occurs at knees and thighs.

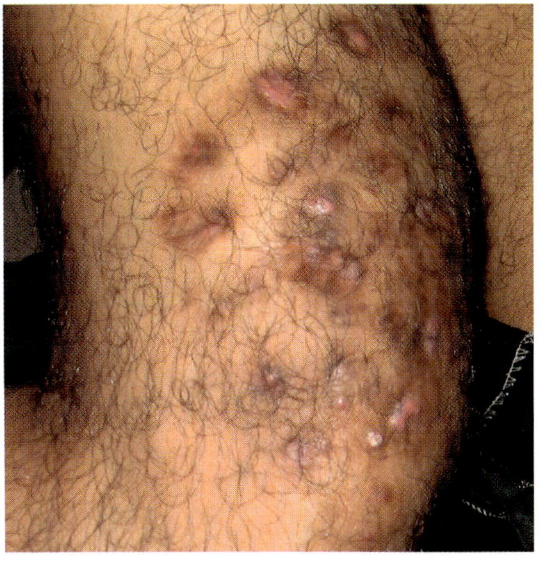

Fig. 52: Multiple discharging sinuses in healing stage at lower thigh and knee in actinomycetoma

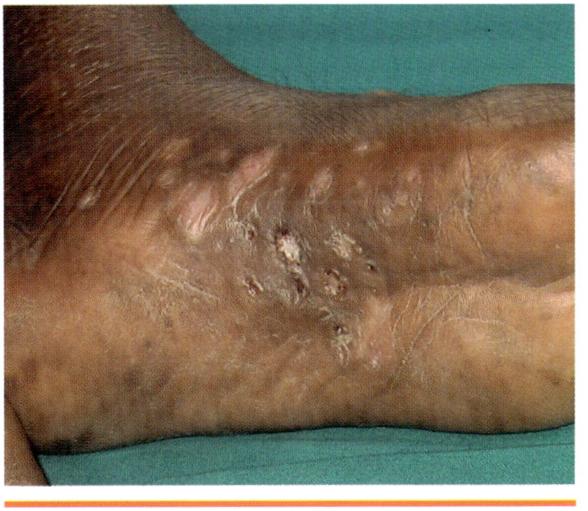

Fig. 53: Multiple sinuses at the sole in eumycetoma

Treatment

- Long term itraconazole (200-400 mg/day), ketoconazole (200 mg/day), voriconazole, fluconazole (400-800 mg/day) for eumycetoma. Duration of treatment is variable from 9-36 months.
- Dapsone, trimethoprim-sulfamethoxasole, amikacin, amoxycillin-clavulanic acid, etc. for actinomycetoma. Average duration of treatment is 9 months.

- Amikacin is usually is given as a pulse therapy (15 mg/kg, im/iv, for 2-3 weeks and then 2-3 weeks rest) for 3 pulses.

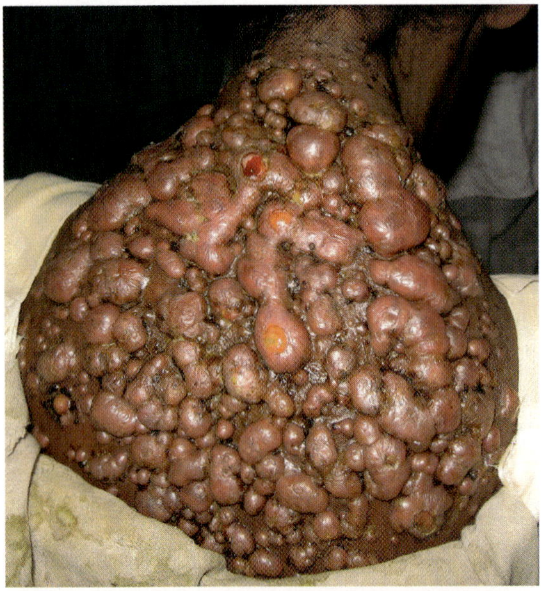

Fig. 54: Multiple edematous and erythematous nodules

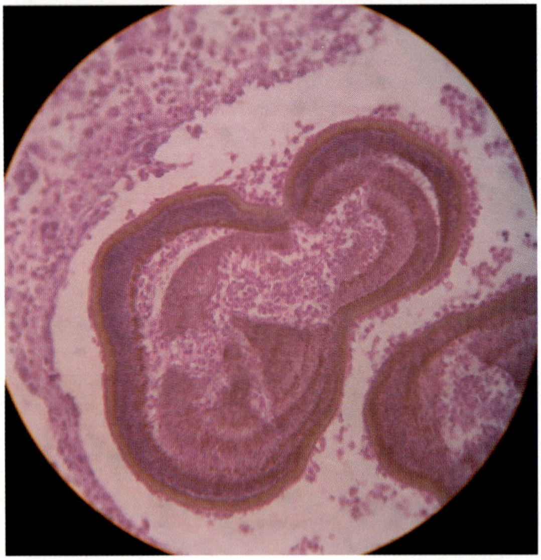

Fig. 55: Spore of eumycetoma

Sporotrichosis

* This is chronic suppurative and granulomatous infective disorder, caused by *Sporothrix schenckii* fungi.
* It affects the skin and spreads through lymphatics.
* Direct microscopy and culture can demonstrate the organism.

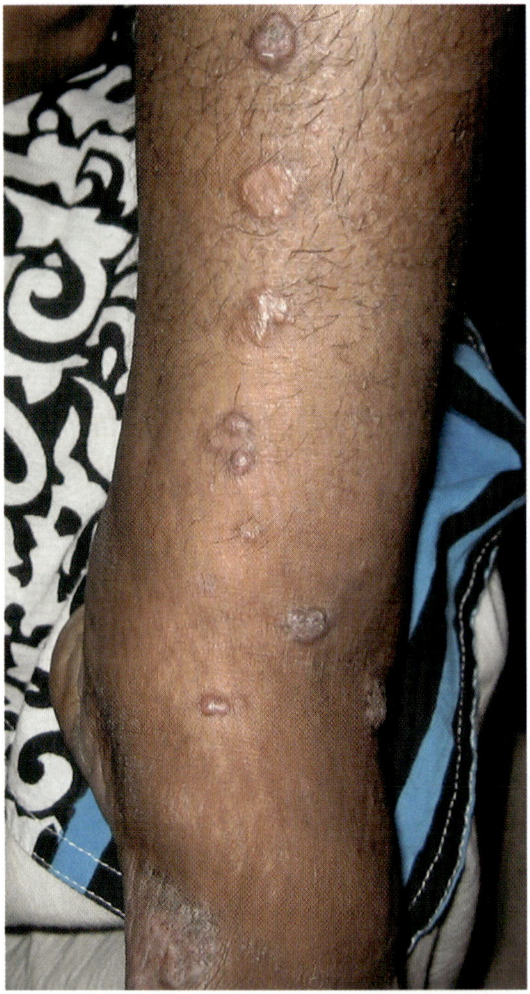

Fig. 56: Erythematous plaques in a linear distribution

Clinical features

- Primary lesions are granulomatous papules and plaques, arranged in a linear fashion due to spreading from distal to proximal parts of the limbs through lymphatics.
- Number is usually few but may be single.
- Lesions are erythematous, painless and firm.
- Very often they become eroded and have mild seropurulent discharge with crusting.

- Fixed type does not spread.
- Extremities are the commonest sites.

Histopathology

- Suppurative infiltration contains neutrophils at the center, surrounded by epithelioid cells and lymphocytes at the periphery.
- Cigar shaped cells and asteroid bodies may be found.

Treatment

- Itraconazole 200 mg/day for 3-6 months.
- Fluconazole 400 mg/day for 6 months.
- Saturated solution of potassium iodide, starting with 5 drops per day to 40 drops thrice daily with fruit juice. At least 4 weeks extra treatment to be given after resolution of the lesions.

Chromoblastomycosis

* It is caused by any of the following dematiaceous or pigmented fungi:
  - Phialophora verrucosa
  - Fonsecaea pedrosoi
  - Fonsecaea compactum
  - Exophiala jeanselmei
  - Cladosporium carrionii
* Infection occurs due to traumatic implantation of the fungi from soil, decaying vegetations and rotten woods.

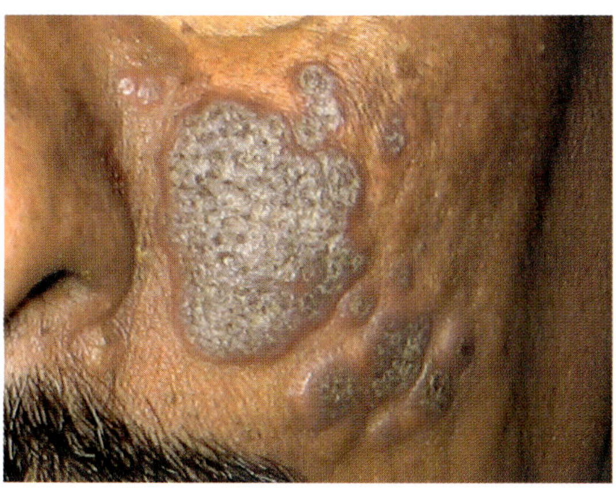

Fig. 57: Erythematous verrucous plaque with satellite lesions

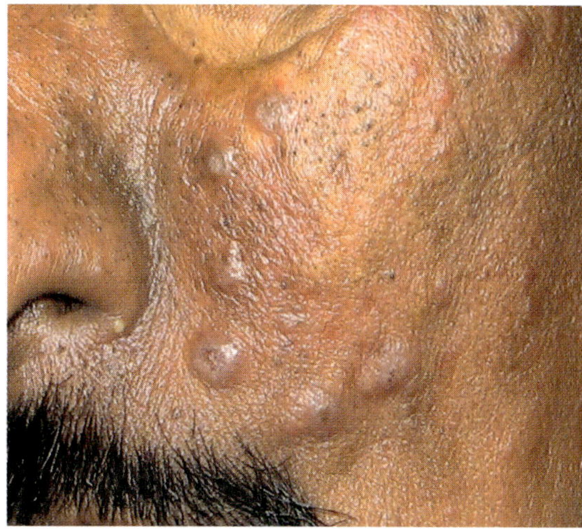

Fig. 58: Lesions almost disappeared following treatment with itraconazole

Clinical feature

* Lower limbs are commonly affected.
* It may present as a papule, nodule or verrucous plaque with varying degree of pruritus. Some lesions may heal by scarring and some are spread by developing new satellite lesions due to auto-inoculation or lymphatic drainage.
* Elephantiasis may occur due to disruption of lymphatics.
* Rarely hematogenous spread may cause numerous skin lesions.

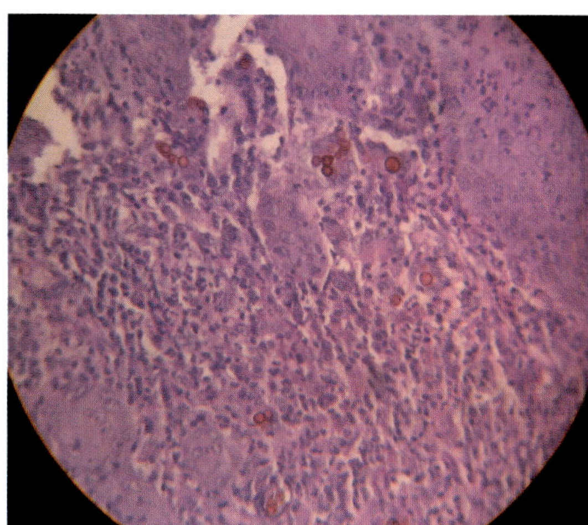

Fig. 59: Multiple pigmented spore within giant cells

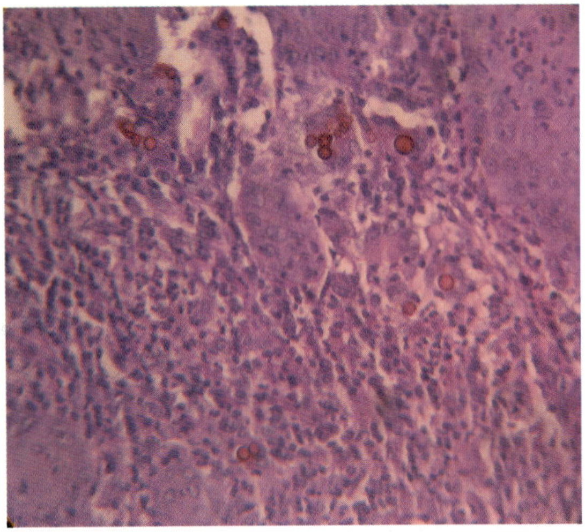

Fig. 60: Copper penny bodies in chromoblastomycosis

Histopathology

- Pseudoepitheliomatous epidermal hyperplasia.
- Lichenoid-granulomatous infiltration in the dermis.
- Infiltration is composed of epithelioid cells forming tuberculoid granulomas, multinucleated giant cells, clusters of neutrophils forming small abscesses, variable amount of lymphocytes, plasma cells and eosinophils.
- Fungi are found within giant cells or freely within the abscesses.
- Fungi appear as thick-walled, dark-brown, oval to round spores. Their size is varying from 6 to 12 μm. They lie singly, or in chain or in cluster. Due to their color, no special stain is required for recognition.

* Treatment is given with systemic itraconazole or terbinafine.

Cryptococcosis

* It is caused by *Cryptococcus neoformans*, naturally found in soil contaminated with excreta of birds, specially pigeon and chicken.
* The fungi infect human through respiratory tract and spread to the skin in 10-15% cases.
* Primary inoculation form is rarely seen in the skin.
* It commonly occurs in presence of immunosuppression, specially in AIDS.

Cutaneous features

- Lesions are variable in number and morphology. These may be papules, pustules, herpetiform vesicles, nodules, indurated plaques and subcutaneous abscess or ulcers.
- Lesions are having an erythematous background and central necrosis. So, such lesion sometimes mimics infected molluscum contagiosum.
- Cellulitis-like lesion may develop in some cases.

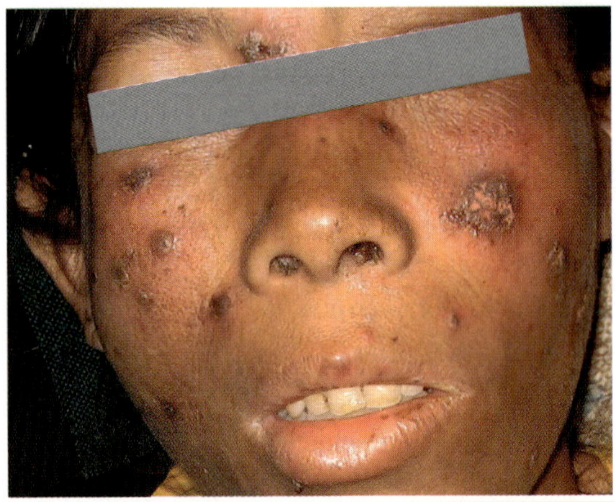

Fig. 61: Few erythematous papules and plaques with central necrosis in HIV seropositive patient

Histopathology

- The dermal reaction may be of two types, gelatinous type and granulomatous type. Any of the two or both may be present in single site.
- The fungi stain black with Fontana-Masson stain. They are also stained with PAS and methenamine silver.

* Gelatinous type:
  - It contains numerous organisms in aggregates with negligible tissue reaction.
  - Size of the spore is little larger, about 5 μm in diameter
* Granulomatous type:
  - It contains few organism but profound tissue reaction in the form of infiltration and fibro-

blastic activity. Infiltration is composed of histiocytes, giant cells, lymphocytes and fibroblasts.

- Size of the spore is smaller, about only 3 μm in diameter. They are found largely within the macrophages and giant cells.

Granuloma pyogenicum/Lobular capillary hemangioma

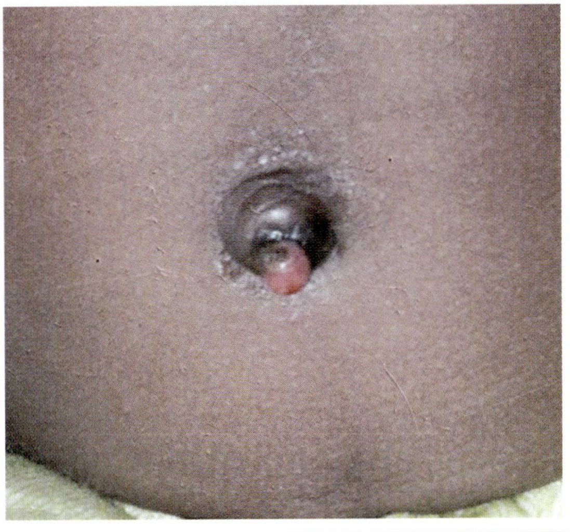

Fig. 62: Circumscribed bright red papular ulcer at the umbilicus

Characteristic features

- It is nothing but excess proliferation of granulation tissue, usually at the site of a persisting pyogenic infection.
- It appears as circumscribed, bright red, soft to firm papule or plaque, from 3 mm to 1 cm in size.
- It is having a tendency of bleeding following minor trauma.
- Common sites are umbilicus of infant/child, lips, fingers, toes and nose.

Histopathology

- Epidermis becomes flattened and may be eroded.
- Dermis contains lobulated masses of angiomatous tissue, mimicking granulation tissue. These are surrounded by a myxoid stroma, containing stellate and spindle-shaped connective tissue cells.
- Angiomatous tissue is composed of dilated blood-filled capillaries and poorly canalized vascular channels.
- Feeding vessels are extended into surrounding dermis.
- Some endothelial cells become larger focally.
- Inflammatory infiltration present in superficial part.

Treatment

- Antibiotic for the infection
- Chemical cautery
- Electrosurgery.

Angiokeratoma

* It is characterized by minute keratotic papules with a bleeding tendency on minor trauma due to their vascular origin.
* Lesion may remain discrete or coalesce to form plaques.

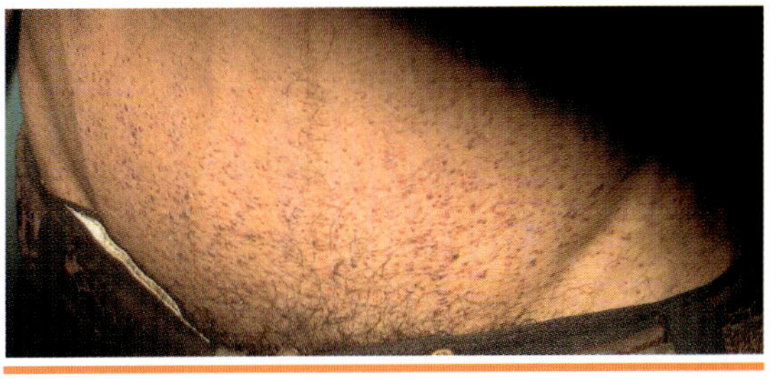

Fig. 63: Diffuse tiny keratotic angiomatous lesion at lower abdomen

Types

- Angiokeratoma corporis diffusum: Symmetrically distributed numerous clusters of tiny red papules in the bathing-trunk area. It may be associated with lysosomal enzyme deficiencies.
- Angiokeratoma of Mibelli: Dark red papules of 3-5 mm size and several in number. Common sites are fingers and toes. Surface may be slight verrucous. Lesion appear in childhood and adolescence.

- Angiokeratoma of Fordyce: Early lesions are red, soft and compressible. But later, they become more keratotic, bluish and noncompressible. They arise in middle or in later life. Number may be multiple. Scrotum is the commonest site and size of the lesion is variable from 2-4 mm. But when vulva is affected size becomes larger and deeper and may be associated with itching.
- Angiokeratoma circumscriptum: Initial discrete lesions coalesce to form circumscribed plaque.
- Solitary angiokeratoma: It commonly occurs in young adult and at lower limbs. Size of the lesion is larger, from 2-10 mm in diameter. Though solitary but sometimes lesion may be multiple.

Histopathology

- Hyperkeratosis with varying degree of acanthosis.
- Papillary dermis contains multiple thin-walled dilated and congested capillaries.

Treatment

- Chemical surgery with 88% phenol or 80% trichloroacetic acid, or electrosurgery.

Angiolymphoid hyperplasia/Epithelioid hemangioma

- Development of cluster of erythematous and translucent papules at and around the ear with history of occasional bleeding from the lesion.
- Peripheral eosinophilia may be present.

Histopathology

- Epidermis may be acanthotic or atrophic due to ulceration.
- Lobular proliferation of small to medium vessels.
- Many of the vascular channels are lined by large endothelial cells. These endothelial cells resemble epithelioid cells and designated as histoid cells.
- Some of the endothelial cells may be projected towards lumen and show a cobblestone appearance.
- Some of the endothelial cells may have prominent intracytoplasmic vacuolation.
- The most abnormal vessels are surrounded by stellate and spindle-shaped cells within a mucoid stroma.
- Perivascular infiltration consist of lymphocytes and eosinophils. Infiltration is loosely scattered around the affected vessels.
- Nodular lymphocytic infiltration rarely forms follicle.

Treatment

- Waiting for spontaneous regression by 3-6 months.
- Electrosurgery.

Keratosis pilaris

- It is a common keratinizing disorder of hair follicles, affecting the adolescents.
- It is often associated with ichthyosis vulgaris.

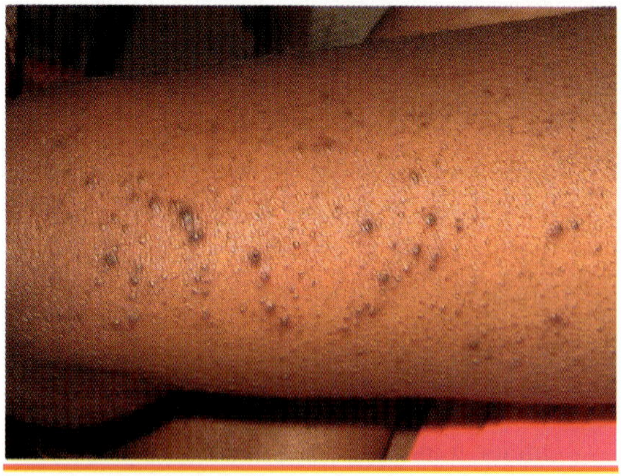

Fig. 64: Keratotic follicular papules with perilesional erythema

Clinical features

- Discrete tiny follicular keratotic papules, often associated with perifollicular erythema.
- Lesions commonly affects the posterolateral aspect of the upper arms, thighs, buttocks and may be widespread also.

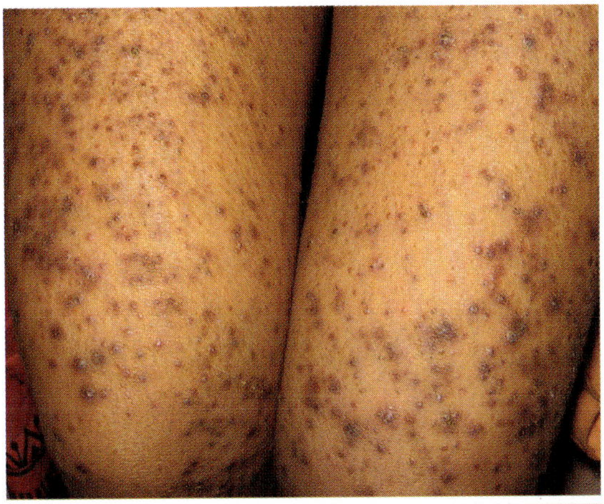

Fig. 65: Keratotic follicular papules with perilesional erythema

Lymphangioma circumscriptum

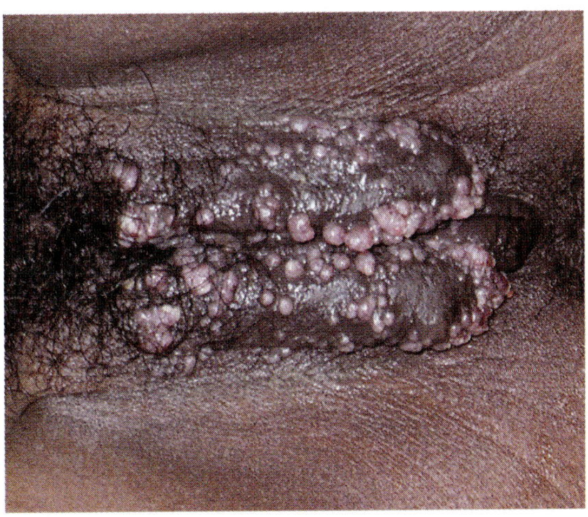

Fig. 66: Circumscribed and irregular swelling of the vulva, studded with reddish vesicles

* This is due to malformation of lymphatic vessels of dermis or subcutaneous tissue and characterized by minute discrete or confluent vesicles.
* Lesions may be translucent or dark colored and some may contain hemorrhagic fluid. Most of the lesion coalesce and form an irregular plaque, studded with the primary lesions. Discharge of clear fluid from the surface is often present and known as lymphorrhea.
* It is usually presented since birth but may appear later.
* Commonly affected sites are buttocks, vulva, trunk and proximal parts of the limbs.
* Treatment is radical surgery.

Flegel's disease/Hyperkeratosis lenticularis perstans

* A defect in the membrane-coating granules in the keratinocytes of the upper spinous layer, is likely to be the cause of the disease.

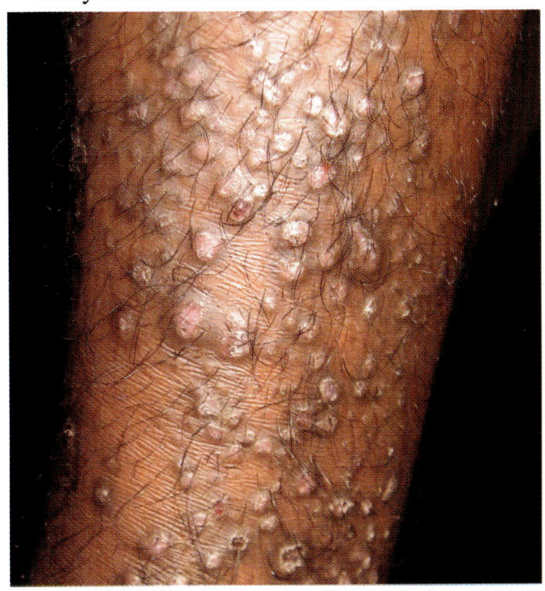

Fig. 67: Hyperkeratotic papules with adherent scale

Clinical features

- Primary lesions are asymptomatic flat hyperkeratotic papules with central horny adherent scale. Slight bleeding occurs following removal of adherent scale.
- Common sites are dorsa of the feet and lower legs. Other sites are thighs, upper limbs and ears. Rarely oral mucosa is affected.
- Size is variable from 1-5 mm.
- Some lesions show collarette of fine scales at the periphery.

Histopathology

- Hyperkeratosis with occasional parakeratosis or strongly eosinophilic compact keratin layer.

- ♦ Acanthosis with papillomatosis, appearing as church spire at the periphery and flattening at the center with thinning or absent granular layer.
- ♦ Lymphoid cells infiltration in the upper dermis as a narrow band.

Kyrle's disease

- ✶ Altered keratinization forms a horny plug.
- ✶ This penetrating plug incites a dermal granulomatous inflammatory reaction.
- ✶ It occurs in young to middle aged persons.
- ✶ A history of diabetes is often present.

Clinical features

- ♦ Primary lesions are follicular and nonfollicular dome shaped papules with central keratin plugs. Some lesions coalesce to form a plaque.
- ♦ Common sites are extremities.
- ♦ Number is usually numerous.
- ♦ Excoriation marks are present close to the lesions.
- ♦ Lesions may be linear due to Koebnerization.

Histopathology

- ♦ Follicular or extrafollicular cornified plug, invaginated by the hyperplastic epidermis.
- ♦ Basophilic material is seen as small collections within the plugs.
- ♦ Altered collagen or elastic tissue is absent.
- ♦ Vacuolated or dyskeratotic cells are present in the epidermis with irregular acanthosis.
- ♦ Presence of granulomatous inflammation with small foci of neutrophilic abscess in the dermis.

Reactive perforating collagenosis

- ✶ It is a form of genodermatosis, inherited as autosomal dominant or recessive pattern.
- ✶ There is an acquired form also, occurring in association with diabetes mellitus and chronic renal failure.
- ✶ Precipitating factors are trauma, arthropod bite, folliculitis and cold exposure.
- ✶ Subepidermal foci of altered collagen, incite a dermal granulomatous foreign body reaction.
- ✶ Altered collagen is extruded through transepidermal elimination.
- ✶ Male and female both are affected.
- ✶ Lesions start to appear in early life.

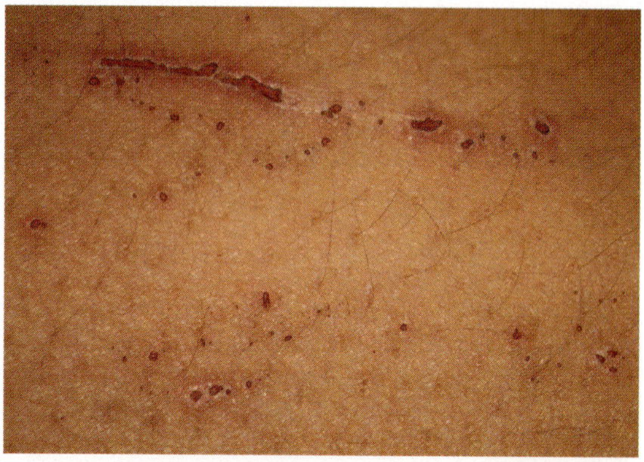

Fig. 68: Multiple papules with necrotic center along a line of excoriation

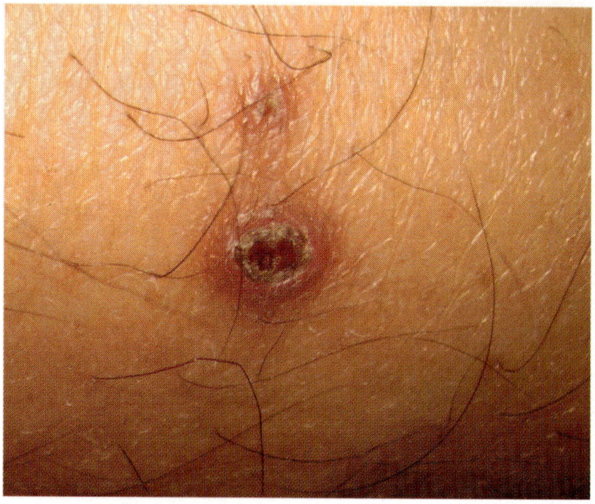

Fig. 69: Single necrotic papule

Clinical features

- ♦ Prmary lesions are umbilicated papules with central keratin plugs. Some lesion may be eroded.
- ♦ Common sites are face and upper limbs. But lower limbs and trunk are also affected.

- Size is variable from 5-10 mm.
- Lesions regress spontaneously and are left by superficial pock like scars.
- Postinflammatory hyperpigmentation may be present.

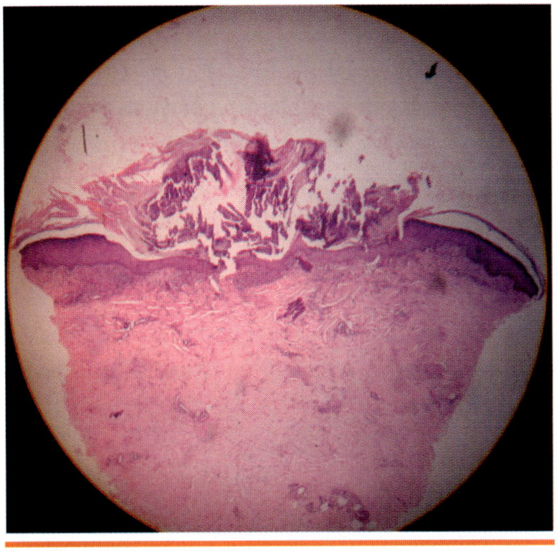

Fig. 70: Central crater with epidermal perforation

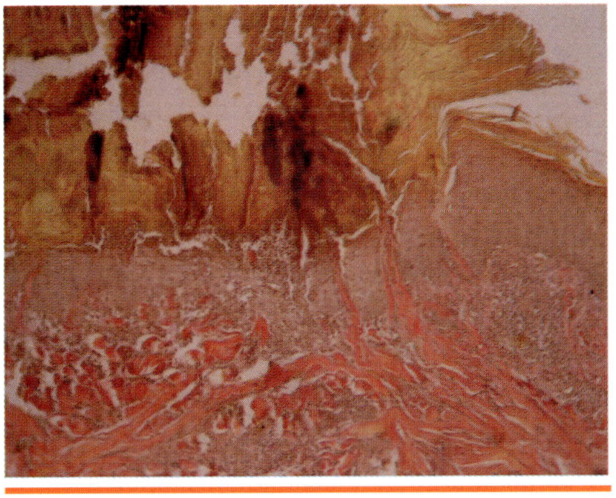

Fig. 71: Expulsion of collagen through epidermal channel (VVG stain)

Histopathology

- Cup-shaped vertically oriented channel, containing degenerated basophilic material and basophilic collagen.
- Vertically oriented perforating bundles of collagen fibers are present at the base of the channel where epidermis is attenuated. Masson trichrome and VVG stains confirm the presence of collagen.

Elastosis perforans serpiginosa

* It is a perforating dermatosis showing classical picture of transepidermal elimination.
* Thickened elastic fibers act as foreign body and incite a dermal reaction.
* Altered elastic tissue is extruded through the epidermis.
* Associated disorders are Down syndrome, Ehler-Danlos syndrome, osteogenesis imperfecta, pseudoxanthoma elasticum and Marfan's syndrome.
* It commonly occurs in young adults and peak age of onset is 2nd decade.
* Males are more affected than females.

Clinical features

- Primary lesions are papules with central keratin plugs. Lesions coalesce and arrange in an arcuate or serpiginous configuration.
- Size is variable from 2-5 mm.
- Common sites are nape of the neck, face and upper extremities.

Histopathology

- Acanthotic epidermis invaginates a narrow channel that contains eosinophilic elastic fibers.
- Elastic fibers are increased in size and number.
- At the base of the channel, elastic fibers maintain the normal staining property but it alters at the epidermal level.

Perforating folliculitis

* Follicular hyperkeratosis due to a primary irritant, results in a mechanical breakdown of the follicular wall which incites an inflammation.
* It usually occurs in 2nd to 4th decade.

Clinical features

- Primary lesions are follicular papules with central keratotic plugs.
- Common sites are extensors of the extremities and the buttocks.
- Size is variable from 2-8 mm.

Histopathology

- Dilated follicular infundibulum containing compact ortho- and parakeratotic plugs.
- Presence of basophilic material, formed by altered collagen and neutrophilic debris within the follicle.
- One or more perforation at the follicular wall.
- Perifollicular mixed inflammatory infiltrate, mostly of neutrophils.
- Near the perforation altered elastic fibers are also seen.

Secondary perforating dermatosis

- It is associated with chronic dermatoses like renal disease and diabetes mellitus.
- Chronic rubbing causes epidermal alteration, leading to follicular hyperkeratosis and perforation.
- In case of renal failure, lesions appear within few months of starting of dialysis.

Clinical features

- Primary lesions are follicular papules with central keratotic plugs.
- Common sites are extensors of the lower limbs.
- Number of the lesion is often numerous.

Histopathology

- Orthokeratotic and parakeratotic plug, invaginated by the follicle.
- Presence of altered collagen or elastin within the follicle.
- Presence of follicular perforation, usually at the base.
- Vertically oriented dermal connective tissue.

Larva currens

- It is caused by infectious larvae of *Srongyloides stercoralis* which penetrate perianal mucosa and migrate to the skin.

Clinical features

- Cutaneous features are band like urticaria, eosinophilic folliculitis, and in severe cases generalized petechiae and purpura or chronic urticaria or thumbprint-like periumbilical ecchymoses.
- Skin lesion start within 30 cm of anus and spreads as much as 10 cm per day. The illness may persist for 40 years.
- General features are abdominal pain, nausea, vomiting, diarrhea or constipation and pneumonitis.

Treatment

- Ivermectin 200 μg/kg/day for two days.
- Thiabendazole maximum 3 g/day for two days.

Erythema annulare centrifugum

- It is a disease of unknown etiology. But sometimes is may be associated with tinea pedis, candidiasis, ascariasis and sarcoidosis.
- It starts as an erythematous and edematous papule which gradually enlarges to form a plaque with flattened center and elevated margin.
- Extension of the lesion may be irregular and forms an archiform plaque.
- Trailing scales and vesicle may be present at the margin.
- Sometimes purpura and pigmentation occur in the center.
- Number of the lesion may be single or multiple.
- Histopathology shows perivascular lymphocytic infiltration with coat sleeves appearance.

Granuloma annulare

- Lesion start as an papule which gradually enlarges with central flattening, resulting in an smoothly elevated border.

- Some of the papules coalesce and enlarge to form an annular plaque with beaded border.
- Some areas of the border of any of the lesion may be flattened, forming an arcuate plaque instead of purely an annular plaque.
- Size of the plaques varies from 1 cm to 5 cm and number may be few or many.
- Common sites are dorsa of the hands, feet and digits and upper limbs and trunk.
- Lesions are usually asymptomatic.
- Histopathology shows lymphohistiocytic palisading granulomas with collagen degeneration.

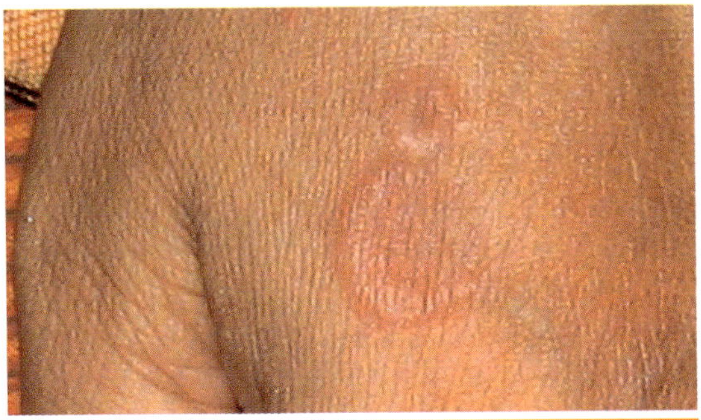

Fig. 72: Arcuate papule and plaque on dorsum of left-hand

Differential diagnosis

- Tuberculoid leprosy
- Sarcoidosis
- Erythema annulare centrifugum.

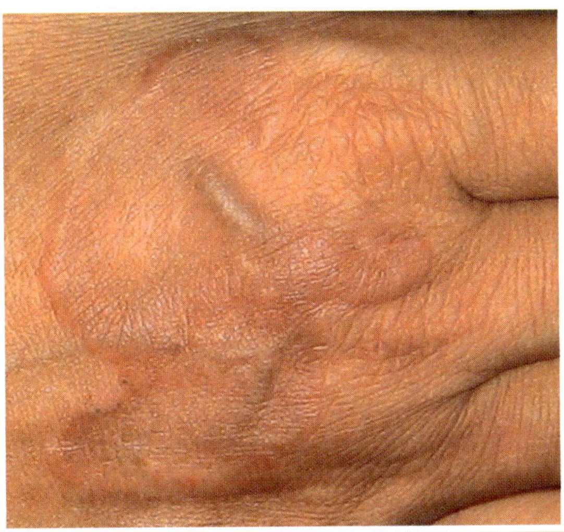

Fig. 73: Annular plaque at dorsum of right-hand

Differential diagnosis

- Borderline tuberculoid leprosy
- Sarcoidosis
- Tinea corporis.

Treatment

- Topical corticosteroid.
- Oral therapy with DDS (dapsone), isotretinoin, potassium iodide and PUVA.
- Intralesional injection with sterile water.
- Cryotherapy for recalcitrant lesion.

Porokeratosis

- It is characterized by hyperkeratotic plaque having thread-like raised keratotic border which histologically corresponds with a column of parakeratosis.
- Lesion starts as crateriform hyperkeratotic papule, gradually evantuates into a plaque of classical appearance.
- Lesions are asymptomatic except pruritus in some variants, specially in disseminated actinic porokeratosis.
- Dysregulated keratinization with premature apoptosis of keratinization is the mechanism of porokeratosis. Lesions are aggravated by UV light.
- Complications are contracture of joints and risk of development of Bowen's disease or squamous cell carcinoma.

Types

- Disseminated superficial actinic porokeratosis
- Disseminated superficial porokeratosis
- Porokeratosis of Mibelli
- Giant porokeratosis
- Linear porokeratosis
- Punctate porokeratosis

Porokeratosis of Mibelli

- It is the commonest form of porokeratosis having single/few/multiple annular plaques.

- Lesions may appear at any age but usually at childhood.
- Common sites are face, neck, forearm, hands, feet, ankles, even at buccal mucosa and glans penis.
- When occurs at scalp, it causes alopecia.

Disseminated superficial actinic porokeratosis

- It is a form of porokeratosis having autosomal dominant inheritance and lesions usually appear at 3rd to 4th decade.
- Peripheral ridges of the lesions are slightly raised and common site are sun-exposed areas like lower legs and forearms.
- Lesions are multiple in number, usually >50 and an average size is 0.5-1 cm, ranging from 0.1-4.5 cm.

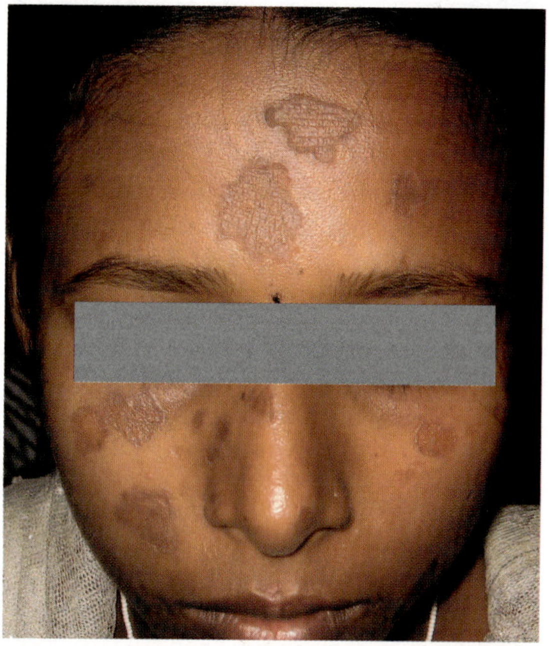

Fig. 75: Pigmented keratotic patches with sharply cut margins in a case of superficial actinic porokeratosis

Disseminated superficial porokeratosis

- This is an autosomal dominant subtype of porokeratosis having a late onset like 3rd to 4th decade.
- Lesions are bilateral symmetrical and mainly affect the extremities without sparing sunprotected areas.

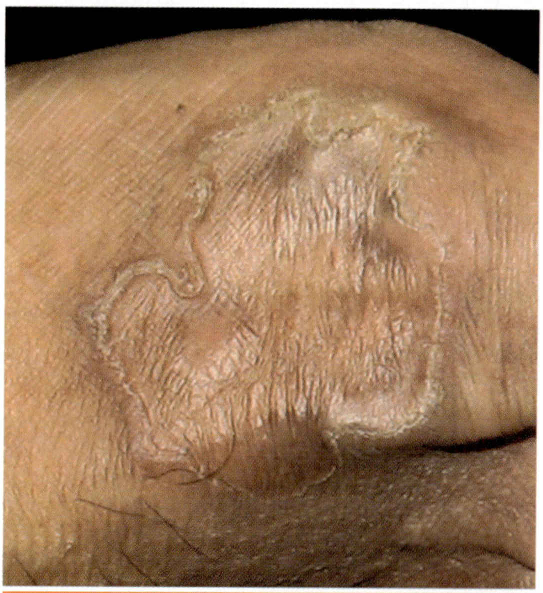

Fig. 74: Irregular plaque having thread-like raised keratotic border

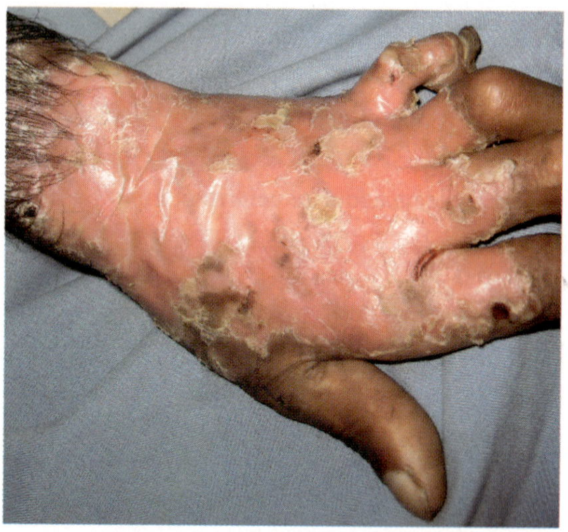

Fig. 76: Erythematous scaly plaque of giant porokeratosis with deformity of the hand

Differential diagnosis

- Psoriasis
- Bowen's disease
- Lupus vulgaris

Lichen striatus

- It starts as a group of minute pink, lichenoid or hypopigmented papules which spread in a linear fashion and affect mostly the age between 5-15 years.
- Gradually the lesions coalesce to form an irregular linear plaque.
- It commonly involves limbs and trunk.
- It usually resolves within 3-6 months.
- Absence of Wickham's striae and umbilication helps to differentiate it form linear lichen planus and absence of Auspitz sign differentiates it form linear psoriasis.
- Linear epidermal nevus is presented since childhood and it is persistent in nature. It is more hyperkeratotic and dark colored and non-itchy. But inflammatory linear epidermal nevus is pruritic and closely mimics lichen striatus.
- Lesion of linear porokeratosis is having double edged margin.
- Treatment includes reassurance and topical steroid.

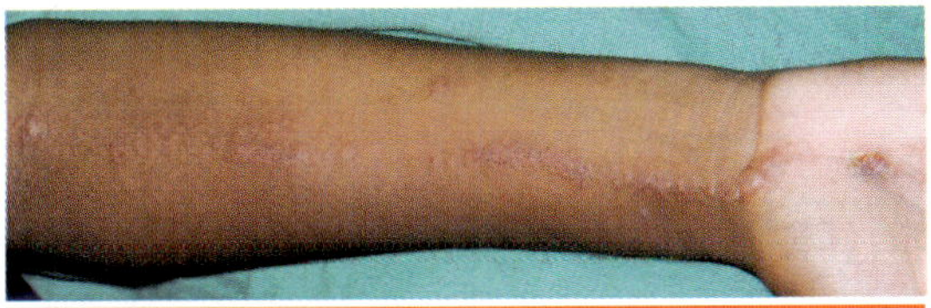

Fig. 77: Linear lesions along the right forearm extending from elbow to wrist

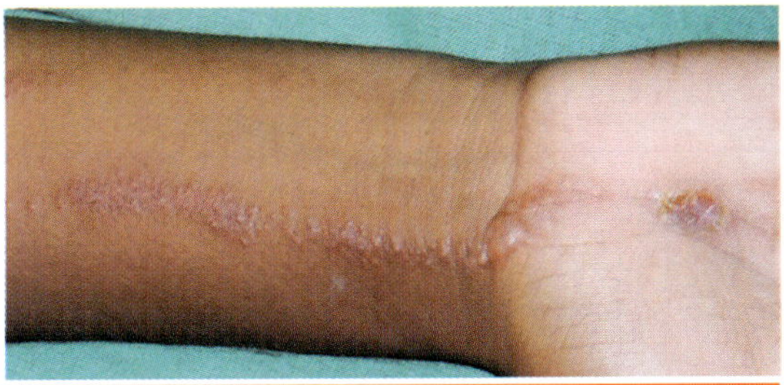

Fig. 78: Linear and confluent minute papules in close up view

Differential diagnosis

- Linear lichen planus
- Linear psoriasis
- Inflammatory linear verrucous epidermal nevus.
- Psoriasiform epidermal nevus (PEN).
- Psoriasiform epidermal nevus with congenital ipsilateral limb defects (PENCIL).

Inflammatory linear verrucous epidermal nevus (ILVEN)

- Extremely pruritic linear erythematous and scaly plaque, develops along the Blaschko's line.
- Common sites are vulva, scrotum, penile shaft and limbs.
- It usually appears in childhood and occasionally at birth or in adulthood.
- Lesion progresses for months to years.
- It responds poorly to anti-inflammatory drugs and rarely resolves spontaneously.

Linear porokeratosis

- Linear lesion but composed of multiple small annular plaques of superficial porokeratosis.
- Lesions start at infancy or childhood and follow Blaschko's line.
- Sometimes squamous cell carcinoma may develop.

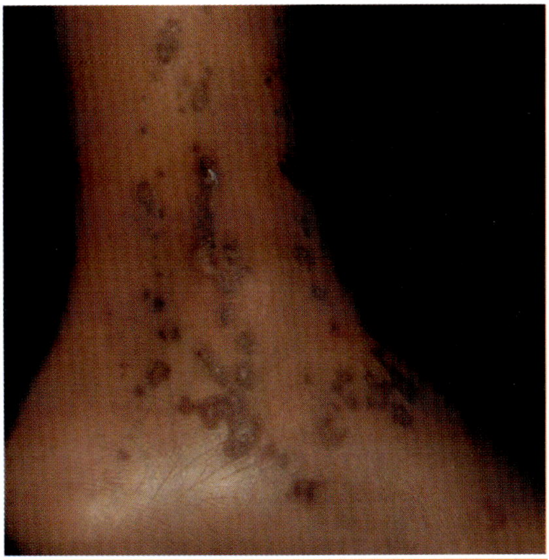

Fig. 79: Superficial porokeratotic lesions distributed in a linear pattern

Verrucous epidermal nevus

- Primary lesion is linear plaque, composed of verrucous or warty papules. But surface may be smooth or barely palpable.
- Color of the lesion varies from dark brown, pink, yellow to tan. At birth color is whitish and may not be noticed by the parents.
- Lesion is usually localized and unilateral but may be extensive and systematized.

Porokeratotic eccrine osteal and dermal duct nevus (PEODDN)

- Primary lesions are umbilicated keratotic papules, resembling comedonal nevus, distributed in a linear fashion.
- It occurs at palms and soles where no sebaceous gland is present.
- Adjacent hairy area contains verrucous and pitted papules.

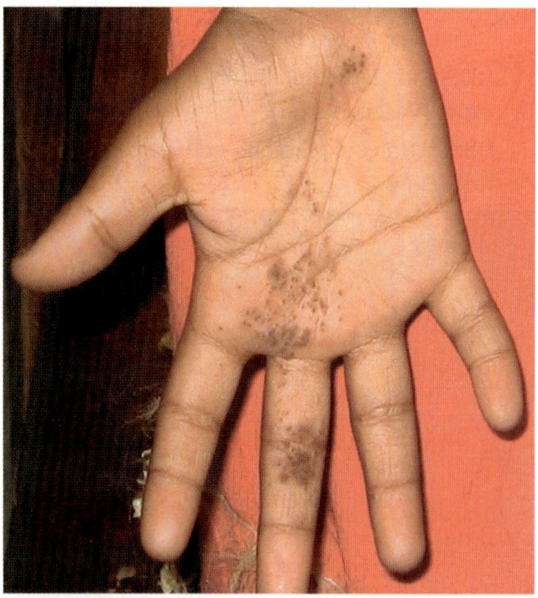

Fig. 80: Linear porokeratotic lesions at palms

Differential diagnosis

- Nevus comedonicus.

Syringocyst adenoma papilliferum

* This is a tumor of apocrine differentiation.
* At scalp it frequently arises in association with nevus sebaceous.

Clinical features

- It presents as single or several papules in a linear fashion or as a plaque at birth or in early childhood.
- During puberty, lesions increase in size to become papillomatous and crusted.
- Commonest sites are face and scalp. But in 25% cases it develops elsewhere.

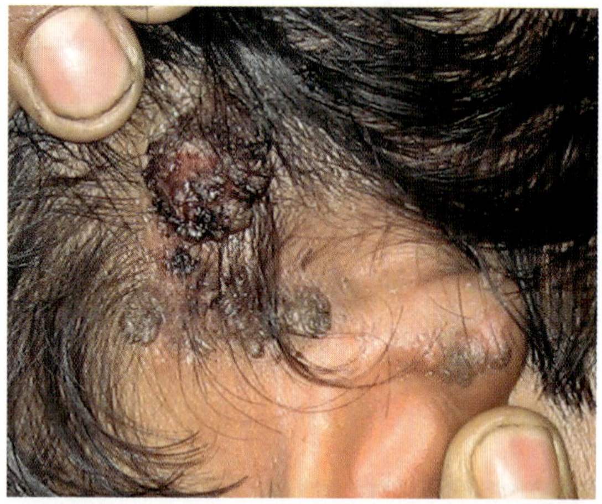

Fig. 81: One large ulcerated plaque with few hyperkeratotic brownish papules, arranged in a linear fashion

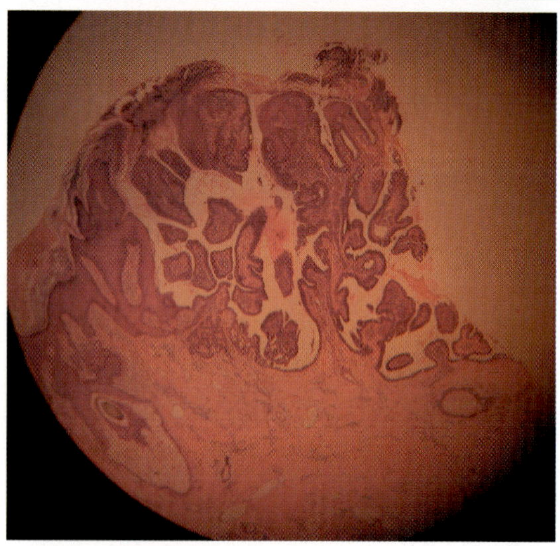

Fig. 82: Multiple villi–like proliferations within the cystic cavity under low power

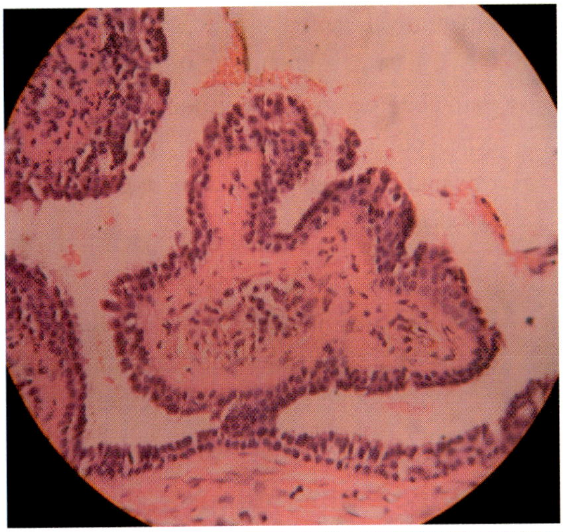

Fig. 83: Villi-like proliferation within the cystic cavity

Histopathology

- Papillomatosis
- Single or several cystic invaginations, extending from epidermis to dermis.
- Upper part of the invagination is lined by keratinizing epithelium like the epidermis.
- Lower part is having multiple papillary projections extending into the lumen of the cystic invagination, lined by glandular epithelium.
- This glandular epithelium consists of two rows of cells.
- Luminal layer or inner layer cells are columnar with oval nuclei and sometimes may be multilayered resulting in a lace-like pattern.
- Outer layer contains small cuboidal cells with round nuclei.
- Stroma contains a dense infiltrate, mostly composed of plasma cells.

Treatment

- Surgical excision or electrosurgery.

Punctate porokeratosis

- Lesions start between age of 15-25 years at palms and soles as asymptomatic, small seed like keratotic papules and slightly elevated peripheral rim.
- Lesions are bilateral and almost symmetrical.
- It should be differentiated from arsenical keratosis and punctate keratoderma.

Erythema ab igne

- It is characterized by reticular telangiectasia, hyperpigmentation, atrophy and hyperkeratosis.
- It particularly occurs at sites which are repeatedly exposed to heat, like inner and anterior sides of legs exposed to domestic heat during cooking by sitting near the oven.
- Sometimes lesions may be pruritic.

Chilblains

* Commonest victims are females around 35 years of age. But it may occur in children and older persons.
* The peak time of onset is between last week of December to first week of January.

Clinical features

- It is characterized by erythematous swelling of the fingers and toes in association with moderate to severe itching or burning sensation, classically occurring in winter season.
- In severe cases, blisters and ulceration may develop.
- Other involving sites are earlobes, tip of the nose and side of the thighs in early morning horse-riders.

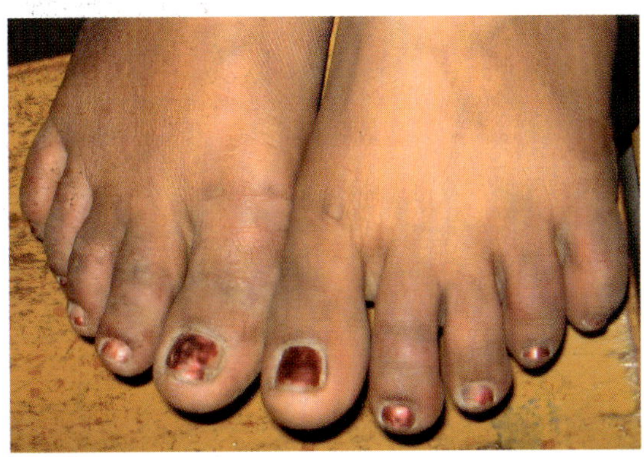

Fig. 84: Erythema and swelling of the toes

Treatment

- Avoidance of cold and proper clothing to protect cold.
- Oral nifedipine 10 mg twice daily for two weeks.
- In resistance cases, systemic steroid like oral triamcinolone 8 mg daily for two weeks.

Erythema nodosum

* This is a form of panniculitis, occurs mostly in middle aged female between 20-30 years of age and male/female ratio is 1:3-6.

Etiology

- Infections like bacteria, virus, protozoa or fungus
- Sarcoidosis in 30% cases
- Drugs like sulphonamides, bromides and oral contraceptive pills
- Malignancy like adenocarcinoma, lymphoma, leukemia
- Miscellaneous causes like pregnancy, radiotherapy acne fulminans, ankylosing spondylosis, Reiter's disease, Sweet's syndrome and Behcet's syndrome.

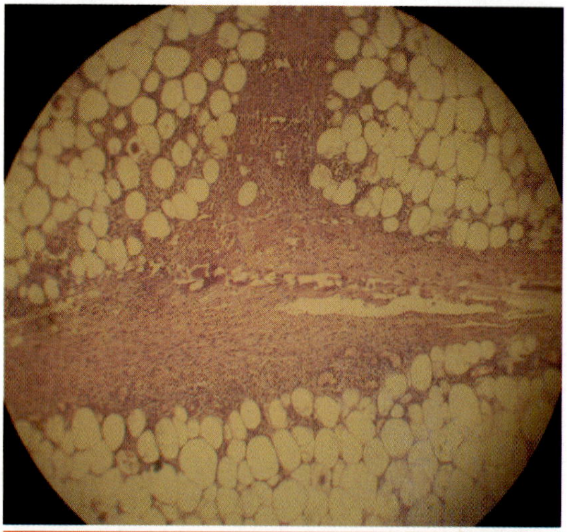

Fig. 85: Inflammation at the septum

Characteristic freatures

- Presence of erythematous, tender, evanescent nodules or erythema multiforme like lesions or lichenoid lesions.
- Fever, myalgia, malaise, arthralgia present in 60-70% cases and arthritis in 30% cases.
- Pain abdomen, vomiting, diarrhea and headache, episcleritis, retro-orbital optic nerve neuritis and phlyctenular conjunctivitis, may be associated.

Histopathology

- Septal panniculitis, Miescher's radiating granuloma and sometimes lobular panniculitis, vasculitis, superficial thrombophlebitis are present.

Tumid lupus erythematous

* It is form of chronic cutaneous lupus erythematosus.
* Lesions are very much photosensitive.

Clinical features

- Primary lesions are erythematous and edematous papules and plaques, developing at face and trunk.
- Overlying skin is shiny and smooth.

Histopathology

- Profuse dermal lymphocytic infiltration with abundant mucin deposition.

Treatment

- Intralesional triamcinolone
- Oral chloroquine.

Lupus profundus/Lupus panniculitis

* This is form of chronic cutaneous lupus erythematosus, affecting the subcutaneous fat.

Clinical features

- Primary lesions are firm subcutaneous nodules, developing at face, extremities and trunk.
- Overlying skin is usually smooth; but may have DLE like changes.
- Healing results in sunken, cosmetically disturbing scars.

Pyoderma gangrenosum

* It is a form of chronic nonhealing ulcerative dermatosis of unknown etiology, having a lot of diagnostic and therapeutic challenge.
* It is a form of vasculopathy with neutrophilic infiltration and tissue destruction.
* It may be associated with many other dermatoses including Crohn's disease in 5% cases.
* It is not a true leukocytoclastic vasculitis except the central zone where some amount of leukocytoclastic vasculitis is seen.
* It commonly occurs in 30-50 years of age.
* In children commonly affected sites are buttocks, pereneal region, head and neck.
* Lesions develop at the sites of trauma including intravenous puncture sites, surgical wounds and periostomal sites as a **pathergy phenomenon** in 20% cases.
* Perivascular deposition of IgM and C3 is seen in more than 50% cases.
* In 10% cases monoclonal gammopathy is seen.
* Vesiculopustular type is commonly associated with ulcerative colitis or hepatitis.
* It is also associated with some drugs like interferon α, GM-CSF and antipsychotic drug sulpiride.
* Patients present with chronic nonhealing and painful ulcer, usually at lower limbs.
* Initially these patients attend general or homeopathic practitioners or even surgeons or medicine specialists.
* Following a poor result often after trial of various antibiotics, they attend to the dermatologists.
* Though the disease is termed as pyoderma, there is no relation with pyogenic bacterial infection.
* In 50% cases it is not associated with any other internal diseases, but in remaining 50% cases it may be associated with Crohn's disease, ulcerative colitis, leukemia, chronic active hepatitis, lupus erythematosus and rheumatoid arthritis.
* Practically the cases which directly come to the dermatologist, usually they do not have any internal disease; but who attend Medicine specialist, usually they are associated with some form of internal diseases.

Types

- Acute type: Sudden onset with more painful lesions and rapid progress.
- Chronic type: Slow onset and progress with less painful lesion.

Variants

- Vesiculopustular
- Superficial granulomatous

Clinical features of acute PG

- Lesion starts as superficial hemorrhagic pustule, surrounded by an erythematous halo.
- Pustule breaks down to form an ulcer.
- Border of the lesion is dusky red or purple, boggy and raised. It is studded with pustules and sinuses with purulent discharge.
- Edge is undermined and irregular.
- Floor contains purulent and hemorrhagic exudates with or without granulation tissue.
- Pustules may present at the floor also.
- Around the border an advancing halo of erythema is seen.
- In some cases disseminated vesicles and pustules are seen. Some are follicular pustules.
- Healing of the ulcer produces a cribriform scar.

Clinical features of chronic PG

- Ulcer progresses slowly but spreads over a larger area.
- Lesions contains a lot of granulation tissue, often an exuberant proliferation, exhibiting massive granulation tissue.
- Margin is hyperkeratotic and crusted.

- In untreated cases, lesions may persist for months to years before spontaneous healing.
- Commonest sites are lower extremities and trunk.

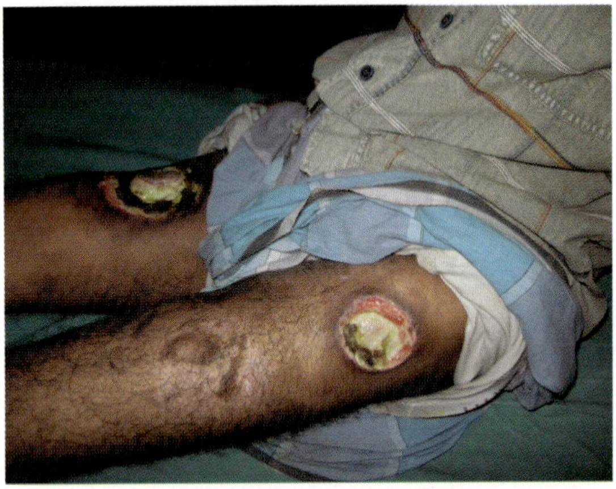

Fig. 86: Well defined and undermined ulcer with necrotic slough at the floor

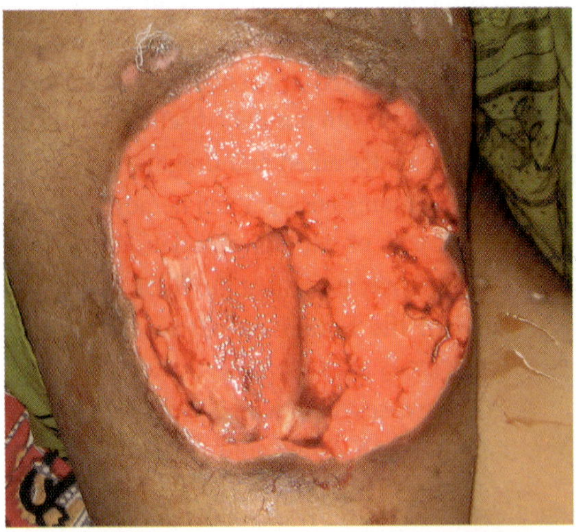

Fig. 87: Nonhealing ulcer at back of the upper thigh with clean floor and sharp margin and undermined edge

Differential diagnosis

- Furuncle or carbuncle or ecthyma gangrenosum due to severe pseudomonas infection.
- Tubercular ulcer
- Ulcerative deep fungal infection
- Vascular ulcer
- Diabetic ulcer
- Tropical ulcer
- Trophic ulcer or bed-sore
- Medium vessel vasculitis.

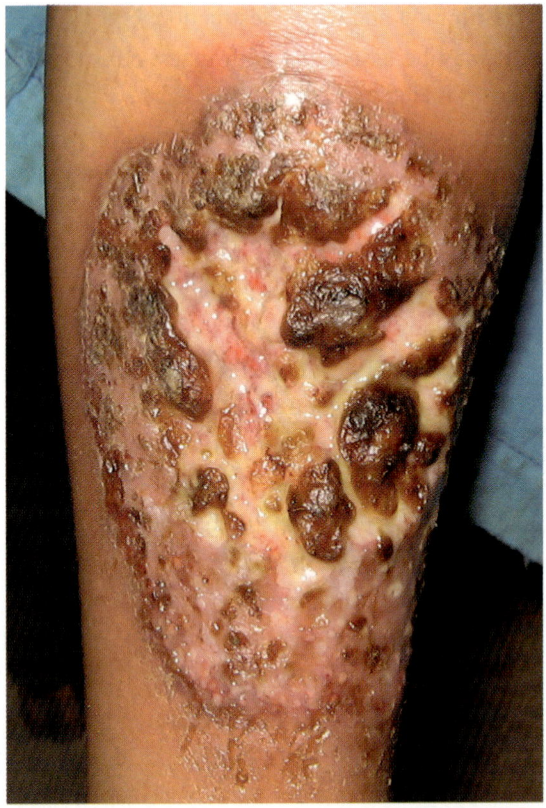

Fig. 88: Ulcer at lower leg with ragged margin and undermined edge and necrotic floor

Histopathology

- Central necrotizing suppurative inflammatory reaction with ulceration.
- Peripheral perivascular and intramural lymphocytic infiltration.
- Mural necrosis or fibrin deposition does not occur.
- Intermediate zone shows perivascular neutrophilic infiltration around the lymphocytic infiltration.
- Mixed infltration is known as Sweet-like vascular reaction.

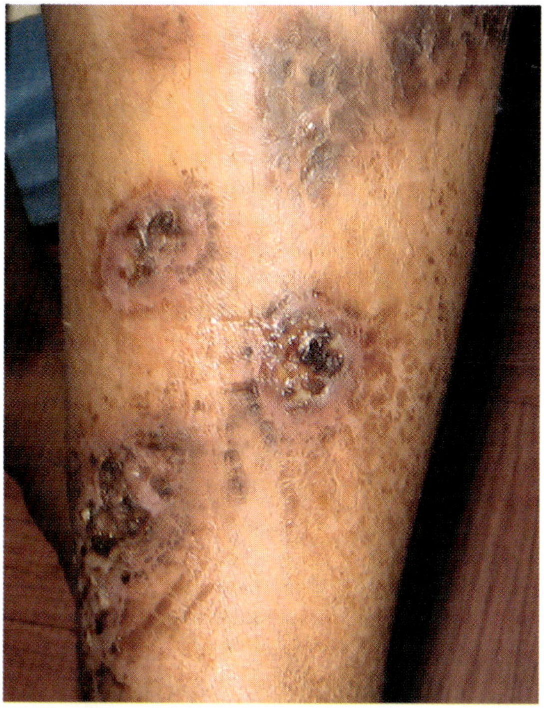

Fig. 89: Multiple healing ulcers of acute pyoderma gangrenosum

Treatment

- ♦ Intralesional triamcinolone and topical tacrolimus for solitary lesion.
- ♦ Pulse steroid therapy for extensive involvement.
- ♦ Sulfasalazine
- ♦ Cyclosporine
- ♦ Cyclophosphamide
- ♦ Azathioprine
- ♦ Clofazimine
- ♦ DDS
- ♦ Infliximab, etanercept, adalimumab, etc.

Sweet's syndrome/Acute febrile neutrophilic dermatosis

- ✶ It is an idiopathic inflammatory dermatosis.
- ✶ Women are commonly affected than male and commonly affected age group is 30-60 years.
- ✶ Bullous lesions are associated with leukemia.
- ✶ It is associated with peripheral leukocytosis and elevated ESR.
- ✶ It is often associated with infection like upper respiratory tract infection, drugs like GM-CSF and malignancy.

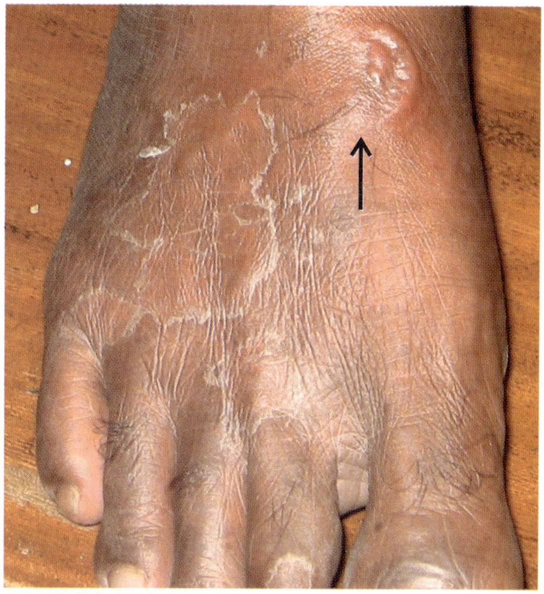

Fig. 90: Pseudovesicular plaque at the dorsum of the foot

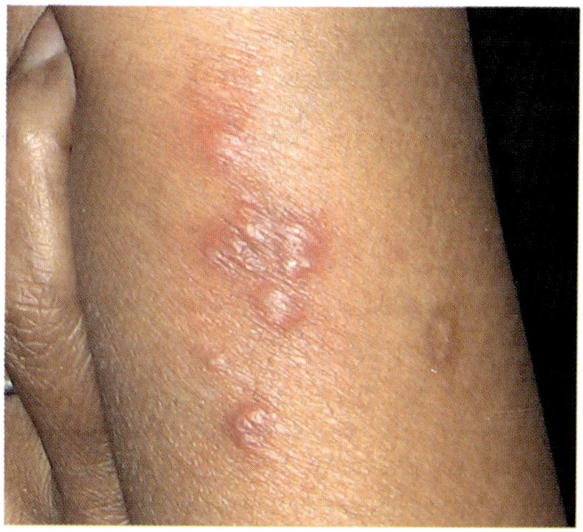

Fig. 91: Erythematous and edematous papules

Clinical features

- ♦ Preceding features like fever, tonsillitis and diarrhea may develop 1-3 weeks prior to onset of primary lesions.

- Primary lesions are painful, tender, edematous, shiny and smooth papules and plaques.
- Plaques are sharply defined but may be irregular in shape when it is formed by coalescence of nearby papules.
- When edema becomes prominent, lesions appear as vesicles and termed as pseudovesiculation.
- But true bullae and pustules may also develop.
- When these pseudovesicular lesions dry up, appear as mammilated.
- When a lesion heals quickly and resolves from the center or periphery, takes an annular or arcuate shape respectively.
- Number of the lesions may be single or multiple and they are distributed asymmetrically.
- Common sites are face, neck, upper extremities and rarely lower limbs.
- Conjunctivitis or episcleritis may be associated.
- Rarely lesions may be generalized.
- Associated features are fever, malaise and arthralgia.
- But fever may not present in every case.
- Over a period of days or weeks lesions may resolve without any scar formation.

Histopathology

- Normal epidermis.
- Profuse papillary dermal edema.
- Dense neutrophilic infiltration in mid dermis with sparse eosinophils and lymphocytes.
- Leukocytoclasia and nuclear dust may present but no endothelial change is seen.
- Neutrophils may also invade the subcutaneous tissue.

Treatment

- Systemic glucocorticosteroids (prednisolone 30-50 mg/day).
- Potassium iodide.
- Dapsone (DDS).
- Colchicine.

Diagnostic criteria of Sweet syndrome

- Major criteria:
  - Abrupt onset of painful erythematous plaque or nodule.
  - Histopathology shows dense neutrophilic infiltrate, without leukocytoclastic vasculitis.
- Minor criteria:
  - Pyrexia > 38°C.
  - Associated with hematologic or visceral malignancy or preceded by respiratory/gastrointestinal infection/vaccination.
  - Excellent response to systemic corticosteroid or potassium iodide.
  - Any three of the four laboratory findings: ESR > 20 mm/hour, positive C-reactive protein, leukocytes >8000 mm^3 and neutrophils >70% in peripheral smear.

Erythema elevatum diutinum

- This is a form of small vessel vasculitis of unknown etiology.

Clinical features

- Persistent reddish-violaceous to brown yellow papules and plaques.
- Symmetrically distributed at extensor surfaces of extremities.
- Consistency initially soft and later becomes firm.

Histopathology

- Predominant neutrophilic infiltration.
- Sparse eosinophils and plasma cells.
- Granulation and fibrous tissue in chronic stage.
- Rarely neutrophilic abscess present at tips of dermal papillae, like dermatitis herpetiformis.
- Fibrotic lesion shows array of spindle cells and collagen bundles parallel to the epidermis.

- Leukocytoclasis, neutrophilic dusts and fibrin deposition present.
- Focal areas of basophilic collagen, mixed with neutrophilic dusts mimic mucin depositon.

Lymphocytoma cutis/pseudolymphoma

- It is a form of reactive dermatosis of various etiology.
- It clinically and histologically resembles cutaneous lymphoma.

Clinical features

- It is characterized by erythematous and edematous or infiltrated nodule or plaque.
- Number of the lesion may be single or multiple.
- It mostly affects the face.

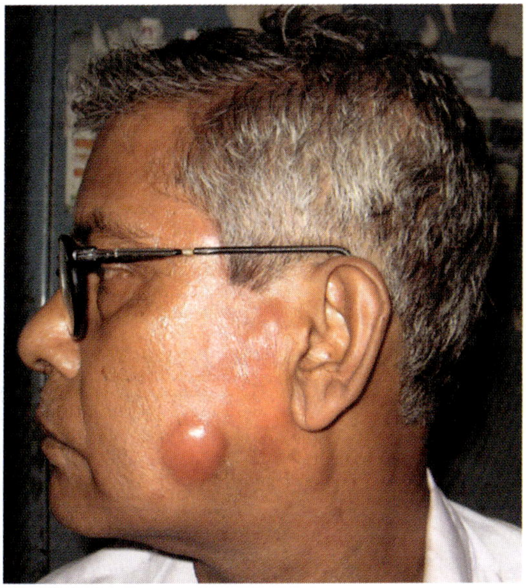

Fig. 92: Erythematous and edematous nodules at left cheek

Histopathology

- Presence of clear interface between epidermis and dermal infiltration (grenz zone).
- Dense nodular lymphohistiocytic infiltrations in the upper dermis, sparing the appendages and vessels.

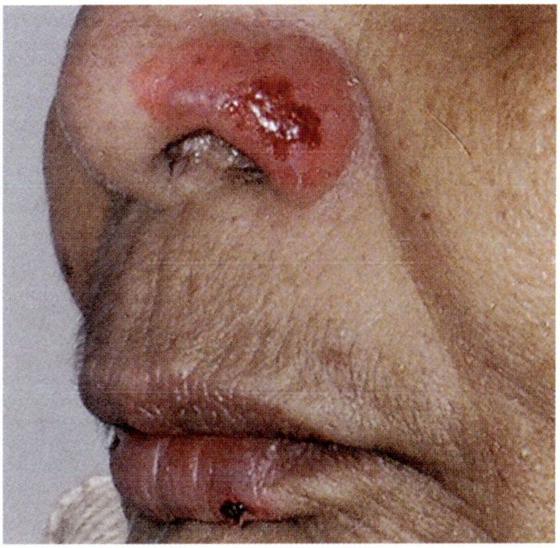

Fig. 93: Erythematous plaque at the nose with minor hemorrhage at the center

Juvenile xanthogranuloma

- Commonest type of non-Langerhans cell histiocytosis and majority of the cases manifest within first year of life.

Clinical features

- Lesions are rubbery and round papules or nodules with a pink to yellow tint.
- Common sites are head and neck.
- Atypical lcsions like hyperkeratotic nodule, flat or pedunculated plaque may be present.
- Atypical sites like lips, genitalia, palms-soles and iris also may be affected.

Histopathology

- Circumscribed noncapsulated dermal infiltration, composed of foam cells, mononuclear cells, eosinophils, and neutrophils. These foam cells may be present as touton giant cells or foreign body giant cells.

Fixed drug reaction

- This is a form of cutaneous drug reaction very often encountered in dermatology clinics.
- Commonest drugs are cotrimoxazole (sulfa drugs), non-steroidal anti-inflammatory drugs

(analgesic-antipyretic) and metronidazole/tinidazole (antiamebic/anti-diarrheal preparations).

* Nonpigmented reaction is seen with pseudoephedrine.

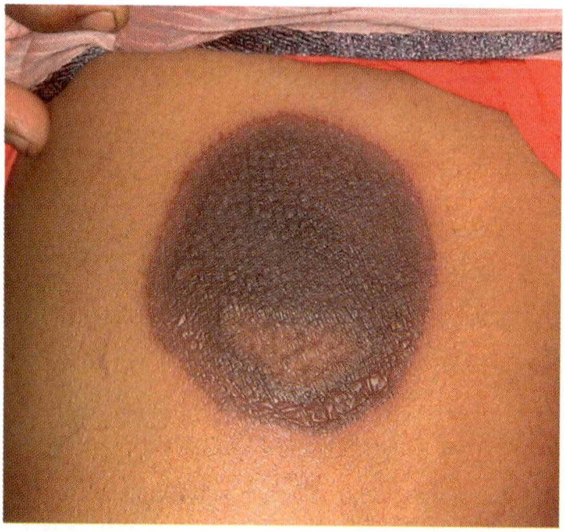

Fig. 94: Well circumscribed coppery color patch studded with tiny vesicles and central erosion

Clinical features

- It is characterized by pruritic, well circumscribed, erythematous, plaque with or without blister or erosion.
- Color of the lesion graudally changes from bright red to brown.
- It occurs repeatedly at same site, usually involving new sites following taking of a particular drug or a group of drugs.
- Any site may be affected but common sites are lips, glans penis, trunk and limbs.
- Lesion develops within variable period from 30 minute to 8 hours following ingestion of the drug.

Histopathology

- Necrosis of the epidermal cells with spongiosis.
- Vacuolar degeneration of basal layer.
- Pigment incontinence.

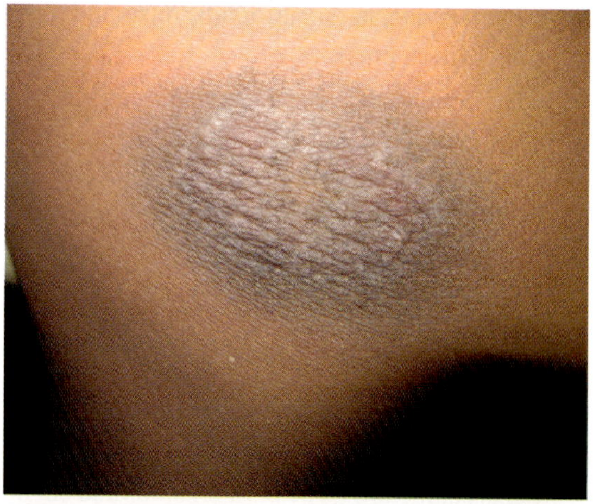

Fig. 95: Partially healed crusted lesion

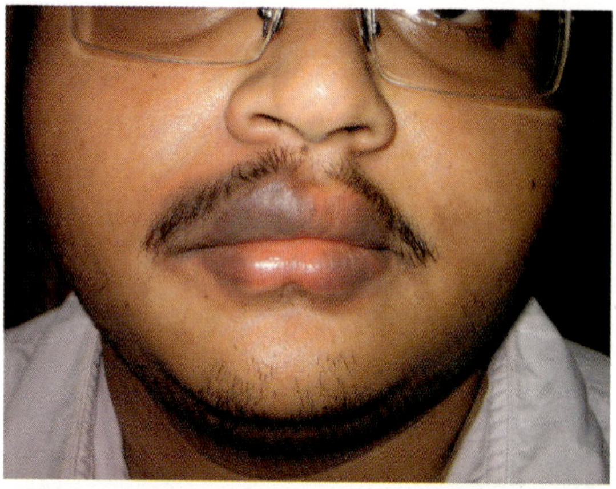

Fig. 96: Reddish brown plaque involving both lips

Delusional parasitosis

* This is a psychological disorder, often encountered by dermatologists.
* It occurs in elderly above the age of 60 years.
* Intellectuals including psychiatrists are commonly affected.
* Sometimes family members may suffer from the similar complaints.
* Patients are self-convinced that they must be infested with parasites.
* They use soap frequently to washout the insects.
* It may associated with pellagra, vitamin B12 de-

ficiency, coronary bypass surgery, renal disease and drugs like phenelzine.

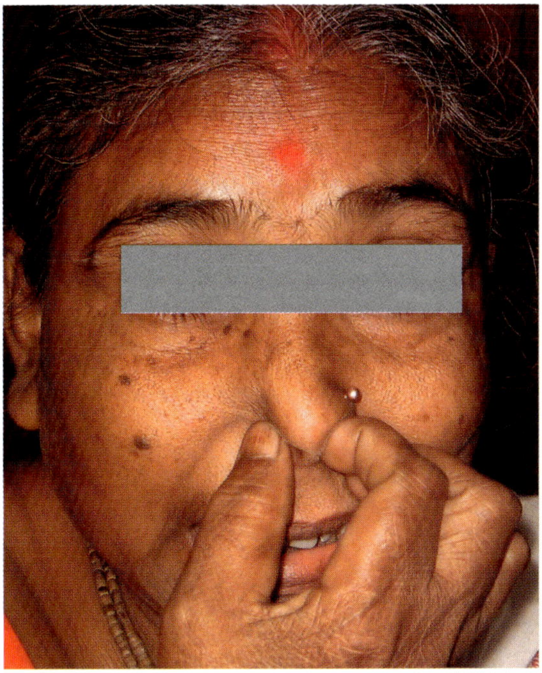

Fig. 97: Patient is trying to bring out the parasite from the nose

Clinical features

- Patients feel crawling of insects and often demonstrate skin debris as insects to the close relatives and to the physicians.
- Excoriation marks may be seen.

Treatment

- Pimozide is the drug of choice. It starts with 2 mg/day with weekly increment upto 12 mg. But practically the drug often becomes intolerable to the patient.

Dermatitis artefacta

- It is induced by self with full conciousness and without any rational motive.
- It occurs at the peak of an emotional outburst following an demand without fulfillment.
- Females are commonly affected.
- Commonest age group is 15-30 years who are having a labile emotion.
- Morphology of the lesions is very much variable but unique in individual case.

Clinical features

- Lesions are excoriations, erosions or ulceration.
- They may be lincar, arciform or angulated.
- Lesions are uniform and distributed haphazardly at easily approachable areas.
- Common sites are face, cheeks, limbs, genitalia, breast and chest.

Treatment

- Counselling.
- Local dressing and antibiotic for ulcers.

Cutaneous horn

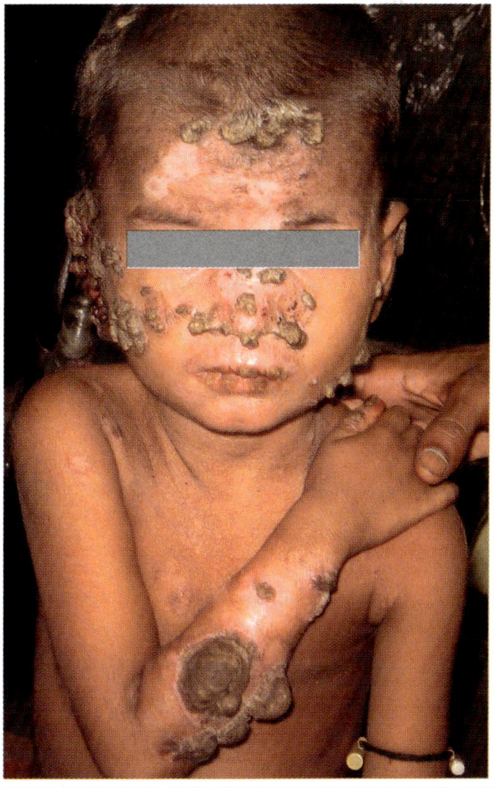

Fig. 98: Multiple horny growth on lesions of discoid lupus erythematosus

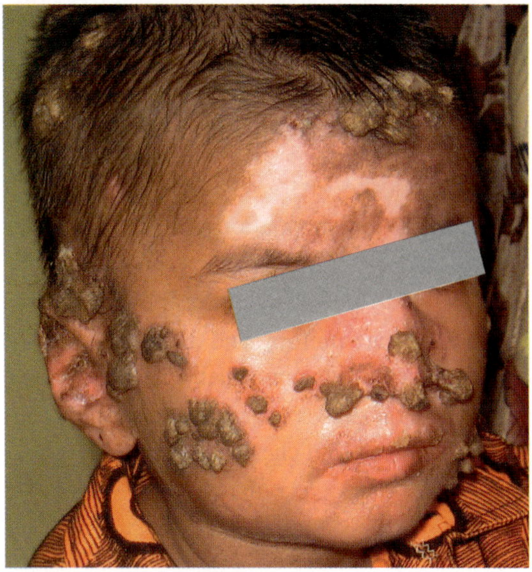

Fig. 99: Multiple plaques with conical horny growth

* The term is used for a conical or elongated keratotic papule or plaque.
* It is formed by deposition of keratin due to some abnormality in the spinous layer.
* Males are commonly affected than females.
* About 20% of cutaneous horns arise from underlying carcinoma in situ.
* Other common causes are verruca and seborrheic keratosis.

Clinical features

- Size of the lesion is variable from few mm to several cm.
- Photo-exposed areas are more frequently affected.
- Color is variable from white-brown to yellowish.

DERMATOSES WITH DIVERSE FEATURES

CHAPTER D2

Chronic arsenic dermatosis

* It is caused by long-time drinking of arsenic containing water and affects almost all organs including skin.

Pathological levels of arsenic

- Water: > 50 μg/L (Indian standard)
- Water: > 10 μg/L (WHO standard)
- Urine: > 50 μg/L
- Hair: > 1 μg/G
- Nail: > 1.5 μg/G

Inorganic arsenic presents in two forms

- Trivalent arsenic or arsenite
- Pentavalent arsenic or arsenate.

* Drinking water mostly contains pentavalent form. But toxicity is related to trivalent form. Pentavalent form is converted into trivalent toxic form by reduction through glutathione reduction system.
* Body tries to inactivate this active form through repeated oxidative methylation and reduction. Methylated compounds excrete through renal system. But this detoxification and excretion is variable from person to person.
* Toxic trivalent arsenic binds with sulfhydryl groups like glutathione and cysteine related to various metabolic systems of the cells.
* The term arsenolysis is used when phosphate is replaced by arsenic during glycolysis, resulting in production of dysfunctional ATP.
* Effects of arsenic toxicity at the molecular level:
  - Chromosomal aberration
  - Impaired DNA repair
  - Inactivation of tumor suppressor genes.
  - Abnormal expression of growth factors and transcription factors.
  - Increased expression of Keratin 16, an indicator of hyperproliferation.
  - Increased expression of Keratin 8 & 18, an indicators of poor differentiation.
  - Increased release of cytokines like IL8, TGFβ, TNFα and GM-CSF.

Clinical features

- It is characterized by presence of diffuse pigmentation, patchy pigmentation and spotted dyspigmentation, known as leukomelanosis or raindrop pigmentation.
- Palmoplantar keratosis is a prominent feature.
- Peripheral vascular disease, manifests as black foot.
- Bowen's disease, squamous cell carcinoma and basal cell carcinoma develop frequently.
- Hematological abnormalities are anemia, leucopenia and thrombocytopenia.
- Non-cirrhotic portal hypertension, hepatocellular carcinoma, cardiovascular disease, diabetes, fertility problem, and malignancies of the bladder, lung, and kidney may develop.

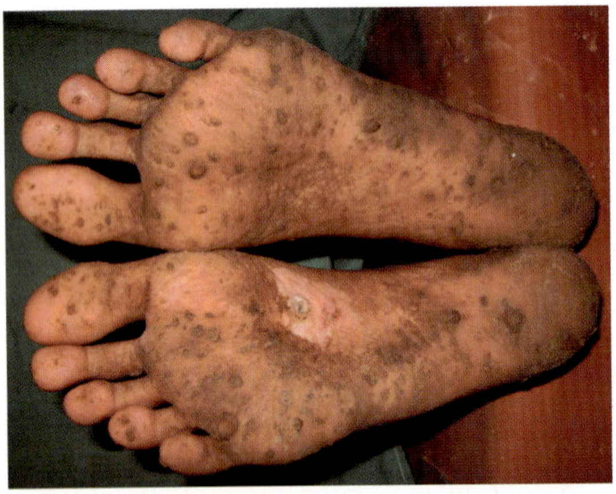

Fig. 1: Keratotic papules at both soles

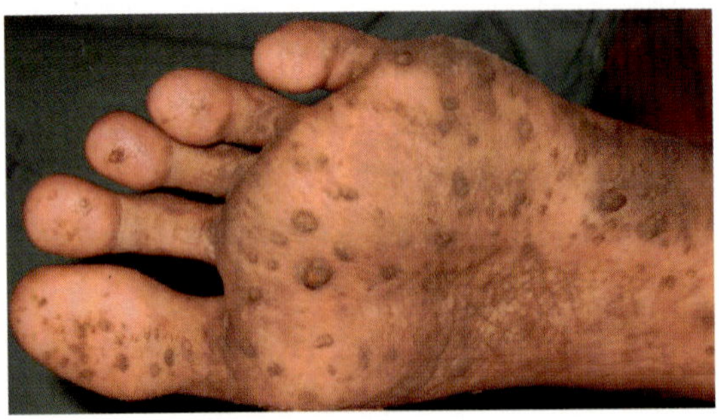

Fig. 2: Keratotic papules at right sole

Primary systemic amylodosis

- It affects many organs like skin, tongue, heart and gastrointestinal tract.

Clinical features

- Waxy and translucent pseudovesicular, smooth, firm and flat-topped papules, affect perinasal, perioral and periorbital areas and mucotaneous junctions.
- Papules may coalesce to form plaques and nodules
- Genital lesions resemble condylomata.
- Purpura and ecchymoses affect eyelids, oral cavity and limbs.
- Purpura, often elicited by trauma (pinch purpura) or following vomiting, coughing, and during proctoscopic examination or pulmonary function test is noted.
- Hemorrhagic bulla may develop at hands and feet.
- Tongue shows gross enlargement (macroglossia) with furrows and dental indentations at lateral sides. Papules, plaques and purpuric lesions may develop at the tongue also.
- Scalp shows diffuse or patchy alopecia and sometimes folded skin (cutis verticis gyrata) may develop.
- Limbs show paresthesia mimicking pure neuritic leprosy, scleroderma/scleromyxedema-like changes, carpal tunnel like features.
- Prominent deltoid muscle, due to deposition of amyloid, is known as shoulder pad sign.
- Nail shows atrophy of nails plates, longitudinal striae, partial anonychia, splitting and crumbling of nail plates.
- Cord-like thickening along the blood vessels may be seen which mimics thrombophlebitis.
- Rheumatoid arthritis like arthropathy, orthostatic hypotension, gastrointestinal bleeding and nephrotic syndrome may develop.
- Cardiac arrhythmia and congestive cardiac failure may occur.
- Cadiac problems are the commonest causes of death.

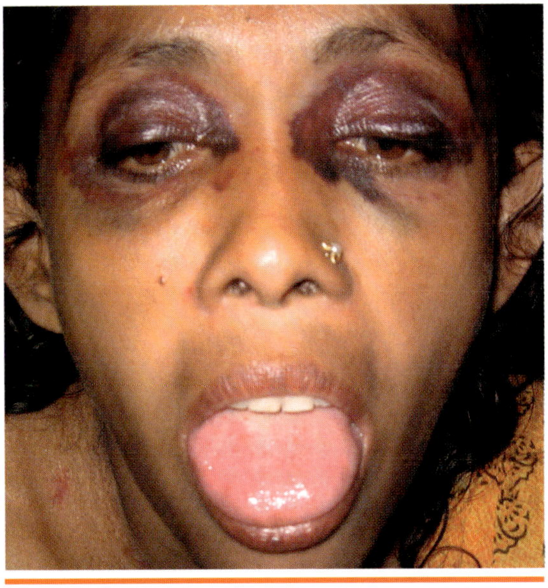

Fig. 3: Periocular ecchymosis with macroglossia

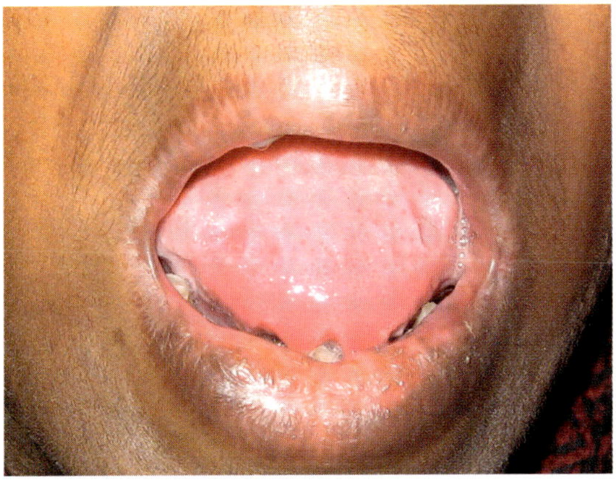

Fig. 4: Grossly enlarged tongue with indentations of teeth at margin of the tongue

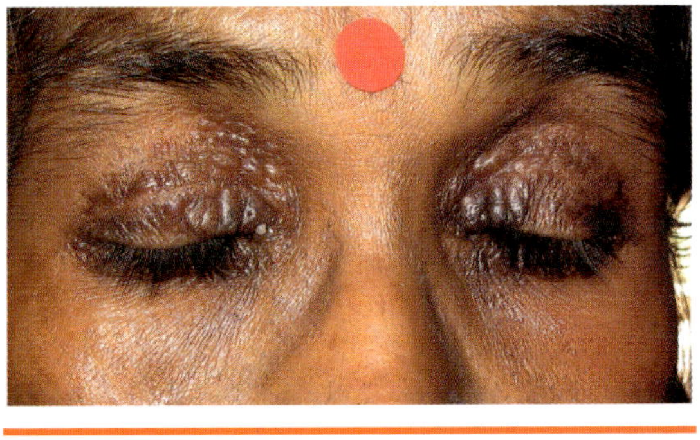

Fig. 5: Waxy papules at the eyelids

Treatment

- Systemic chemotherapy, mainly with melphalan.

Dysmorphophobia/dermatological non-disease/body dysmorphic disorders

- It is one of the frequently encountered disorder at every branch of medical sciences including dermatology.
- Patient often presents with lot of complaints without any organic base.
- It is commonly seen in divorced, poorly socialized, solitary and unmarried males and females.
- It often develops following reading of some ordinary medical journals or by observing the sufferings of some close relatives, specially from cancers.
- They visit one after another consultants without any satisfaction and simply they are called doctor shoppers.
- After a consultation, they ask to repeat the advice, already told.
- Same thing they may do after returning home over telephone.
- Their complaints are usually restricted to some particular areas like scalp, face, oral cavity, tongue, perineum and genitalia.
- Scalp and facial complaints predominantly affect the females.
- Perineal complaints are more in males.
- The term scalp dysesthesia is used for complaint related to scalp.
- The term orodynia is used for complaints related to oral cavity.
- The term glossodynia is used for complaints related to tongue.
- The term vulvodynia is used for complaints related to vulva.
- The term scrotodynia is used for complaints related to scrotum.
- The term penodynia is used for complaints related to penis.
- Oral cavity, tongue, urethral opening are frequently examined by mirror or directly if com-

plaints are related to oral cavity, tongue and penis respectively.

* Some patients admitted to me that they examined the oral cavity 5-15 times per day.
* Most of the patients suffer from anxiety, depression and sleeplessness.
* Patients often wake up early and are not able to sleep further.

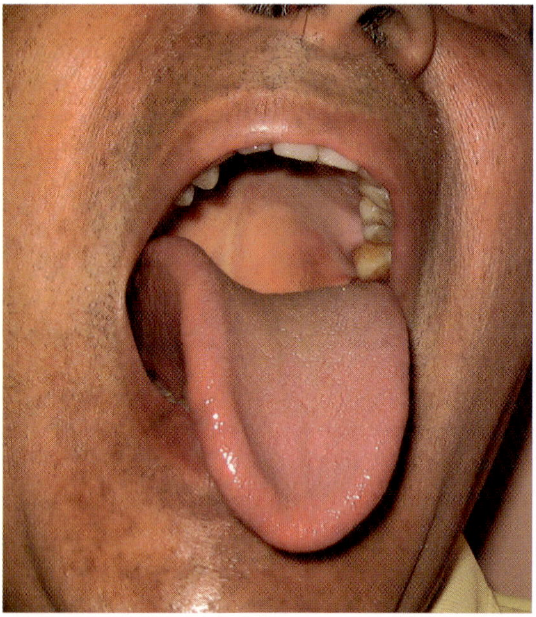

Fig. 6: Trying to show oral ulcer. He was successfully treated with amitriptyline

Facial complaints

- Excessive redness.
- Burning sensation.
- Feeling of scarring or pigmentation.
- Greasiness or dryness.
- Excessive hair growth.

Complaints related to oral cavity and tongue

- Pain or burning sensation.
- Overconsciousness about the taste buds.
- Presence of ulcers.

Complaints related to scalp

- Feeling of heat or burning sensation in older patients.
- Excessive hair loss in younger patients.

Complaints related to perineum and genitalia

- Presence of urethral discharge, excessive redness of the scrotum and ulcer at the urethral opening in males.
- Pruritus and burning sensation in females.

Treatment

- Anxiolytic and antidepressive.
- Counselling.

Dermatomyositis

* It is a dermatosis of skin and muscles without any exact etiology. Immune dysregulation has a confirmed role.
* Proximal muscle weakness is the most common presenting feature and characteristic skin lesions are seen in 40% cases during first evaluation. But skin lesions may precede muscle weakness even more than a year.
* It affects all age groups and affects male and female equally.
* Malignancy is associated in 25-30% cases.

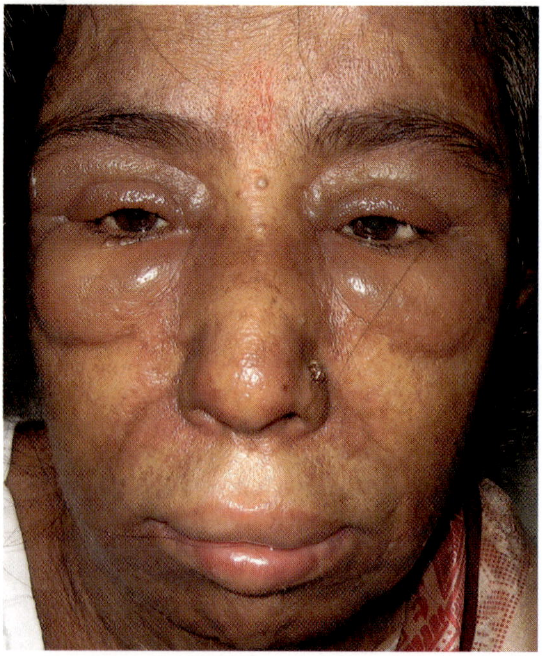

Fig. 7: Heliotrope erythema of eyelids

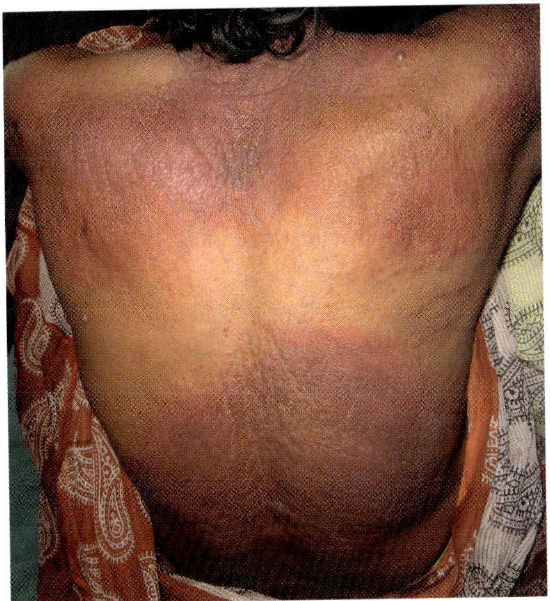

Fig. 8: CMVE at the back

Pathognomonic signs

- ***Heliotrope erythema of eyelids***: Periorbital edema with violet discoloration may be an earliest cutaneous sign or a residual of subsided diffuse facial edema.
- ***Gottron's papules***: These are smooth, flat-topped papules. Size ranges from 0.2-1 cm, and color varies from violet to red. Lesions may have central depression like a scar, lacy scale and telangiectasia. Commonest sites are dorsolateral aspects of interphalangeal/metacarpophalangeal joints of hands; but rarely knees and elbows are also affected. These are seen 60-80% cases during the course of the disease.

Hallmark skin lesions

- ***Confluent macular violaceous erythema (CMVE)***: These may be localized or diffuse and may be minimally raised and scaly. Localized form affects bony prominences like interphalangeal joints, metacarpophalangeal joints (knuckles), elbows, knees and ankles. Though knuckles and interphalangeal joints are classically affected, the intervening part of the phalanges are spared but in SLE these parts are characteristically involved. Diffuse form affects sun-exposed areas of face, neck, back, arms, buttocks, thighs and legs.
- Periungual erythema and telangiectasia.
- Poikiloderma vasculare atrophicans.
- Calcinosis cutis.

Epidermodysplasia verruciformis/Lewandowsky-Lutz disease

- It is an autosomal recessive disorder with mutation of EVER1 and EVER2 genes, encoding membrane proteins of endoplasmic reticulum and it is associated with various HPV serotypes like HPV3, –5, –8, –9 and –10.
- It manifests since childhood.
- Presence of immunosuppression probably causes viral infection.

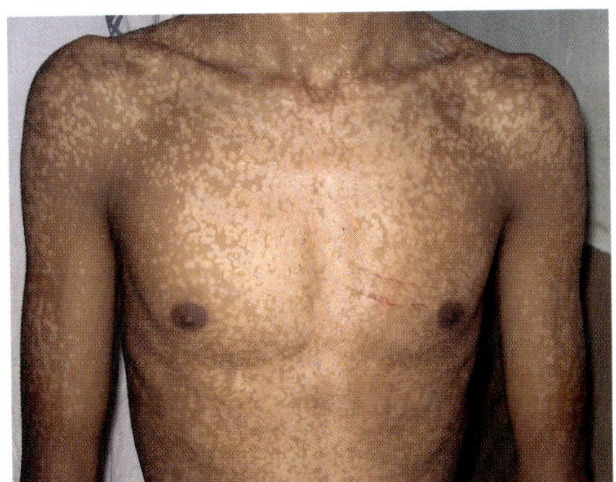

Fig. 9: Pityriasis versicolor like hypopigmented mild elevated lesions

Clinical features

- Primary lesions are numerous pityriasis versicolor like macules and patches. Lesions may be discrete, confluent and coalesced.
- Lesions show no tendency to regress spontaneously.
- Multiple warty papules and plaques are developed.
- Trunk and proximal extremities are the common sites.

- In later life, Bowen's disease or frank squamous cell carcinoma develops at sun-exposed areas.

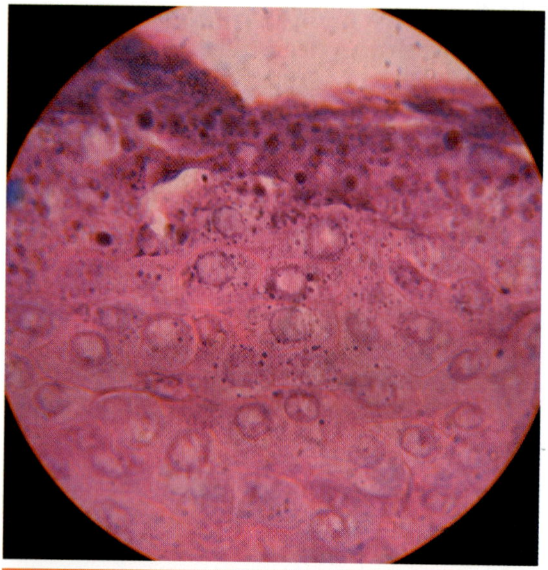

Fig. 10: Large keratinocytes with coarse keratohyaline granules

Histopathology

- Swollen and irregularly shaped keratinocytes in the upper layers.
- Basophilic cytoplasm with numerous round keratohyaline granules.
- Few dyskeratotic keratinocytes in the lower epidermis.

Erythema multiforme

- This is a reactive disorder of various etiology with a recurrent episodes of crops of lesions.
- Morphology of lesions is variable in same episode.

Variants

- Erythema multiforme (EM) minor
- Erythema multiforme (EM) major
- Steven-Johnson syndrome (SJS).

- The term erythema multiforme minor is used when all the lesions are discrete with or without mucosal involvement and target lesions barely turn into bullae.
- The term erythema multiforme major is used when many lesions coalesce, many target lesions show central vesicle and mucosal involvement is not more than one site.
- The term SJS is used when most of the lesions coalesce and target lesions are converted into bullae and more than one mucosal surfaces are involved.
- Some consider EM major and SJS as same.
- Some prefer to classify according to area of involvement and consider toxic epidermal necrolysis (TEN) as last manifestation of the disease spectrum. That classification is as follows:
  - SJS is < 10% body surface area involvement.
  - SJS-TEN overlap is 10-30% body surface area involvement.
  - TEN is > 30% body surface area involvement.
- In 50% cases of EM minor is caused by herpes simplex viral infection.
- In 70-90% cases of SJS is caused by drugs.
- More than 90% cases of TEN are caused by drugs. Whatever cases of TEN, so far I have seen, all were caused by drugs.

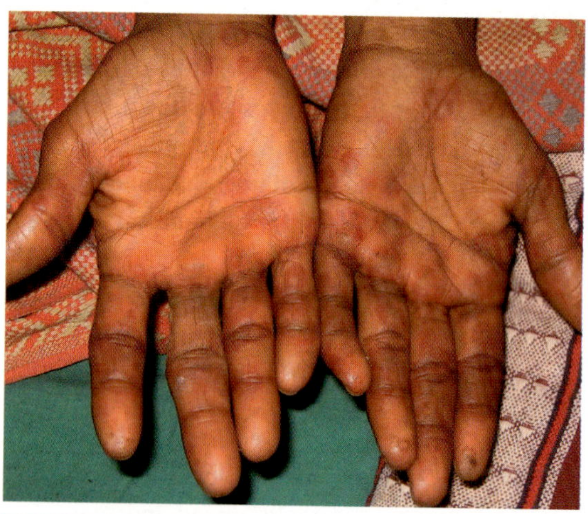

Fig. 11: Multiple erythematous and edematous target lesions at palms

Clinical features

- Lesions start as crops of papules or vesicles or papulovesicles with an erythematous base.

- The most characteristic lesion is known as **target lesion** which is comprised of three different zones as dusky erythema in the center, edematous zone at the middle and erythematous zone at the periphery.
- **Herpes iris of Bateman** is another erythematous plaque with central bullae. Sometimes a ring of vesicles may be present at the periphery of central bulla. It is characteristically seen in erythema multiforme associated with herpes infection.

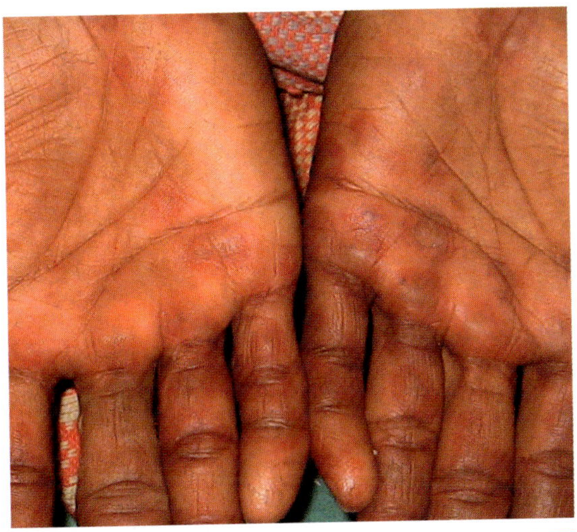

Fig. 12: Target lesions on palms

Treatment

- Treatment of the active herpetic infection.
- Removal of the offending drug.
- Antihistaminics for pruritus.
- Calamine lotion for soothing effect.
- Short term systemic corticosteroid for recalcitrant or progressive cases. Dose of prednisolone is ranging from 30-60 mg/day.

Mastocytosis

- It is a disorder of mast cells.

Types

- Mastocytoma
- Urticaria pigmentosa
- Diffuse cutaneous or bullous mastocytosis
- Telangiectasia macularis eruptiva perstans.

- Mastocytoma is the most common form of cutaneous mastocytosis in children.

Clinical features of Diffuse cutaneous mastocytosis

- It is manifested as grossly thickened doughy, reddish brown skin with peau d' orange appearance.
- Occasionally extensive bullous lesions develop with generalized pruritus, flushing and elevated temperature.
- General features are vomiting, diarrhea, abdominal pain, gastrointestinal ulceration, respiratory distress and even shock.

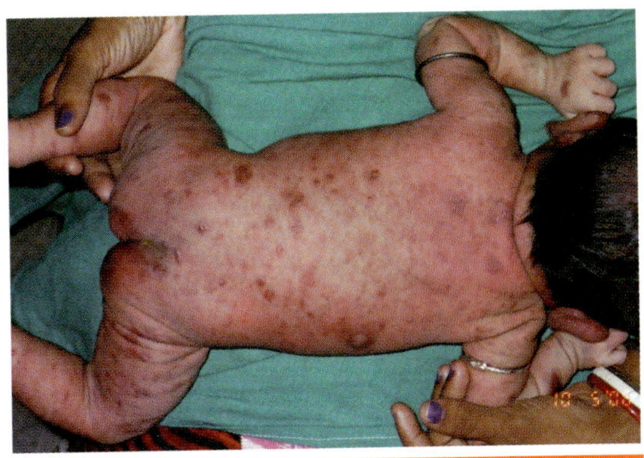

Fig. 13: Multiple erythematous macules and papules

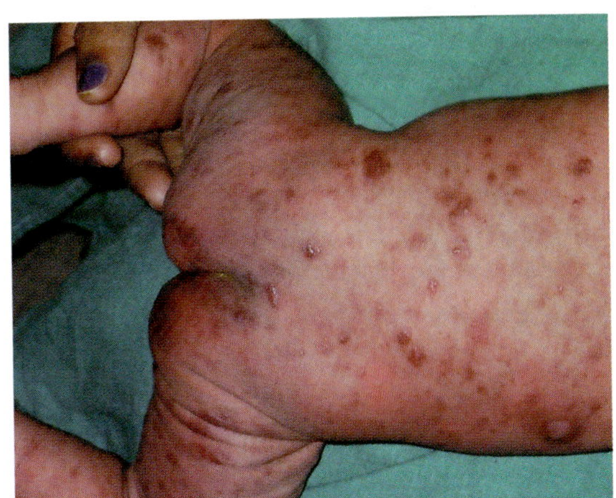

Fig. 14: Close-up view of the lesions

Clinical features of mastocytoma

- It presents with solitary or multiple flesh colored to yellow-orange papules and plaques. Surface of the lesion may be bruised or peau d' orange-like. Intermittent blister may develop, mimicking bullous impetigo or herpes simplex. But the tendency of vesiculation disappears by 1-3 years. Lesions usually involute after several years.
- Size is varying from few mm to several cm. Common sites are arms, neck and trunk or it may develop at any site.
- **Darier sign** is strongly positive. Even stroking or rubbing of the lesion may give rise to flushing or colic.

Pityriasis lichenoides

- It is characterised by successive crops of skin eruption with a wide range of morphology.
- Etiology is not yet clear.
- Adolescent and young adults are commonly affected.

Types

- Acute form is known as pityriasis lichenoides et varioliformis acuta (PLEVA/Mucha-Habermann disease). This is the severest form.
- Pityriais lichenoides chronica (PLC/Guttate parapsoriasis of Juliusberg). This is the mildest form.
- Overlapping of both.

Clinical features of PLEVA

- Primary lesions are bright red edematous papules.
- Sometimes vesicular lesions develop.
- Center of the lesion becomes necrosed and forms hemorrhagic crusts.
- Lesions evolve by central necrosis to form papulonecrotic lesions within a period of few weeks.
- Lesions may be asymptomatic or pruritic or painful.
- Lesions appear in crops.
- Number of the lesions are usually numerous but may be few.
- Some lesions become 1-2 cm in size.
- In some cases lesions suddenly flare up with numerous coalescent ulcers associated with fever and systemic features.
- Lesions heal with scar and postinflammatory hyperpigmentation.
- Lesions are distributed randomly. Mostly present at trunk and proximal extremities but may be generalized, including palms and soles.
- Associated features are fever, malaise and headache.

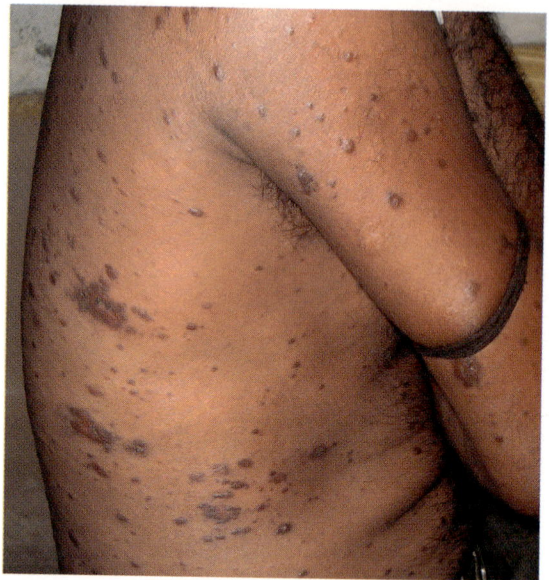

Fig. 15: Brownish papules and plaques

Clinical features of PLC

- Primary lesions are reddish-brown papules with central mica-like scale.
- Size 4-10 mm.
- Lesions resolve with postinflammatory hypo- or hyperpigmented macules.
- Lesions are distributed randomly. Mostly present at trunk and proximal extremities but may be generalized, including palms and soles.
- Lesions evolve by 3-6 weeks.

- Lesions may resolve spontaneously after 6-12 months.

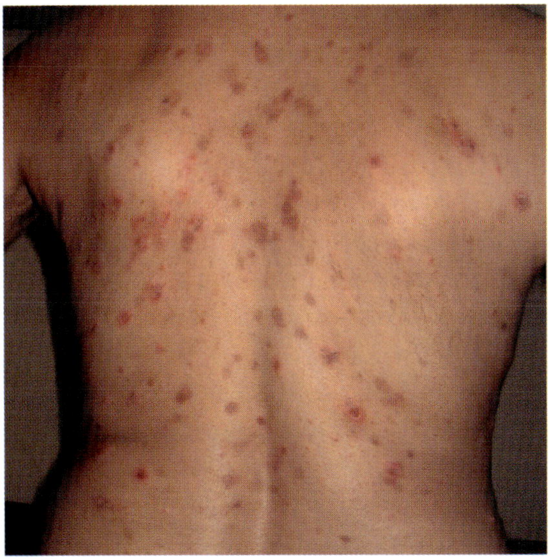

Fig. 16: Pleomorphic lesions consist of erythematous papules with central necrosis, erythematous papules and postinflammatory hyperpigmentation at the back

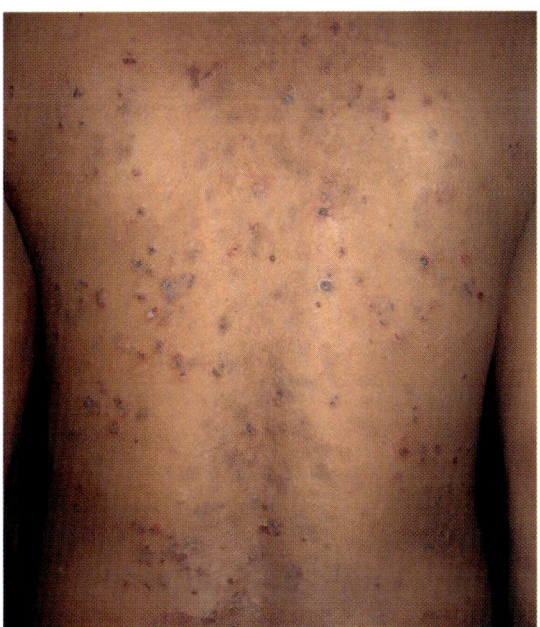

Fig. 17: Pleomorphic lesions consist of erythematous papules with central necrosis, erythematous papules and postinflammatory hyperpigmentation at the back

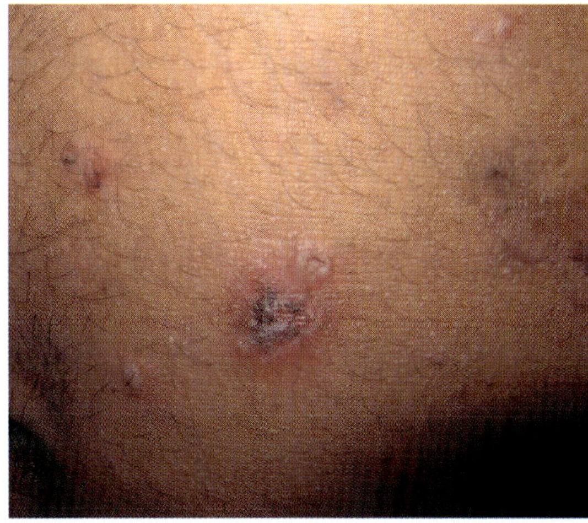

Fig. 18: Individual necrotic lesions of PLEVA

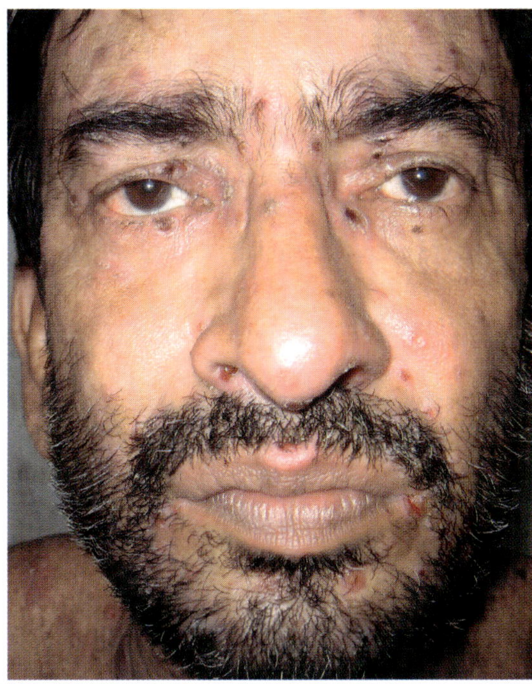

Fig. 19: Necrotic lesions of PLEVA

Histopathology of PLC

- Confluent parakeratosis.
- Spongiosis, exocytosis and necrosis of keratinocytes.
- Vacuolar degeneration of basal layer
- Extravasated erythrocytes and few melanophages in the papillary dermis.

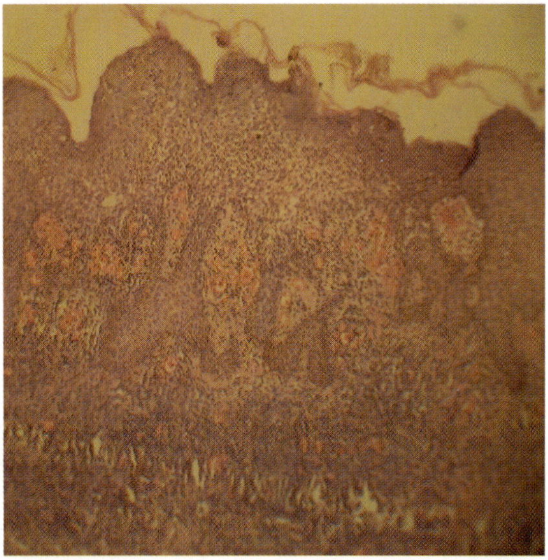

Fig. 20: Presence of erosion, acanthosis, spongiosis, exocytosis, dilated vessels and extravasation of RBCs

Histopathology of PLEVA

- Variable amount of epidermal necrosis leading to erosion and ulceration.
- Dense band-like papillary dermal and perivascular infiltration.
- Infiltration predominantly contains lymphocytes.
- Basal layer degeneration and obliteration of basement membrane zone.
- Wedge-shaped extension of the infiltration to deep dermis.
- Dermal edema, chronic inflammatory infiltrates, extravasated erythrocytes in the papillary dermis, sometimes in the epidermis.
- Swelling of the endothelial cells, congestion of vessels and hemorrhage.

Treatment

- Doxycycline or minocycline
- Systemic PUVA

Sarcoidosis

- **Sarcoidosis**, the term derived from **Sarkoid**, which was first introduced by *Caesar Boeck* in 1899 and probably due to resemblance with sarcoma.
- It is a multisystem granulomatous disease; but lungs, skin, eye, liver, peripheral lymph nodes are commonly affected.
- Lungs are affected in 90% cases.
- All ages and sexes are affected. But ages around 30 years and above 50 years are more involved.
- Females are slightly more suffered than males.
- It is most frequently seen in areas away from equator, like Denmark and Sweden.
- Most common cutaneous sites are head and neck. It also may affect scar at any site.
- Erythema nodosum, a nonspecific feature, seen in about 30% cases. It indicates a good prognosis.
- It is also more common in life-time nonsmokers.
- Most common cutaneous lesions are translucent, red-brown to yellow-brown, papules with apple jelly appearance on diascopy.
- Noncaseating, naked granuloma, is suggestive but not specific.
- Symptoms and signs depend on the affected organ. But 30-60% of pulmonary sarcoidosis are asymptomatic.
- Cytokines released with the granulomatous inflammation is responsible for constitutional symptoms like fever, night sweats, malaise, and weight loss.
- Specific cutaneous lesions are usually asymptomatic and pruritus or pain is rare.
- It may have acute onset, presenting with erythematous tender nodules, known as **erythema nodosum**, or insidious onset, presenting with asymptomatic papules and plaques of the skin or pulmonary infiltrate found accidentally during routine X-ray of the chest.
- General features includes fever, fatigue, weight loss and arrhythmia.
- Increased level of serum angiotensin converting enzyme, hypergamma globulinemia and hypercalcemia, may be associated.

Cutaneous lesions

- Primary lesions are macules/patches, papules, plaques and nodules. These may affect any part of the skin and mucosae, distributed symmetrically or asymmetrically.
- Size varies from few mm to several cm and shape is also variable from round/annular to bizarre.
- Surface may be scaly, telangiectatic or atrophic.
- **Lupus pernio** is violaceous in color and affects nose, earlobe, cheeks and digits. Lesions may extend to nasal sinuses leading to crusting and bleeding.
- **Angiolupoid** lesions are more pink but less in number in color with prominent telangiectasia and affect the face.
- **Darier-Roussy sarcoid** is a form of painful or painless, persistent subcutaneous nodules which commonly affect the extremities.
- Scarring or non-scarring alopecia develops if scalp is affected. Reversibility of hair growth depends on degree of hair follicle destruction.
- Nail changes are rare due to either nail bed or adjacent bone involvement. These are clubbing, dystrophy, discoloration and subungual hyperkeratosis.
- Tongue, oral mucosa, lacrimal/parotid glands, sublingual/submandibular lymph glands may be affected. **Mikulicz syndrome** may also be caused by sarcoidosis.
- **Atypical lesions:**
  (a) Psoriasiform lesions, discoid lupus-like lesions, lichen nitidus-like lesions, prurigo nodularis-like lesions and morphea form/ verrucous plaques.
  (b) Folliculitis-like pustular lesions and ulcerations.
  (c) Polymorphous light eruption-like lesions and nongranulomatous exanthematous eruptions.
  (d) Faint erythema, palmar erythema and erythroderma.
  (e) Ichthyosis and lower limb edema.
  (f) Penile or vulvar lesions.

Systemic features

- **Lofgren syndrome:** Characterized by bilateral hilar adenopathy, arthralgia and fever. This is also known as acute sarcoidosis with eventual resolution.
- **Lungs:** Symptoms are dyspnea, cough, chest pain and wheezing. Bilateral hilar adenopathy are seen in 50-90% cases and parenchymal involvement is seen in 25-60% cases. Pulmonary function is diminished in abnormal and normal chest radiograph in 50-70% and 20-40% respectively.
- **Eyes:** Involved in 25-75% cases and symptoms vary from asymptomatic to threatening of vision. Burning, itching, dryness and redness are main symptoms. Most common form is uveitis which may complicate to cataracts and glaucoma. Conjunctivitis, keratoconjunctivitis sicca (dry eyes) and loss of vision due to optic nerve neuritis are other features.
- **Heerfordt syndrome:** Fever, parotid glands swelling, facial palsy and anterior uveitis are the main features.

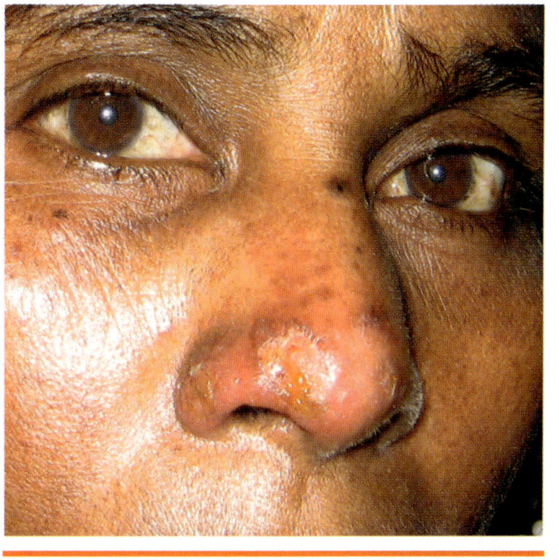

Fig. 21: Erythematous, edematous and eroded plaque at the nose

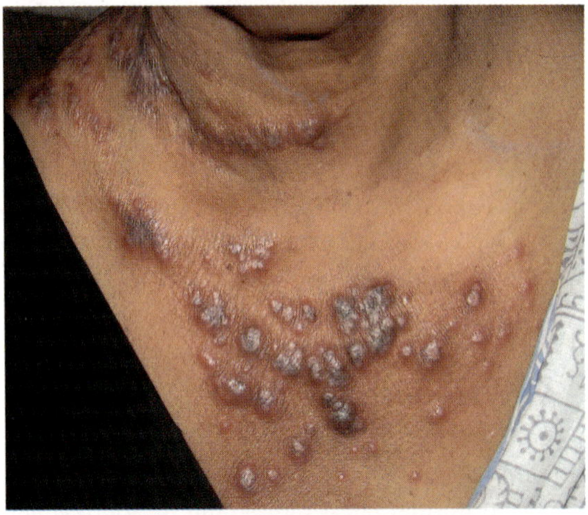

Fig. 22: Multiple erythematous and violaceous papules at chest

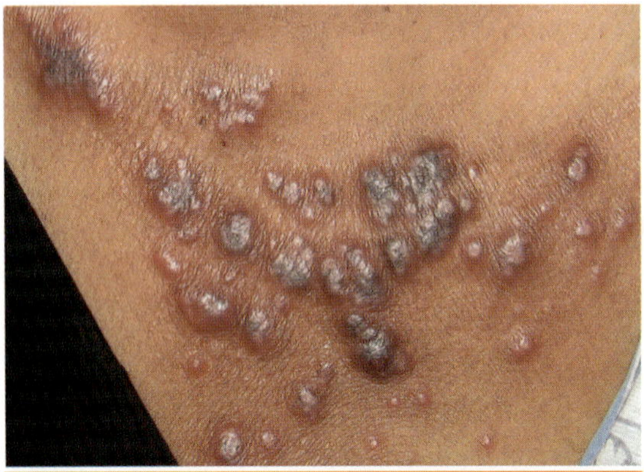

Fig. 23: Confluent erythematous to violaceous papules at chest

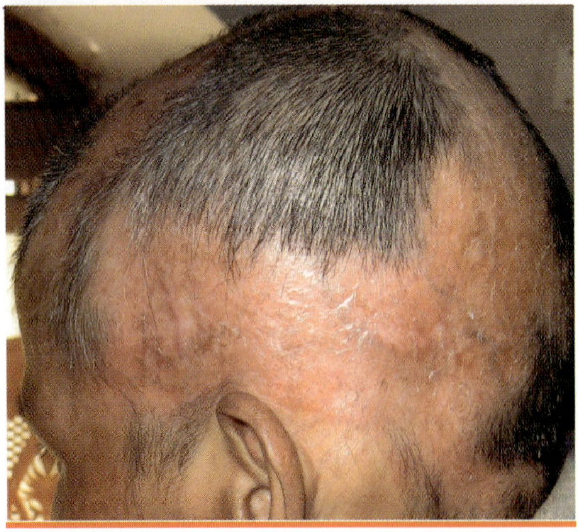

Fig. 24: Scalp sarcoidosis with scarring alopecia

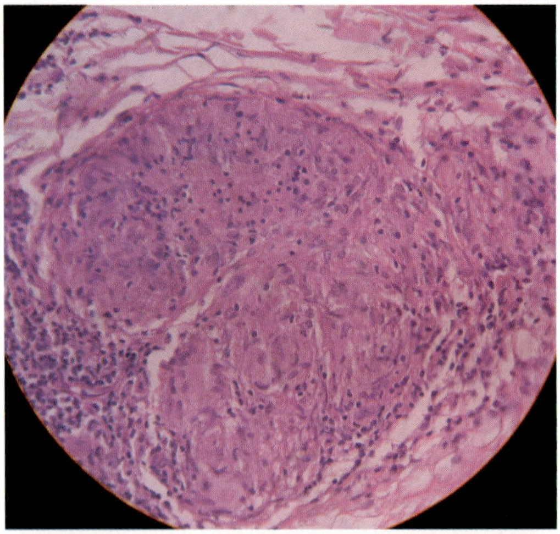

Fig. 25: Naked and noncaseating granuloma

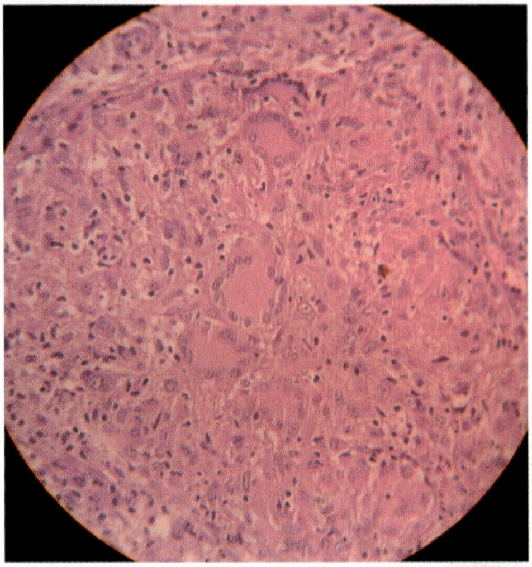

Fig. 26: Epithelioid granuloma with multiple giant cells

Histopathology

- Dermis contains granuloma with epithelioid cells at the center and scanty lymphocytes at the periphery.
- Giant cells of variable shape and size are often present. Some of these may contain asteroid bodies.
- Caseation is usually absent but rarely fibrinoid necrosis may be present.

Treatment

- Intralesional triamcinolone (3 mg/ml) for single or few lesions.

- ♦ Systemic corticosteroid for multiple lesions, disfiguring lesions, active ocular lesion, cardiac arrhythmia, CNS involvement and hypercalcemia.
- ♦ Hydroxychloroquine 100 mg twice daily, but only partially effective.
- ♦ Methotrexate 5-7.5 mg/week, also partially effective.

Cutaneous vasculitis

- ✶ **Vasculitis** is a pathological term but equally used for clinical description.
- ✶ It is characterized by invasion of the vessel wall by neutrophils, swelling of the endothelial cells, disruption of the vessel wall, and extravasation of red blood cells. Most of neutrophils are destroyed and turned into neutrophilic dusts, known as **leukocytoclasia** and for this, cutaneous vasculitis is also called **leukocytoclastic vasculitis**.
- ✶ Clinical features depend on:
  - ♦ Types of blood vessels affected.
  - ♦ Types of organs involved, including skin.
- ✶ Most of the patients are **asymptomatic** but common symptoms are burning, pain and pruritus.
- ✶ If the lesion persists more than 72 hours, gradually neutrophils are replaced by lymphocytes and if persists for several days or weeks, damaged vascular walls show **fibrinoid degeneration**.
- ✶ Features of vasculitis are directly reflected on the skin when **small vessels** (arterioles, capillaries and post capillary venules) in papillary/mid dermis are involved or when **medium sized vessels** in lower dermis or hypodermis are involved.
- ✶ But when large vessels like aorta and temporal arteries are affected, cutaneous features are the results of indirect effect and known as **vasculotides**.
- ✶ **Site of involvement** has a predilection for lower limbs where hydrostatic pressure is more or at waist area where compression occurs due to tight clothing.
- ✶ Livedo reticularis and livedo racemosa are features of vasculitis.

Livedo reticularis	Livedo racemosa
• Bilateral symmetrical	• Unilateral
• Regular	• Broken/irregular
• Reversible	• Irreversible

Etiopathogenesis: Though the exact etiology is not yet known, following facts are noted:

- ♦ Basically vasculitis is an immune complex mediated disease where antigens are more than antibodies. Some cases antibodies are formed against a specific antigen, but not in many cases.
- ♦ Specific antibodies are diffuse cytoplasmic antineutrophilic cytoplasmic antibody (**cANCA**) against **proteinase 3** and perinuclear antineutrophilic cytoplasmic antibodies (**pANCA**) against **myeloperoxidase**.
- ♦ Both the antigens are present in neutrophils. But the mechanism of antibody formation is still in dark.
- ♦ Antigen-antibody complexes at vessel wall activate complement system to produce C3a/5a and membrane attack complex (MAC).
- ♦ MAC damages the vessel wall directly and C3a/5a attract neutrophils for consumption of the immune-complexes. But during consumption neutophilic granules are degranulated to produce collagenase, elastase and oxygen free radicals. These are responsible for further vascular damage.
- ♦ Upregulation of adhesive molecules at the endothelial cells as well as at the neutrophils. This helps in marginalization as well as extravasation of neutrophils.
- ♦ Release of chemotactic cytokines like IL_1, IL_6, IL_8, TNFα and G-CSF maintain the inflammation.
- ♦ Mast cells also play a role, specially in urticarial vasculitis. Release of histamine causes dilatation of blood vessels and thus helps in extravasation of red blood cells.
- ♦ Aggregation of platelets slows the microcirculation and thus the interaction among im-

mune-complexes, neutrophils, endothelium will be going on for longer time.

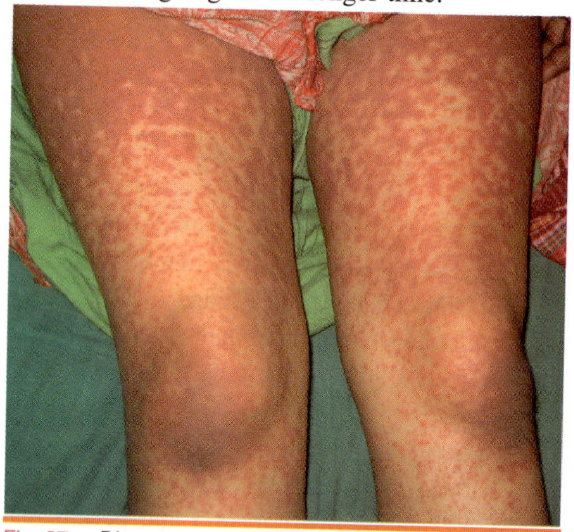

Fig. 27: Discrete, confluent and coalesced erythematous mild elevated papules and plaques

Cutaneous features of small vessels vasculitis in general

- Palpable purpura
- Ecchymoses
- Erythema multiforme-like lesions.
- Urticarial papules
- Vesicles.
- Pustules.

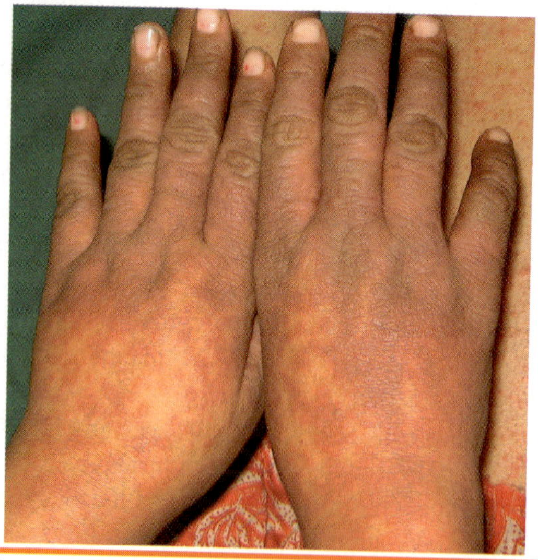

Fig. 28: Discrete, confluent and coalesced erythematous mild elevated papules and plaques

Cutaneous features of small to medium vessel vasculitis in general

- Palpable purpura
- Ecchymoses

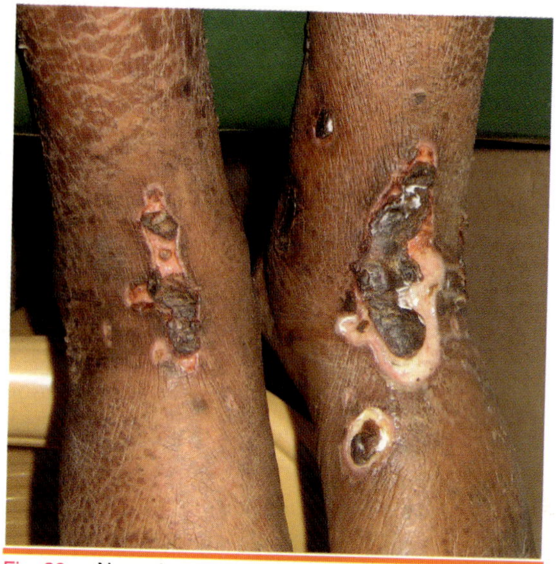

Fig. 29: Necrotic ulcers with hemorrhagic crusts in medium vessel vasculitis

- Erythema multiforme-like lesions
- Urticarial papules
- Nodules
- Vesicles
- Pustules
- Necrotic superficial ulcers.

Cutaneous features of medium vessel vasculitis in general

- Nodules
- Necrotic deep ulcers

General and systemic features

- Fever, arthralgia, arthritis
- Pain or burning sensation, rarely pruritus
- Pulmonary, renal, gastrointestinal and neural manifestations.

Systemic lupus erythematosus (SLE)

* It is a form of lupus erythematosus, affecting most of the internal organs with variable cutaneous manifestations.

* Patient may develop SLE as de novo or may be converted from acute LE, subacute LE or DLE.
* Bullous SLE is a variant of SLE.
* Acute LE is always associated with SLE.
* Cutaneous lesions is variable from patient to patient, or in same patient from time to time.
* There are 11 criteria, including 4 for skin, 5 for internal organs and 2 for immunological irregularities. Among these, at least 4 are required to diagnose SLE. These 4 criteria may be found simultaneously or subsequently.
  1. Malar rash
  2. DLE-like lesions
  3. Painless palatal ulcers.
  4. Photosensitivity
  5. Neurological disorders like psychosis or seizure.
  6. Serositis like pleuritis and carditis.
  7. Renal involvement with persistent proteinuria (> 0.5 gm/day) or presence of cellular casts in urine.
  8. Non-erosive arthritis.
  9. Hematological features like anemia, leucopenia and thrombocytopenia.
  10. Immunological disorders like LE cell phenomenon, anti-DNA antibody, anti-Sm antibody, positive VDRL for more than 6 months.
  11. Antinuclear antibody.

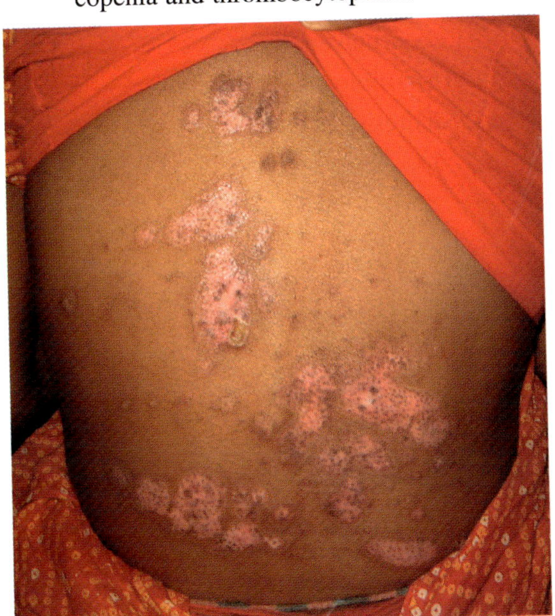

Fig. 30: DLE-like lesions in SLE

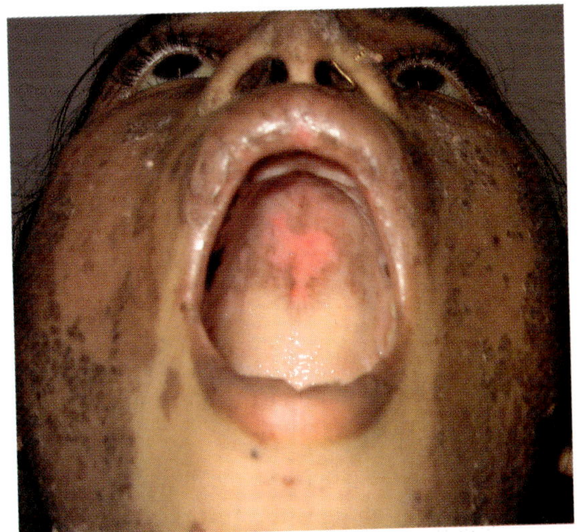

Fig. 31: Palatal erosion

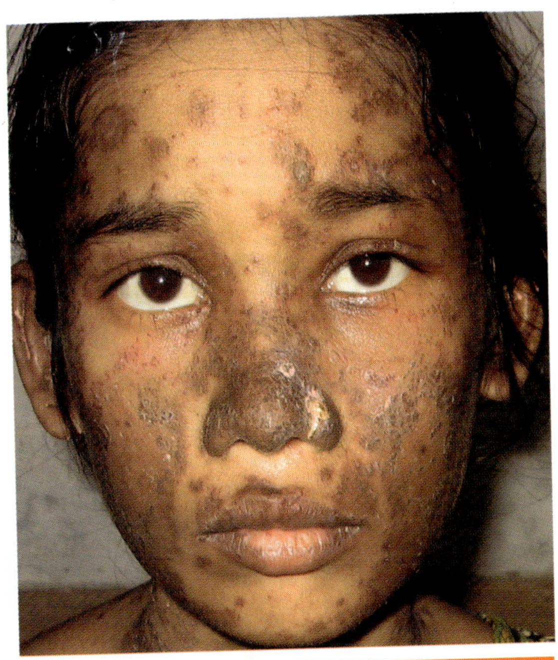

Fig. 32: Malar rash sparing nasolabial fold

Immune reconstitution inflammatory syndrome (IRIS)

* It is a pathologic inflammatory response to pre-existing microbial, host, or other antigens that results in clinical deterioration in HIV infected persons after initiating highly active antiretroviral therapy (HAART).
* The suppression of HIV replication allowing gradual restoration of immune status is the central feature of IRIS pathogenesis.

Incidence

- It is seen in 15-25% of all HIV patients on HAART.

Risk factors

- Presence of opportunistic infections at initiation of HAART.
- Shorter interval between the initiation of treatment for opportunistic infections and starting of HAART.
- Lower baseline CD4 count and higher baseline viral load.
- More rapid changes in CD4 cell count and viral load during HAART.

Background of IRIS manifestation

- Unmasking of previously untreated opportunistic infection: It shows an atypical presentation.
- Paradoxical reaction: It is best seen with tuberculosis and cryptococcal meningitis.
- Development of autoimmune disease: Best example is development of Grave's disease or sarcoidosis.

Dermatologic manifestation

- Herpes simplex viral infection 1 & 2., herpes zoster, Kaposi's sarcoma due to HSV8, cytomegalovirus infection, wart and molluscum contagiosum.
- Mycobacterium avium complex infection and other atypical mycobacterial infection.
- Mycobacterium tuberculosis and leprosy.
- Cryptococcosis, histoplasmosis, tinea corporis and candidiasis.
- Eosinophilic and inflammatory folliculitis and acne vulgaris.
- Reiter's syndrome.
- Leishmaniasis.
- Sarcoidosis and foreign body reactions, SLE and lupus tumidus.
- Alopecia universalis.
- Dermatofibroma.
- Dyshidrosis.

REGIONAL DERMATOSES

CHAPTER D3

Alopecia areata

* It is characterized by focal loss of hair without any scarring. Though exact etiology is not known, probably it has a T cell mediated autoimmune etiology. Genetic background and anxiety are common precipitating factors.
* Sometimes it may be associated with other autoimmune disease like diabetes, vitiligo and thyroid disease.

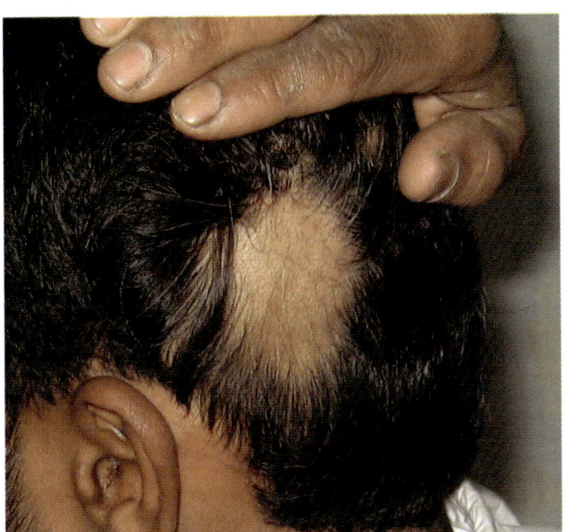

Fig. 1: Patchy loss of hair

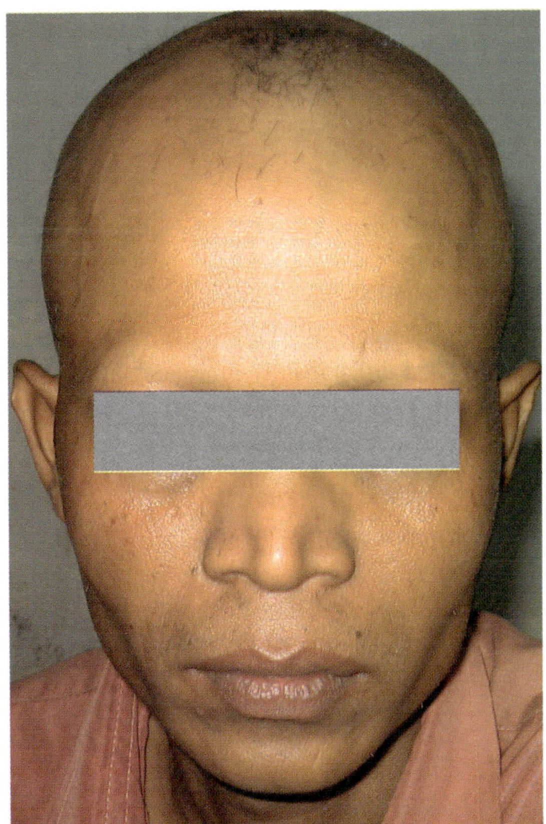

Fig. 2: Alopecia universalis with generalized hair loss

Clinical features

- Any hair bearing area may be affected but in 90% cases scalp is involved.
- Early lesion is well circumscribed and coin-like size. Gradually size enlarges and takes variable shape. Usually hair loss is complete but later few hair may grow within the lesion. Presence of short hair with broad distal end and thin proximal end, appearing as **exclammation sign**, at the periphery of the lesion indicates that the disease is active and its prognosis is not favourable.

Variants

- Alopecia totalis: Whole scalp is affected.
- Alopecia universalis: Whole body is affected.
- Ophiasis: Broad hair lines at occipital and temporal regions are affected.

Histopathology

- Diagnostic feature is peribulbar lymphocytic infiltration as **swarm of bees appearance**, around the anagen follicle.

Treatment

- Potent topical corticosteroid like clobetasol or halobetasol ointment.
- Minoxidil (2-5%) solution.
- Topical immunotherapy with diphencyprone.
- Topical inflammatory drug like anthralin.
- Intralesional triamcinolone (10 mg/ml) injection at 1-3 weeks interval.

Androgenetic alopecia

- It occurs due to influence of androgen and has a familial tendency.
- It occurs in 50% of men by the age of 50 years.
- It affects both males and females.

Clinical features

- Pattern of involvement is different in male and female.
- In males, it usually starts at temporal region and gradually progresses to vertex.
- In females, there is a diffuse involvement.

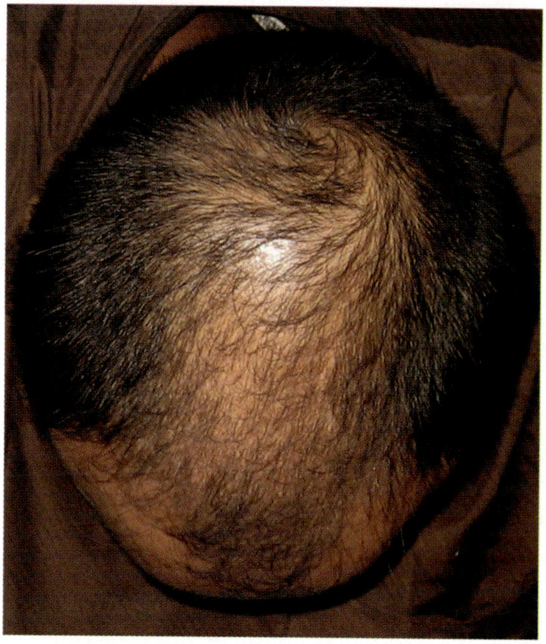

Fig. 3: Androgenetic alopecia

Histopathology

- Miniaturization of hair follicles is the hall mark.

Treatment

- Oral finasteride 1 mg daily and topical minoxidil 2-10% for males and 2% minoxidil for females.

Pseudopelade

- It is a common form of cicatricial alopecia of unknown etiology.
- It occurs in adults.

Clinical features

- It is characterized by irregularly defined shiny depressed patches of alopecia with loss of follicular markings. Nearby patches often coalesce to form a bizarre shaped lesion.
- This type of presentation is designated as **footprints in the snow**.
- Loss of follicular markings helps to differentiate it from pelade or alopecia areata.

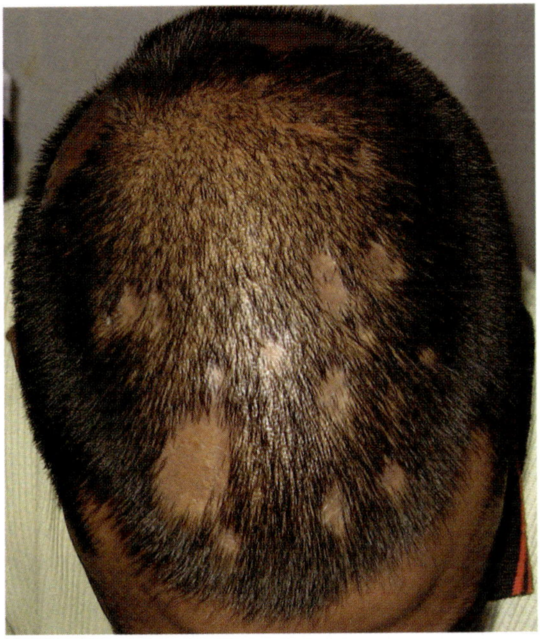

Fig. 4: Patches of alopecia with atrophic and depressed skin

Differential diagnosis

- Alopecia areata

Trichotillomania

- Patients feel an irresistable impulse to pluck hair and also feel a sense of relief after doing it.
- This is also associated with nail biting, known as **onychotillomania** and nail eating, known as **onychophagia**.
- Other associated features are dysthymia or loss of interest in normal activities, anxiety, learning disability and stressful life.
- Alopecia is the main feature due to forceful plucking.
- Children as well as adults are affected.
- Trichomalacia is the pathognomonic feature, seen in histopathology.

Clinical features

- Variable amount of alopecia occurs.
- Hairs are short, irregularly broken and distorted.
- Follicular openings become hyperkeratotic and pigmented.
- Scalp hair and eyelashes are commonly involved but eyebrows and pubic hairs are also involved.
- Commonest sites of scalp are temporal and vertex areas.

Treatment

- Clomipramine is the drug of choice.

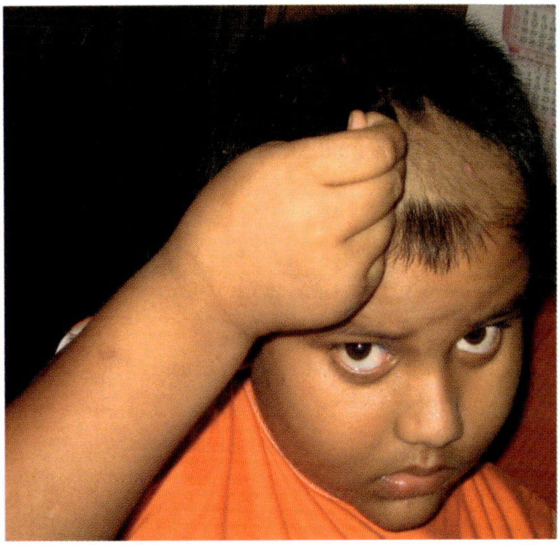

Fig. 5: Forceful traction of hair

Piedra

- Asymptomatic fungal infection of the hair shaft, caused by *Piedraia hortae* in black piedra and *Trichosporon biegelii* in white piedra.

a. **Black piedra** is characterized by adherent, small, hard, brown to black nodules along the hair shaft of the scalp. These nodules are composed of honey-comb like masses of fungal asci and ascospores containing calcium, phosphorus and sulfur. Oral terbinafine, may be useful.

b. **White piedra** is characterized by white to tan, soft, elongated nodules along the hair shaft of the scalp, eyelash, eyebrow, beard, axillary hair and pubic hair. These closely mimic nits or hair casts. These are composed of yeasts like fungi which completely encircle the hair shaft. These fungi may cause disseminated systemic infection in immunocompromized person including skin involvement with purpuric papules, nodules and necrosis. Oral itraconazole may be useful.

Pityriasis amiantacea

* A form of reactive dermatosis of the scalp, without any definite cause.
* It is seen in association with seborrheic dermatitis, psoriasis, contact dermatitis, atopic dermatitis, etc.

Clinical features

- It is characterized by massive white adherent scales with matted hair. Sometimes their arrangement appears as tiles of the roof.

Treatment

- Whole night 10% acetic acid soak for 3-4 days.
- Daily cleaning with coal tar and salicylic acid shampoo.
- Therapy of primary cause.

Syringoma

* It is an adenoma of the intraepidermal part of the eccrine ducts.
* It commonly occurs in females during puberty or later life.

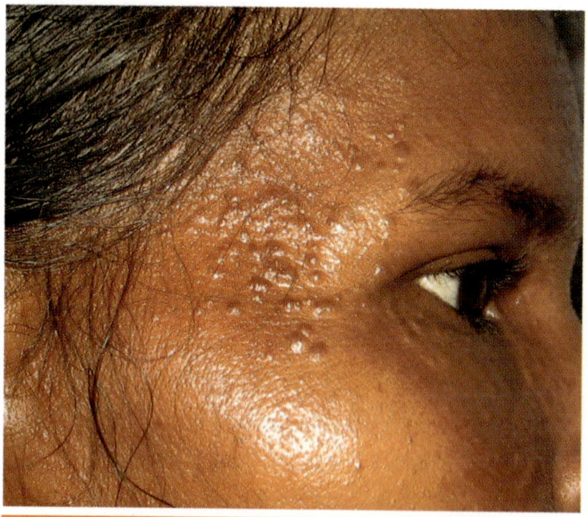

Fig. 6: Multiple skin colored pinhead papules

Clinical features

- Lesions are soft to firm, small, skin colored or slight yellowish papules.
- Number is usually multiple but may be numerous or even few.
- Lesions are discrete or confluent and rarely may be unilateral and linear.
- Common sites are lower eyelids, cheeks, thighs, axillae, abdomen and vulvae.
- Lesions in eruptive syringoma appear in successive crops at anterior trunk of young adults.
- Rarely scalp lesions may be associated with diffuse thinning of the hair or with cicatricial alopecia.

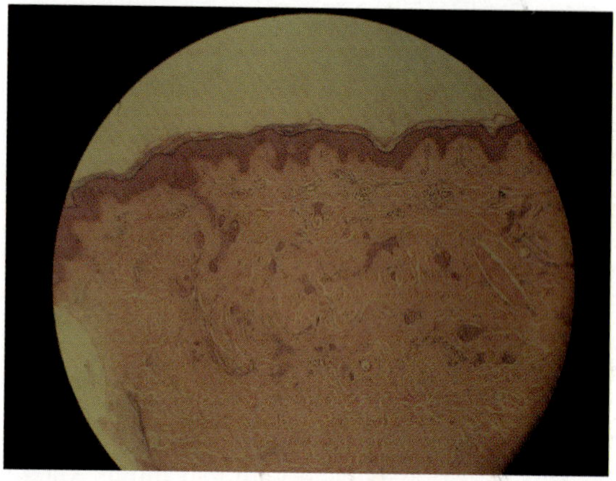

Fig. 7: Multiple ductal structures in the dermis

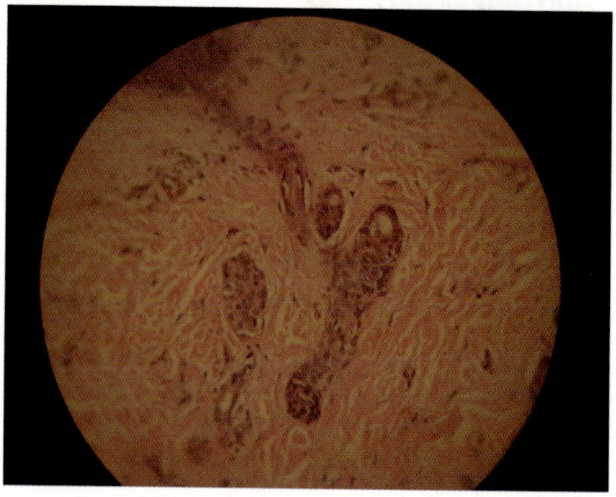

Fig. 8: Ductal proliferation leading to tadpole appearance

Histopathology

- Numerous small ducts embedded in fibrous stroma. Ductal wall is lined by two layers of flattened epithelial cells. Sometimes inner layer cells appear vacuolated. Lumen of the duct is filled up with amorphous debris.
- Some of ducts show elongated proliferation to appear as comma shaped configuration or like a **tadpole**.
- Keratin cysts may be present near the epidermis and epithelial cells of the wall may have keratohyaline granules. If they rupture, a foreign body reaction develop in the dermis.
- Multiple islands of epithelial mass are present. Most of the cells are clear cells except the peripheral ones. Cells appear clear due to glycogen.

Treatment

- Electro- or laser surgery.
- Dermabrasion.

Trichoepithelioma

- It is a benign hair follicle tumor.
- Number of the lesions may be single or multiple.
- Solitary trichoepithelioma is more common than multiple one. It is characterized by firm and flesh-colored nodule and less than 2 cm in diameter.
- Giant solitary trichoepithelioma is more than 2 cm in diameter.
- Trichoepithelioma with multiple lesions has an autosomal dominant inheritance.

Clinical features of multiple trichoepithelioma

- First lesion usually appear in childhood and gradually number increases.
- Lesions are numerous rounded, skin colored, firm papules and nodules. Lesions may ulcerate or transform into basal cell carcinoma in rare occasion.
- Size varies from 2 mm to 8 mm.
- Common sites are nasolabial folds, nose, forehead and upper lips. But rarely scalp, neck and upper trunk may be affected.

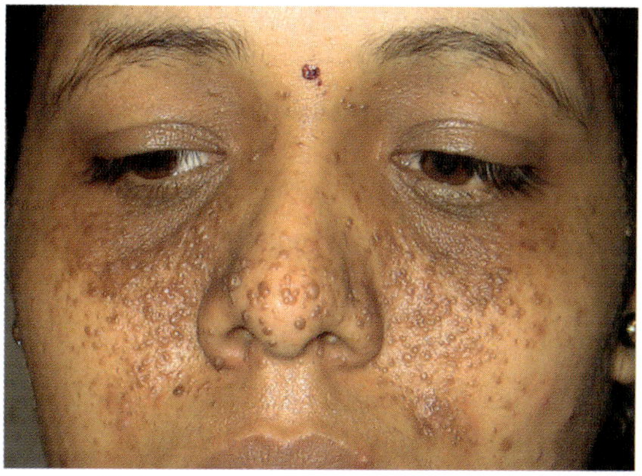

Fig. 9: Brownish papules at central face

Histopathology

- Presence of horn cysts with central abrupt and complete keratinization and peripheral basaloid cells as in basal cell carcinoma. But these epithelial cells show less atypia and mitoses than basaloid cells of basal cell carcinoma. In squamous cell carcinoma, keratinization is gradual and incomplete.
- Often, one or few layers of cells with eosinophilic cytoplasm and large, pale, oval, vesicular nuclei, may be present between basophilic cells and horn cyst.
- Multiple islands of basophilic cells are arranged in an adenoid pattern or lace-like pattern or as solid masses.
- Peripheral cells of these islands show a palisading arrangement and surrounded by a fibrous stroma. Fibroblasts remain as a tight collar, so that retraction artifact does not develop which is commonly seen in basal cell carcinoma.
- Islands of epithelial cell may invaginate fibroblasts and appear as follicular papillae.
- Sometimes horn cysts may rupture and produce a foreign body type of granulomatous reaction in the dermis.

Treatment

- Electro- or laser surgery.
- Dermabrasion.

Seborrheic keratosis

- It is a very common dermatosis, presented often with multiple lesions and rarely with single lesions.
- Lesions usually do not appear before middle age.
- It affects almost 20% of elderly persons.

Clinical features

- Lesions are sharply demarcated, brownish, slightly raised papules and plaques.
- Lesions appear as stuck on the skin.
- Surface is verrucous and having a soft friable consistency.
- Size is variable from few mm to several cm.
- Lesions may be erythematous and crusted due to local trauma.
- Some of the lesions may be pedunculated like soft fibroma.

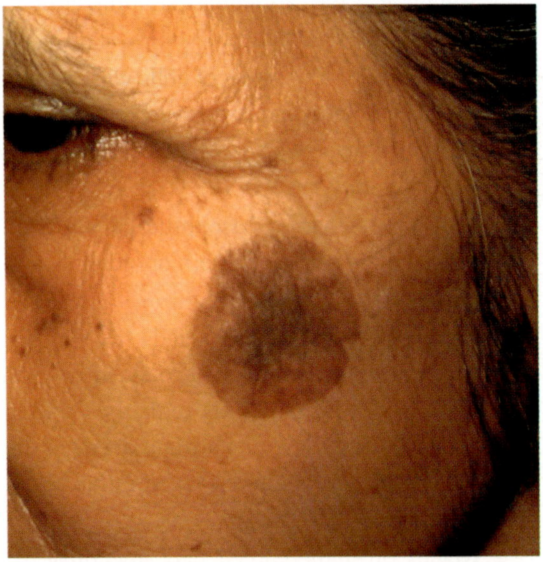

Fig. 10: Mild elevated well defined brownish plaque

Histopathology

- Hyperkeratosis, acanthosis and papillomatosis.
- Acanthosis occurs upwards fashion and so lower border of the tumor is even as it lies on a straight line, extending from one end to other end.
- Tumor cells are of two types: squamous cell type and basaloid type.
- Squamous cells are like normal keratinocytes but basaloid cells are small and uniform.
- Mild intercellular edema may be present which makes the intercellular space clear to some extent.

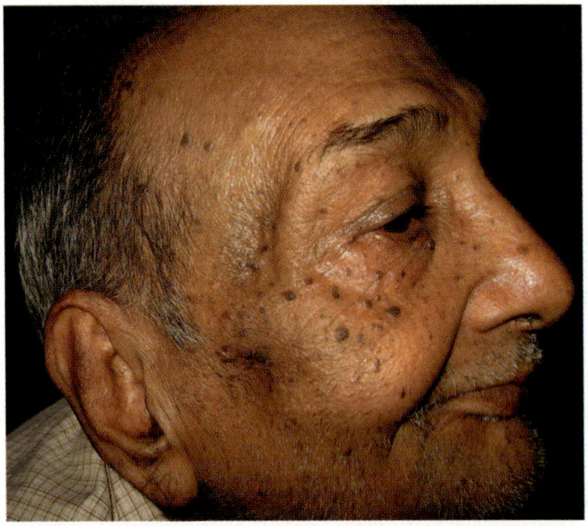

Fig. 11: Dark brown papules in an old person

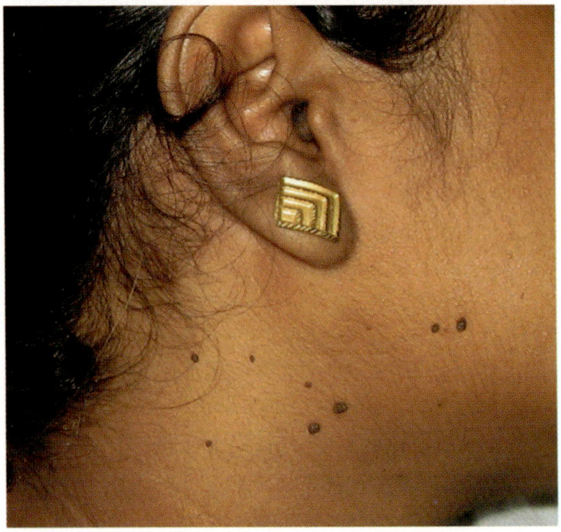

Fig. 12: Dark brown pinhead papules of dermatosis papulosa nigra in a middle aged female

Histopathological variants

- Adenoid or reticulated type
- Acanthotic type
- Hyperkeratotic type
- Clonal type
- Irritated or activated type
- Melanoacanthoma
- Benign squamous keratosis

Granuloma faciale

- It occurs predominantly in adult males and females with a mean age of presentation as 52 years.
- Its etiology is not yet clear, probably a localized form of fibrosing vasculitis.

Clinical features

- Primary lesions are single or more asymptomatic soft brown-red and slowly progressive papules or plaques.
- Surface shows an orange peel appearance.
- It exclusively occurs at face.

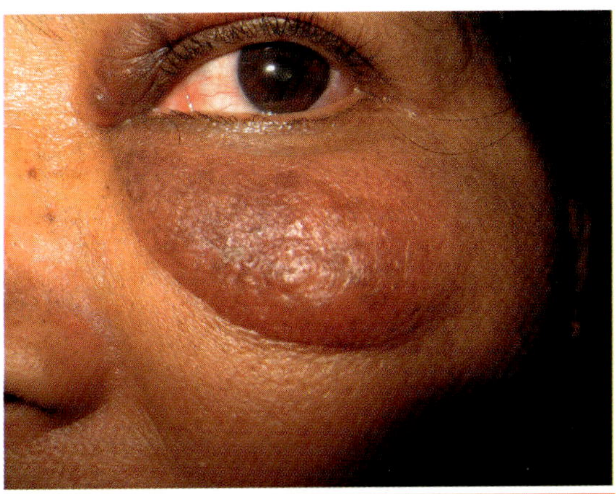

Fig. 13: Reddish-brown plaque with prominent follicular ostea

Histopathology

- Upper half of the dermis is densely infiltrated with neutrophils.
- Infiltration may extend upto subcutaneous tissue.
- Infiltrations spare the epidermis and pilosebaceous appendages.
- Pilosebaceous structures remain normal.
- Infiltrations also contain eosinophils, lymphocytes, plasma cells and mast cells.
- Grenz zone, the narrow interface between the epidermis and dermal infiltrates, is usually present.
- Mild vascular damage with deposition of fibrinoid material in and around the vessel walls may be seen.
- Leukocytoclasia and nuclear dusts may be present around the capillaries.
- Extravasation of RBCs is seen. Older lesion shows foam cells and fibrosis.

Xanthelasma palpebrarum

- This is a dermatosis of lipid metabolism.
- Hyperlipidemia is not associated in more than 50% cases.
- Following successful treatment, it recurs after 1-2 years.
- Normalization of hyperlipidemia does not change the course of the disease.

Clinical features

- These are asymptomatic, soft, yellowish and flat papules or plaques.
- Lesions usually develop bilaterally and symmetrically at upper eyelids, around inner and outer canthus, and infraorbital region.

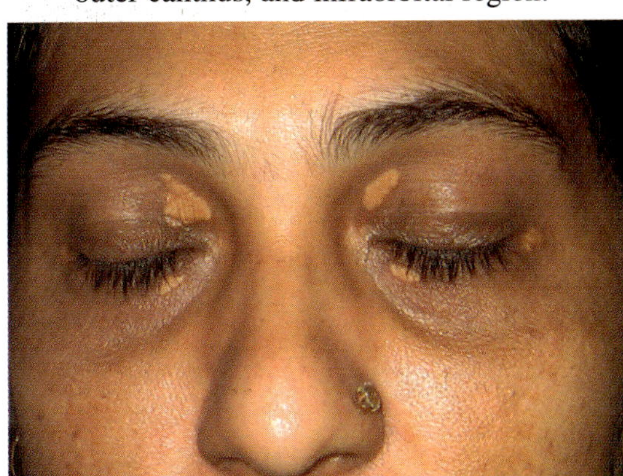

Fig. 14: Yellowish flat papules and plaques at upper and lower eyelids, and at outer canthus

Treatment

- Electrosurgery, cryosurgery or laser surgery.
- Chemical cautery with 50-70% trichloroacetic acid.

Circumscribed follicular keratosis of chin and cheek (CFKCC)

* This is an asymptomatic benign but neglected entity with a lot of cosmetic concern.
* It commonly occurs in older children and adolescents. But it also may develop in adults.
* Commonest age group is 10-20 years.
* It occurs due to chronic friction.
* Patients are having a habit to rest the chin or cheek on their palms.

Clinical features

- A circumscribed plaque formed by confluent tiny follicular papules.
- Papules of the central part are more pigmented and more keratotic.
- Size of the plaque is variable from 2-4 cm.
- It commonly occurs unilaterally, but may be bilateral, depending on the patients' habit.

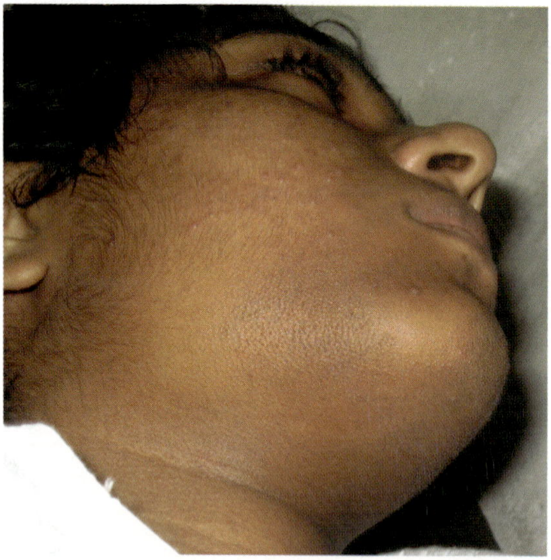

Fig. 15: Confluent follicular horny papules at mandibular region

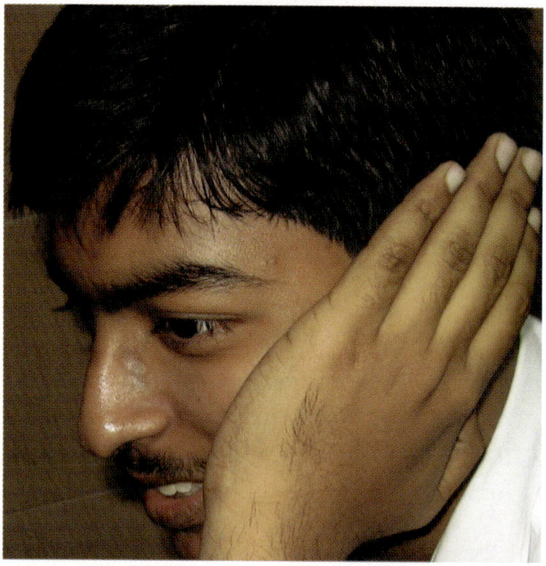

Fig. 16: Habit of taking rest on the palm

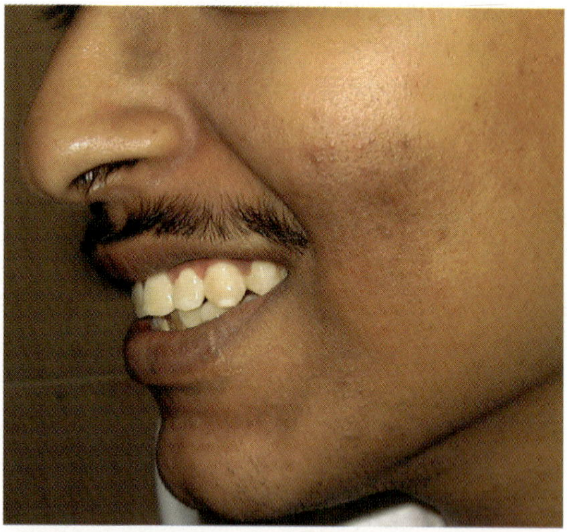

Fig. 17: Lesions at the cheek

Treatment

- Avoidance of friction.
- Application of topical retinoic acid.

Acne agminata/Lupus miliaris disseminata faciei

* It is an acneiform dermatosis occurring in central face of the young adults.

Clinical features

- Primary lesions are bright red soft papules. They gradually turn into brown and appear as apple jelly color on diascopy.
- Some lesions may turn into pustules, followed by crust and scar formation.
- Lesions are discrete and 2-5 mm in size.
- Commonest site is central part of the face including eyelids, cheeks, angles of the mouth, paranasal and mental areas. Periorbital areas are the favoured sites and rarely neck is affected.

Histopathology

- Granulomatous infiltration with central necrosis.

Treatment

- Dapsone is the treatment of choice.

Chronic actinic dermatitis/Actinic reticuloid

* It is a chronic photosensitive dermatosis, caused by ultraviolet as well as visible light.
* Older persons are commonly affected.
* It is exaggerated in summer.
* Lesions may persist for years, such as 10% for 5 years, 20% for 10 years and 50% cases for 15 years.
* Severe form is known as **actinic reticuloid**.
* Pruritus is the commonest symptom.

Clinical features

- Primary lesions are erythematous and shiny papules, appearing as pseudolymphomatous lesions.
- Initially lesions are discrete; but gradually they coalesce to form irregular plaque.
- Sometimes lesions start as erythematous patches and later turn into lichenified plaques.
- Sun-exposed areas are commonly affected with a sharp cut off line between covered and uncovered areas. Spared areas are depth of furrows, upper eyelids, finger-webs and retroauricular areas. Palms and soles are rarely affected. Though thickly covered hairy scalp is spared, bald scalp is often affected.
- Scalp hair or eyebrows may be lost.

Histopathology

- Acanthosis.
- Spongiosis with exocytosis and Pautrier-like microabscess formation.
- Focal epidermal necrosis.
- Superficial and deep perivascular infiltration with lymphohistiocytes, eosinophils and plasma cells.
- Deposition of fibrin at dermoepidermal junction.
- Vertical orientation of papillary dermal collagen.

Treatment

- Azathioprine 100 mg/day is the drug of choice.

Aphthous stomatitis

* It is a chronic and recurrent oral ulcer disease of unknown etiology. It is often precipitated by local trauma.
* Labial mucosa, gums, margins of the tongue and buccal mucosa are commonly affected.
* Ulcers are extremely painful and may be single or multiple and are having well defined margin, erythematous halo and whitish floor.
* Individual ulcer persists for 1-4 weeks before spontaneous healing.

Types

- **Minor ulcer** or **Mikulicz ulcer:** Number of the ulcer is 1-6 but size is only 2-4 mm in diameter.
- **Major aphthous ulcer** or **Sutton's ulcer:** Number of the ulcer is > 6, size is > 4 mm in diameter. They are more painful and occur more frequently.

- **Herpetiform ulcer:** Lesions start as vesicles and rapidly turn into extremely painful ulcers. These ulcers then increase in size and coalesce to form a larger ragged ulcer.

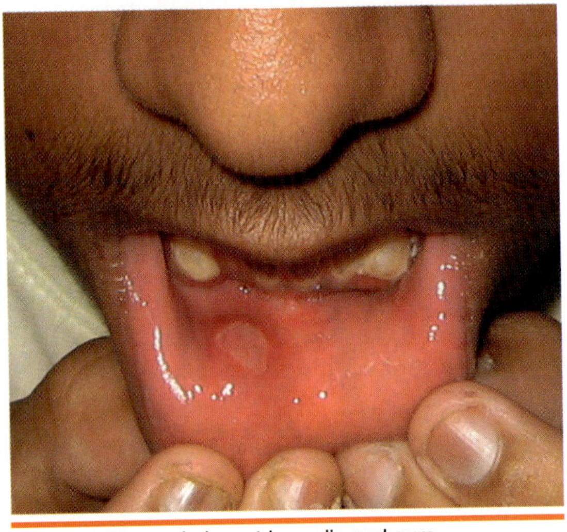

Fig. 18: Mucosal ulcer at lower lip and gum

Treatment

- Topical corticosteroid as triamcinolone in orabase
- Tetracycline or corticosteroid mouth wash.
- Systemic corticosteroid for an acute attack and for recalcitrant groups.
- Dapsone, colchicine and thalidomide are used to prevent recurrence.

Differential diagnosis

- **Behcet's ulcer:** It is having orogenital ulcers along with joint and eye involvement.
- **Hand-foot-mouth disease:** Usually children are affected with fever, followed by painful oral ulcers and development of vesicles at palms-soles, dorsa of hands and feet, knees, elbows and buttocks. Lesions start to heal within a week. Pruritus may be associated in some cases.
- **Herpetic ulcer:** Lesions start as vesicles in a group and form superficial painful ulcers. It is difficult to differentiate from herpetiform aphthous ulcers. Serology may help.

Geographic tongue

- It is a benign, asymptomatic, erosive dermatosis of the tongue, having a lot of psychological impact.
- It is an abortive form of pustular psoriasis of the tongue, characterized by asymptomatic, benign erosion/ulcer.
- It often takes a geographic configuration and there is tendency to change the configuration from time to time.

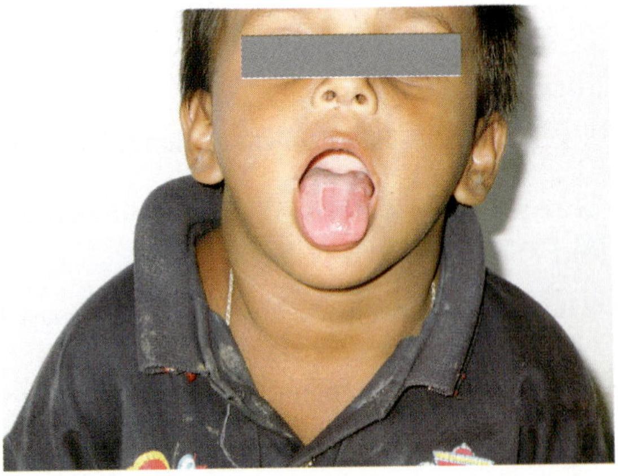

Fig. 19: Two erosions at tongue

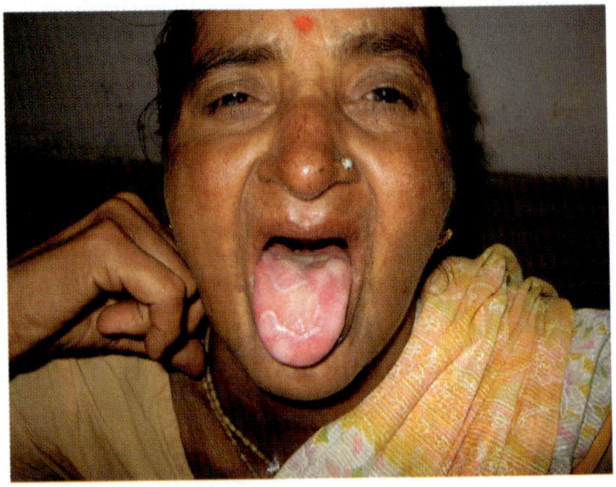

Fig. 20: Geographic ulcer at the tongue

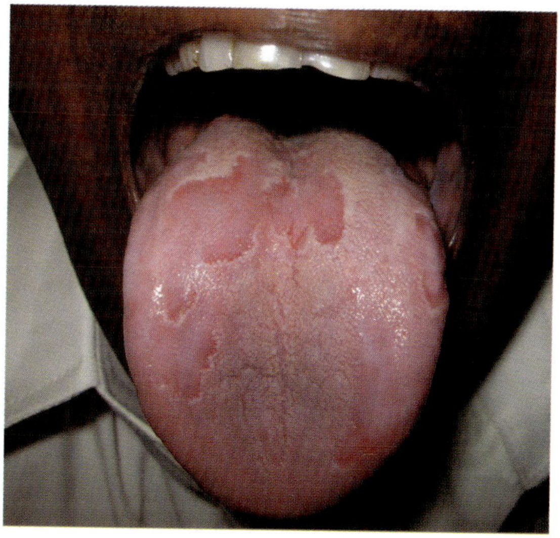

Fig. 21: Polycyclic erosions on the tongue

Treatment

- Reassurance.

Burning mouth syndrome

- It is an intraoral painful or burning sensation, unaccompanied by clinical signs. Peri- and post menopausal women are commonly affected.
- Usually onset is insidious but may be acute.
- Associated other features are feeling of stickiness or dryness and altered taste.
- In large number of patients psychological aspects such as anxiety, depression or neurosis like hysteria may be related.
- Some studies found significant increase of substance P or decrease of serotonin, estrogen and progesterone levels.

History

- Repeated examination with mirror is revealed in history of almost all cases.
- Patients feel burning sensation at waking which worsen as the day passes on and may be relieved by eating or drinking.
- Whole mouth and distal parts of the tongue may be affected.
- Patients try to convince normal posterior taste-buds as abnormal to the physician.

On examination

- No abnormality will be found.

Diagnosis

- It is diagnosed by ruling out other possible causes of burning mouth like nutritional deficiency, candidiasis, xerostomia, stomatitis medicamentosa, esophageal reflux and antibiotic.

Differential diagnosis

- Burning tongue may be an early sign of temporal arteritis or damage of chorda tympani and loss of inhibition of trigeminal nerve.

Treatment

- Reassurance.
- Management of psychological impairment.

Actinic cheilitis

- It is a chronic dermatosis of the lips due to prolonged sun exposure.
- Adults are commonly affected.
- Allergic or irritant contact dermatitis often causes similar picture. But vermilion border in these cases remains intact.
- Histopathology is required to rule out malignant transformation.
- Malignant transformation occurs in 1% cases per year.

Clinical features

- Lip becomes dry, scaly, erythematous and edematous.
- Gradually fissuring, crusting and atrophy develop.
- Vermilion border is obliterated.
- Lower lip is commonly affected.

Treatment

- Application of water proof sunscreen.

- Application of 5-Fluorouracil (5%) cream 2-3 times daily for 10 days and then to wait for 3 weeks to heal the erosion.

Chronic granulomatous cheilits

- It may be a component of Melkersson-Rosenthal syndrome when associated with facial paralysis and scrotal or plicated tongue.

Characteristic features

- Its onset is sudden but the course is progressive. It is characterized by painless swelling of the lips, usually not associated with scaling, fissuring or ulceration.
- Often upper lip is affected first, followed by lower lip.

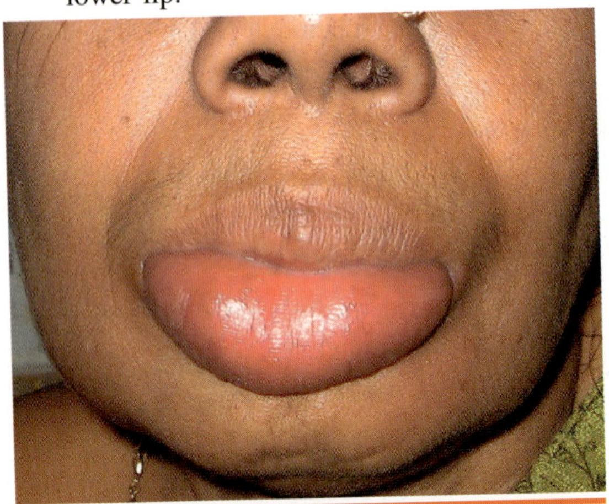

Fig. 22: Persistent swelling of the lower lip

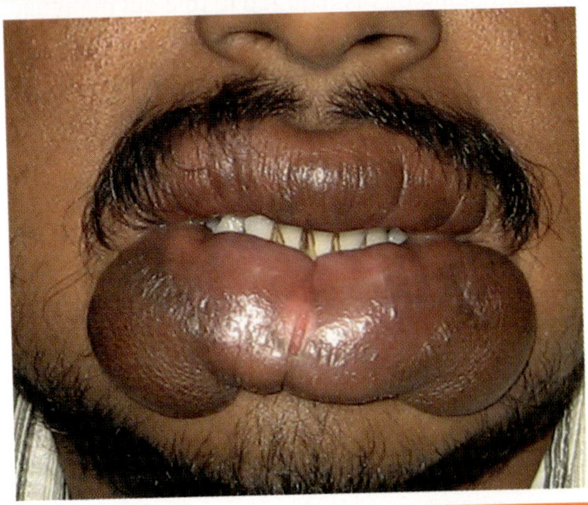

Fig. 23: Well defined brownish plaque at both lips

Histopathology

- Dermis contains noncaseating granuloma, composed of epithelioid cells, Langhans' giant cells and lymphocytes.
- Dermal infiltrate also contains plasma cells and histiocytes.

Treatment

- General measures include cold compress and oral antihistamines to reduce erythema, and emollient to protect from fissuring.
- Corticosteroids in the forms of topical, intralesional or systemic may be used.
- Clofazimine, thalidomide, hydroxychloroquine and sulfasalazine may be used.
- Minocycline 200 mg/day or tetracycline 500 mg/day may be used to prevent rebound phenomenon after improvement with corticosteroid.
- Biologicals like infliximab and adalimumab are also useful in resistant cases.
- Surgical intervention is needed when all conservative approaches are failed. It improves aesthetic deformity or functional impairment.

Differential diagnosis

- Cheilitis glandularis
- Crohn's disease
- Sarcoidosis
- Hereditary angioedema
- Lupus vulgaris, BT leprosy with type 1 downgrade reaction and deep fungal infection.

Cheilitis glandularis

- It is a chronic inflammatory reaction due to chronic irritation, atopy, factitious or actinic damage of the lips.

Clinical features

- Diffuse swelling of the lips with eversion of lower lip.
- Patulous openings of the ducts of the mucous glands.

- History of sticking of the lips during sleep, due to glue-like secretion from the labial glands.
- Pebble-like feeling when lips are palpated between thumb and index finger.
- More aggressive affection of lower lip is often noted.
- Rarely abscess formation may occur due to infection of the mucous glands, known as **glandularis apostematosa**.

* Histopathology shows moderate infiltration of lymphocytes, histiocytes and plasma cells in and around the mucous glands.

Treatment

- Treatment of the cause, if found.
- Intralesional corticosteroid.
- Surgical debulking.

Cheilitis exfoliativa

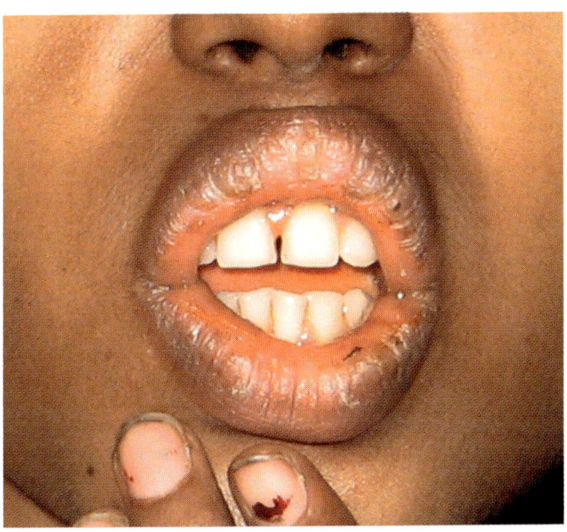

Fig. 24: Scaly thickened lips

* This is a mild inflammatory, desquamative dermatosis of the lips without any known cause.
* It is recurrent in nature and characterized by scaling, crusting, fissuring and pain. A glazed surface is seen when crust is removed.
* It is aggravated in winter.
* Similar feature is seen secondary to many causes, such as lip licking, seborrheic dermatitis, atopic dermatitis, psoriasis, retinoid/5-fluorouracil therapy and prolonged sun exposure.

Treatment

- Application of emollient.
- Mild topical corticosteroid/topical tacrolimus/pimecrolimus.

Fordyce's spot

* These are asymptomatic pinpoint whitish to creamy colored smooth papules which are basically ectopic sebaceous glands.
* Lesions are usually coalesced to form an irregular plaque, but discrete lesions are also seen surrounding the plaque.

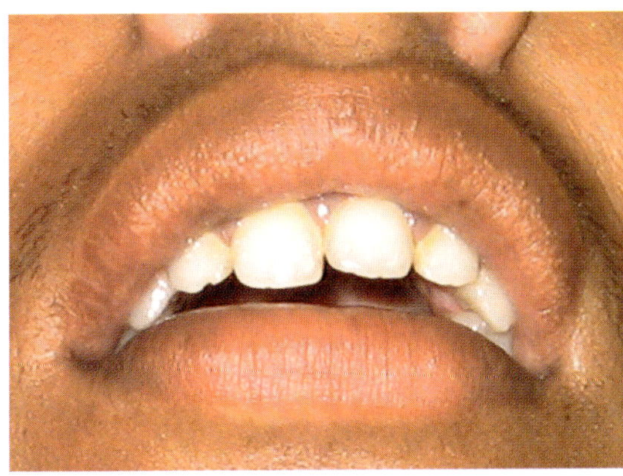

Fig. 25: Tiny whitish papules at upper lip

Hirsutism

* It is defined as presence of male pattern excess terminal hair in a women at unwanted areas of face.
* It often produces a cosmetic problem leading to lot of mental stress.
* Androgen plays a major role but not in all cases.
* Usually it is idiopathic but may be related to excess androgen, originated from various sources like hypothalamus, pituitary gland, adrenal cortex, ovary, and failure of peripheral conversion

of androgen to non-androgen or peripheral increased sensitivity to androgen.

* Common conditions, related to hirsutism are pregnancy, polycystic ovary, stress, congenitial adrenal hyperplasia and adrenal carcinoma.

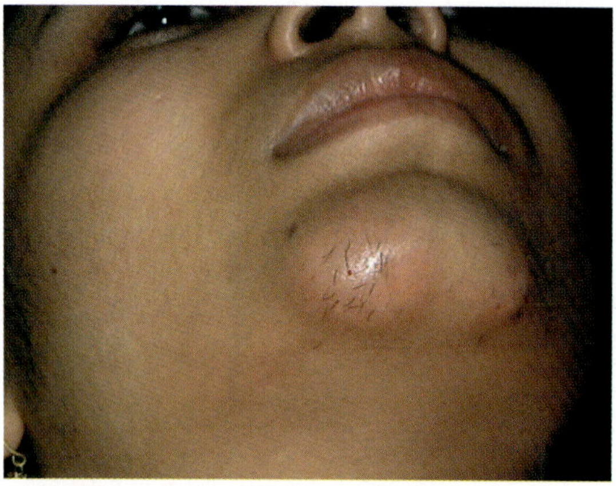

Fig. 26: Terminal hairs at chin in a young girl

Differential diagnosis

- Hypertrichosis

Treatment

- Removal of the cause
- Topical and systemic antiandrogen therapy.
- Physical removal by electrolysis.

Erythrasma

* It is a chronic bacterial infection, caused by *Corynebacterium minutussimum*. These are spore-bearing Gram-positive diphtheroid bacteria. They are found in normal skin flora and cause disease in certain conditions.
* Adults are commonly affected.
* Wood's lamp examination shows **coral-red** fluorescence due to presence of **coproporphyrin III**.

Predisposing factors

- Hot and humid climate.
- Occlusive clothings or shoes
- Obesity
- Hyperhidrosis.

Clinical features

- Well demarcated reddish-brown patch affects the axillae, groins and submammary regions.
- Lesions are usually asymptomatic.
- Whitish, macerated and hyperkeratotic lesions present at toe-webs.

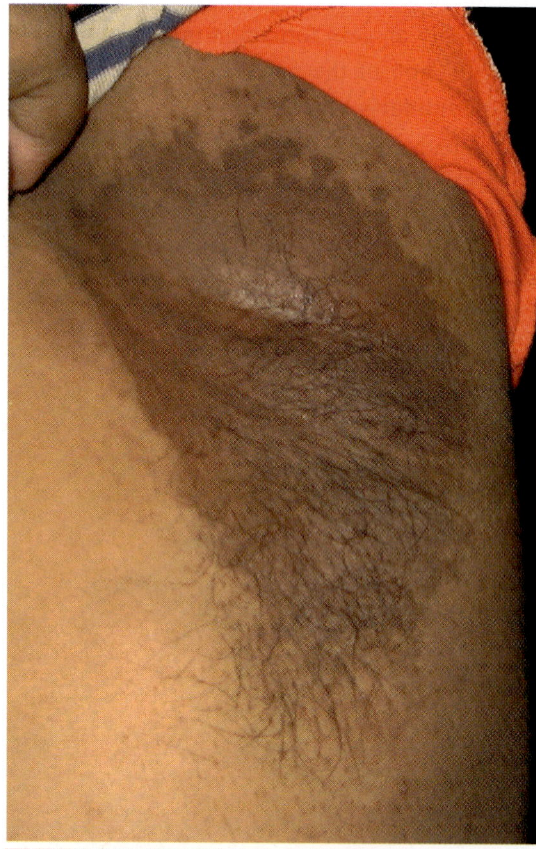

Fig. 27: Reddish-brown patch at axilla

Differential diagnosis

- Pityriasis versicolor
- Seborrheic dermatitis.

Treatment

- Topical sodium fusidate.
- Topical clotrimazole.
- Topical 2% clindamycin solution.
- Benzoyl peroxide (5%).
- Oral azithromycin or erythromycin.

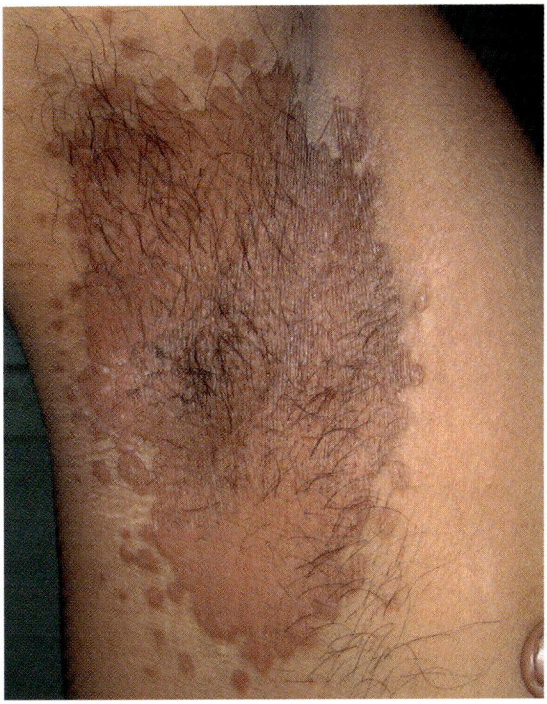

Fig. 28: Reddish-brown patch at axilla

Hidradenitis suppurativa

- It is a chronic suppurative disorder of unknown etiology.
- It commonly affects axillae, groin and buttocks, the sites rich with apocrine glands.
- Propably it originates following follicular occlusion, though previously thought that it is solely developed from apocrine glands.
- Lesions frequently become infected with pyogenic bacteria.
- Commonly middle aged persons are affected.
- Histopathology is not diagnostic but helps to differentiate other disorders.

Characteristic features

- Lesions start as boil like tender nodules which gradually suppurate and rupture to form sinuses. Subsequently number of lesion increases and they communicate with each other by interconnecting sinuses.
- Some of the lesions healed spontaneously with cord like puckered scar but simultaneously new lesions appear and thus the disease remains active.

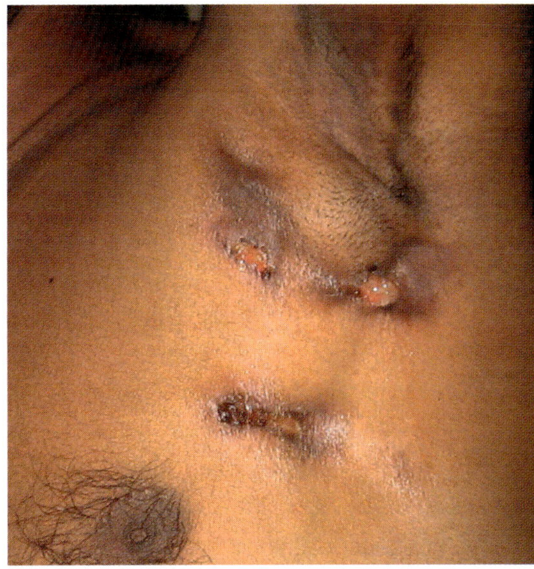

Fig. 29: Multiple interconnected sinuses and cord like scars at left axilla

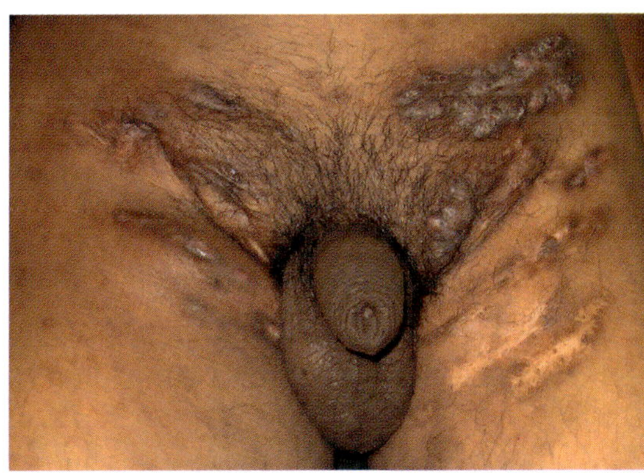

Fig. 30: Multiple interconnected sinuses and cord like scars at groins

Differential diagnosis

- Scrofuloderma
- Mycetoma.

Treatment

- Systemic antibiotics like minocycline, lincomycin and clindamycin.
- Intralesional triamcinolone 10 mg/ml.

Papular purpuric gloves and socks syndrome (PPGSS)

* It is caused by Parvovirus B19, occurring in young adult during summer and spring.
* It is associated with leucopenia and thrombocytopenia.
* It resolves spontaneously by 1-2 weeks.

Clinical features

- Acute onset of rapidly progressive symmetric erythematous and pruritic swelling of hands and feet with petechial or purpuric component.
- Lesions are sharply demarcated at wrists and ankles.
- A widespread papular exanthema may present at skin of the other parts of the body.
- An enanthem including hyperemia, petechiae and erosions may be associated. These are seen at soft and hard palate, pharynx, lungs and inner lips.
- Associated symptoms are fever, arthralgia and malaise.

Unilateral laterothoracic exanthema

* Exact etiology is not known, probably there is a viral cause.
* Unilateral axilla and lateral trunk are commonly affected at initial stage; but gradually may be generalized.
* Resolve spontaneously by 3-6 weeks.
* Histopathology reveals clusters of lymphocytic infiltration around the eccrine ducts.

Clinical features

- Lesions are polymorphic including macules, papules, morbilliform, scarlatiniform and eczematous.
- Lesions may be discrete, confluent, coalesced and annular or reticulate pattern.
- Some red papules may have a pale halo.

Bromhidrosis/Malodorous sweat

* It is an embarrassing malodorous entity in which often an excessive and offensive odor comes out from the skin and produces a social problem.
* Plantar bromhidrosis is often associated with pitted keratolysis.

Types

* Apocrine bromhidrosis
  - It results from bacterial degradation of apocrine sweat.
  - It is seen in all postpubertal individual, originating only from axillae.
* Eccrine bromhidrosis
  - It originates from microbiologic degradation of stratum corneum, softened by excessive eccrine sweat.
* Special type of smell and relevant association
  - **Boiled cabbage odor** in methionine adenosyltransferase deficiency.
  - **Fishy odor** in trimethylaminuria and dimethylglycine dehydrogenase deficiency.
  - **Mousy** or **musty** odor in phenylketonuria.
  - **Sweaty feet odor** in isovaleric acidemia.
  - **Sweet odor** in maple syrup urine disease.
  - Nonspecific odor due to garlic, penicillin, bromides and dimethyl sulfoxide.
  - Only axillary apocrine glands produce malodorous sweat and no odor billows from apocrine apparatus of other areas.

Pitted keratolysis

* It is caused by small cocci and filamentous bacilli, of which commonest organism is *Kytococcus sedentarius*.
* It is associated with hyperhidrosis of soles and humid weather.

Clinical features

- It is characterized by shallow or sometimes deeper, round pits of 1-3 mm in size.
- Lesions are often discrete but sometimes may coalesce to form irregular furrows.

- ♦ Lesions are usually asymptomatic but often produce malodor.
- ♦ It occurs at thick and weight-bearing parts of the sole and rarely at palms.

Treatment

- ♦ Topical erythromycin, clindamycin, clotrimazole, miconazole and 5% benzoyl peroxide are effective.

Keratoderma of palms and soles (PPK)

- ✶ This is a group of disorders having focal or diffuse thickening of palms and soles along with some other associated features.

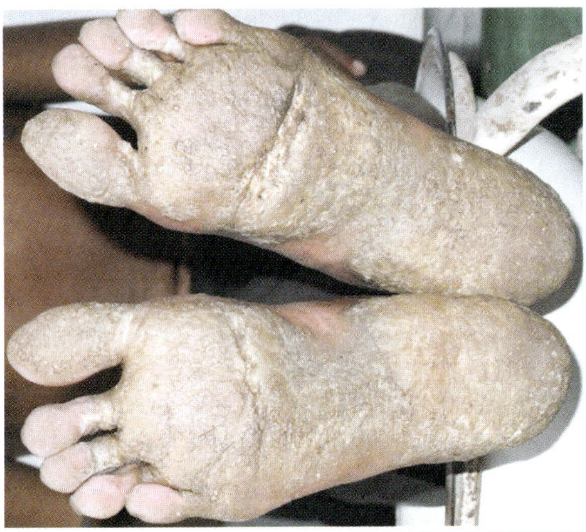

Fig. 31: Sharply defined diffuse and gross hyperkeratosis of both soles

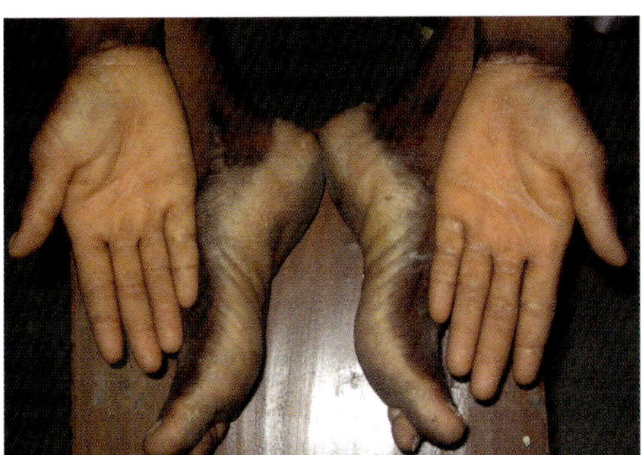

Fig. 32: Keratoderma of palms and soles with transgradiens

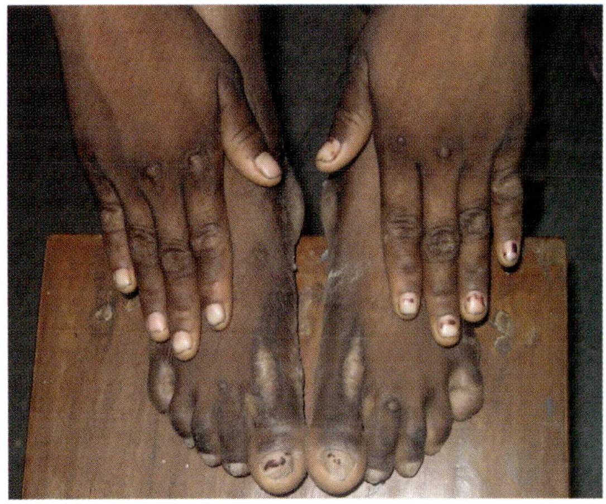

Fig. 33: PPK involving dorsa of hands and feet

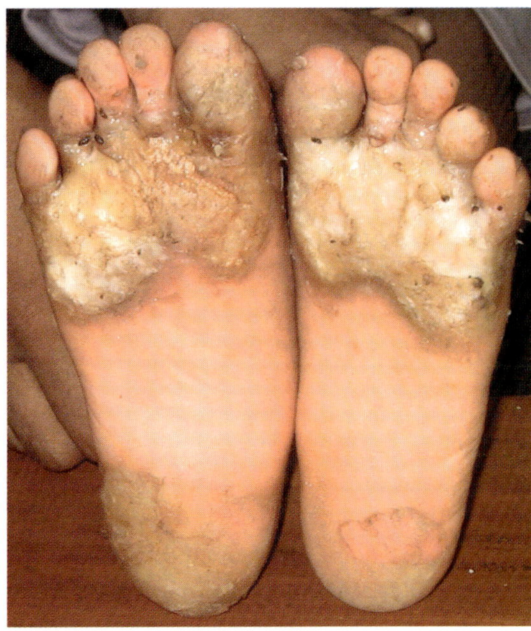

Fig. 34: Focal keratoderma

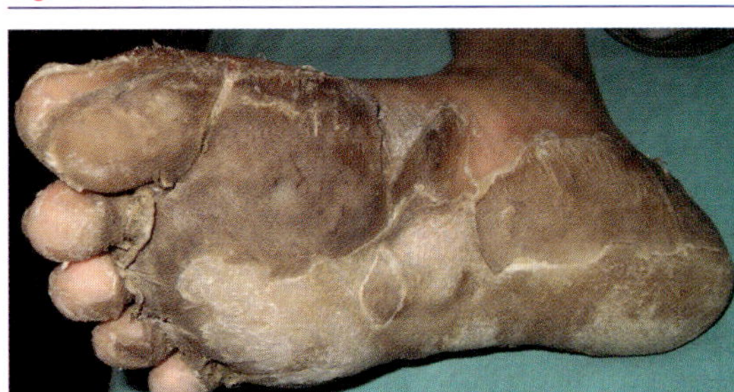

Fig. 35: Acquired keratoderma due to chemical contact

Epidermolytic palmoplantar keratoderma

- Autosomal dominant condition with diffuse but sharply circumscribed congenital thickening of palms and soles.
- Associated with hyperhidrosis, fissuring and maceration.
- Waxy hyperkeratosis, limited to palms and soles, surrounded by **erythematous border**.
- Histopathology shows epidermolytic hyperkeratosis as in bullous ichthyosiform erythroderma.

Non-epidermolytic palmoplantar keratoderma

- Similar to epidermolytic keratoderma, except histopathology shows no epidermolysis.

PPK with deafness

- Onset, between 5-15 years of age.
- Intensive plantar involvement in comparison to palmar involvement and also involvement of knees, elbows, achilles tendons and dorsal surface of toes.
- Intensive palmar involvement in manual workers.
- Hearing loss in 60% cases.

Mal de Maleda

- Autosomal recessive condition with diffuse hyperkeratosis of palms and soles, **perioral erythema** hyperhidrosis and superinfection.
- PPK, extending to dorsal aspects of hand and feet, and overlying joints.
- Nail abnormality including spontaneous amputation of digits.

Naxos disease

- Autosomal recessive condition with cardiac abnormalities including EKG change and ventricular arrhythmia.
- Diffuse keratoderma and wooly hair.

Sclerotylosis/Huriez syndrome

- Autosomal dominant disorder with diffuse PPK, appearing at birth.
- Pseudoslerodermatous fingers.
- Longitudinal ridging, hypoplasia and clubbing of nails.
- Risk of developing squamous cell carcinoma at palms and soles between 3rd and 4th decade of life.

Pachyonychia congenita (PC)

- A group of autosomal conditions, having nail dystrophy, pachyonychia, focal PPK, oral leukoplakia, follicular keratosis and steatocystoma.
- Oral leukoplakia, characteristic of PC type 1.
- Steatocystoma multiplex, appearing after 1st decade of life and characteristic of PC type 2.

Striate PPK

- Autosomal dominant condition with streaks of keratoderma developing at palms and soles since infancy.
- Autosomal recessive type has dilated cardiomyopathy. Histopathology of this type shows large intercellular spaces.

Keratosis punctata palmaris et plantaris

- Autosomal dominant entity with discrete keratotic papules at palms and soles, specially at palmar creases and volar aspect of fingers.
- Central keratinous plugs may be lost or can be picked out to form shallow depressed pits.
- Painful walking for plantar lesions and painful hand for palmar lesions during manual work.

Keratolysis exfoliativa

- It occurs in young adults during the end of winter or early summer season; but some patients suffer irrespective of season.
- Lesions appear as tiny white rings or air bubbles which rupture and peeled off.
- Treatment is frequent application of emollient.

Keratolytic winter erythema

- It is characterized by cyclical centrifugal peeling of the hands and feet with erythematous background.
- It occurs in winter season.
- Sometimes lower legs and limbs are affected.
- Treatment includes application of emollient and systemic retinoids.

Plasma cell balanitis of Zoon

- It starts as a single lesion which may enlarges or a few small lesions may develop and coalesce to form a single larger lesion.
- It affects uncircumcised penis and age group between 25-80 years.
- It affects the inner surface of prepuce and glans penis.
- Rarely it affects vulvae in women which is characterized by erosions, studded with punctate hemorrhage and development of synechia.
- It may also affect oral mucosa, lips, cheeks and tongue, designated as plasmacytosis circumorificialis.

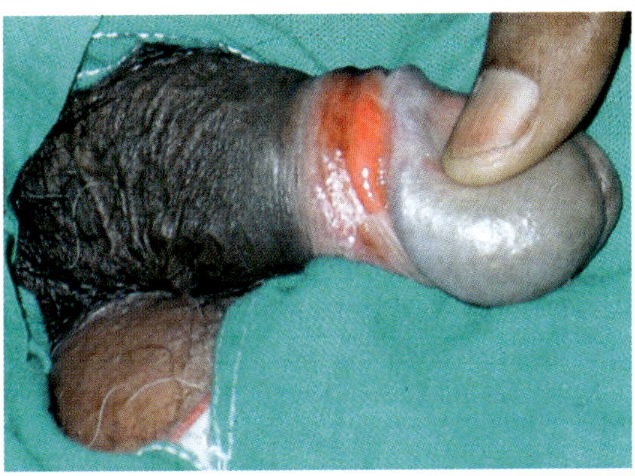

Fig. 36: Erythematous and well defined glassy patch at inner prepuce

Differential diagnosis

- Cadidal balanoposthitis
- Fixed drug reaction.
- Erythroplasia of Queyrat
- Purpuric allergic contact dermatitis.

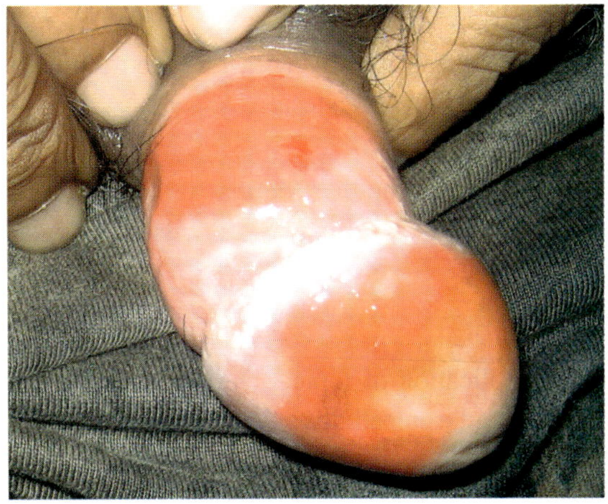

Fig. 37: Erythematous and well defined glassy patches at glans and inner prepuce

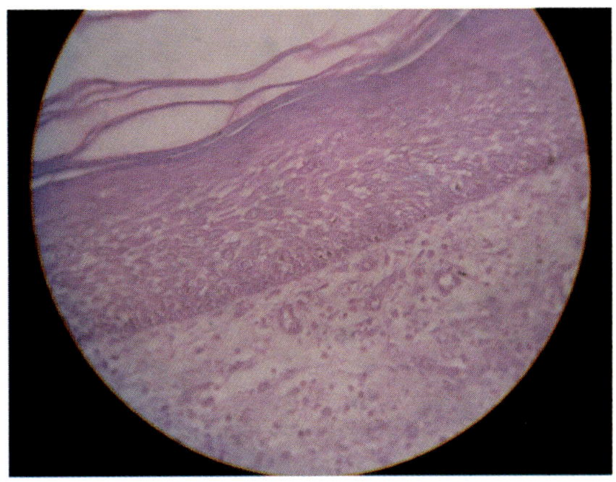

Fig. 38: Flattened epidermis with mild lichenoid upper dermal infiltration

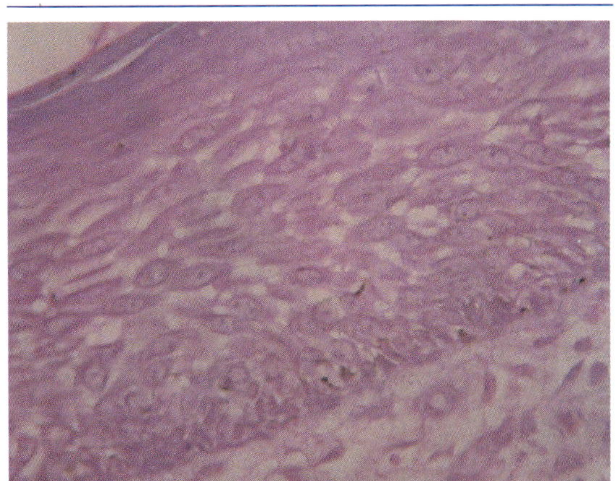

Fig. 39: Lozenge shaped keratinocytes with mild spongiosis

Histopathology

- Epidermal atrophy with flattened diamond shaped keratinocytes.
- Mild spongiosis.
- Band-like papillary dermal infiltration with varying degree of plasma cells and dilated vessels.

Treatment

- Application of topical steroid and systemic steroid as a palliative therapy.
- Circumcision is curative.

Postphlebitic syndrome

- It occurs at legs following deep vein thrombosis.
- The thrombus commonly develops at the cusps of the deep veins which may be dissolved by plasmin.
- But the thrombus and the residual effect of the resolved thrombus make the valves incompetent.
- So, the calf muscle-pump fails to send the blood to the heart and the consequences that happens at the legs, known as **postphlebitic syndrome**.
- **Stage 1**
  - The blood volume of the deep veins produces a back pressure and capillary hydrostatic pressure is increased.
  - Patient starts to feel aching or burning sensation at the feet following long standing and pain during examination of any pitting edema.
- **Stage 2**
  - Dilated capillaries leak out and fluid containing fibrin and RBCs come out at the extravascular spaces. The legs become swollen due to pitting edema and the RBCs become degraded to form hemosiderin. Iron of the hemosiderin makes the skin pigmented.
- **Stage 3**
  - Due to increased hydrostatic pressure at venous ends of the capillaries diffusion of nutrients from arterial ends become compromised. Moreover fibrin gets deposited around the capillaries and diffusion of oxygen is also compromised. Both the conditions lead to a malnourished skin. The skin initially becomes dry and scaly and later becomes oozy and crusted. Sometimes blisters form. These changes are designated as stasis dermatitis. Patients start to apply various medications containing paraben preservative, lanolin, neomycin etc. which very often produce an allergic contact dermatitis. This is further complicated by secondary infection including cellulitis. Sometimes dermatitis in an acute stage and cellulitis are difficult to differentiate.
  - This compromised skin easily gets traumatized leading to ulceration. Ulcer may be single or few in number and superficial or deeper. Margin of the ulcer may be sharp or sloping. Base of the ulcer is formed with granulation tissue and very often the floor remains covered with crusts and oozing.
- **Stage 4**
  - Repeated inflammation due to dermatitis and infection, subcutaneous tissue is also affected. A fibrosing panniculitis develops where fat is gradually replaced by fibrous tissue. So, the skin of the lower third of the legs becomes indurated and bound down. These changes are known as **lipodermatosclerosis**. Microvessels are further compromised due to strangulation with the fibrous tissue.
  - Parts proximal and distal to this firm area become swollen due to obstruction of the lymphatic flow. So, lymphatic fluid leaks out which gradually organizes and the skin becomes brawny. After a long time, multiple brown to reddish papules develop which become confluent to form verrucous plaques. These are known as **stasis papillomatosis**.
- **Stage 5**
  - Due to stagnation of blood flow and sludging of platelets, microthrombi are formed. This leads to infarction and formation of multiple

small ulcers. These ulcers heal spontaneously with white scars. Sometimes telangiectasia and hyperpigmentation are also present along with scars. These changes are known as **atrophie blanche**.

- **Stage 6**
  - Due to continuous back pressure, superficial vessels like medial and lateral saphenous veins become dilated and tortuous. Largest perforator is situated just above the ankle and sometimes the tortuous and dilated veins are seen only at this area. This is known as **ankle blow-out**.

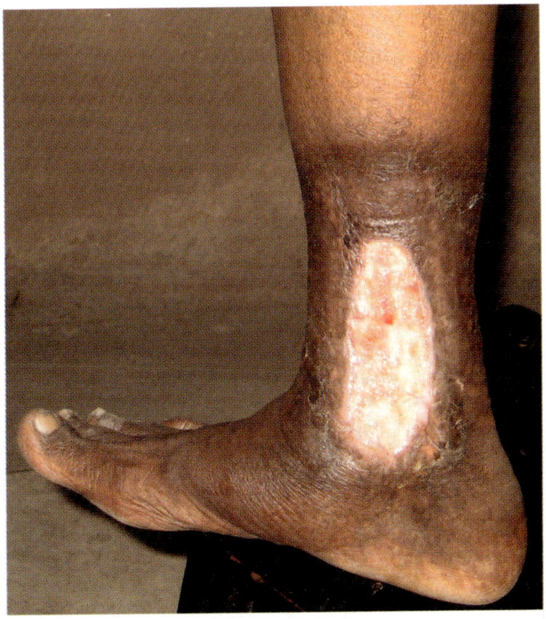

Fig. 40: Lipodermatosclerosis of the lower leg with large stasis ulcer and swollen proximal leg

Treatment

- Physiological:
  - Rest: As much as possible.
  - Leg elevation: During day time, leg to be kept elevated minimum for 30 minutes at 3-4 hours interval. At night footend of the cot is to be kept elevated 15-20 cm during sleep.
  - Occupation: Prolonged standing or even sitting to be avoided.
  - Food habit: Smoking and alcohol must be avoided. Nutritious food containing zinc, vitamin C and E should be taken.
- Physical
  - Compression: To maintain venous pressure 30-40 mm Hg at the ankle, compression is given in following ways:
  - Multilayer bandage: This is the cheapest and easy to put at place. But this maintains only a fixed pressure. So it should be kept only around the ankle.
  - Graded elastic stocking: It maintains desired pressure from ankle to knee. It is costly and after a few days elasticity is lost and so frequent change is required.
  - Nonelastic bandage (Unna's/Duke's boot): Zinc oxide impregnated bandage is used to control the venous pressure as well as to dress the venous ulcer.
  - Pneumatic pump.
  - Debridement.
  - Occlusive dressing with hydrogel, hydrocolloid, alginate, foam and film.

Palmo-plantar pustular psoriasis

- Chronic pustular eruption with or without presence of psoriasis at other sites.

Clinical features

- Lesions start as vesicles, surrounded by erythema at palms and soles and they quickly turn into pustules of 2-4 mm in size.
- Pustules are sterile and deep-seated. They gradually dry up to form dark yellow or brown scales and crusts.
- Stages of relapse and remission are frequent.
- Often crops of fresh pustules appear before shedding of previous one.

Histopathology

- Presence of large unilocular intraepidermal pustules containing neutrophils, known as **spongiform pustule of Kogoj**.

Pustular bacterid

- Symmetric and grouped vesicular or pustular or vesiculopustular eruptions at palms and soles due to distant focus of infection which may be cured following treatment of the infective focus.
- Tiny hemorrhagic puncta may be intermingled with pustules.
- When numerous lesions coalesce, a honey comb like structure is formed.
- Lesions start at center portions of the palms and soles and then spread centrifugally. Web spaces are spared.
- Exacerbation and remission are common and continue for a long time.
- Dry, tough and adherent scales are formed when lesions start to dry up.
- During exacerbations crops of lesions develop with severe pruritus and leukocytosis.
- Tenderness is present in full blown state.

Acrodermatitis continua/acrodermatitis perstans/acrodermatitis repens

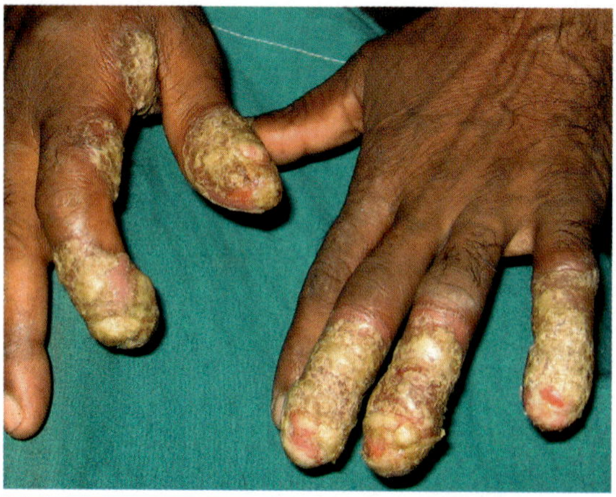

Fig. 41: Pustular lesions with crusting at fingers

- Usually the lesions remain localized at palms and soles, but may be generalized.
- They start at distal parts of the digits as pustules of nail beds or as paronychia.
- Lesions are unilateral initially and later become bilateral with asymmetrical distribution.
- New crops of pustules develop proximally which are dried up and become crusted.
- Nails turn dystrophic and float away on lake of pus.
- Even in localized lesions mucous membrane may be affected with painful, round and white plaques.
- Histopathology shows hyperkeratosis, parakeratosis and spongiforms pustules.

Callosity and corn

- In these conditions, lesions develop characteristically at pressure points like knuckles, lateral malleolus, heel, balls of the toes, lateral side of the little toe, elbow, knee, forehead, and at any area associated with chronic friction.
- Chronic and repeated pressure give rise to the lesion.
- Callosity is having a focal thickening of the skin and corn is having a central thorn-like core surrounded with a thickened collar.

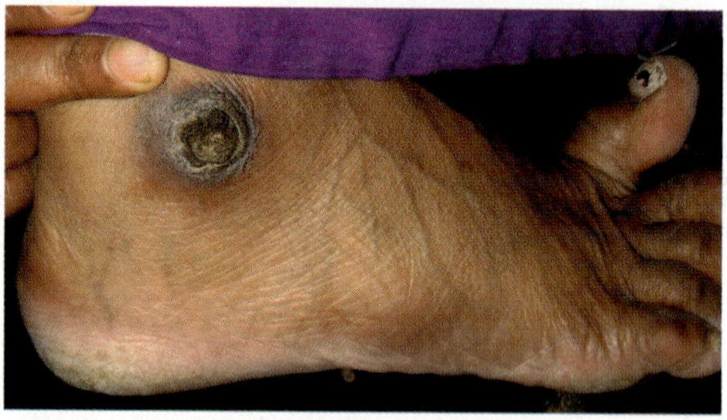

Fig. 42: Complicated callosity

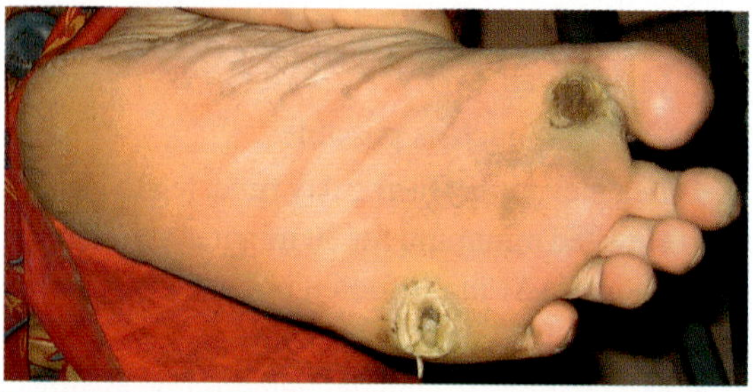

Fig. 43: Corn with hyperkeratotic collar at the margin

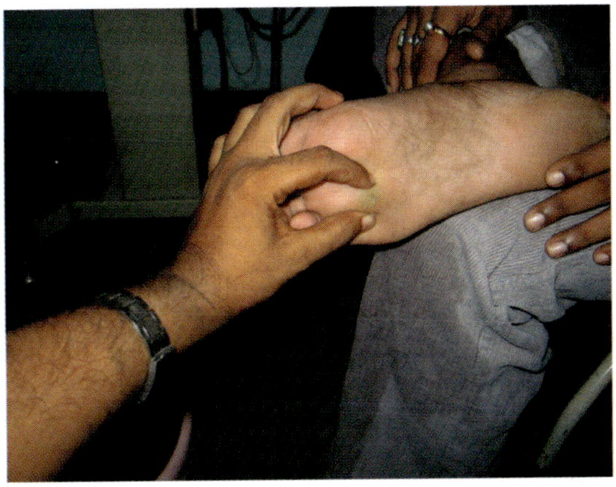

Fig. 44: Demostrating pressure from the sides

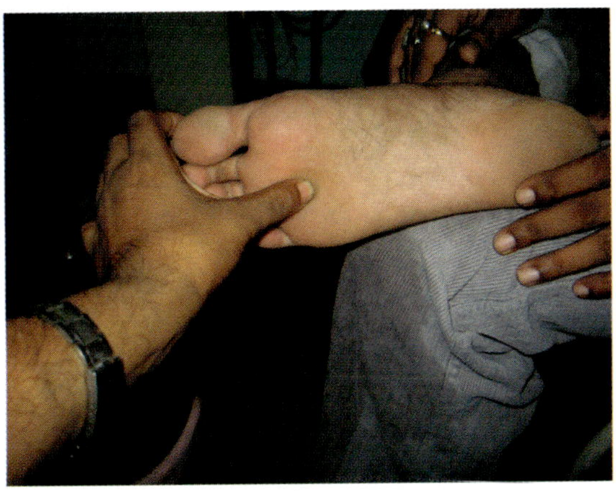

Fig. 45: Demonstrating direct pressure

- When a direct pressure is given on the center of the corn, it elicits an excruciating pain and this test helps to differentiate it from that of plantar wart, which elicits more pain by pressing from sides than pressing at the center.
- In case of corn, the central core acts as a thorn where pressure is concentrated at a point and in case of wart, nerve endings are compressed between downward projections when pressed from the sides.
- Lesion itself is painless but during any work when a lesion is pressed, it produces pain. Initially the patients ignore it and compromise with it by changing the mode of walking. But after a certain period this gives rise to new lesions at new sites. So, gradually patient is forced to restrict walking when multiple lesions are developed at soles.
- Callosity at lateral malleolus becomes profoundly thickened. Underlying tissues are damaged and overlying skin becomes ulcerated and secondarily infected.
- Treatment
  - Avoidance of pressure and regular paring of the lesion.
  - Application of keratolytic agents like salicylic acid.
  - Surgical removal by laser/electrosurgery.

CHAPTER D4

MENTAL BLOCK

Q1. Features

- Cutis marmorata telangiectatica congenita.
- Congenital aplasia cutis.
- Distal transverse limb defect.

Diagnosis?

Q2. Features

- Rare slowly progressive autosomal dominant pigmentary disorder, occurring in adolescents or in adults.
- Presence of reticular, brown to black patches with peripheral similar but discrete pigmented macules.
- Common sites are flexurals including axilla, neck and inframammary regions.
- Hidradenitis suppurativa-like lesions at axillae and groins associated with or without pigmented pitted scars around the mouth.

Diagnosis?

Q3. Features

- Presence of ichthyosis and leiomyoma.
- Sensorineural deafness.
- Eye, renal and parathyroid abnormalities.
- Thrombocytopenia.

Diagnosis?

Q4. Features

- Livedo racemosa
- Severe headache
- Abortion
- Thromboembolism.

Diagnosis?

Q5. Features

- Autosomal dominant condition.
- Acne vulgaris, cutaneous or osseous syndactyly.
- Broad and flat face, hypoplastic nose and maxilla, prominent eyes in shallow orbit and downward palpebral fissure.
- Premature and irregular fusion of cranial sutures.

Diagnosis?

Q6. Features

- Chronic and recurrent non-pruritic urticarial lesion in adults. Angioedema in 15% cases.
- Associated with recurrent fever, arthralgia and bone pain.
- IgM gammopathy and predominant neutrophilic infiltration.

Diagnosis?

Q7. Features

- Occurs in children below 5 years.
- Fever > 39°C, not responding to antipyretics.
- Skin eruption in 80% cases with maculopapular or morbilliform or scarlatiniform eruptions. Sometimes lesions may be erythema multiforme-like or pustular or vesiculobullous.
- IgA producing plasma cells are deposited at coronary arteries, pancreas, kidneys and upper respiratory tract.

Diagnosis?

Q8. Features

- Solitary, skin colored dome shaped small nodule having a central pore.
- Occurs in adults with involvement of face, scalp and neck.
- A tuft of immature wool-like white hairs emerge from the central pore.
- Histopathology shows large cystic space lined by squamous epithelium, containing horny material and fragments of hair shaft.

Diagnosis?

Q9. Features

- Autosomal dominant inheritance and associated with keratitis, congenital ichthyosis and sensorineural deafness.
- At birth skin is erythematous, gradually becomes thickened and leathery, and later palmoplantar keratoderma develops.
- There may be generalized tiny stippled papules, verrucous plaques at face and limbs, variable degree of congenital alopecia, dystrophic nails and reduced sweating.
- Other features are photophobia, recurrent infection of skin, eye and ear.

Diagnosis?

Q10. Features

- It is caused by prototheca, a genous of algae.
- Single/multiple papules, plaques or nodules are primary lesions.
- Surface may be smooth/verrucous/ulcerated.
- Organisms are stained with methenamine silver or PAS as a spherical structure (6-10 μm) within giant cell or tissue and these may have endospores due to septation. Further division of daughter cell leads the parent cell into a *sporangia*.
- A cluster of 50 cells or more form a sporangia, known as *morula*-like structure.

Diagnosis?

Q11. Features

- Knuckle pad.
- Leukonychia.
- Sensory nerve deafness.
- Palmoplantar keratoderma.

Diagnosis?

Q12. Features

- Localized absence of skin at legs.
- Mucocutaneous blister.
- Autosomal dominant variant of epidermolysis bullosa.

Diagnosis?

Q13. Features

- An autosomal dominant condition.
- Follicular atrophoderma at dorsa of hands and feet since birth.
- Multiple basal cell carcinoma since adolescence.
- Facial hypohidrosis and with/without generalized hypohidrosis.
- Sparse hair.

Diagnosis?

Q14. Features

- Fine, thin, dry skin with mottled leukoderma (leopard skin).
- Facies having flat, saddle nose, thick lips and fine wrinkling around mouth and eyes.
- Stunted growth, bird-like legs, delayed and incomplete dentition and severe mental retardation.

Diagnosis?

Q15. Features

- An autosomal recessive disorder due to helicase gene mutation.
- Clinical features are telangiectatic facial erythema resembling lupus erythematosus, distinctive facies, abnormal immune response, predisposing for malignancy and short stature.
- The facies include narrow head, prominent nose, hypoplastic malar areas and receding chin.
- Other features are café-au-lait macules, syndactyly, congenital heart disease, high pitch voice, high arched palate and azoospermia.

Diagnosis?

Q16. Features

- Hereditary universal melanosis progresses since early infancy.
- It is initially diffuse but later becomes mottled.

Diagnosis?

Q17. Features

- Autosomal recessive condition and common in Amish/Finnish population.
- Soft doughy skin due to degeneration of elastic tissue, and sparse and fine scalp/body hair.
- Prone to develop viral infections due to reduced cell mediated immunity and sometimes neutropenia.
- Other features are short limbs, hyperextensible digits, Diamond-Black anemia, toxic megacolon and lymphoreticular malignancy.

Diagnosis?

Q18. Features

- Recurrent infection.
- Partial albinism
- Nystagmus.

Diagnosis?

Q19. Features

- Chondrodysplasia punctata.
- Congenital hemidysplasia.
- Unilateral ichthyosiform erythroderma.
- Limb defects.

Diagnosis?

Q20. Features

- Thickened, dry and ichthyosiform skin at birth.
- Fine and sparse hair, may be associated with trichorrhexis nodosa.
- Pruritus develops within first few month of life.
- Characteristic facies includes hypertelorism, broad and flat nasal bridge, upslanting palpebral fissure, epicanthic fold, long columella and short philtrum, macrostomia, full lips, cupped ears, and rolled helices.
- Other features are coloboma of the eye, heart defect, brachydactyly, mental retardation, etc.

Diagnosis?

Q21. Features

- Autosomal dominant condition with nail and hair abnormalities.
- Slowly growing, thickened/thinned, striated, discolored, brittle or hypoplastic nails.

- Chronic paronychia, complete destruction of nail matrix and pseudoclubbing of digits.
- Sparse body hair with thinned or absent eyebrows and eyelashes and normal scalp hair at infancy but fragile and sparse at puberty.
- Smooth texure of the skin.

Diagnosis?

Q22. Features

- Autosomal recessive condition with scalp hypotrichosis.
- Hypoplastic or absent fifth finger nails and distal phalanges.
- Mental retardation.

Diagnosis?

Q23. Features

- Occurs due to consumption of food supplement containing L-tryptophan and taking of pacitran, an antidepressant drug.
- Papular and urticarial lesions.
- Localized or generalized morphea-like lesions.
- Myalgia, arthralgia, neuralgia and dyspnea.
- Eosinophilia.

Diagnosis?

Q24. Features

- Shortening of digits with dimple (Albright sign) and frontal bossing.
- Dyskeratosis and pitting at palms and soles, calcinosis cutis and milia formation.
- Medulloblastoma.
- Basal cell carcinoma.
- Cyst of ovary, heart and mandible.
- Fibroma of ovary and heart.
- Mental retardation.

Diagnosis?

Q25. Features

- Linear or reticular pigmentation.
- Dermal hypoplasia and fat just under epidermis.
- Telangiectasia.

Diagnosis?

Q26. Features

- In 50% cases the disoder is familial with autosomal dominant inheritance and in remaining 50% cases are sporadic.
- Mutation of loricrin gene/connexin causes the disease.
- Clinical features are large, fixed, geographic and symmetrical fine, scaly erythematous plaques distributed at knees, elbows, hands and feet.
- It starts at an early childhood, progresses for next few years and then remains stable over time in respect of color, morphology and site of involvement.
- Palmoplantar keratoderma is associated in 50% cases.
- Histopathology shows focal parakeratosis and well-preserved granular layer.
- Most common differential diagnosis is circumscribed juvenile pityriasis rubra pilaris.

Diagnosis?

Q27. Features

- Scarring alopecia due to lichen planopilaris.
- Nonscarring alopecia at axillae and groins.
- Rapidly progressive keratosis pilaris.

Diagnosis?

Q28. Features

- Hypotrichosis of scalp, eyebrows and eyelids.
- Scalp alopecia is prominent at frontal and parietal regions.
- Dwarfism, beaked nose and brachycephaly.

Diagnosis?

Q29. Features

- After 1-2 days of abrasions, plantar surface of foot develops red and tender nodules, due to pseudomonas infection.

Diagnosis?

Q30. Features

- Autosomal recessive condition with late onset of palmoplantar keratoderma by 6-12 years of age at pressure points.
- Follicular hyperkeratosis and frictional keratosis at elbows and knees.
- By age of 65 years, in 95% cases squamous cell carcinoma develops at mucosal surfaces including esophagus.

Diagnosis?

Q31. Features

- Type II mucopolysaccharide metabolic disorder.
- Distinctive, firm, flesh colored papules and nodules at buttocks are its cutaneous marker.

Diagnosis?

Q32. Features

- Autosomal dominant entity, associated with red and atrophic skin at dorsal aspect of hands and feet since birth.
- Mild but diffuse palmo-plantar keratoderma.
- Sclerodactyly and nail changes include ridging, fissuring, hypoplasia and koilonychia.
- Risk of developing squamous cell carcinoma in areas of atrophic skin.
- Histopathology of keratoderma: Orthohyperkeratosis, acanthosis and increased granular layer.
- Electron microscopy: Clumped keratohyalin granules and *absence of Langerhans cell.*

Diagnosis?

Q33. Features

- Autosomal dominant inheritance and associated with keratitis, congenital ichthyosis and sensorineural deafness.
- At birth skin is erythematous and gradually becomes thickened and leathery, and develops palmoplantar keratoderma.
- There may be generalized tiny stippled papules, verrucous plaques at face and limbs, variable degree of congenital alopecia, dystrophic nails and reduced sweating.
- Other features are photophobia, recurrent infection of skin, eye and ear.

Diagnosis?

Q34. Features

- A rare autosomal recessive disorder appears at early infancy.
- Features are photosensitivity, acral blistering, generalized progressive poikiloderma and marked cutaneous atrophy.
- Sometimes it is associated with long cuticles of nails.

Diagnosis?

Q35. Features

- An autosomal recessive condition, associated with ichthyosis, atopy and hair shaft deformities, and prematurity.
- Generalized scaling and erythema present at neonatal or early infantile period, often in premature babies.
- Skin is characterized by polycyclic, scaly, migratory, ichthyotic patches, known as *ichthyosis linearis circumflexa.* Periphery of the lesion is having double edged scale. These lesions are seen in 70% cases and usually do not develop before age of 2 years.
- Hairshaft deformities are *trichorrhexis invaginata (bamboo hair/ball & socket deformity)* due to defect in keratinization of

inner root sheath (IRS), early breakage and lusterless poorly manageable hair.

- Other features are atopic diathesis with raised serum IgE level and have a poor skin barrier function.

Diagnosis?

Q36. Features

- Progressive development of mutilating palmoplantar keratoderma with erythematous border and starting at infancy to childhood.
- Autoamputation of digits due to progressive constriction.
- Varying degree of thickening and fissuring of periorificial areas.
- Alopecia and nail dystrophy.

Diagnosis?

Q37. Features

- Autosomal recessive condition with erythematous diffuse to focal palmoplantar keratoderma since infancy or childhood.
- Keratoderma extending towards dorsal aspect of palms and soles and psoriasiform lesion at elbows and knees.
- Rapidly progressive periodontitis and periosteal changes of alveolar bones, resulting in loss of both deciduous and permanent teeth.
- Gingival changes, starting at age of 3 years.
- Calcification of falx cerebri.

Diagnosis?

Q38. Features

- An autosomal inherited disorder due to mutation of SKT 11 gene.
- Mucocutaneous hyperpigmentation as dark blue or brown macules in and around the mouth, eyes, nostrils, perianal areas, fingers and feet.
- Macules on face fade in puberty but oral lesions persist in adulthood.
- Histologically increased number of melanocytes at dermoepidermal junction and increased melanin at basal cells.
- Hamartomatous polyps are often present in small intestine, stomach and large intestine which may cause chronic bleeding, anemia and recurrent obstruction or intussusceptions.
- Gonadal tumor may develop.

Diagnosis?

Q39. Features

* Common manifestations
  - Asymmetric overgrowth of any part of the body.
  - Verrucous epidermal nevus.
  - Infantile hemangiomas.
* Other features
  - Pigmentary changes: linear or whorled and hypo- or hyperpigmentation.
  - Tuberous/cerebriform hyperplasia of skin, specially at soles.
  - Skeletal abnormality.
  - Ocular abnormality.
  - Testicular tumor.
  - Normal IQ.

Diagnosis?

Q40. Features

- It is characterized by inflammation and chronic enlargement of salivary glands, keratoconjunctivitis sicca, xerostomia and fatiguability.
- Dryness and scaling of the skin.
- Sparse, dry, and brittle hair.
- Hypergammaglobulinemic purpura, annular erythema and erythema nodosum.
- Lipodystrophy
- Raynaud's phenomenon
- Laboratory abnormalities are positive ANA, rheumatoid factor and anti-La antibody, and reduced tear formation and salivary flow.

Diagnosis?

Q41. Features

- An autosomal recessive disorder due to deficiency of fatty aldehyde dehydrogenase.
- Non-bullous ichthyosiform erythroderma type of congenital ichthyosis.
- Spastic paralysis.
- Mental retardation.

Diagnosis?

Q42. Features

- Livedo racemosa
- CNS thromboembolic features

Diagnosis?

Q43. Features

- Associated with internal malignancy in about 21% cases and commonest malignancy is acute myeloid leukemia.
- Excessive amount of G-CSF secreted by malignant cells is the cause behind recruitment of neutrophils.
- Lesions may spontaneously resolve over 1-3 months.

Diagnosis?

Q44. Features

- A form of localized scleroderma.
- Characteristic feature is presence of *calcinosis* at extremities.

Diagnosis?

Q45. Features

- Autosomal dominant entity with **honeycomb pattern palmoplantar** keratoderma.
- Pseudoainhum leading to amputation of distal digits.
- **Starfish like** keratoderma at knuckles.
- Sensorineural deafness.

Diagnosis?

Q46. Features

- An autosomal recessive disorder due to defect in transport of neutral amino acids in the small intestine and kidney.
- An abnormality in tryptophan transport leads to niacin deficiency which is responsible for the pellagra-like eruption and photosensitivity.
- Amino acids like tryptophan which retained within the intestinal lumen are converted by bacteria to indolic compounds. These products are toxic to the nervous system.
- Presenting features are pellagra-like skin eruptions, cerebellar ataxia, and gross aminoaciduria.
- Skin rashes resemble seborrheic dermatitis, pellagra, congenital poikiloderma with photosensitivity, lupus erythematosus and carcinoid syndrome.

Diagnosis?

Q47. Features

- Focal epithelial hyperplasia due to infection with human papilloma virus (HPV) 13 & 32.
- Characteristic lesions are soft papules and plaques and lower lip is commonly affected.
- It regresses spontaneously over several months.

Diagnosis?

Q48. Features

- It is characterized by acquired elastic tissue degeneration of unknown etiology.
- It is having asymptomatic, well-circumscribed or diffuse larger areas of fine wrinkling. Wrinklings follow the usual lines of cleavage. Due to wrinkles skin appears aged. Some cases have discrete perifollicular papules.
- Other features are erythematous patches and telangiectasia.

- Lesion are not associated with scaling, induration or herniation.
- Common sites are trunk, lateral neck and upper limbs.
- Histopathology shows selective loss of elastic tissue at mid-dermal level.

Diagnosis?

Q49. Features

- Exclusively occurs in adult and very rarely in children.
- Firm, red brown papules, mostly distributed at fingers, hands, lips, ears and nose.
- **Coral beads sign** may present as chain of papules along with the cuticle.
- Nodular lesions may present at arms, elbows and knees.
- Facial disfigurement due to cartilaginous damage and **leonine facies**.
- Mucous membrane may be involved in 50% cases, mostly the oral cavity.
- Joint involvement is highly destructive and mostly affects interphalangeal joints in the form of **telescopic/opera glass** deformity.
- May regress spontaneously after 6-8 years.
- May be associated with internal malignancy in 10-30% cases.

Diagnosis?

Q50. Features

- Autosomal recessive disorders with phenylalanine hydroxylase deficiency and accumulation of phenylalanine.
- Symptoms and signs appear within first 4-24 months of age and usually normal at birth.
- **Guthrie test** is done for screening.
- **Musty odor** of urine and sweat is due to decomposed products like phenyl acetic acid and phenyl acetaldehyde.
- General features include mental retardation, seizure, hyperactivity, hypertonicity, hyperreflexia, peculiar gait and self-destructive behavior.
- Dermatological features are atopic dermatitis and sclerodermoid changes with sparing of hand and feet.
- Skeletal features are microcephaly, short stature, pes planus and syndactyly.
- Serum phenylalanine level increases 10-50 times (> 20 mg/dl).
- Presence of phenylalanine in urine is detected with pouring 10% ferric chloride with few drops of urine which turns green/blue color.
- Serum tyrosine level remains normal or may increase.
- Low phenylalanine rich diet should be maintained.

Diagnosis?

Q51. Features

- A rare and localized subcutaneous or intramuscular fungal infection.
- There are about 100 species of these **dematiaceous** fungi, such as *Exophiala jeanselmei, Exophiala dermatitidis*, etc.
- It begins with a firm, sometimes tender nodule which gradually converts into a large cyst.
- Histopathology shows a cystic cavity full of necrotic material. The wall of the cyst contains dense fibrous tissue, epithelioid cells, numerous Langhans' and foreign body types of giant cells and lymphocytes.
- Fungi can be seen at the granulomatous lining of the cyst wall with PAS/Grocott's stain.
- Commonest differential diagnosis is Baker's cyst.

Diagnosis?

Q52. Features

- It is rare autosomal dominant trait, having congenital absence of melanocytes in affected areas of the skin and hair, and this is due to mutation of c-kit proto-oncogene which is responsible for differentiation and migration of melanoblasts.
- The main clinical feature is relatively stable depigmented patches with depigmented hairs presenting at birth.
- Partially repigmented areas may present within and around the depigmented patches.
- White forelock of hair, often triangular in shape may be the only manifestation in 80-90% cases.

Diagnosis?

Q53. Features

- Chronic granulomatous disorder, caused by *Rhinosporidium seeberi* which is endemic in South India and Sri Lanka.
- The infection usually occurs through contact with stagnant fresh water like swimming pools and commonly affects the mucosae of nose, eyes, larynx and penis, and rarely other parts of the body such as skin.
- Characteristic cutaneous and mucosal lesions are pedunculated or sessile polypoid mass.
- Subcutaneous form is extremely rare and presents as asymptomatic lobular swelling at lower limbs, back and abdomen and the lesions resemble lipoma, sebaceous cyst, fibroma, and disseminated pheohyphomycosis.
- Histopathology shows sporangia at various stages of development.
- Treatment mainly DDS (dapsone) therapy, surgical excision and electro-surgery.

Diagnosis?

Q54. Features

- It is probably due to the circulating autoantibody formation against type II collagen, a component of cartilage.
- Most common clinical features are erythema, swelling and pain involving the auricle sparing ear lobe and resembling cellulitis where ear lobe is also being affected. In chronic cases ear cartilage is damaged to form a **cauliflower ear**.
- **Saddle nose deformity** is seen when nasal cartilage is involved.
- **Hoarseness of voice**, dyspnoea, cough, wheezing develop when respiratory tract is involved.
- Ocular involvement causes conjunctivitis, episcleritis, uveitis, corneal ulceration and even inflammation of optic nerve.
- Non-erosive arthritis is seen at sternoclavicular, sternomandibular and costochondral joints.
- Other associated cutaneous features are aphthous stomatitis, palpable purpura, livedo reticularis, panniculitis and neutrophilic dermatoses like Sweet syndrome.
- Systemic steroid is the main treatment.

Diagnosis?

Q55. Features

- It is a form of calcinosis cutis where calcium salts are deposited in the skin due to an unknown mechanism.
- A large periarticular deposits of calcium resembling a tumor is often found around hip, shoulder, and elbow joints.
- Number of the lesions is usually multiple and commonly affects young adults and males are more affected than females.

Q56. Features

- It occurs in infant or young children, having diffuse cutaneous mastocytosis when a massive amount of histamine is released from infiltrating mast cells.

- It is characterized by bronchospasm, headache, diarrhea, hypotension, flushing and pruritus.
- Death may occasionally be happen.

Diagnosis?

Q57. Features

- Recurrent epistaxis since childhood or infancy or at early adult life is the usual presenting feature.
- Telangiectasia appears at 3rd-4th decade, not before puberty.
- Telangiectatic lesions are punctate or linear.
- Rarely non-pulsatile spider nevus-like lesions develop.
- Sometimes nodular lesions are seen.

Diagnosis?

Q58. Features

- History of strenuous exercise or trauma present.
- Children and adults both are affected; but males suffer more than females.
- Painful and tender indurated swellings are usually present at lower limbs.
- Limited movement of hands and feet.
- Rarely face and abdomen are involved.
- Eosinophilia upto 30% is a striking feature.
- Increased ESR and hypergammaglobulinemia may be present.
- Histopathology shows dermal sclerosis, inflammation upto deep fascia and presence of **flame figure**.

Diagnosis?

Q59. Features

- Frequent abortion.
- Cerebrovascular attack.
- Erythema and edema/postphlebitic syndrome.
- Leg ulcers may be painful superficial star-shaped ulcer, pyoderma gangrenosum-like and Degos-like.
- Necrotizing purpura.
- Digital gangrene.
- Fingertip cyanotic spot.
- Nonfading acral microlivedo.
- Subungual splinter hemorrhage.

Diagnosis?

Q60. Features

- It is a rare disease with fatal outcome and characterized by necrotizing granulomatous inflammation and vasculitis.
- It predominantly affects the small to medium sized arteries and veins.
- Initially it remains limited to certain organs but gradually affects other organs like upper and lower respiratory tract, kidney and skin.
- Facial skin is commonly affected.
- Skin involvement may precede many months before involving other internal organs.
- Common skin lesions are papules, plaques and ulcers.

Diagnosis?

Q61. Features

- An X-linked dominant disorder, starts within first few weeks of life and passes through three stages of skin eruptions.
- Bullous stage contains recurrent crops of tense vesicles and bullae in a linear fashion, mostly along the **Blaschko's lines** of the limbs.
- Papular stage contains erythematous smooth papules and plaques developing along with the vesiculo-bullous lesions or following them. Lesions may be warty at dorsa of the hands.

- Pigmentary stage contains gray to brown pigmentation developing following healing of the previous lesions or rarely developing earlier as the sole lesion without any other lesion.
- Other associated features are telangiectasia, and defects in the nervous system, dental system and skeletal system.

Diagnosis?

Q62. Features

- It is a congenital disorder, having unilateral or bilateral depigmented patches in a whorled pattern along the Blaschko's lines.

Diagnosis?

Q63. Features

- It is disease of childhood, due vasculitis.
- Erythema multiforme-like skin lesions.
- Red lips and strawberry tongue.
- Red and swollen palms-soles.
- Generalized lymphadenopathy.
- Conjunctiva is nonpurulent in comparison to SJS syndrome.
- Treatment includes intravenous gamma globulin 2 gm/kg body weight, as a single infusion over a period of 10 hours.

Diagnosis?

Q64. Features

- It is characterized by erythematous urticarial plaques with intermittent and migratory nature, caused by *Gnathostoma dolorosa* or *Gnathostoma spinigerum*, a nematode.
- It usually occurs at every 2-6 weeks interval and each episode persists for 7-10 days. Total duration of the illness may be for 10 years.
- The underlying parasite moves about 1 cm per hour.
- Histopathology shows eosinophilic panniculitis and then designates as **larva migrans profundus**.
- Treatment includes albendazole 400 mg once or twice a day for 21 days, or ivermectin 200 μg/day for two days.

Diagnosis?

Q65. Features

- An autosomal dominant disorder due to defect in genes for keratin 4 and keratin 13.
- It may appear at birth or anytime from infancy to adolescence and maximum size reaches by early adulthood.
- It is characterized by asymptomatic, exuberant, white plaque. Sometimes it becomes thickened with fissures, folds and erosions.
- It commonly affects oral mucosa, along with other mucosae.

Diagnosis?

Q66. Features

- Autosomal recessive entity, with deficiency of hepatic tyrosine aminotransferase, causing accumulation of tyrosine.
- At age of 1 year, it is presented with sharply demarcated, yellowish keratotic papules at palms and soles.
- Gradually lesions become more erythematous, erosive and painful.
- Nail dystrophy.
- Photophobia and bilateral tearing within first 3 months of life.

Diagnosis?

Q67. Features

- It is a rare disease with fatal outcome and characterized by necrotizing granulomatous inflammation and vasculitis.
- It predominantly affects the small to medium sized arteries and veins.

- Initially it remains limited to certain organs but gradually affects other organs like upper and lower respiratory tract, kidney and skin.
- Facial skin is commonly affected.
- Skin involvement may precede many months before involving other internal organs.
- Common skin lesions are papules, plaques and ulcers.

Diagnosis?

Q68. Features

- An autosomal recessive entity, associated with severe intrauterine growth retardation and edematous appearance.
- Ichthyosis is present at birth with variable severity from mild to Harlequin ichthyosis.
- Characteristic facies includes protuberant eyes, flattened nose, slanted forehead, micrognathia, deformed ears and short neck.
- Other features are syndactyly, digital hypoplasia, limb contracture, poor bone mineralization, microcephaly and agenesis of corpus callosum.

Diagnosis?

Q69. Features

- Mostly occurs in young women.
- Presence of livedo racemosa and Raynaud's pheneomenon.
- Presence of thromboembolic complications, history of abortion and unexplained headache.
- Persistent acral ulceration, necrosis and gangrene.
- May be associated with drugs, SLE, lymphoma, chronic viral infection.
- Antiphospholipid antibodies target β 2-glycoprotein and antigen-antibody complex activates T-cells, thrombocytes and endothelial cells.

Diagnosis?

Q70. Features

- Presence of asthma.
- Presence of granulomatous vasculitis of skin and lungs.
- Eosinophilia of tissue and blood.
- Presence of mononeuritis multiplex and affection of kidneys, heart and gastrointestinal tract.
- Urticarial vasculitis lesions, purpura and nodular lesions at skin.
- Histopathology of skin lesion showing palisading granuloma and necrosis with eosinophilia, nuclear dusts and giant cells at a distance.
- In 20% cases both cANCA and pANCA are positive.

Diagnosis?

Q71. Features

- Acanthosis nigricans
- Palmoplantar hyperkeratosis
- Hypotrichosis
- Hypohidrosis
- Nail dystrophy
- Early loss of adult teeth
- Mental retardation.

Diagnosis?

Q72. Features

- Occurs in presence of short gut, malabsorption, parenteral nutrition, multiple carboxylase deficiency, biotinidase deficiency, antibiotic therapy and raw egg ingestion.
- Skin and nervous system are primarily affected.
- Patchy red eroded and crusted dermatitis mimicking acrodermatitis enteropathica and essential fatty acid deficiency, is the cutaneous manifestation.
- Periorificial regions and groins are commonly affected.
- Candidal infection is frequently found in the lesion.

- Alopecia of the scalp, eyebrows and eyelashes is commonly found.
- Conjunctivitis may be associated.
- Neurologic manifestations in adults are depression, lethargy, hallucination and paresthesia of the limbs.
- Neurological manifestations in children are hypotonia, lethargy, withdrawal behavior, ataxia, seizure, deafness and developmental delay.

Diagnosis?

Answers

1. Adam's-Oliver syndrome.
2. Dowling-Dego's disease/Dark dot disease.
3. Alport syndrome.
4. Antiphospholipid syndrome.
5. Apert's syndrome.
6. Schnitzler's syndrome.
7. Kawasaki disease
8. Trichofolliculoma
9. KID syndrome
10. Protothecosis
11. Bart-Pumphrey syndrome
12. Bart's syndrome
13. Bazex syndrome
14. Berlin syndrome
15. Bloom syndrome
16. Carbon baby syndrome
17. Cartilage hair hypoplasia syndrome
18. Chediak-Higashi syndrome
19. CHILD syndrome
20. CHIME syndrome
21. Clouston syndrome
22. Coffin-Siris syndrome
23. Eosinophilia-myalgia syndrome
24. Gorlin/Multiple basal cell nevus syndrome
25. Goltz syndrome
26. Gottron's syndrome (Progressive symmetrical erythrokeratoderma)
27. Graham-Little syndrome
28. Hallerman-Streiff syndrome
29. Hot foot syndrome
30. Howel-Evans syndrome (Tylosis)
31. Hunter syndrome
32. Hurriez syndrome
33. KID syndrome
34. Kindler syndrome
35. Netherton syndrome
36. Olmsted syndrome
37. Papillon-Lefevre syndrome
38. Peutz Jegher's syndrome
39. Proteus syndrome
40. Sjogren's syndrome
41. Sjogren-Larsson syndrome
42. Sneddon syndrome
43. Sweet's syndrome
44. Thibierge-Weissen syndrome
45. Vohwinkel syndrome
46. Hartnup disease
47. Heck's disease
48. Mid-dermal elastolysis
49. Multicentric reticulohistiocytosis
50. Phenylketonuria (PKU)
51. Pheohyphomycosis
52. Piebaldism
53. Rhinosporidiosis
54. Relapsing polychondritis
55. Tumoral calcinosis
56. Mastocytosis syndrome
57. Hereditary hemorrhagic telangiectasia
58. Eosinophilic fasciitis/Shulman syndrome
59. Antiphospholipid syndrome
60. Wegener's granulomatosis
61. Incontinentia pigmenti
62. Incontinentia pigmenti achromians of Ito
63. Kawasaki's disease
64. Gnathostomiasis
65. White sponge nevus
66. Richner-Hanhart syndrome
67. Wegener's granulomatosis

68. Neu-Laxova syndrome
69. Antiphospholipid syndrome
70. Churg-Strauss disease
71. Lelis syndrome, a form of ectodermal dysplasia
72. Biotin deficiency.

DERMAQUIZ

1. Robert Koch isolated M. tuberculosis in ____________.
2. In 1953, ________ differentiated bullous pemphigoid from pemphigus.
3. In 1841, _________ separated psoriasis from leprosy.
4. The chemical, ______ is responsible for smell in bromhidrosis.
5. In chromhidrosis, minimal amount of sweat required for color is __________/per follicle.
6. SSKI works in sporotrichosis as ____________________________.
7. Hallmark of Griselli syndrome is __________________________________.
8. Facial skin appears as pig-skin leather in _______________.
9. Lobomycosis can affect animal other than human is ___________.
10. Natural source of glycolic acid is ______ and salicylic acid is _____________.
11. Pseudo-ochronosis is seen among ____________________ workers.
12. Treatment of choice in scrub typhus is ______________________.
13. Predominant palmar finding in Costello syndrome is _______________.
14. Lichen aureus commonly occurs in age group __________________.
15. Pattern of dermal necrosis in Degos disease is ___________________.
16. Linezolid inhibits __________ subunit of 50s ribosome.
17. Unilateral laterothoracic exanthema is commonly seen in age group ___________ years.
18. Tigecycline is a derivative of ____________________________________.
19. Ehrlichiae has tropism for ____________ and Anaplasmodiae has tropism for __________.
20. Rash in Rocky Mountain fever spreads centrifugally or centripetally, which one? ______________________.
21. Inflammation in Muckle Well syndrome is induced by _____________.
22. Follicular dendritic cell membrane bound iccosome bodies contain _______________.
23. Rituximab antagonizes _______________ on __________ cells.
24. Which part of upper limb is classically affected in Erysipelas? _________________________.
25. Childhood Melioidosis is commonly present as acute unilateral suppuration of _________.
26. Anakinra antagonizes ___________________.
27. Tufts of wooly hair at the pore is diagnostic of ________________________.
28. Facial pigmentation in hereditary hemachromatosis is largely due to _______________.
29. Pigmentation in acanthosis nigricans is due to __________________________.
30. Reticular pigmentation in Partington syndrome is due to _______________________.
31. Red color in erythroplakia is due to ___________________________________.
32. White color in leukoplakia is due to ______________________.
33. Syphilitic angina affects ___________________________________.
34. Commonest site of Merkel cell carcinoma is __________________________.
35. Rocky island pattern of plaques are seen in _____________________.
36. Sreptococcus iniae causes hand cellulitis following handling of _____________, a fresh water fish.
37. Absorption of Itraconazole is reduced in AIDS due to ______________________.
38. Toxin part of Denileukin diftitox is derived from ______________________.
39. __________________ biochemical content is

common in all: Gordona, Corynebacterium, Nocardia and Rhodacoccus.

40. In photodynamic therapy, cytotoxic action of singlet oxygen is > ____________ and half life is < ____________.
41. Normal basal cell cycling is 10%, but in psoriasis ____________%.
42. ____________ is common in all: Crohn's disease, herpes genitalis, rheumatoid arthritis, pyoderma gangrenosum and Behcet's disease.
43. Chracteristic cutaneous feature of dysbetalipoproteinemia is ____________.
44. To detect cryoglobulinemia, serum is refrigerated at ____________ temperature.
45. ____________ atypical mycobacterial infection histopathologically mimics LL/histoid leprosy.
46. ____________ atypical mycobacteria found on the surface of leprosy lesion.
47. LL like globi of AFB is also found in ____________ atypical mycobacterial infection.
48. Rock hard thigh is seen in ____________.
49. Main antigen in Dermatitis herpetiformis is ____________.
50. Walking dandruff at the back of dogs and cats is caused by ____________ mite.
51. Spontaneous onset of one or more painful hematoma in middle aged female is a feature of ____________.
52. A form of Ehler- Danlos syndrome, characterized by extreme skin fragility, bruising, droopy skin, joint laxity, umbilical hernia and blue sclera is ____________.
53. Pitted, scarry and songy skin along with chronic ulceration in skin are features of ____________.
54. Acrogeria manifests with dry, thin, transparent and wrinkled skin at hands and feet at ____________.
55. Progeria manifests with profound growth failure, reduced subcutaneous fat at face and limbs, and appearing as fledgling bird at age of ____________.
56. Pangeria manifests at age between ______ to ____ years.
57. Earliest manifestation of pangeria is ____________.
58. Lepechaunism affects ____________ of skin.
59. Bouchard's node affects ____________ joints.
60. Bean bag cells are characteristically seen in ____________.
61. Primitive brown fat is seen in ____________.

Answer

1. 1882, **2.** Lever, **3.** Hebra, **4.** 3Methyl-2 hexenoic acid, **5.** 0.001 ml, **6.** Immunomodulator, **7.** Silvery hair, **8.** Lipoid proteinosis, **9.** Dolphin, **10.** Sugarcane, wilow bark, **11.** Jewelry, **12.** Doxycycline, **13.** Deep creases, **14.** 2nd and 3rd decade, **15.** Wedge shaped, **16.** 23s, **17.** 1-5, **18.** Minocycline, **19.** Monocyte, granulocyte, **20.** Centripetally, **21.** Cryopyrin, **22.** Antigen-antibody complex, **23.** CD20, B, **24.** Wrist to DIPJ (distal interphalangeal joints), **25.** Parotid gland, **26.** IL1, **27.** Trichofolliculoma, **28.** Melanin, **29.** hyperkeratosis, **30.** Melanin, **31.** absence of keratin, **32.** Hyperkeratosis, **33.** Tonsils, **34.** Face, **35.** Sweet syndrome, **36.** Tilapia, **37.** Hypochlorhydria, **38.** Diphtheria toxin, **39.** Mycolic acid, **40.** 0.02 μm and 0.04s, **41.** 100, **42.** Pathergy phenomenon, **43.** Palmar xanthoma, **44.** 4°C, **45.** MAC, **46.** M. scrofulaceum, **47.** M. hemophilum, **48.** Stiff skin syndrome, **49.** Epidermal trans glutaminase, **50.** Cheyletiella, **51.** Achenbach's syndrome, **52.** Dermatosparaxis, **53.** Prolidase deficiency, **54.** Birth, **55.** 2 years, **56.** 14-18 years, **57.** Grey hairs at temporal region, **58.** Subcutaneous tissue, **59.** Proximal interphalangeal joints, **60.** Cytophagic histiocytic panniculitis, **61.** Hibernoma.

PART E

DERMATOSURGERY

CHAPTER E1

DERMATOSURGERY

Electrosurgery

Principle

- Electric current passes through the transformer within the electrosurgery machine to get reaquired amount of voltage and then passes through an oscillating circuit to increase frequency as 500-3500 KHz.
- When this high frequency current is brought near a lesion through the handpiece electrode, it faces a sudden resistance resulting in production of heat energy.
- Quality of heat depends on wave pattern/type of oscillation and this heat may be used for electrodessication, electrofulguration, electrocoagulation and electrosection/cutting.
- In electrodessication, the electrode touches the lesion.
- In **electrofulguration**, an air interface persists between the electrode and the lesion.
- In **electrosection**, wave pattern is fully rectified and the electrode sharply cuts the tissue like a hot knife cuts the butter.

Types of electrodes

- Loop for electrodessication
- Needle for electrofulguration
- Ball for electrocoagulation
- Wire for electroepilation
- Blade for electrosection.

* When loop is used, charred tissue often adheres to it and prevents further use. This charred tissue can be easily removed by wrapping the electrode with wet gauge piece and switch on the machine for 10 seconds only.

Precaution

- Caution should be taken in patients with pacemaker.
- To enquire about hypersensitivity to local anesthesia.
- To use non-alcoholic cleanser as alcoholic cleanser may catch fire.

Hazards

- There is a chance of electric shock.
- There may be a disturbance with pacemaker.

- There is a risk to catch fire, specially when working at perianal area due to passage of flatus, containing methane.

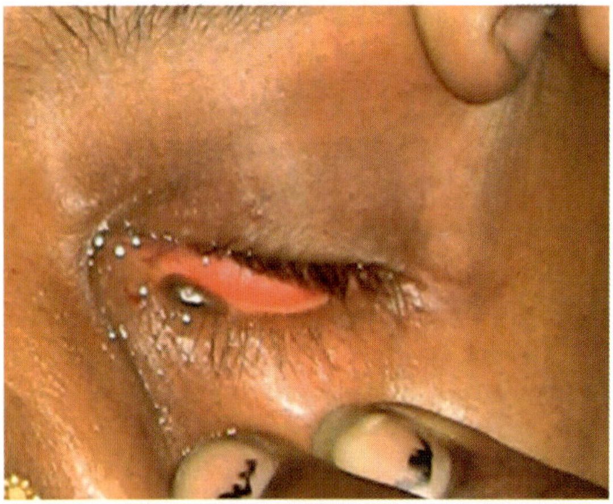

Fig.1 A tiny lesion of acquired compound melanocytic nevus at the margin of the lower lid

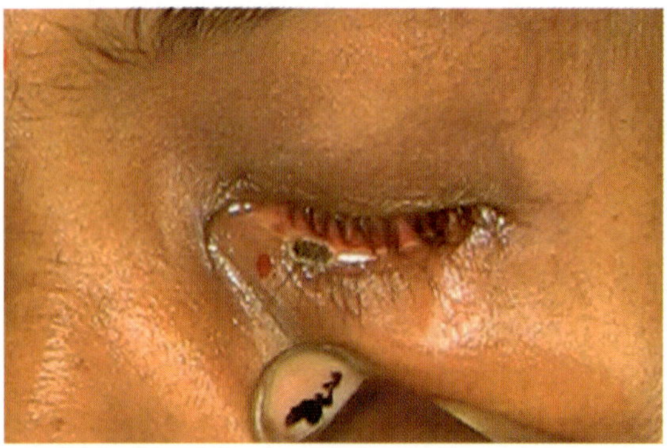

Fig.2 Though risky but electrofulguration done sucess-fully

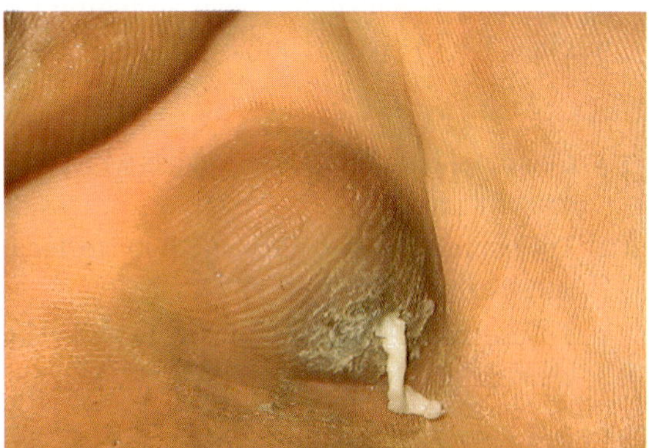

Fig. 3 A discharging epidermoid cyst at sole eligible for electrofulguration

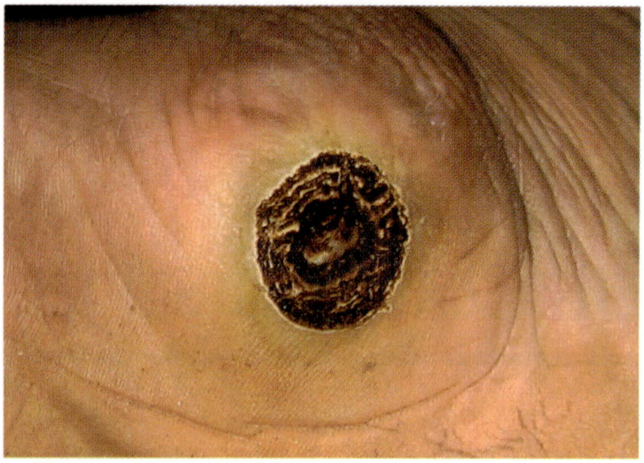

Fig.4 A corn at sole, treated after electrofulguration

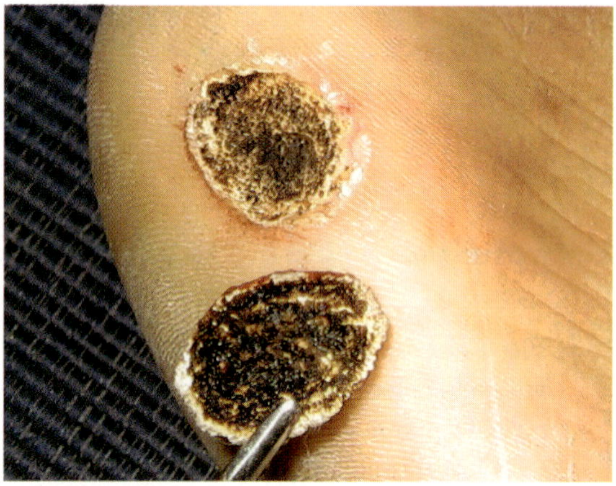

Fig.5 Plantar wart is removed successfully following electrosurgery

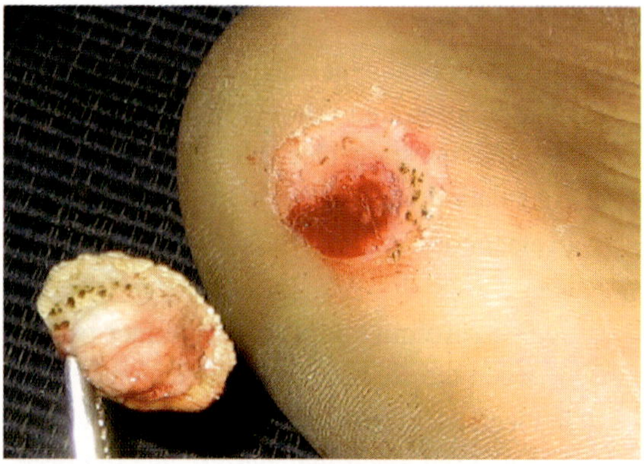

Fig.6 A plantar wart, treated by electrofulguration

Cryosurgery

- Tissue is destroyed by deep freezing
- The freezing agent is called cryogen.
- Freezing starts at the center of the application and forms a sphere, called **iceball**.
- For a large lesion, multiple contiguous ice-ball formation is required.
- For a smooth lesion, cryogen is touched with a probe.
- For a rough surface, cryogen is sprayed on the surface.

Types of cryogen

- Liquid nitrogen (–196°C).
- Carbon dioxide (–80°C).
- Nitrous oxide (–75°C).

Complications

- Development of urticaria, edema or vesiculation.
- Headache when it is used at forehead.
- Periorbital edema when it is used at eyelids.
- Rarely depigmentation and scarring develop.

Laser surgery

Principle

- LASER stands for light amplification by stimulated emission of radiation.
- It requires a medium.
- Laser light is monochromatic and waves are coherent and collimated.
- The rays show convergence by convex lens.
- Laser light interacts with skin and causes photothermal reaction, photochemical reaction and photomechanical action.
- Photothermal reaction causes destruction of tissue and hemostasis.
- Photochemical reaction causes selective destruction depending on type of laser and type of tissue.
- Photomechanical action causes disruption of tissue.

Types of medium

- Solid: Ruby crystal
- Liquid: Rhodamine dye
- Gas: Argon.

Laser safety and precautions

- Eyes must be protected with shield or glass for both patient and operator.
- Operating room should be closed.
- Smoke is to be evacuated immediately.
- Inflammable objects like spirit should be kept away.
- Care must be taken during working at perianal area with invisible carbon dioxide laser. Flatus may contain methane which may ignite by laser light.
- Switching off the machine after therapy.

Chemical surgery

* This is suitable for patients with fair complexion.
* There is a chance of postinflammatory hyperpigmentation.

Commonly used chemical

- Trichloroaceticacid (30-90%)
- Phenol (88%).
- Salicylic acid (30-60%).
- Potassium hydroxide (10-20%).

Tricholoroacetic acid

- 30% Is used for pigmentary disorders. This should be used only in fair patients.
- 50-70% Is used for xanthelasma.
- 80-90% Is used for wart, specially genital wart in pregnancy or recalcitrant genital wart.
- 90-100% Is used for seborrheic keratosis.

Phenol (88%)

- Commonly used for freckles and dermatosis papulosa nigra (DPN).

Salicylic acid (30-60%)

- It is used for skin rejuvenation and for profuse freckles.

Potassium hydroxide (10-20%)

- It is used for molluscum contagiosum.

PART F

MULTIPLE CHOICE QUESTIONS (MCQs)

MULTIPLE CHOICE QUESTIONS (MCQs)

CHAPTER F1

1. All statements are true about autoerythrocyte sensitization syndrome (AES), except
   a) Also known as Gardner-Diamond syndrome/psychogenic purpura
   b) Commonly occurs in females
   c) Disturbances in blood coagulation system
   d) No abnormalities of vessel walls
   e) Surgical operations are contraindicated
   f) Painful, erythematous, indurated and edematous plaques progress to annular ecchymoses
   g) Hysterical personality traits
   h) Positive intracutaneous test with autoerythrocytes
2. Single hypoaesthetic patch, probable diagnosis is
   a) Morphea
   b) Lichen sclerosus et atrophicus
   c) Idiopathic guttate hypomelanosis
   d) Ashleaf macule
   e) Cafe-au-lait macule
3. Rule out the incorrect statement regarding confluent and reticulate papillomatosis
   a) Hyperkeratosis and papillomatosis without acanthosis
   b) Infection may be an etiology
   c) Teenagers and young adults are rarely affected
   d) Characterized by flat dry papules up to 5 mm in diameter
   e) Common sites are neck, upper chest, between the breasts, interscapular area and the axillae
4. Crowe's sign is associated with
   a) Neurofibromatosis
   b) Tuberous sclerosis
   c) Hailey Hailey disease
   d) Dowling-Degos disease
   e) Chagas' disease
5. Rule out the wrong statement regarding tripe palm
   a) Velvety and rugose thickening of palms
   b) Almost always associated with internal malignancy
   c) Serum epidermal growth factor may be elevated
   d) Commonly associated with pulmonary and bronchial carcinoma
   e) It is not a variant of acanthosis nigricans

6. Drug does not cause acanthosis nigricans
   a) Triazinate, a folic acid antagonist
   b) Fusidic acid
   c) Protease inhibitors
   d) Retapamulin
   e) Nicotinic acid
7. Find out the wrong statement regarding malignancy associated acanthosis nigricans
   a) Lesions are more severe and extensive
   b) Nails may be brittle and ridged and hair may shed
   c) Warty papillomatous thickening around the lips and eyes
   d) Rapid progress and mucous membrane involvement are useful warning signs.
   e) Commonest underlying malignancy is gastric adenocarcinoma.
   f) It never precedes other symptom of the underlying malignancy.
8. Butterfly erythema may be seen in all except
   a) Bloom syndrome
   b) Systemic lupus erythematosus
   c) Netherton syndrome
   d) Pemphigus erythematosus
9. Herald patch is seen in
   a) Pityriasis asteatoides
   b) Pityriasis rotunda
   c) Pityriasis amiantacea
   d) Pityriasis nigra
   e) Pityriasis lichenoides chronica
   f) Pityriasis rosea
10. All statements are correct regarding pityriasis alba, except
   a) A pattern of dermatitis where hypopigmentation is the most conspicuous feature
   b) Mild erythema and scaling may precede the development of hypopigmentation
   c) Reduced number of active melanocytes and decreased number and size of melanosomes
   d) Children between ages of 3 and 16 are commonly affected.
   e) Commonest sites are cheeks
   f) Trunk and limbs are never affected
   g) Individual lesion is ill defined oval or round hypopigmented patch.
11. Ear lobe infiltration is not seen in
   a) PKDL
   b) Leprosy
   c) Relapsing polychondritis
   d) Polymorphic light eruption
   e) Chilblains
12. Incorrect statements about Netherton's syndrome is
   a) Episodic peeling of the skin as migratory double-aged annular scaly patches or ichthyosis linearis circumflexa
   b) Associated hair shaft defect, known as trichorrhexis invaginata
   c) Mutation of serine protease inhibitor kazal type 5 (*SPINK5*)
   d) Premature lamellar body and abnormal lipid processing in the intercellular spaces, leading to impairment of epidermal permeability barrier
   e) Increased epidermal DNA synthesis and turnover
   f) Failure to convert sulphydryl groups to disulphide bonds in the cortical cells of the hair at the level of keratogenous zone contributes to focal softening.
   g) Retinoid therapy improves most of the cases
13. Acantholysis is not seen in
   a) Actinic keratosis
   b) Hailey Hailey disease
   c) Grover's disease
   d) Warty dyskeratoma
   e) Darier's disease
   f) Acanthosis nigricans
14. Find out the wrong statement regarding ichthyosis hystrix
   a) Encompasses a number of rare conditions
   b) Development of dark warty scaling
   c) Absence of blistering and skin fragility

d) Sparing of face, palms and soles
e) Orthohyperkeratosis, patchy parakeratosis, acanthosis and papillomatosis
f) Scattered vacuolated and binucleate keratinocytes in the upper epidermis
g) Symmetric porcupine-like scaling
h) Systemic retinoids never becomes beneficial

15. Probable cause of itching at night in scabies
a) Crawling of the female mite within the burrow
b) Crawling of the female mite outside the burrow
c) Crawling of the male partner of the female mite
d) Movement of the mites during copulation
e) Hypersensitivity reaction to egg and excreta of mite

16. Dermatological feature not present in Noonan's syndrome
a) Lymphedema of feet and legs
b) Leukokeratosis of the lips and gingiva
c) Light colored coarse curly hair with low posterior hair line
d) Downy hypertrichosis may occur on the cheeks and shoulder
e) Pubic hair is scanty and beard growth is poor in male
f) Ulerythema oophryogenes never occurs

17. Munro's microabscess is not seen in
a) Psoriasis
b) Candidiasis
c) Geographic tongue
d) Pellagra
e) Parapsoriasis

18. Statement incorrect in ataxia telangiectasia
a) Abnormally raised serum α-fetoprotein in more than 90% cases
b) Prophylactic antibiotic is essential to reduce morbidity
c) Presence of defective DNA repair
d) Telangiectases usually appear between 2 and 8 years of age
e) Hypo- or hyperpigmented patches
f) Radiosensitivity is uncommon

19. Annular lesion is not seen in
a) Subcorneal pustular dermatosis
b) Granuloma annulare
c) Granuloma multiforme
d) Discoid lupus erythematosus
e) Psoriasis
f) Lichen planus

20. Find out the wrong statement about Mal de Meleda
a) Grossly thickened stratum corneum, increased stratum lucidum, marked acanthosis and pseudospongiosis
b) Patches of ivory-yellow hyperkeratosis of whole palms and soles crossing over to dorsal surfaces
c) Onset is in early childhood
d) Hyperkeratosis is followed by erythema
e) Angular cheilitis and superficial fungal infection are common

21. Dory flop sign is associated with
a) Primary syphilis
b) Secondary syphilis
c) Tertiary syphilis
d) Late congenital syphilis
e) Tubercular gumma

22. Which is not a transgradient keratoderma?
a) Loricrin keratoderma
b) Greither's syndrome
c) Sybert's keratoderma
d) Thost-Unna keratoderma

23. Tzanck cell is basically a
a) Macrophage
b) Merkel cell
c) Keratinocyte
d) Plasma cell
e) Dermal dendritic cell

24. Find out the wrong statement regarding the features of Thost-Unna keratoderma
a) Very thick yellow hyperkeratosis initially appears at soles, followed by palms

b) Sharp cut-off at wrist and no tendency to spread at dorsal surfaces
c) Livid red border to outcry the hyperkeratosis
d) Hyperhidrosis with fungal infection and pitted keratolysis is common
e) Nails may be normal but hair and teeth are always abnormal.

25. Anatomical keratinocyte-melanocyte ratio at interfollicular skin is
a) 10:1
b) 50:1
c) 17:1
d) 100:1
e) 5:1

26. Physiological keratinocyte-melanocyte ratio at interfollicular skin is
a) 10:1
b) 36:1
c) 17:1
d) 100:1
e) 5:1

27. Anatomical keratinocyte-melanocyte ratio at hair follicle is
a) 10:1
b) 50:1
c) 17:1
d) 100:1
e) 5:1

28. Which feature is not seen in pachyonychia congenita?
a) Hyperkeratosis of nail bed appears in first or second year of life
b) Frictional blisters may occur on the foot in childhood, specially in hot weather
c) In adult focal hyperkeratosis causes marked pain during walking
d) Palmoplantar keratoses are more severe in type 2 than type 1
e) Hoarseness of voice is a feature of type 1
f) Development of cysts is a feature of type 2

29. Dermatosis not associated with hidradenitis suppurativa
a) Ulcerative collitis
b) Crohn's disease
c) Fox-Fordyce disease
d) Steatocystoma multiplex
e) Pityriasis rubra pilaris
f) Acanthosis nigricans
g) Dowling-Degos disease
h) SAPHO

30. False about hairy malformation of palms and soles
a) Transmitted as an autosomal dominant trait
b) Asymptomatic areas of skin with somewhat altered texture and bearing hairs
c) Areas on the palms near the wrist and medial aspect of the the longitudinal arch of the foot are commonly affected
d) Histopathology shows no abnormality other than the presence of hair follicles
e) Only palms without sole involvement is never seen

31. Linear lesion is not seen in
a) Lichen scrofulosorum
b) Lichen planus
c) Psoriasis
d) Pederus dermatitis
e) Rhus dermatitis

32. Lesion does not occur in secondary syphilis
a) Pustule
b) Macule
c) Plaque
d) Vesicle
e) Erosion

33. Coral-beads like lesions are seen in
a) Hypertrichosis lanuginosa acquisita
b) Xanthogranuloma
c) Multicentric reticulohistiocytosis
d) Mycosis fungoides
e) Dermatomyositis

34. Dermatoses having 100% association with internal malignancy in all, except
a) Tripe palm

b) Hypertrichosis lanuginosa acquisita
c) Paraneoplastic pemphigus
d) Necrolytic migratory erythema
e) Bazex syndrome

35. Leser-Trelat sign is associated with
a) Systemic scleroderma
b) Internal malignancy
c) Chronic arsenicosis
d) Crohn's disease
e) Ulcerative colitis

36. Staphne's sign is associated with
a) Systemic scleroderma
b) Internal malignancy
c) Chronic arsenicosis
d) Crohn's disease
e) Bacterial endocarditis

37. Janeway lines in bacterial endocarditis is seen at
a) Heel
b) Tip of the toes
c) Tip of the fingers
d) Thenar and hypothenar areas of the palms
e) Arch of the foot

38. Which is not a differential diagnosis of pityriasis versicolor?
a) Epidermolysis dysplasia verruciformis
b) Acrokeratoelastoides of Costa
c) Lepromatous leprosy
d) Early vitiligo
e) Late lesions of pityriasis lichenoides chronica

39. Which is not a premalignant condition?
a) Actinic keratosis
b) Bowen's disease
c) Erosive lichen planus
d) Epidermolysis dysplasia verruciformis
e) Acrokeratoverruciformis of Hoff

40. Surface of the lesion may be umbilicated in all, except
a) Cryptococcosis
b) Lichen planus
c) Molluscum contagiosum
d) Racouchot-Fabre disease
e) Papulonercotic tuberculid
f) Erythema nodosum

41. Ulceration or erosion never occurs on the lesion of
a) Erythema nodosum
b) Erythema induratum of Bazin
c) Scrofuloderma
d) Plasma cell balanitis
e) Lichen planus

42. What is the incorrect statement about phakomatosis pigmentovascularis?
a) There are five types from type I to type V.
b) Type II is the commonest type
c) Nevus flammeus (port-wine stain) is a component in all types except type v
d) Nevus anemicus may or may not be associated in type II, III and IV
e) Dermal melanosis is a component in type II, III and V
f) Cutis marmorata telangiectatica congenita is not a feature of type V.

43. Which statements or statements is/are not correct regarding impact of HIV infection on leprosy?
a) Decreased incidence of type 1 reaction
b) Increased incidence of TT leprosy
c) Increased bacterial index
d) None of the above

44. Herald patch is seen in
a) Pityriasis amiantacea
b) Pityriasis rosea
c) Pityriasis lichenoides chronica
d) Pityriasis versicolor
e) Pityriasis sicca
f) Pityriasis rubra pilaris
g) None of the above
h) All of the above

45. Dermatosis not related with mycobacterial infection
a) Lichen spinulosa
b) Lichen scrofulosorum

c) Erythema induratum of Bazin
d) Buruli ulcer
e) Scrofuloderma

46. Lupus pernio is a form of
a) Lupus vulgaris
b) Chilblains
c) Lupus erythematosus
d) Sarcoidosis
e) Rosacea

47. Mad hatter's disease is related with poisoning of
a) Arsenic
b) Mercury
c) Lead
d) Zinc
e) Salicylic acid

48. All statements are true about green nail syndrome, except
a) Color is due to pyoverdin
b) Caused by *Pseudomonas aeruginosa*
c) Absence of onycholysis
d) Paronychia is often associated
e) 1% Acetic acid is helpful

49. All statements are true about malakoplakia, except
a) Granulomatous disease of the genitourinary tract.
b) Unresistable infection with *Pseudomonas aeruginosa, Staphylococcal aureus* and *Escherichia coli*
d) Foamy eosinophilic Hansemann macrophages contain intracytoplasmic calcified Michaelis-Gutmann bodies
e) Periurethral and perianal areas are the uncommon sites.

50. Exogenous ochronosis is not related with
a) Clofazimine
b) Hydroquinone
c) Hydroxychloroquine
d) Potassium permanganate
e) Phenol
f) Picric acid
g) Resorcinol
h) Levodopa
i) Mercury

51. All statements are the features of erythrasma, except
a) Sharply defined reddish-brown scaly patches at intertriginous areas.
b) Caused by *Corynebacterium minutissimum*.
c) Coral red fluorescence is seen under Wood's lamp examination
d) Organisms are spore-forming and rod shaped.
e) Topical tolnaftate and miconazole both are effective.

52. Find out the odd one
a) Civatte bodies
b) Sclerotic bodies
c) Mauriform cells
d) Copper penny bodies
e) Medlar bodies

53. A 10 year-old boy presented with single asymptomatic ill defined hypopigmented macule at face. What could be the diagnosis?
a) Pityriasis alba
b) Post kala-azar dermal leishmaniasis
c) Seborrheic dermatitis
d) Previtiligo
e) Nevus hypochromicus
f) Indeterminate leprosy

54. Find out the odd one
a) Lobomycosis
b) Keloidal blastomycosis
c) Acne keloidalis

55. In Mal-de-Meleda, Meleda is named after
a) Name of an Island
b) Name of first patient
c) Dermatologist who first described
d) Name of the river along which most of the cases were found

56. Bowen's disease is not associated with
a) Chronic UV radiation
b) Chronic arsenicosis

c) Acute arsenic poisoning
d) Lead exposure
e) Mercury exposure

57. A 11 year-old girl suddenly develops a linear hypopigmented mild elevated lesion extending from the shoulder to wrist of left hand. What could be the possible diagnosis?
a) Lichen planus
b) Lichen striatus
c) Lichen nitidus
d) Lichen spinulosa
e) Lichen scrofulosorum

58. Polilosis is associated with
a) Piebaldism
b) Waardenburg syndrome
c) Albinism
d) Alkaptonuria
e) PIBIDS

59. Single well defined erythematous and scaly plaque. Which is not a differential diagnosis?
a) Bowen's disease
b) Bowenoid papulosis
c) Psoriasis
d) Discoid lupus erythematosus
e) Nummular dermatitis

60. In infants, hypoglycemia may be induced by
a) Psoralen
b) Isotretinoin
c) Cyclosporine
d) Propranolol
e) Methotrexate

61. Fordyce spots are basically
a) Ectopic sebaceous glands
b) Ectopic apocrine glands
c) Ectopic eccrine glands
d) Ectopic hair follicles
e) None of the above

62. Drug does not cause hypoglycemia
a) Methotrexate
b) Quinine
c) Salicylates
d) Propranolol
e) Isotretinoin

63. Fox-Fordyce disease originates from
a) Ectopic sebaceous glands
b) Eccrine sweat glands
c) Apocrine sweat glands
d) Hair follicles
e) None of the above

64. Hypopigmented lesion is not a feature in
a) Waardenburg syndrome
b) Piebaldism
c) Tuberous sclerosis
d) Neurofibromatosis
e) Post kala-azar dermal leishmaniasis

65. Wrong statement about Degos' disease
a) A potentially fatal obliterative arteritis syndrome
b) More frequently found in females than males
c) Age of presentation between 20-40 years
d) Presence of reddish edematous papules which later become umbilicated with porcelain-white center and red telangiectatic periphery
e) Death is usually due to fulminant peritonitis following multiple intestinal perforations

66. Meffert's sign is related with
a) Geographic tongue
b) Fordyce's disease
c) Hand-foot-mouth disease
d) Kyrle's disease
e) Pyostomatitis vegetans

67. Wrong statement about Dowling-Degos disease
a) Inherited as an autosomal dominant trait
b) Presence of pigmented patches with confluence at the center and reticular pattern at the periphery
c) Acneiform pitted scars and cysts may be found
d) Hidradenitis suppurativa like lesions may be present at axillae and groin
e) Squamous cell carcinoma never develops

68. Rapamycin or sirolimus is a promising drug for
   a) Neurofibromatosis
   b) Tuberous sclerosis
   c) Organoid nevus syndrome
   d) Inflammatory verrucous epidermal nevus
   e) Klippel-Trenaunay syndrome

69. Riehl melanosis does not present with
   a) Pruritus
   b) Erythema
   c) Pigmentation
   d) Lichenification

70. Find out the incorrect statement about Melkersson-Rosenthal syndrome
   a) Attacks usually start during adolescence
   b) Permanent or transitory paralysis of one or both facial nerves
   c) Repeated migraine attacks
   d) Swelling of lips and circumoral area
   e) Scrotal tongue is not a feature

71. Effective drug for angiofibroma in tuberous sclerosis
   a) Mycophenolate mofetil
   b) Tacrolimus
   c) Calcipotriol
   d) Acitretin
   e) Rapamycin

72. Pock-like scars are seen in all, except
   a) Papulonecrotic tuberculid
   b) Reactive perforating collagenosis
   c) Elastosis perforans serpiginosa
   d) Acne vulgaris
   e) Acne agminata

73. Antibody deposition in palpable purpura of Henoch-Schonlein purpura in adult correlates with renal involvement
   a) IgM
   b) IgG
   c) IgA
   d) IgE
   e) None of the above

74. Cribriform scar may be seen in
   a) Hidradenitis suppurativa
   b) Pyoderma gangrenosum
   c) Chicken-pox
   d) Hand-foot-mouth disease
   e) Granuloma annulare

75. Periocular wrinkles may be treated with topical preparation of
   a) Tacrolimus (0.1%)
   b) Hydroxychloroquine (1%)
   c) Imiquimod (5%)
   d) 5-Fluorouracil (1%)
   e) Nifedipine (0.5%)

76. Koilocytes are seen in
   a) Verruca vulgaris
   b) Lichen planus
   c) Darier's disease
   d) Ichthyosis vulgaris
   e) Pseudoxanthoma elasticum

77. Cells resemble fried eggs in histopathology
   a) Mast cells
   b) Dermal dendritic cells
   c) Langerhans cells
   d) Apoptotic keratinocytes
   e) Keratinocytes

78. Snail-track ulcers of oral mucosa may be seen in
   a) Pyostomatitis vegetans
   b) Secondary syphilis
   c) Lichen planus
   d) Pemphigus vulgaris
   e) Systemic lupus erythematosus

79. Breakbone fever is nothing but
   a) Dengue fever
   b) Psoriatic osteoarthritis
   c) Reiter's disease
   d) Rheumatic fever
   e) Multicentric reticulohistiocytosis

80. All types of skin lesions present in lepromatous leprosy, except
   a) Macules

b) Papules
c) Plaques
d) Nodules
e) Telangiectasia

81. Bacterium can cause miliaria in an experimental setting
a) *Bacillus anthracis*
b) *Staphylococcus epidermidis*
c) *Streptococcus pyogenes*
d) *Pseudomonus aeruginosa*
e) *Propionibacterium acne*

82. Which statement is wrong about Peutz-Jeghers syndrome?
a) Intestinal polyposis present in 60-80% cases
b) Hyperpigmented macules present on the lips and oral mucosa
c) Life-time cancer risk is 10-18 fold greater than general population
d) Half of the patients develop cancer at a mean age of 40 years
e) Capsule endoscopy has no special role to find out the hidden polyps not accessible to routine endoscopy

83. Toasted skin syndrome is another name of
a) Erythema ab igne
b) Poikiloderma of Civatte
c) Xeroderma pigmentosa
d) Bloom syndrome
e) Acrogeria

84. In carotenemia and lycopenemia, which part of the body is spared?
a) Palms
b) Soles
c) Central face
d) Sclerae

85. Percentage of formaldehyde for patch test
a) 35%
b) 10%
c) 5%
d) 1%
e) 0.1%

86. Carotenemia may be associated with
a) Diabetes mellitus
b) Hyperthyroidism
c) Hypothyroidism
d) Cushing syndrome
e) Pseudohyperparathyroidism

87. Myroxylon pereirae is nothing but
a) Glycolic acid
b) Salicylic acid
c) Balsam of peru
d) Gallates
e) Sorbitans

88. Which is incorrect statement regarding von Hippel-Lindau syndrome?
a) Autosomal dominant inheritance
b) Presence of pancreatic and renal cysts
c) Angiomas at occipitocervical region
d) Secondary polycythemia due to erythropoietin produced by cerebellar hemangioblastoma
e) Ocular lesion never leads to retinal detachment

89. Find the odd one
a) Benzophenone-3
b) Lyral
c) Xybenzone
d) Eusolex 4360
e) Uvinal M40

90. Ross Miles test is done to assess
a) Foaming power of shampoo
b) Sweat production in the leprosy-patch
c) Amount of sweat production in hyperhidrosis of palms and soles
d) Corrosive effect of phenol
e) Peeling capacity of glycolic acid

91. Permanent wave solution consists of
a) Propylene glycol
b) Gallates
c) Glyceryl monothioglycolate
d) Paraphenelenediamine
e) Anthralin

92. Lutidine test is used to diagnose allergic contact dermatitis induced by
    a) Neosporin
    b) Chlorhexidine
    c) Detergent
    d) Formaldehyde
    e) Cement

93. Propolis is nothing but
    a) Bee glue
    b) Colophony
    c) Thimerosal
    d) Geraniol
    e) Balsam of Peru

94. Role of Buehler test in allergic contact dermatitis
    a) To assess the sensitization time
    b) To detect the allergen
    c) To assess the severity of itching
    d) To assess the erythema
    e) To assess the tolerance of the subject

95. Wool wax, sebaceous secretion of sheep contains
    a) Coumarin
    b) Cinnamate
    c) Lanolin
    d) Farnesol
    e) Sorbitans

96. The term dyshidrosiform in dyshidrosiform dermatitis
    a) Indicates increase sweating
    b) Indicates decreased sweating
    c) Indicates absence of sweating
    d) Indicates occasional increase or decrease of sweating
    e) Is a misnomer

97. Colophony,a natural resin obtained from
    a) Oak tree
    b) Pine tree
    c) Eucalyptus tree
    d) Sugar cane
    e) Aloe vera

98. Which is the wrong statement about familial cold urticaria?
    a) It is an autosomal dominant disorder
    b) Cryopyrin associated with it is the product of the CAIS1 locus
    c) Characterized by fever, rash, conjunctivitis and arthralgia
    d) Same genetic defect is shared by Muckle-Wells syndrome and chronic infantile neurologic cutaneous and articular syndrome (CINCA).
    e) Arthralgia is not elicited by generalized exposure to cold

99. Draize test is designed to test safety of shampoo for which organ?
    a) Nose
    b) Eyes
    c) Scalp
    d) Genitalia
    e) Nail

100. What is the wrong statement about alopecia areata?
    a) Alternative term is pelade
    b) Sudden whitening of hair may represent widespread alopecia areata
    c) Nails may have irregular pits
    d) May be associated with higher incidence of atopic dermatitis, diabetes mellitus, lichen planus, vitiligo, thyroiditis and myasthenia gravis
    e) Exclamation sign indicates activity of the disease

101. Erysipelas-like lesion is seen in
    a) Familial mediterranian fever
    b) Muckle-Wells syndrome
    c) PAPA syndrome
    d) Tumor necrosis factor receptor associated periodic fever
    e) Polycythemia vera

102. Congress grass or scourge of India is
    a) Parthenium hysterophorus
    b) Hibiscus rosasienensis
    c) Osimum sativum

d) Cocos nucifera
e) Mangifera indica

103. Ballooning or reticular degeneration of epidermis is not seen in
a) Chicken pox
b) Herpes labialis
c) Herpes genitalis
d) Herpes zoster
e) Impetigo herpetiformis

104. Fish odor syndrome may occur with chronic use of
a) Hydroquinone
b) Metronidazole
c) Ornidazole
d) Minocycline
e) Rifampicin

105. Which is not found in Sjogren-Larsson syndrome?
a) Begins by the age of 2-3 years
b) Features are ichthyosis, retinitis, mental retardation, spastic paralysis and oligophrenia
c) Central face is prominently affected whereas extremities are spared
d) Scalp, hair and nails are usually not affected
e) Electron microscopy reveals prominent Golgi apparatus and increased number of mitochondria in the keratinocytes

106. Alkaptonuria is characterized by all except
a) Thickening of the cartilage of pinnae
b) Calcification of aortic valve
c) Dark cerumen
d) Pigmentation of sclera (Osler's sign)
e) Increased intervertebral spaces
f) Calcification of prostate gland

107. A two-year-old child presented with erythrodontia and passing of red urine under sunlight. What could be the diagnosis?
a) Congenital erythropoietic porphyria
b) Erythropoietic protoporphyria
c) Variegate porphyria
d) Hepato-erythropoietic porphyria
e) Porphyria cutanea tarda

108. Pseudo-pseudoxanthoma elasticum may be a complication of
a) Corticosteroids
b) Dapsone
c) Azelaic acid
d) Calcipotriol
e) Tacrolimus

109. A 3-year-old child presented with severe burning sensation on sunexposure. First two years of life was eventless. What could be the diagnosis?
a) Congenital erythropoietic porphyria
b) Erythropoietic protoporphyria
c) Variegate porphyria
d) Hydroa vacciniforme
e) Neonatal systemic lupus erythematosus

110. Homme rouge, an irreversible form of pronounced erythema of skin may be a complication of
a) Mupirocin
b) 5-Fluorouracil
c) Bleomycin
d) Corticosteroid
e) Dithranol

111. Which statement is incorrect about Refsum syndrome?
a) A form of ichthyosis having autosomal recessive inheritance
b) Dietary restriction of phytanic acid-containing vegetables has no role
c) Epidermal cell turnover rate is increased
d) Hypertrophic peripheral neuropathy is a feature.
e) Ataxia, deafness and retinitis pigmentosa are also associated

112. Calomel is nothing but
a) Zinc chloride
b) Ferric oxide
c) Zinc oxide
d) Para-aminobenzoic acid

e) Ferric chloride
f) Mercuric chloride

113. Which statement is wrong about erosio interdigitalis blastomycetica
a) This is a form of cutaneous blastomycosis
b) Third web space between middle and index fingers is commonly involved
c) Moisture and maceration predispose the infection
d) Diabetes is also a predisposing disease

114. Azelaic acid is derived from
a) Pityrosporum ovale
b) Pseudomonas aeruginosa
c) Trichophyton rubrum
d) Epidermophyton floccosum
e) Corynebacterium minutissimum

115. What is the wrong statement regarding Vibrio vulnificus infection?
a) Infection is acquired following ingestion of oyster or other seafoods
b) The bacterium enters the blood stream at the level of duodenum
c) Skin lesion starts within 24-48 hours of exposure
d) Skin lesions are characterized by erythematous, edematous and indurated plaques.
e) Lower extremities are rarely affected
f) Initial plaque is followed by formation of hemorrhagic bullae, ulceration and central necrosis.

116. Leaves of bear-berry plant produce
a) Azelaic acid
b) Salicylic acid
c) Glycolic acid
d) Liquitrin
e) Arbutin
f) Kojic acid
g) Psoralen

117. Which feature is not associated with chronic meningococcemia?
a) Recurrent episodes of fever, arthralgia and skin rash
b) Skin rash contains erythematous macules with central hemorrrhage
c) Patients are generally older
d) Fever lasts for 12 hours followed by 1-4 days of well-being
e) It is a rare variant of meningococcemia

118. Grapes contain
a) Glycolic acid
b) Lactic acid
c) Malic acid
d) Tartaric acid
e) Azelaic acid

119. Skin lesions of gonococcemia may be identical to those seen in all, except
a) Nongonococcal bacterial endocarditits
b) Rheumatoid arthritis
c) Rickettsial disease
d) Systemic lupus erythematosus
e) Periarteritis nodosa
f) Haverhill fever
g) Typhoid fever
h) Chikungunya fever

120. Ear lobe crease is seen in all, except
a) Chondrodermatitis hallucis nodularis
b) Relapsing polychondritis
c) Diabetes mellitus
d) Atherosclerotic arterial disease
e) Primary open angle glaucoma

121. Basal layer degeneration is seen in all except
a) Pemphigus vulgaris
b) Lupus erythematosus
c) Lichen planus
d) Lichen nitidus
e) Dermatomyositis

122. Target sign in emphysema is
a) Circumscribed hyperkeratotic plaque on knees.
b) Lichenified plaque at forehead
c) Pigmented patch at palate
d) Callosity at hypothenar eminences
e) Periorbital ecchymoses

123. Grenz zone is seen in all except
a) Lepromatous leprosy
b) Granuloma faciale
c) Granuloma annulare
d) Lymphocytoma cutis
e) B cell lymphoma

124. Palisade granuloma is seen in
a) Zirconium granuloma
b) Scrofuloderma
c) Erythema nodosum
d) Erythema induratum
e) Granuloma annulare

125. Pseudo-Darier sign is seen in
a) Darier's disease
b) Pseudo-porphyria
c) Leiomyoma cutis
d) Urticaria pigmentosa
e) Dermatofibrosarcoma protuberans

126. A middle-aged woman presented with brownish papules at her umbilicus and scar at the lower abdomen following a gynecologic surgery. What could be the diagnosis?
a) Metastatic ovarian carcinoma
b) Cutaneous endometriosis
c) Leiomyoma cutis
d) Leiomyosarcoma
e) Carcinoid tumor

127. Ecthyma gangrenosum is caused by
a) *Pseudomonas aeruginosa*
b) *Staphylococcal aureus*
c) *Streptococcus pyogenes*
d) *Nocardia aesteroides*
e) *Escherichia coli*
f) *Klebsiella*

128. Which is not a feature of transient acantholytic dermatosis or grover's disease?
a) Asteatotic dermatitis occurs several times more than normal
b) Fragile vesicles rapidly turn into crusted and keratotic erosions
c) Males above 50 years are commonly affected
d) Chest, shoulder girdle and upper abdomen are the common sites
e) Direct immunofluorescence (DIF) test is confirmatory
f) Histopathology may mimic Darier's disease, pemphigus foliaceous,Hailey Hailey disease, pemphigus vulgaris and spongiotic dermatitis

129. Anti-hyperglycemic drugs having anti-psoriatic action
a) Insulin
b) Metformin
c) Fenformin
d) Troglitazone
e) Pioglitazone

130. Which is not used for rosacea as topical therapy?
a) Sodium sulfacetomide-sulfur
b) Tacrolimus
c) Benzoyl peroxide
d) Azelaic acid
e) Neomycin

131. Natural source of tartaric acid is
a) Gauva
b) Grape
c) Orange
d) Banana
e) Mango

132. Which systemic drug is not used in rosacea?
a) Cyclosporine
b) Metronidazole
c) Isotretinoin
d) Minocycline
e) Erythromycin

133. Alfa hydroxyl acid in green apple is
a) Citric acid
b) Glycolic acid
c) Lactic acid
d) Malic acid
e) Azelaic acid

134. A 10-year-old child presented with firm flesh color to white pebbly papules and nodules at the angles of the scapulas. What could be the diagnosis?
  a) Hunter syndrome
  b) Hurler syndrome
  c) Farber disease
  d) Lafora's disease
  e) Cadasil syndrome

135. Jellinek sign is seen in
  a) Hypothyroidism
  b) Hypoparathyroidism
  c) Hyperthyroidism
  d) Hyperparathyroidism
  e) Primary systemic amyloidosis

136. Which is not a feature of Hurler syndrome?
  a) Mental retardation, hepatosplenomegaly, umbilical and inguinal hernia, genital infantilism, corneal opacities
  b) Broad saddle nose, thick lips and large tongue
  c) Skin is thickened with ridges and grooves, specially affecting the upper half of the body
  d) Widely distributed course hair at trunk and fine lanugo hair at extremities
  e) Presence of dermal melanocytosis

137. Jellinek sign is the conspicuous pigmentation at
  a) Flank
  b) Periumbilical region
  c) Glans
  d) Eyelids
  e) Ear lobe

138. Which is not a feature of Farber disease?
  a) Rubbery subcutaneous nodules of 1-2 cm in diameter with a yellowish hue at joint, lumbar spine, scalp and weight-bearing areas
  b) Presence of weak hoarse cry
  c) Mental retardation
  d) Onset is during first month of life and death is expected before the age of 2
  e) Painful joint deformities never occurs
  f) Farber bodies (curvilinear bodies) are present within cytoplasm or phagosomes of fibroblasts, histiocytes or endothelial cells and banana shaped bodies are present within Schwann cells and zebra bodies are present within endothelial cells and neuron

139. Rule out the odd one
  a) Bulla spreading sign
  b) Lutz sign
  c) Asboe-Hansen sign
  d) Nikolsky sign

140. Which is not a feature of Lafora's disease?
  a) Papulonodular lesions on the ears
  b) Indurated thickened plaques at arms
  c) Progressive epilepsy begins at puberty
  d) Dysphagia
  e) Death in late adulthood

141. The scale identifies a person's position in homosexual-heterosexual scale is
  a) Kinsely
  b) Huxely
  c) Henle
  d) Langhans
  e) Langerhan

142. Sudamina is nothing but
  a) Miliaria rubra
  b) Miliaria crystalina
  c) Miliaria pustulosa
  d) Miliaria profunda
  e) Milia

143. Juvenile melanoma is nothing but
  a) Nevus anemicus
  b) Spitz nevus
  c) Nevus achromicus
  d) Lentigo maligna
  e) Pseudomelanoma

144. Interface dermatitis is not seen in
  a) Lichen planus
  b) Discoid lupus erythematosus
  c) Pityriasis lichenoides

d) Acute dermatitis
e) Flexural psoriasis

145. Erosion of sigmoid notch of ulna is seen in
a) Early congenital syphilis
b) Tertiary syphilis
c) Relapsing polychondritis
d) Multicentric reticulohistiocytosis
e) Juvenile rheumatoid arthritis

146. Auspitz sign may be positive in all, except
a) Psoriasis
b) Darier's disease
c) Seborrheic keratosis
d) Actinic keratosis

147. Wide follicular pits at concha or triangular fossa of the ear in lupus erythematosus are known as
a) Shuster's sign
b) Carpet-tack sign
c) Dorry-Flop sign
d) Higomenaki's sign
e) Brocq sign

148. Which is not a feature of atypical adult type of pityriasis rubra pilaris?
a) Ichthyotic changes
b) Eczematous changes
c) Alopecia
d) Chronic course as >20 years
e) Associated with malignancy

149. Rule out the odds
a) Lipschutz ulcer
b) Ulcus molle
c) Cold sore
d) Fever blister
e) Herpes labialis

150. Which is the wrong statement about atypical juvenile type of pityriasis rubra pilaris?
a) Most of the cases are familial
b) Sclerodermoid changes of the palms and soles
c) Early onset and chronic course
d) Hyperkeratotic follicles
e) Frequent erythema

151. Barlow disease is
a) Hartnup disease
b) Infantile psoriasis
c) Early congenital syphilis
d) Infantile scurvy
e) Adult-onset atopic dermatitis

152. Which is not a feature of HIV associated atypical pityriasis rubra pilaris?
a) Presence of cystic and pustular acneiform eruptions
b) Elongated follicular plugs or lichen spinulosa-like lesions
c) Resistant to usual treatment
d) Responding to HAART
e) Palmoplantar erythema is a diagnostic feature

153. Rubbing of feet in infantile scabies is known as
a) Dennie's sign
b) Osler's sign
c) Prayer sign
d) Brocq sign
e) Gottron's sign

154. Which variant of porokeratosis never turns into malignancy?
a) Porokeratosis of Mibelli
b) Disseminated superficial actinic porokeratosis
c) Linear porokeratosis
d) Porokeratosis Palmaris, plantaris et disseminata
e) Giant porokeratosis

155. Wimberger ring is a feature of
a) Secondary syphilis
b) Congenital syphilis
c) Tertiary syphilis
d) Scurvy
e) Acute pancreatitis

156. Which variant of porokeratosis has highest risk to turn into malignancy?
a) Porokeratosis of Mibelli
b) Disseminated superficial actinic porokeratosis

c) Linear porokeratosis
d) Porokeratosis Palmaris, plantaris et disseminata
e) Giant porokeratosis

157. Drug does not induce dermatomyositis
a) NSAIDs
b) D-penicillamine
c) Omeprazole
d) Griseofulvin

158. Increased risk of drug reactions occurs in HIV infection when CD4 cell count is between
a) 0-25
b) 25-200
c) 200-400
d) 400-500

159. Statement does not fit with vitamin C
a) Humans can convert glucose into ascorbic acid
b) Helps in iron absorption
c) Reduces free radicals
d) Important for collagen synthesis

160. What type of drug reaction occurs when an AIDS patient having *Pneumocystis carinii* infection being treated with sulfamethoxazole-trimethoprim?
a) Morbilliform
b) Vesiculobullous
c) TEN-like
d) Lichenoid
e) Erythema multiforme-like

161. Not true about Bazex syndrome
a) Constitutes of two different geneodermatoses.
b) One is inherited as X-linked dominant trait.
c) Another one is also known as acrokeratosis paraneoplastica
d) Generalized hyperhidrosis is a feature of X-linked one.
e) Psoriasiform lesion is the feature of paraneoplastic one

162. Severe bullous reaction, SJS and TEN occur in AIDS. How many time the risk is increased than non-AIDS patients treated with same medicines?
a) 10-100 times
b) 100-1000 times
c) 1000-10000 times
d) None of the above

163. Trichodynia is a painful sensation at scalp during
a) Hair loss
b) Sensitization to hair dye
c) Hair-pull test
d) Hair cutting
e) Lanthilization

164. Nevirapine, a non-nonucleoside reverse transcriptase inhibitor commonly used drug in HIV infection causes
a) Morbilliform eruption
b) Lichenoid reaction
c) SJS/TEN
d) Pyoderma gangrenosum-like eruption
e) Lipodystrophy

165. Acupuncture has been shown to be effective in
a) Urticaria
b) Pruritus
c) Wrinkle
d) Senile comedone
e) Idiopathic guttate hypomelanosis

166. Source of kojic acid is
a) Japanese rice wine (sake)
b) Sugarcane
c) Bamboo shoot
d) Tulip
e) Aloe vera

167. Source of liquitrin is
a) Licorice extract
b) Curd
c) Rotten egg
d) Tulip
e) Aloe vera

168. Cutaneous eruption with lymphocyte recovery following chemotherapy is associated with all, except
  a) Maculopapular eruptions
  b) Fever
  c) Nonspecific superficial perivascular mononuclear cell infiltrate
  d) Infiltrate primarily contains B lymphocytes
  e) Treatment is not required as it resolves spontaneously

169. Component of henna causes allergic contact dermatitis
  a) Paraphenelenediamine
  b) Paraben
  c) Mercaptobenzothiazole
  d) Cobalt chloride
  e) p-Tertiary butyl phenol

170. Flagellate hyperpigmentation is associated with
  a) 5-Fluorouracil
  b) Capecitabine
  c) Bleomycin
  d) Cytosine arabinoside
  e) Doxorubicin

171. Threading does not cause
  a) Herpes simplex
  b)Verrucae
  c) Impetigo
  d) Molluscum contagiosum
  e) AIDS

172. Palmoplantar erythrodysesthesia syndrome or acral erythema may be caused by all, except
  a) Cyclosporine
  b) 5-Fluorouracil
  c) Doxorubicin
  d) Cytosine arabinoside

173. Role of Th_{17} cells in the pathogenesis of psoriasis is
  a) To produce cytokines such as IL_{17} and IL_{22}.
  b) To produce IFN-γ,TNFα,IL-2 and IL-12
  c) To induce expression of TGF-α,IL-8 and VEGF
  d) To synergize the stimulation of IFN-γ release.
  e) To produe IL_{23}.

174. Cyclophosphamide can cause pigmentation of
  a) Hair
  b) Nail
  c) Genital mucosa
  d) Palms
  e) Soles

175. The role of dendritic cells in the pathogenesis of psoriasis is
  a) To recognize and capture an as yet unidentified antigen and stimulate T cells by presenting them the said antigen
  b) To produce several mediators which can cause further migration of immune cells in the dermis helping in angiogenesis.
  c) To produce IL_{17} and IL_{22}
  d) To release proteases like elastase and cationic proteins like lactoferrin

176. Exudative hyponychial dermatitis may be caused by
  a) Docataxel
  b) Doxorubicin
  c) Isotretinoin
  d) Mycophenolate mofetil
  e) Systemic corticosteroid

177. Role of keratinocytes in pathogenesis of psoriasis is
  a) To produce several mediators which can cause further migration of immune cells in the dermis and stimulate stromal cells helping in angiogenesis.
  b) To produce IL_{17} and IL_{22}
  c) To release proteases like elastase and cationic proteins like lactoferrin
  d) To recognize and capture an as yet unidentified antigen and stimulate T cells by presenting them the said antigen

178. Diffuse erythema, pruritus, aphthous-like stomatitis, glossitis and flushing may be caused by infusion of
a) IL_1
b) IL_2
c) IL_3
d) IL_4
e) IFNα

179. Role of IL_{23} in pathogenesis of psoriasis is
a) To expand Th_{17} cells reflected by increased production of IL_{17} and IL_{22}
b) To help in angiogenesis
c) To promote neutrophil mobilization and degranulation
d) To regulate transcription of IFNα

180. Acute diffuse indurated edema of extremities and head may be caused by
a) Docataxel
b) Paclitaxel
c) Imatinib
d) G-CSF
e) Infliximab

181. Explanations of the crucial role of IL_{23}/Th_{17} axis in pathogenesis of psoriasis except
a) Its inhibition is central to the modern therapeutic achievement
b) Its vital role in hyperplasia of keratinocytes
c) Its role in neutrophil chemotaxis by production of IL_8
d) Its role in regulation of IFNγ

182. Importance of neutrophil activation product is
a) To mediate inflammation and tissue damage
b) To regulate the transcription of IFNγ
c) To increase the expression of the specific receptor chain for IL_{12}
d) To increase the expression of intercellular adhesion molecule-I promoting skin infiltration of T cells

183. Possible explanations of the vital role of cytokines for the pathological changes in psoriasis, except
a) IL_8 promotes neutrophil infiltrations
b) IL_{22} promotes acanthosis and dermal infiltration
c) VEGF promotes the vascularization of the lesion, contributing erythema of the lesion
d) IL-23 promotes suprapapillary thinning

184. Importance of manipulation of VEGF in therapeutic challenge of psoriasis
a) Angiogenenesis is particularly depends on VEGF
b) VEGF induces psoriatic hyperplasia of keratinocytes
c) Neutrophil infiltration depends on VEGF
d) VEGF induces acanthosis and dermal infiltration

185. Probable explanations of therapeutic success of anti-TNF drugs, except
a) They modulate regulatory T cells
b) They decrease the expression of cellular adhesion molecules
c) They reduce the macrophages and dendritic cells
d) They reduce the mast cells

186. Explanation of the therapeutic success of anti-IL_{23}/IL_{12}
a) They block Th_1 and Th_{17} pathways
b) They prevent the binding of TNF to its receptors
c) They induce deviation of the Th_1 to the Th_2 immune response
d) They inhibit chemotaxis of neutrophils

187. Inappropriate methods to diagnose acute Chagas disease
a) Serological test
b) Inoculation into mice
c) Direct smear
d) PCR
e) Intradermal test

188. Percentage of asymptomative seropositive patients progress to symptomatic chronic Chagas' disease
   a) 10-15%
   b) 15-30%
   c) 30-40%
   d) 40-50%
   e) >50%

189. Worst prognostic feature of acute Chagas' disease
   a) A new bundle branch block in ECG
   b) Presence of trepanosomes in CSF
   c) Presence of Chagoma at right hand
   d) Fever
   e) Arthritis

190. Typical laboratory abnormalities in acute Chagas' disease, except
   a) Eosinophilia
   b) Elevated liver enzymes
   c) Anemia
   d) Thrombocytopenia

191. Possible route of large-scale outbreak of acute Chagas' disease
   a) Contaminated food and drink
   b) Blood transfusion
   c) Fecal-oral route
   d) Invasions by the insect vector into non-native habitat

192. Nifurtimox in Chagas' disease may cause
   a) Peripheral neuropathy
   b) Aplastic anemia
   c) Xerosis
   d) Pulmonary edema
   e) Leukotrichia

193. A 72-year-old male presented with slowly progressive pruritic plaques at neck for 5 years and no improvement following topical corticosteroid. These could be the differential diagnosis, except
   a) Primary cutaneous B-cell lymphoma
   b) Mycosis fungoides
   c) Pseudolymphoma
   d) Metastatic adenocarcinoma
   e) Granuloma annulare

194. Most appropriate method to evaluate reactivation of Chagas' disease
   a) Skin biopsy for histopathological examination
   b) Serum ELISA
   c) Serum PCR
   d) Inoculation of blood into mice

195. Unlikely to develop Chagas' disease following
   a) Sexual contact with a woman who subsequently develop Chagas' cardiomyopathy
   b) Consumption of raw guava juice during a trip to brazil 20 years back
   c) Receipt of a blood transfusion 15 years back
   d) Exposure to Reduviid bugs as a child in rural Tennesse

196. Drugs causing systemic lupus erythematosus, rarely associated with skin lesions
   a) Hydralazine
   b) Procainamide
   c) Hydrochlorthiazide
   d) Diltiazem
   e) Terbinafine

197. Drugs causing subacute lupus erythematosus, frequently associated with skin lesions
   a) Hydralazine
   b) Procainamide
   c) Hydrochlorthiazide
   d) Diltiazem
   e) Terbinafine

198. Dermatomyositis-like skin lesions may be caused by chronic use of
   a) Cyclosporine
   b) Isotretinoin
   c) Hydroxyurea
   d) Iodide
   e) Bromide

199. Doughnut sign is associated with
   a) Scleromyxedema
   b) Scleredema
   c) Scleroderma
   d) Dermatomyositis
   e) Rheumatoid arthritis

200. Leonine facies is seen in all except
   a) Multicentric reticulohistiocytosis
   b) Actinic granuloma
   c) Lepromatous leprosy
   d) Scleromyxedema
   e) Chronic actinic dermatosis

Answers

1. c; 2. a; 3. c; 4. a; 5. e; 6. d; 7. f; 8. c; 9. f; 10. f; 11. c; 12. g; 13. f; 14. h; 15. e; 16. f; 17. e; 18. f; 19. d; 20. d; 21. a; 22. d; 23. c; 24. e; 25. a; 26. b; 27. e; 28. d; 29. a; 30. e; 31. a; 32. d; 33. c; 34. a; 35. b; 36. a; 37. d; 38. b; 39. e; 40. f; 41. a; 42. f; 43. a, d; 44. b; 45. a; 46. d; 47. b; 48. c; 49. e; 50. a, c, d; 51. d; 52. a; 53. a; 54. c; 55. a; 56. c, d, e; 57. b; 58. a, b; 59. b; 60. d; 61. a; 62. a, e; 63. c; 64. d; 65. b; 66. b; 67. e; 68. b; 69. d; 70. e; 71. e; 72. c; 73. a; 74. a, b; 75. e; 76. a; 77. a; 78. a, b; 79. a; 80. e; 81. b; 82. e; 83. a; 84. d; 85. d; 86. c; 87. c; 88. e; 89. b; 90. a; 91. c; 92. d; 93. a; 94. b; 95. c; 96. e; 97. b; 98. e; 99. b; 100. c; 101. a; 102. a; 103. e; 104. a; 105. c; 106. e; 107. a; 108. a; 109. b; 110. d; 111. b; 112. f; 113. a; 114. a; 115. e; 116. e; 117. c; 118. d; 119. h; 120. a, b; 121. a; 122. a; 123. c; 124. e; 125. c; 126. b; 127. a; 128. e; 129. d, e; 130. e; 131. b; 132. a; 133. d; 134. a; 135. c; 136. d; 137. d; 138. e; 139. d; 140. e; 141. a; 142. b; 143. b; 144. e; 145. a; 146. c; 147. a; 148. e; 149. a, b; 150. e; 151. d; 152. e; 153. a; 154. d; 155. d; 156. c; 157. d; 158. b; 159. a; 160. a; 161. d; 162. b; 163. a; 164. c; 165. a, b; 166. a; 167. a; 168. d; 169. a; 170. c; 171. a, e; 172. a; 173. a; 174. b; 175. a; 176. a; 177. a; 178. b; 179. a; 180. a, b; 181. d; 182. a; 183. d; 184. a; 185. d; 186. a; 187. a, e; 188. b; 189. a; 190. a; 191. a; 192. a; 193. e; 194. a; 195. a; 196. a, b; 197. c, d, e; 198. c; 199. a; 200. b.

INDEX